The Peroneal Tendons

Mark Sobel

Editor

The Peroneal Tendons

A Clinical Guide to Evaluation and Management

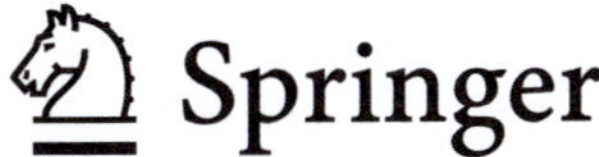

Editor
Mark Sobel
Private Practice
Atlantic Highlands, NJ
USA

ISBN 978-3-030-46648-0   ISBN 978-3-030-46646-6   (eBook)
https://doi.org/10.1007/978-3-030-46646-6

This Springer imprint is published by the registered company Springer Nature Switzerland AG
The registered company address is: Gewerbestrasse 11, 6330 Cham, Switzerland

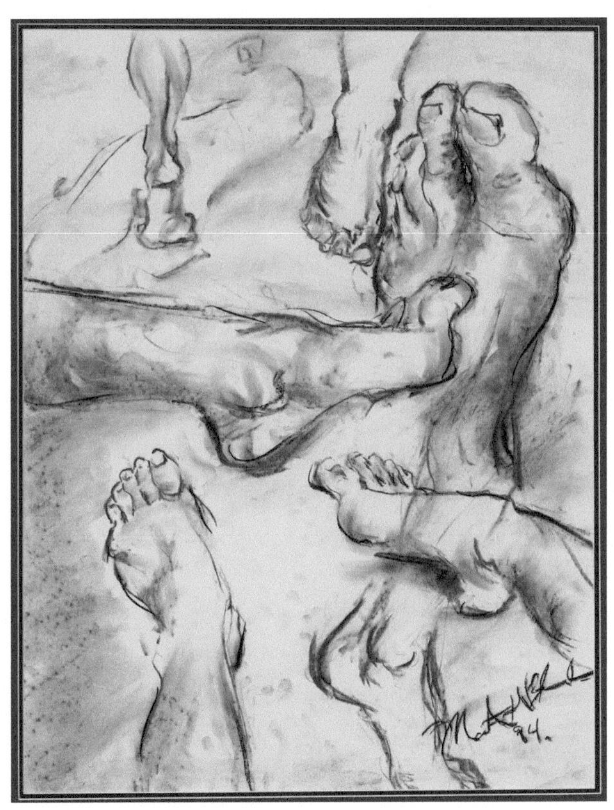

"Foot Study" Martin Blank Studios, Seattle WA.

To my parents Jane Ann and Murray, my wife Mary Grace, and my children Mark Jr., Jay Michael, and Grace Ann.

With love,

Mark Sobel

In loving memory
Mark Sobel, Jr.
12/15/1993 – 7/16/2011
Determination. Motivation. Success.

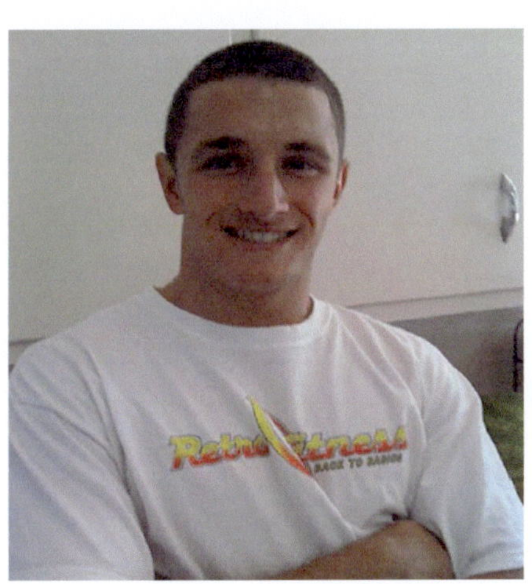

Foreword

Peroneal Passion

Of all the tendons that cross the ankle, the peroneal tendons may be considered the least well loved. The Achilles is adored by all – general orthopedists, sport specialists, pediatric orthopedists, and foot and ankle aficionados. It has been esteemed throughout history by ancient man and its status was even elevated by connection to one of the great heroes in Greek mythology. In the literature, and in these days, more commonly, in Google citations of the Achilles tendon, the search yields 22,500,000 results. Next in line, but more forward in orientation, is the anterior tibial tendon, which gets 3,290,000 results. Third, we find the posterior tibialis. It gets 3,270,000 results on Google. This tendon has "popped" into popularity in the last 70 years with its dysfunction and creation of the adult acquired collapsed foot or pes planovalgus. Thereafter, we find the peroneal tendons, which, despite being two distinct tendons, selflessly cohabit the same sheath, getting 878,000 search results. The tendons both evert the foot and ankle to hold us from falling to the floor. But there is more! Unlike the brevis, the longus also plantarflexes the first ray to give us push off, turning, and cutting power. How cool is that? So why do the peroneals just beat the flexor digitorum longus (868,000 results)? It is understandable that they readily surpass the toe movers: the flexor hallucis longus (460,000 results), the extensor digitorum longus (413,000 results), and the extensor hallucis longus tendon that gets a paltry 141,000 results. My sense is that the peroneals deserve greater recognition. When it comes to our mobility, we need to appreciate our lateral sinews that fight with fervor and zeal to keep us upright!

While the Achilles has had dedicated textbooks, it is my understanding that Sobel's tome is the first one devoted to the less well-loved lower leg tendons, the peroneals. It is interesting to reflect that 30 years ago there was very little novel scientific literature on the peroneals. In fact, about 150 papers were on pub med between 1960 and 1990. That changed between 1987 and 1995 when Mark Sobel, former Varsity football player at the University of Maryland (1982) and graduate at Case Western Reserve University School of Medicine (1987), launched his exploration into the topic. During anatomy lab, his curiosity was peeked about a random finding of a peroneus brevis tear. To determine whether this was common, he asked for permission to explore his class's cadavers. During this deep dive into the lateral ankle, he noted tears of the peroneus brevis in some of the 80 specimens. Perplexed by this finding, he went to the stacks (a.k.a. library) and found the AW Meyer paper on attrition in the body and saw the peroneal tendon tears in this 1924 article [1]. His mission was now fully launched. This then grew to a broader exploration of cadavers at Cleveland's Ohio College of Podiatric Medicine and the University of Toledo College of Medicine and Life Sciences. At these two institutions, he added another 120 cadavers. Thus, armed with data and a strong footing in form and function, he began his life as an MD with an internship at Mt. Sinai (1988), residency at Hospital for Special Surgery, fellowship with foot and ankle guru Roger Mann (1992), and AO Scholarship with the trailblazer Sigvard Hansen (1993). During this time, he managed to research, collaborate, and write, establishing a firm and unique expertise on the peroneal tendons. By 1995 he had written 14 peer-reviewed innovative articles on the peroneals, presented lectures, and written textbook chapters on the topic.

In the early part of his successful career as an orthopedic surgeon, his motivation was to create a platform of literature to enhance the level of understanding of the peroneal tendons. Now, three decades later, he is motivated to complete his magnum opus and gather the world's experts on the topic to create a new foundation for the next generation of clinicians and scientists. It is important to note that Mark's effort was driven purely by his overwhelming passion for the peroneals and desire to make the world a bit better. If he can inspire the readers to be more enlightened, creative, and innovative, his goal will be fulfilled. Let us hope that through his text, subsequent efforts will advance the status of these worthy tendons and our patients will benefit through better comfort and function!

Reference

1. Meyers AW. Further evidence of attrition in the human body. Am J Anat. 1924;34:241–267.

Lew Schon

Director of Orthopedic Innovation, Institute of Foot and Ankle Reconstruction, Mercy Medical Center, Baltimore, MD, USA

Faculty, MedStar Union Memorial Hospital, Baltimore, MA, USA

Professor of Orthopedic Surgery, New York University Langone, New York, NY, USA

Associate Professor of Orthopaedics and BME, Johns Hopkins School of Medicine, Baltimore, MA, USA

Associate Professor of Orthopaedics, Georgetown School of Medicine, Washington, DC, USA

Fischell Literati Faculty, University of Maryland Fischell Department of Bioengineering, College Park, MD, USA

Preface

My start with the Peroneal Tendons began in the cadaver lab when I was a medical student at Case Western Reserve University School of Medicine in Cleveland, Ohio, in 1983. It continued in Dr. Arnoczky's Laboratory For Comparative Orthopaedic Research at the Hospital for Special Surgery in New York while I was an orthopedic resident.

Since my initial anatomical observations and writings on this topic published in the early 1990s, the keen interest and advancement in this area of foot and ankle surgery has been substantial. Many of the key contributors to the furtherance of this topic in the literature have agreed to contribute to this book, which is what makes it extraordinary. The author for each chapter shares a passion for treating patients with Peroneal Tendon Injury.

It is my hope that this publication serves as a foundation for the future development and advancement of this field of Peroneal Tendon Injury and its treatment.

Atlantic Highlands, NJ, USA Mark Sobel

Acknowledgments

Approximately 33 years ago I when I was a medical student at Case Western Reserve University School of Medicine, I began studying the anatomy of the Peroneal Tendons. This work continued during my residency at the Hospital For Special Surgery. I was very fortunate to collaborate with many wonderful illustrators, medical students, residents, fellows, orthopedic surgeons, radiologists, pathologists, and scientists during this time. In addition to the authors in this book, I would like to thank the following individuals for sharing my passion for the Peroneal Tendons:

Matthew E. Levy, MD; Steven A. Arnoczky, DVM; Mark J. Geppert, MD; W. Hodges Davis, MD; Jo A. Hannafin, MD, PhD; Walter H.O. Bohne, MD; Russell F. Warren, MD; Steven Brourman, MD; Stephen J. O'Brien, MD; John Markisz, MD; Leslie Collins, MD; Mark S. Mizel, MD; Eric J. Olsen, MD; Francesca M. Thompson, MD; Jonathan T. Deland, MD; M.B. Patel, MD; Helane Pavlov, MD; and Edward. F. DiCarlo, MD.

Illustrations: Nancy Laverne, Pauline Thomas.

Contents

Contributors

Samuel B. Adams, MD Foot and Ankle Division, Department of Orthopedic Surgery, Duke University Medical Center, Durham, NC, USA

Robert B. Anderson, MD Titletown Sports Medicine and Orthopedics, Green Bay, WI, USA

Associate Team Physician, Green Bay Packers, WI, USA

Nick Casscells, MD Medstar Georgetown University Hospital, Washington, DC, USA

Christy M. Christophersen, MD Department of Orthopaedic Surgery, Mayo Clinic, Rochester, MN, USA

Daniel J. Cuttica, DO The Orthopaedic Foot and Ankle Center, Center for Advanced Orthopedics, Falls Church, VA, USA

C. W. DiGiovanni, MD Massachusetts General Hospital, Harvard Medical School, Boston, MA, USA

Newton-Wellesley Hospital, Newton, MA, USA

Department of Orthopedic Surgery, Massachusetts General Hospital, Harvard Medical School, Boston, MA, USA

Department of Orthopedic Surgery, Newton-Wellesley Hospital, Newton, MA, USA

P. A. D. Van Dijk, BSc (Med) Department of Orthopedic Surgery, Academical University Medical Centers, Amsterdam, The Netherlands

Surgical Department, Onze Lieve Vrouwe Gasthuis, Amsterdam, The Netherlands

Orthopedic Research Department, Academisch Medisch Centrum, Universiteit van Amsterdam, Amsterdam, The Netherlands

Osama Elattar, MD Department of Orthopaedic Surgery, University of Toledo Medical Center, Toledo, OH, USA

Ezequiel Palmanovich, MD Meir Medical Center, Department of Orthopaedic Surgery, Affiliated with the Sackler Faculty of Medicine and Tel Aviv University, Kefar Sava, Israel

Nicholas P. Fethiere, BS University of Florida College of Medicine, Gainesville, FL, USA

Eric Folmar, PT, DPT Department of Physical Therapy, Movement & Rehabilitation Sciences, Northeastern University, Boston, MA, USA

Rabun Fox, MD Anchorage Fracture and Orthopedic clinic, Anchorage, AL, USA

Daniel J. Fuchs, MD Sidney Kimmel Medical College, Thomas Jefferson University, The Rothman Institute, Philadelphia, PA, USA

Michael Gans, PT, DPT PTSMC Orthopedic Residency Program, West Hartford, CT, USA

Physical Therapy and Sports Medicine Centers, Guilford, CT, USA

Glenn Garrison, LPO, CPO Hospital for Special Surgery, New York, NY, USA

Mark J. Geppert, MD Department of Orthopedic Surgery, Wentworth Health Partners Seacoast Orthopedics & Sports Medicine, at Wentworth-Douglass Hospital, Dover, NH, USA

Jasen Gilley, MD Foot and Ankle Orthopedics, Signature Orthopedics, St. Louis, MO, USA

Gregory P. Guyton, MD Department of Orthopaedic Surgery, MedStar Union Memorial Hospital, Baltimore, MD, USA

Andrew E. Hanselman, MD Duke University Department of Orthopaedics, Durham, NC, USA

Rajshree Hillstrom, PhD, MBA Tandon School of Engineering, New York University, New York, NY, USA

Howard J. Hillstrom, PhD Hospital for Special Surgery, New York, NY, USA

Syed H. Hussain, MD Wake Orthopaedics, Raleigh, NC, USA

Joseph E. Jacobson, MD Department of Orthopedics, Indiana University, Indianapolis, IN, USA

Jon Karlsson, MD, PhD Department of Orthopaedics, Sahlgrenska University Hospital, Sahlgrenska Academy, Gothenburg University, Gothenburg, Sweden

Louise Karlsson, MD Department of Orthopaedics, Sahlgrenska University Hospital, Sahlgrenska Academy, Gothenburg University, Gothenburg, Sweden

Armen S. Kelikian, MD Professor of Orthopedics, Northwestern University Medical Center and Intructor at North Shore University, Chicago, IL, USA

Gokhan Kuyumcu, MD Department of Medical Imaging, University of Arizona College of Medicine, Tucson, AZ, USA

Peter Kvarda, P MD Department of Orthopedic Surgery, Massachusetts General Hospital, Harvard Medical School, Boston, MA, USA

Department of Orthopedics and Traumatology, University Hospital of Basel, Basel, Switzerland

L. Daniel Latt, MD, PhD Department of Orthopaedic Surgery, University of Arizona College of Medicine, Tucson, AZ, USA

Nicola Maffulli, MD, PhD, FRCS, (Orth) Department of Musculoskeletal Disorders, School of Medicine and Surgery, University of Salerno, Salerno, Italy

Queen Mary University of London, Barts and the London School of Medicine and Dentistry, Centre for Sports and Exercise Medicine, Mile End Hospital, London, UK

Matias Vidra, MD Tel Aviv Medical Center, Department of Orthopaedic Surgery, Affiliated with the Sackler Faculty of Medicine and Tel Aviv University, Tel Aviv-Yafo, Israel

Jeremy J. McCormick, MD Department of Orthopedic Surgery, Washington University School of Medicine, St Louis, MO, USA

Meir Nyska, MD Meir Medical Center, Department of Orthopaedic Surgery, Affiliated with the Sackler Faculty of Medicine and Tel Aviv University, Kefar Sava, Israel

Dominic Montas, BS University of Florida, Gainesville, FL, USA

Oliver Morgan, BSc Faculty of Science and Engineering, Anglia Ruskin University, Chelmsford, Essex, UK

Steven K. Neufeld, MD The Orthopaedic Foot and Ankle Center, Center for Advanced Orthopedics, Falls Church, VA, USA

Nissim Ohana, MD Meir Medical Center, Department of Orthopaedic Surgery, Affiliated with the Sackler Faculty of Medicine and Tel Aviv University, Kefar Sava, Israel

James A. Nunley, MD Duke University Department of Orthopaedics, Durham, NC, USA

Francesco Oliva, MD, PhD Department of Musculoskeletal Disorders, School of Medicine and Surgery, University of Salerno, Salerno, Italy

David I. Pedowitz, MS, MD Sidney Kimmel Medical College, Thomas Jefferson University, The Rothman Institute, Philadelphia, PA, USA

David A. Porter, MD Methodist Sports Medicine, Indianapolis, IN, USA

Steven M. Raikin, MD Anchorage Fracture and Orthopedic clinic, Anchorage, AL, USA

Ran Atzmon, MD Assuta Medical Center, Department of Orthopaedic Surgery, Affiliated with the Faculty of Health and Science and Ben Gurion University, Ashdod, Israel

Johannes B. Roedl, MD Division of Musculoskeletal Imaging and Intervention, Department of Radiology, Thomas Jefferson University Hospital, Philadelphia, PA, USA

Clelia Rugiero, MD Orthopaedic and Traumatology Department, University of Roma Tor Vergata, Tor Vergata Hospital, Rome, Italy

Kevin A. Schafer, MD Department of Orthopedic Surgery, Washington University School of Medicine, St Louis, MO, USA

Lew Schon, MD Mercy Medical Center, Baltimore, MD, USA

Eric Hamrin Senorski, PT, PhD Department of Orthopaedics, Sahlgrenska University Hospital, Sahlgrenska Academy, Gothenburg University, Gothenburg, Sweden

Rachel Shakked, MD Sidney Kimmel Medical College, Thomas Jefferson University, The Rothman Institute, Philadelphia, PA, USA

Tom Sherman, MD Orthopedic Associate of Lancaster, Lancaster, PA, USA

Mark Sobel, MD Private Practice, New York, NY, USA

Lenox Hill Hospital – Northwell Health, Orthopaedic Surgery, New York, NY, USA

Jay M. Sobel, BS Icahn School of Medicine at Mount Sinai, Biomedical Sciences, New York, NY, USA

Jinsup Song, DPM, PhD School of Podiatric Medicine, Temple University, Philadelphia, PA, USA

Kristopher Stockton, MD Texas Orthopedics, Sports & Rehabilitation Associates, Austin, TX, USA

Department of Orthopaedics, Dell Medical School – The University of Texas at Austin, Austin, TX, USA

Eleonor Svantesson, MD Department of Orthopaedics, Sahlgrenska University Hospital, Sahlgrenska Academy, Gothenburg University, Gothenburg, Sweden

Mihra S. Taljanovic, MD, PhD Department of Medical Imaging, University of Arizona College of Medicine, Tucson, AZ, USA

A. Tanriover, MD Department of Orthopedic Surgery, Massachusetts General Hospital, Harvard Medical School, Boston, MA, USA

Rull James Toussaint, MD The Orthopaedic Institute, Gainesville, FL, USA

Alessio Giai Via, MD Orthopaedic and Traumatology Department, Sant'Anna Hospital, Como, Italy

Keith L. Wapner, MD Department of Orthopaedic Surgery, Penn Medicine, Philadelphia, PA, USA

G. R. Waryasz, MD Massachusetts General Hospital, Harvard Medical School, Boston, MA, USA

Newton-Wellesley Hospital, Newton, MA, USA

Department of Orthopedic Surgery, Massachusetts General Hospital, Harvard Medical School, Boston, MA, USA

Department of Orthopedic Surgery, Newton-Wellesley Hospital, Newton, MA, USA

Normal Anatomy of the Peroneal Tendons

Jasen Gilley and Armen S. Kelikian

Myology

The peroneus longus originates from the proximal lateral fibula and the brevis at middle lateral aspect of the fibula. In the distal third of the fibula, the lateral border twists posteriorly with both peroneus following as it becomes continuous with the posterior aspect of the lateral malleolus. At the level of the lateral malleolus, the tendons lie directly posterior with the brevis against the fibula and the longus on top of it (Fig. 1.1) [1].

At the inferior aspect of the lateral malleolus a sulcus is formed. Edwards' cadaveric study on 178 specimens found that 82% had a concave sulcus while 11% were flat and 7% actually had a convex surface [2]. Ozbag et al. also looked at this region, and in their study of 93 specimens, they found 68% had a concave sulcus and 32% had either convex or flat [3]. The peroneus are evertors and are responsible for 3.7% of plantarflexion power and 87% of eversion power in meter/kg [1]. (#1585–6).

Peroneus Longus

Along the track of the peroneus longus tendon, there are three tunnels and three turns taken before eventually attaching to the plantar aspect of the foot. The first tunnel is the superior peroneus retinaculum that is shared by both the longus and the brevis and is retromalleolar. At the tip of the lateral malleolus, the tendon takes an anterior and downward directed turn as it heads toward and through the inferior peroneus retinaculum. The second tunnel is located at the processus trochlearis at

J. Gilley (✉)
Foot and Ankle Orthopedics, Signature Orthopedics, St. Louis, MO, USA

A. S. Kelikian
Professor of Orthopedics, Northwestern University Medical Center and Intructor at North Shore University, Chicago, IL, USA
e-mail: armen@kelikian.com

© Springer Nature Switzerland AG 2020
M. Sobel (ed.), *The Peroneal Tendons*,
https://doi.org/10.1007/978-3-030-46646-6_1

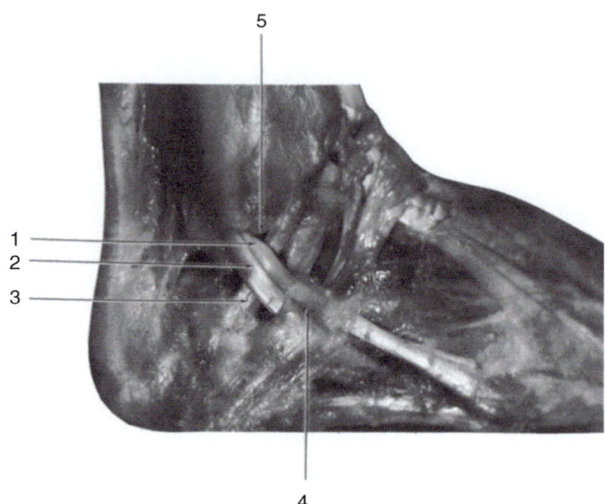

Fig. 1.1 Peroneus longus tendon. (1. Peroneus brevis tendon; 2. peroneus longus tendon; 3. calcaneo fibular ligament; 4. inferior peroneus retinaculum; 5. tip of lateral malleolus, free of insertion.) (From: Sarrafian SK [23], P. 235)

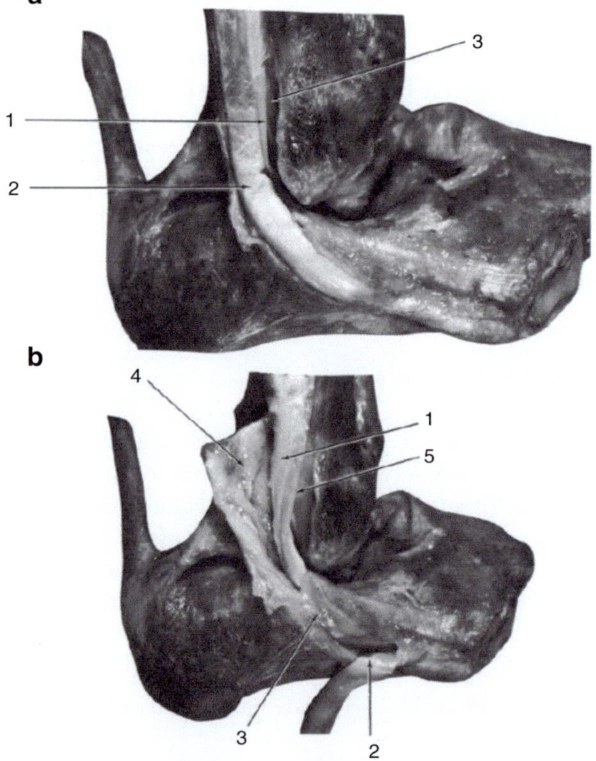

Fig. 1.2 Peroneus longus tendon. (**a**) SPR split. (1. peroneus brevis tendon; 2. peroneus longus tendon; 3. sulcus of peronei.) (**b**) Peroneus longus tendon reflected. (1. peroneus brevis tendon; 2. reflected peroneus longus tendon; 3. septum dividing inferior peroneus retinacular tunnel into two; 4. deep surface of superior peroneus retinaculum; 5.sulcus of peronei.) (From: Sarrafian, P. 235)

the os calcis, and this is also the site of the second directional turn as it now heads inferiorly and medially (Fig. 1.2). Finally, it makes its final turn as it traces around the lateral border of the foot between the cuboid and the base of the fifth metatarsal.

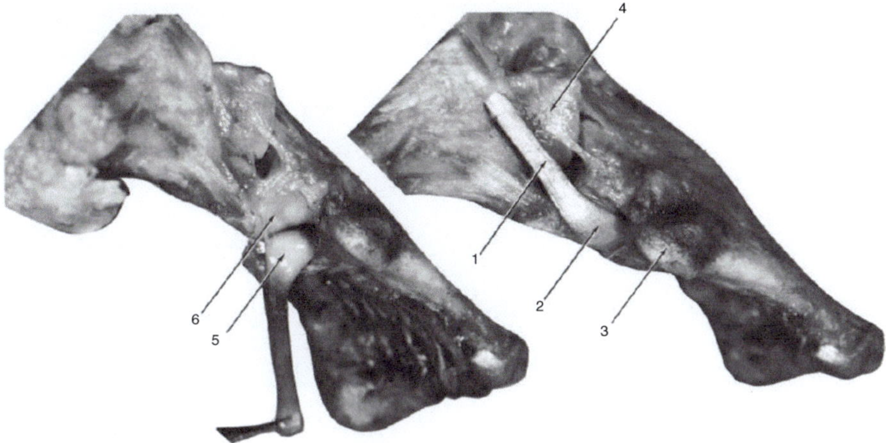

Fig. 1.3 Peroneus longus tendon. (1. peroneus longus tendon; 2. portion of [1] reflected on tuberosity of cuboid and entering sole of foot; 3. tuberosity of fifth metatarsal base; 4. anterior segment or greater apophysis of os calcis; 5. intra-articular sesamoid of peroneus longus tendon; 6. cuboidal tuberosity for reflection of peroneus longus tendon.) (From: Sarrafian [23], P. 236)

This is also where it enters the final tunnel, the plantar tunnel after gliding over the anterior convex slope of the cuboid tuberosity (Fig. 1.3) [1].

On the plantar aspect of the foot, the peroneus longus tendon heads lateromedially and attaches on the lateral tubercle of the base of the first metatarsal. Occasionally, there are accessory attachments to the medial cuneiform, base of the second metatarsal and/or the first dorsal interosseous. The plantar peroneus tunnel is fibrous at the level of the cuboid with fibers that extend from the crest of the cuboid tuberosity to the anterior ledge of the cuboid. The fibers run deep to the long cuboideometatarsal ligament. The inferior aspect of the tunnel is also reinforced by the long plantar ligament to the base of the fourth and third metatarsals. The roof of the tunnel comprises this fibrous layer of the tissue.

At the level of the cuboid tubercle, there is commonly a sesamoid that can be either osseous or fibrocartilaginous within the substance of the tendon. The sesamoid (os peroneum) glides along the plantar oblique articulation of the lateral aspect of the cuboid [4]. Though the sesamoid is usually a single round piece, it can also have multiple segments or be oblong [5]. There can also be a sesamoid within the tendon in the retromalleolar region, but this is rare (Fig. 1.4) [1].

Smith and Brandes looked at 22 patients with surgical or MRI findings of peroneus longus tendinopathy and used this information to define three zones of the peroneus longus tendon where injuries were most likely to occur (Fig. 1.5). These included the following:

- Zone A: From the retromalleolar area, the tip of the lateral malleolus in the region of tendon covered by the superior retinaculum.
- Zone B: The portion of tendon covered by the inferior retinaculum at the level of the lateral calcaneal trochlear process.

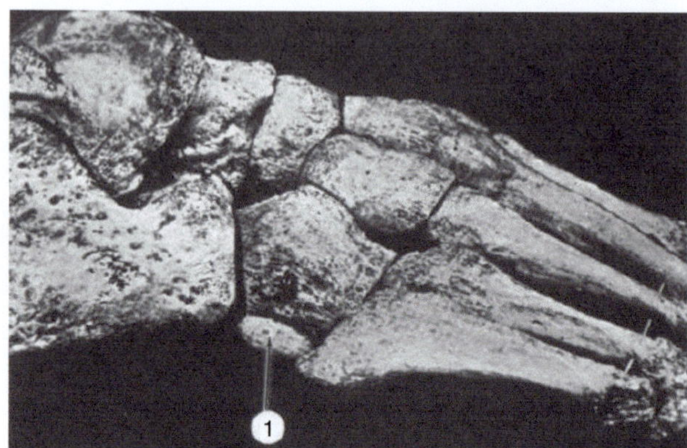

Fig. 1.4 Os peroneum. (From: Sarrafian [23], P. 99)

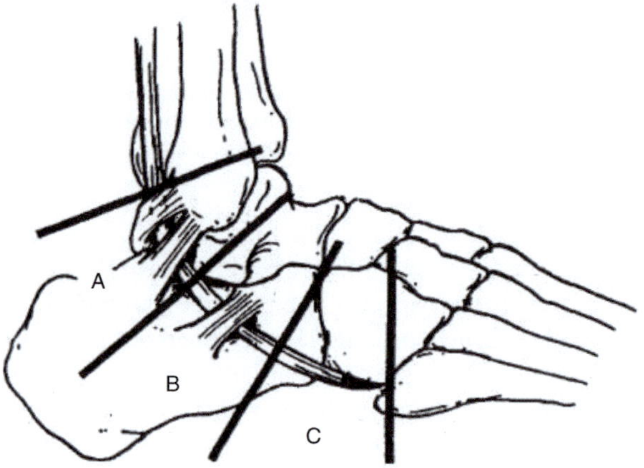

Fig. 1.5 The three zones of the peroneus longus tendon where injuries were most likely to occur as described by Brandes and Smith. These are described above. (From: Brandes and, Smith [6])

- Zone C: The region of tendon that changes direction to the plantar aspect of the foot at the level of the cuboid notch.

In their study, all complete ruptures occurred in Zone C, at the cuboid notch (6 patients), while almost all of the partial ruptures (8 of 9 patients) occurred in Zone B. They then tried to correlate onset of symptoms with the specific zones in regard to insidious versus acute. Though there was a trend toward patients with acute symptoms having a complete rupture in zone C and patients with insidious symptoms having partial tears in Zone B, they could not reach statistical significance [6].

The normal insertions of the tendon are on the plantar first metatarsal base, the plantar aspect of the medial cuneiform, and the superior lateral aspect of the first metatarsal head. The slip to the medial cuneiform arises from the dorsal surface of the longus tendon at the level of the sesamoid in the cuboid tunnel. This fan-shaped slip extends medially and eventually attaches on the anterior aspect of the plantar surface of the medial cuneiform [7].

The slip to the lateral aspect of the first metatarsal head arises from the anterior portion of the tendon. It begins its path toward the base of the second metatarsal where it is adhered very weekly and is braced by transverse ligament that acts as a fibrous bridge. From there the tendinous slip changes direction toward the first metatarsal head as it passes through the first interosseous space. In the interosseous space, there are insertions on both sides of the tendon to the first dorsal interosseous muscle. This slip eventually attaches 1 cm proximal to the first metatarsal head on the lateral aspect of the bone. This slip also forms an arcade along the lateral border of the first metatarsal filled with adipose tissue that gives passage to the dorsal vessels going to the sole of the foot [1]. Picou described the prevalence of these various slips in a 54-specimen cadaveric study. He found that 95% inserted on the cuneiform and metatarsal base, 89% inserted on the metatarsal head, and 5.5% inserted on the metatarsal base alone [7].

Other aberrant attachments include an insertion to the base of the fifth metatarsal at the level of the cuboid sesamoid. There can also be a small connection to the short flexor of the fifth toe, and this forms the anterior frenular ligament. A posterior frenular ligament can exist as well from the sesamoid to the cuboid. The prevalence of these structures have been reported in various cadaveric studies to be 63–80% for the anterior frenular ligaments and 10–13% for the posterior frenular ligaments [7, 8]. Finally, Picou found that the peroneus longus tendon can receive a slip from the posterior tibialis tendon 22% of time [7].

Patil et al. looked at the insertion of the peroneus longus more recently in a study of 30 preserved specimens. The tendon attached to the first metatarsal base in all specimens and the medial cuneiform in 23 feet (86.6%). The attachment to the neck of the first metatarsal was found in 3 feet (10%). Accessory attachments to the bases of the lesser metatarsals were found to the second metatarsal in 20% (6 feet), fourth metatarsal in 16.6% (5 feet), and fifth metatarsal in 23.3% (7 feet). The anterior frenular ligament was present 83.3% (25 feet) of the time while the posterior frenular ligament was present in 13.3% (4 feet) of the specimens [9]. Finally, Patil et al. interestingly found "an additional band and quite similar to the anterior frenular ligament, was observed close to the first metatarsocuneiform joint in nine specimens (30%). This band gave origins of the first and second dorsal interossei and first plantar interosseous muscles" (Figs. 1.6 and 1.7). [9]

Peroneus Brevis

The peroneus brevis glides in the retromalleolar grove along the posterior surface of the lateral malleolus. The tendon alters direction anteriorly just distal to the tip of the lateral malleolus along the contour of bone. The fibrous sheath of the peroneus contains the tendon at this level. From here, the tendon heads anteriorly downward and slightly laterally as it crosses over the calcaneofibular ligament. It eventually fans out and inserts to the apophasis of the base of the fifth metatarsal after passing superiorly to the calcaneal processus trochlearis and through the inferior peroneus retinaculum [1].

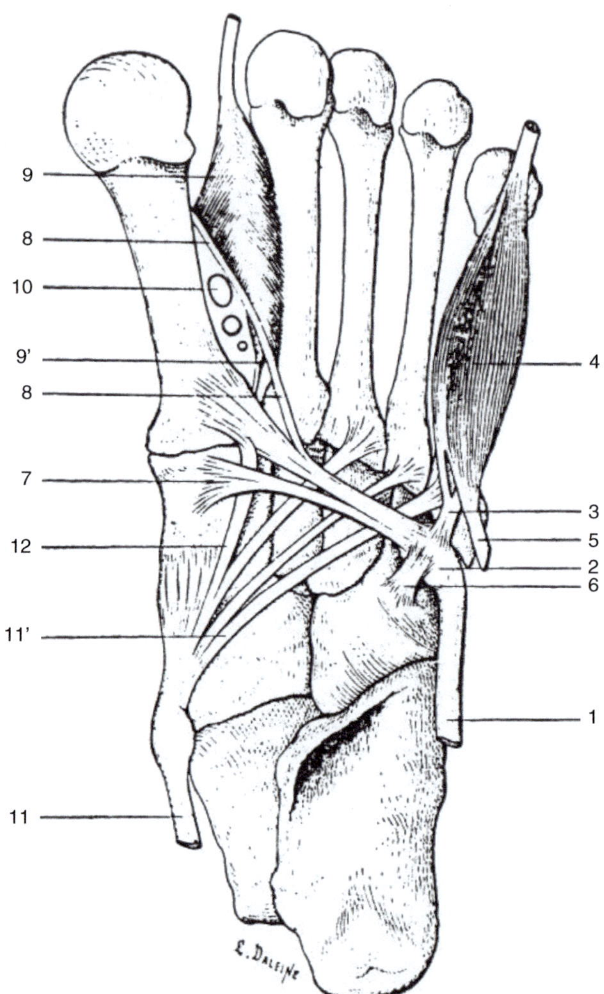

Fig. 1.6 Normal insertions of peroneus longus tendon. (1. peroneus longus tendon; 2. Sesamoid; 3. anterior frenulum of sesamoid; 4. short flexor muscle of fifth toe; 5. expansion of 4 that inserts on fibrous tunnel of peroneus longus tendon; 6. posterior frenulum of sesamoid [inconstant]; 7. attachment of 1 on medial cuneiform; 8. expansion of 1 forming an arcade of origin to the first dorsal interosseous muscle [9] and inserting on the superolateral corner of the first metatarsal neck; 9. origin of first dorsal interosseous from base of first metatarsal; 10. dorsalis pedis vessels; 11. tibialis posterior tendon; 11′. expansion of 11 to base of fifth metatarsal [inconstant]; 12. expansion of 11 to peroneus longus tendon [inconstant].) (From: Sarrafian [23], P. 238)

Peroneus Tertius

The peroneus tertius tendon runs lateral to the extensor digitorum longus and runs under the inferior extensor retinaculum. The tendon tracks anteriorly and laterally and fans out to a broad insertion on the superior aspect of the fifth metatarsal base [1]. The tendon can be absent in a portion of the population with LeDouble showing in a 1890's study that there was a 8.5% [65 of 759] rate of peroneus tertius deficiency [8]. This was reaffirmed by Reimann who showed peroneus tertius absence in 10% of his 200 cadaveric foot study (Fig. 1.8) [10].

There are also insertional variations of the tendon with an additional slip being present in some. An additional slip can attach to the fifth metatarsal shaft, on the interosseous space, the fifth toe at the level of the phalange, or the fifth long

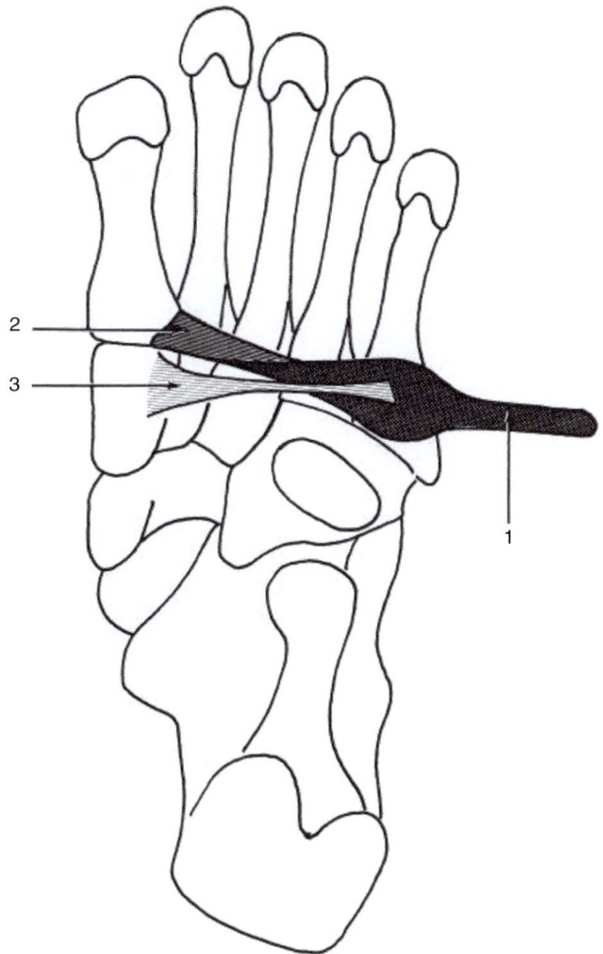

Fig. 1.7 Slip of peroneus longus tendon to the first cuneiform. (1. deep surface of peroneus longus tendon; 2. Superficial surface of 1 inserting on base of first metatarsal; 3. deep slip arising from deep surface of 1 and inserting on first cuneiform.) (From: Sarrafian [23], P. 238)

extensor. There can also be an additional slip to the fourth metatarsal base. This slip can be as long as, if not longer than the main insertion and in rare cases can be the sole attachment of the peroneus tertius [1].

Variations of the Lateral Peronei

There are multiple variations in the lateral peroneus, and with variations in even the descriptive terminology used to describe them, there is "a regrettable confusion." [11] In order to clear the confusion, Testus utilized comparative anatomy and referred specifically to the peroneus digiti quinti in bears and cats. In bears, there are three lateral tendons, a long tendon, short tendon, and then the peroneus digiti quinti which runs in the middle of the other two. It arises at the distal

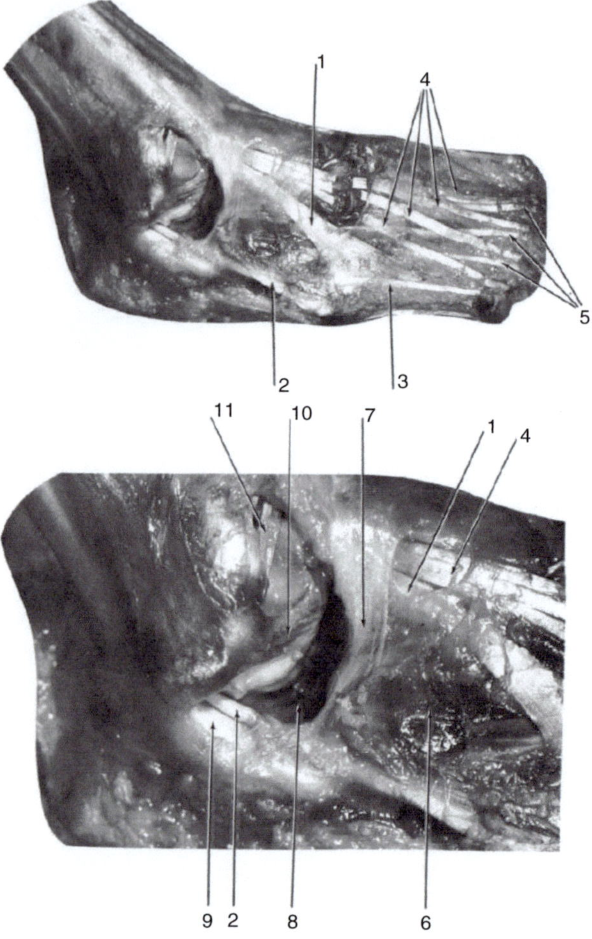

Fig. 1.8 Peroneus tertius tendon. (1. peroneus tertius tendon; 2. peroneus brevis tendon; 3. supplementary slip of 2; 4. extensor digitorum longus tendons; 5. extensor digitorum brevis tendons 2, 3, 4; 6. extensor digitorum brevis muscle origin; 7. stem of inferior extensor retinaculum occupying middle and anterior segments of sinus tarsi [8]; 9. peroneus longus tendon; 10. anterior talofibular ligament; 11. lower band of anterior tibiofibular ligament) (From: Sarrafian [23], P. 234)

fibula, turns around the tip of the lateral malleolus, follows along the dorsum of the fifth metatarsal shaft and eventually inserts on the proximal phalanx of the fifth toe. In humans, he suggested that humans also have a peroneus digiti quinti in some capacity and suggested the following classification for the multiple variations [11].

A. Complete
   - Inserts on the proximal phalanx of the fifth toe and has a complete, independent muscle belly
   - Inserts on the proximal phalanx of the fifth toe and has a shared muscle belly with the peroneus brevis
   - Inserts as a tendon slip of the peroneus brevis on the proximal phalanx of the fifth toe with no muscle belly

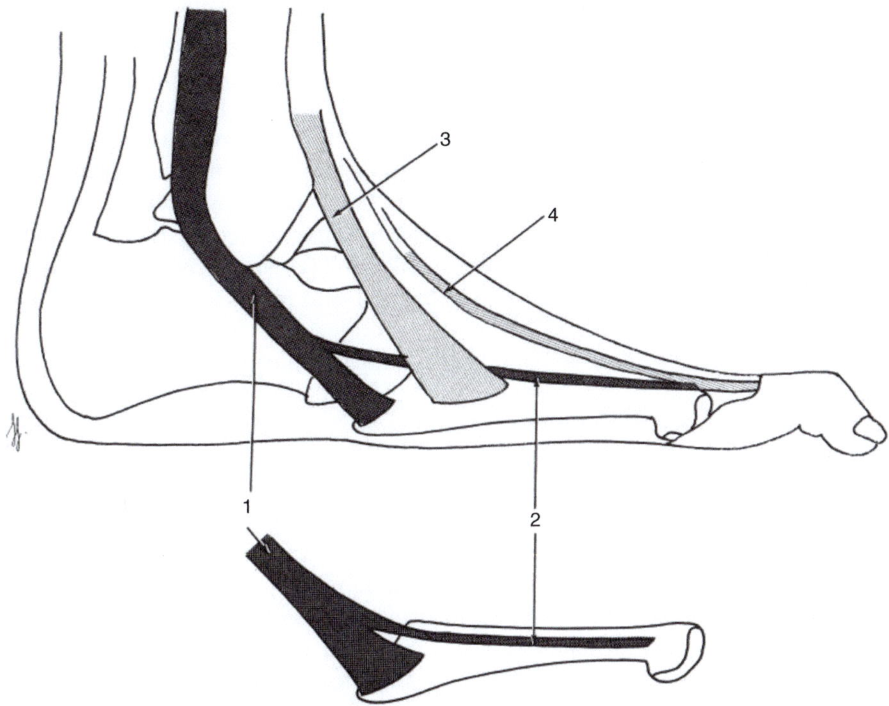

Fig. 1.9 Variation of lateral peronei. (1. peroneus brevis tendon; 2. accessory slip passing through peroneus tertius (3) insertion and attaching to fifth metatarsal shaft (4) or long extensor of fifth toe.) (From: Sarrafian [23], P. 239)

B. Incomplete
- Type I – Peroneometatarsal muscle, the tendon inserts on the fifth metatarsal head, neck or shaft
- Type II
  - Peroneocuboidal muscle, the tendon inserts on the cuboid
  - Peroneoperoneus longus muscle, the tendon inserts to the peroneus longus tendon (the accessorius of Henle)
- Type III – External peroneocalcaneal muscle, tendon inserts on the lateral calcaneus (peroneus quartus of Otto)
- Type IV – Peroneomalleolar muscle, tendon inserts on the lateral malleolus

The peroneus digiti quinti of Huxley is the most common sub-variety and is a slip from the peroneus brevis that pierces the peroneus tertius and then attaches to the fifth toe proximal phalanx, extensor tendon/aponeurosis, or fifth metatarsal, head neck, or base. Various studies have reported on the occurrence of this tendinous slip. In his 102-foot cadaveric series, Wood found a well-developed slip in 23% and a vestigial slip in 13% for a total of 36% [12]. LeDouble's 100-foot series found a well-developed slip in 21% and a vestigial slip in 13% for a total of 34% (Fig. 1.9) [8].

In a study of 200 specimens, Reimann found a tendinous slip for the peroneus brevis in 79.5% of feet. The variable insertions of this slip include the peroneus tertius, extensor aponeurosis of the fifth and fourth metatarsal shaft, extensor aponeurosis fifth toe, fifth metatarsal shaft, fourth and fifth metatarsal shafts, fourth metatarsal shaft, extensor aponeurosis of the fifth toe and peroneus tertius tendon, extensor aponeurosis of the fifth toe with a loop around the tertius and insertion on the fourth metatarsal shaft, fifth metatarsal shaft and peroneus tertius tendon, and finally, the fourth and fifth metatarsal shafts and extensor aponeurosis of the fifth toe [10]. Bareither et al. studied 298 cadaveric limbs and found that 59.7% of the specimens demonstrated a tendinous slip from the peroneus brevis to the aponeurosis of the fifth toe [13].

In 1816, Otto first described the peroneus quartus muscle that originated from the distal fibular, follows the groove within the sheath and then attaches to the lateral calcaneus [14]. A study by Gruber looking at 982 specimens found the peroneus quartus present in 12% [15]. Conversely, Wood found a 3% incidence of the quartus in a series of 70 extremities [12].

Hecker also looked at the variations in the lateral tendons and formed three groups: lateral peroneocalcaneal muscle, peroneocuboid muscle, and finally the peroneoperoneolongus muscle. This study also sought to determine the prevalence of these muscle variations in both adult and embryotic specimens and found them to be 13% (study of 47 feet) and 20% (study of 16 feet) respectively. Within these groups, the most diverse was the lateral peroneocalcaneal, which was found to have 6 subtypes: [16]

- Type I – A muscle that originates from the peroneus longus and brevis, becomes tendinous (4 mm diameter), and passes through the superior retinaculum as it goes around the tip of the lateral malleolus before splitting into two slips. The thin anterior slip attaches above the peroneus brevis tendon to the origin of the inferior peroneus retinaculum. The more robust posterior slip attaches below the brevis tendon on the lateral calcaneus creating a passage for the brevis tendon to traverse.
- Type II – A muscle that originates from the peroneus brevis belly then forms a 5-cm long tendon cylindrical tendon that is 2.5 mm in diameter. It eventually inserts on the lateral calcaneus posterior to the inferior peroneus retinaculum and posterior to the peroneus longus in a broad fan shape.
- Type III – A muscle that originates from the distal peroneus brevis belly then forms a thin tendon that attaches to the lateral calcaneus at the inferior aspect of the inferior retinaculum.
- Type IV – A muscle that originates from the fibula and the posterolateral intramuscular septum then forms a thin tendon with a similar attachment to the type III.
- Type V – A muscle that arises from the peroneus brevis and three fingerbreadths above the tip of the lateral malleolus, a small myotendinous branch diverges and becomes the peroneocalcaneal ligament. The body of the muscle belly then becomes tendinous, forms three distinct branches, and then all branches attach to the lateral calcaneus in line with fibula.
- Type VI – (RARE) A muscle that originates from the middle third of the lateral surface of the fibula, the anterior crest of the fibula, and the lateral intramuscular

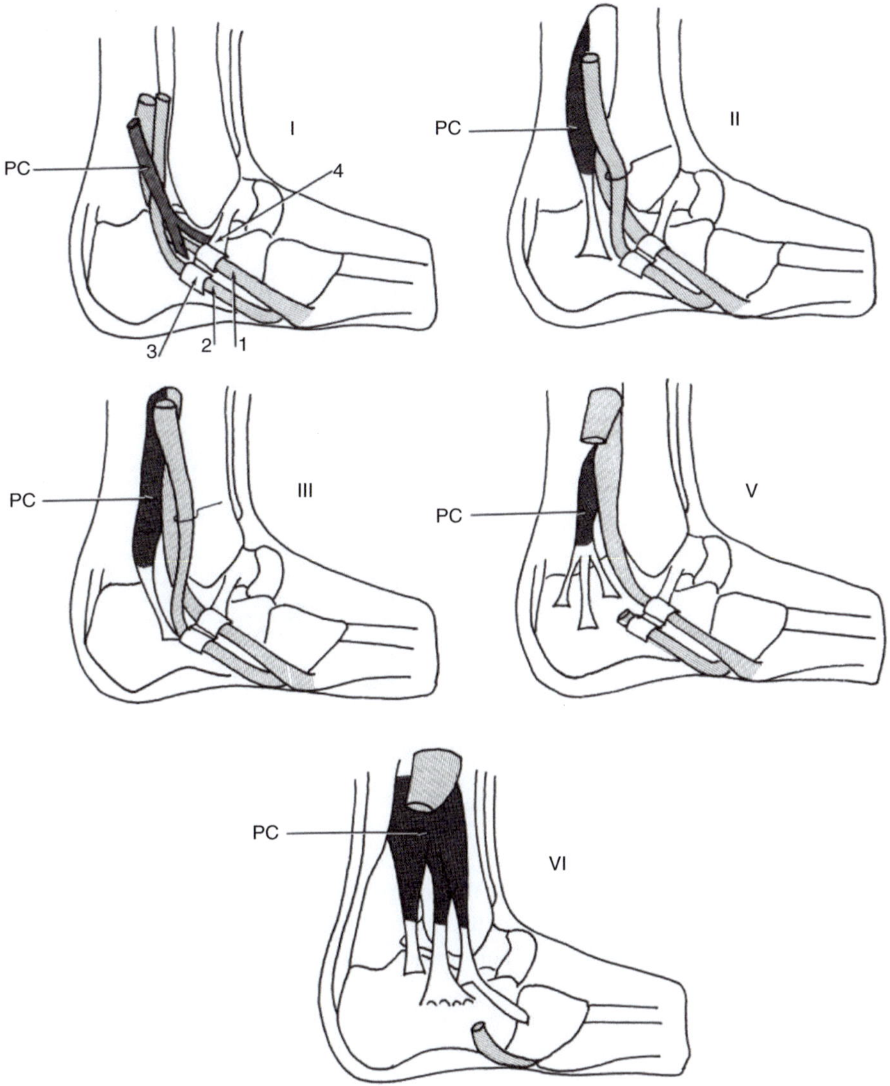

Fig. 1.10 Types of variation of lateral peronei. (PC. peroneocalcaneal muscle; 1. peroneus brevis tendon; 2. peroneus longus tendon; 3. inferior peroneus retinaculum; 4. stem of inferior extensor retinaculum.) (From: Sarrafian [23], P. 241)

septum. This muscle replaces the peroneus brevis and forms three distinct tendons as it tracts inferiorly. The posterior branch is thin and attaches to the lateral calcaneus inferior to the lateral malleolus. The middle branch attaches in a broad fan-shape on the lateral calcaneus. The anterior branch attaches to the lateral calcaneus, the calcaneocuboid ligament, and the lateral aspect of the cuboid (Fig. 1.10).

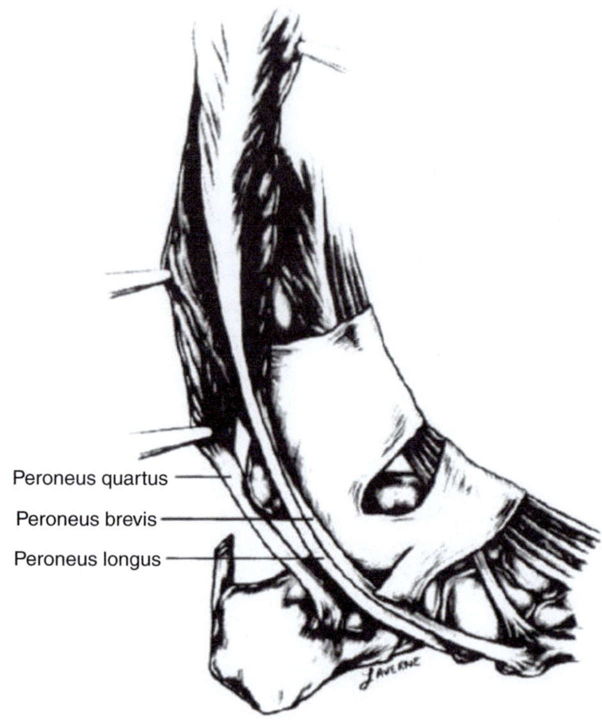

Fig. 1.11 The peroneus quartus takes origin from the lower one-third portion of the peroneus brevis and inserts into the peroneus tubercle of the calcaneus. Hypertrophy of the peroneus tubercle is evident. (From: Sarrafian [23], P. 242)

Other rare variations:

- Peroneocuboid muscle – A muscle that originates from the inferior lateral compartment that forms a tendon that attaches to the lateral aspect of the cuboid.
- Bifid peroneus longus tendon – This tendon forms a bottom hole that the brevis tendon traverses.
- Peroneoperoneolongus muscle – A muscle that originates from the inferior lateral septum and forms a tendon that inserts into the peroneus longus tendon.

More recently, Sobel et al. looked at the peroneus quartus and its variations in a study of 124 feet. They found the quartus to be present in 21.7% of the specimens and also of note, when the quartus was present, there was attrition of the peroneus brevis in the fibular groove 18% of the time [17]. Sobel et al. found the following eight variations listed by most common:

- 63% – Peroneus quartus originates from the peroneus brevis belly and attaches to the peroneus tubercle of the calcaneus (Fig. 1.11).
- 11.1% – Peroneus quartus originates from the peroneus brevis and inserts into the lateral retinaculum.

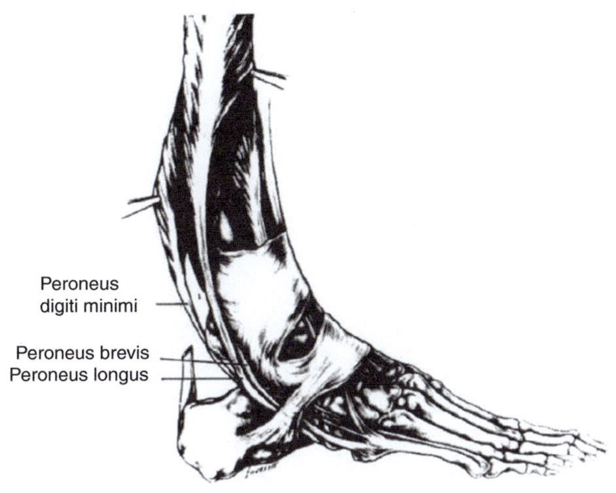

Fig. 1.12 The peroneus digiti minimi quinti takes origin from the peroneus brevis and the tendinous portion splits into two tendons. One slip inserts dorsally at the base of the fifth metatarsal and the long slip inserts into the dorsum of the head of the fifth metatarsal. (From: Sarrafian [23], P. 243)

- 7.4% – Peroneus quartus originates from the peroneus brevis, and then the tendinous portion splits into two slips. One slip attaches to the dorsum of the fifth metatarsal shaft and the other to the fifth metatarsal head (Fig. 1.12).
- 7.4% – Peroneus quartus originates from the proximal peroneus longus and attaches to the peroneus tubercle of the calcaneus (Fig. 1.13).
- 3.7% – Peroneus quartus originates from the peroneus brevis and attaches to the peroneus longus tendon after it exists the retromalleolar groove (Fig. 1.14).
- 3.7% – Peroneus quartus originates from the peroneus brevis belly and attaches back to the brevis tendon after it exists the fibular groove (Fig. 1.15).
- 3.7% – Peroneus quartus originates from the proximal peroneus longus and reattaches to longus tendon after it exists the fibular groove (Fig. 1.16).
- 3.7% – Peroneus quartus originates from the peroneus longus and inserts on the peroneus brevis.

Sonmez et al. reported on the presence in some cases of bilateral peroneus quartus and the peroneus digiti. They also found that when the peroneus quinti muscle was present bilaterally, there was also a slip of tendon from the tibialis anterior tendon to the base of the proximal phalanx of the great toe bilaterally (Figs. 1.17, 1.18, and 1.19) [18].

A study of 102 cadaveric legs and 80 MRI studies of symptomatic ankles by Zammit and Singh showed the prevalence of the peroneus quartus to be 5.9% and 7.5%, respectively, with and overall occurrence of 6.7% [19].

An MRI study of 65 asymptomatic ankles by Saupe et al. found the presence of a peroneus quartus muscle in 17% of their ankles. There was a variable insertion of the tendon to the lateral calcaneus, the cuboid, or the peroneus longus tendon [20].

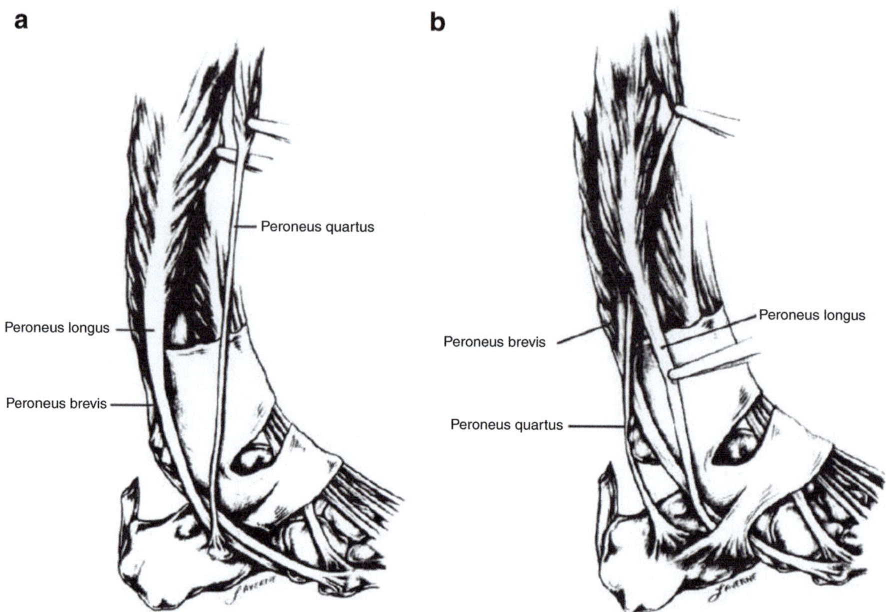

Fig. 1.13 (**a**) The peroneus quartus takes origin high in the leg from the peroneus longus and inserts into the peroneus tubercle of the calcaneus. Hypertrophy of the peroneus tubercle is evident. (**b**) The peroneus quartus takes origin high in the leg from the peroneus longus, courses under the tendon of the peroneus longus, and inserts into the peroneus tubercle of the calcaneus. (From: Sarrafian [23], P. 243)

Fig. 1.14 The peroneus quartus takes origin from the peroneus brevis and inserts into the peroneus longus just distal to the fibular groove. (From: Sarrafian [23], P. 242)

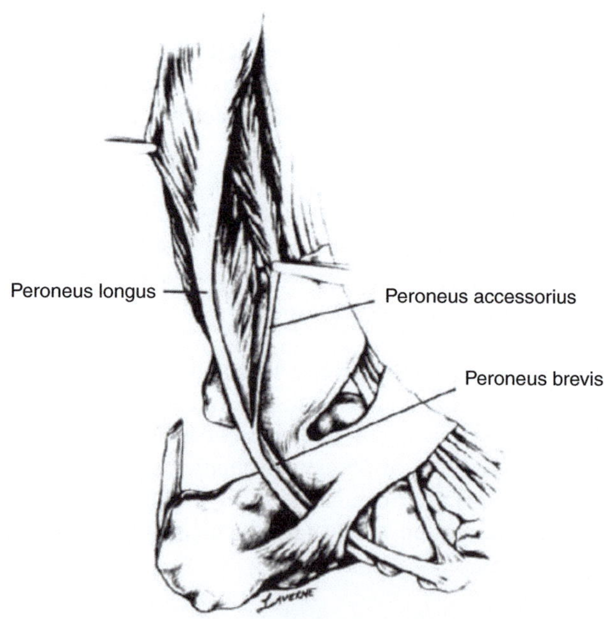

Fig. 1.15 The peroneus quartus takes origin from the peroneus brevis and inserts back into the peroneus brevis just distal to the fibular groove. (From: Sarrafian [23], P. 242)

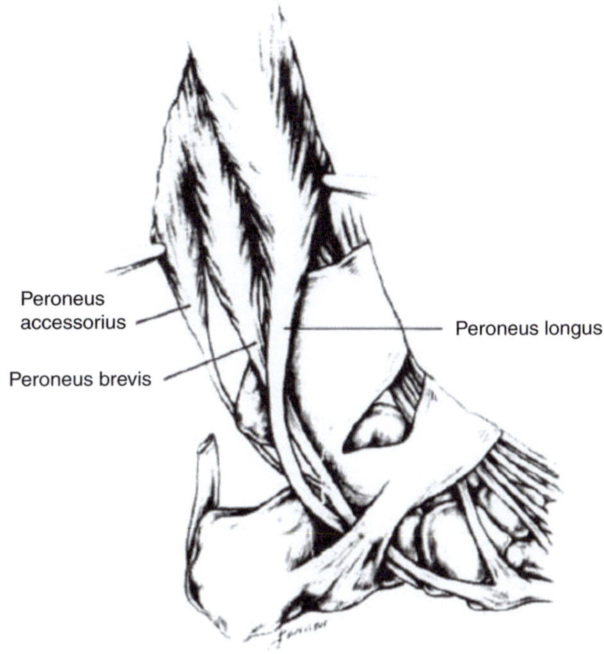

Fig. 1.16 The peroneus quartus takes origin high in the leg from the peroneus longus and inserts back into the peroneus longus just distal to the fibular groove. (From: Sarrafian [23], P. 244)

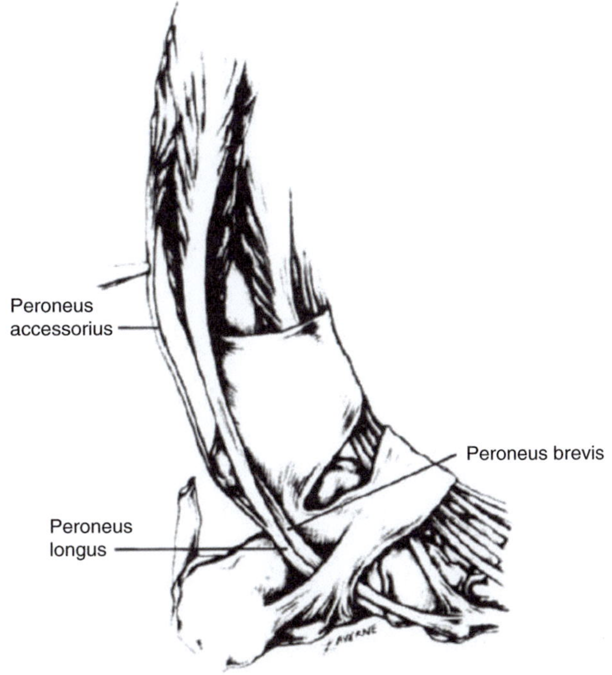

Fig. 1.17 Lateral view of the right foot showing the tendon of the peroneus quartus inserting in the peroneus trochlea on the calcaneus (arrowhead). (From: Sarrafian [23], P. 244)

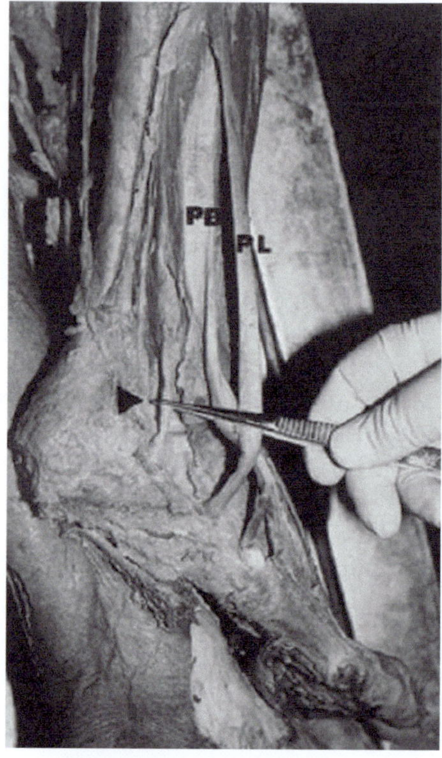

Fig. 1.18 Lateral view of the foot showing the tendon of the peroneus digiti quinti inserting into the aponeurosis of the fifth toe (arrowhead). (From: Sarrafian [23], P. 245)

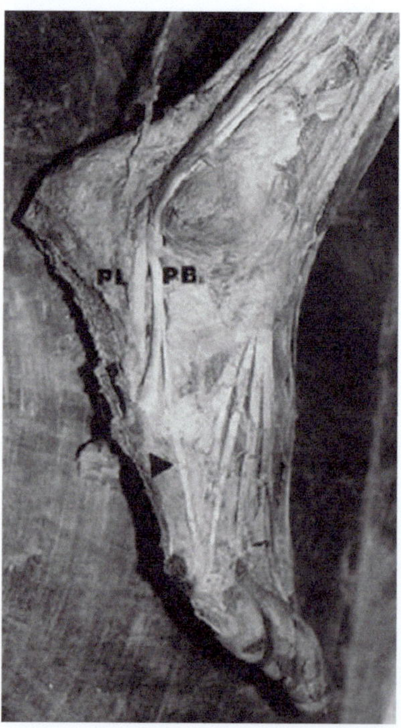

Fig. 1.19 Superomedial view of the right foot showing the accessory tendon of tibialis anterior inserting into the base of the proximal phalanx of the big toe (arrowhead). (From: Sarrafian [23], P. 245)

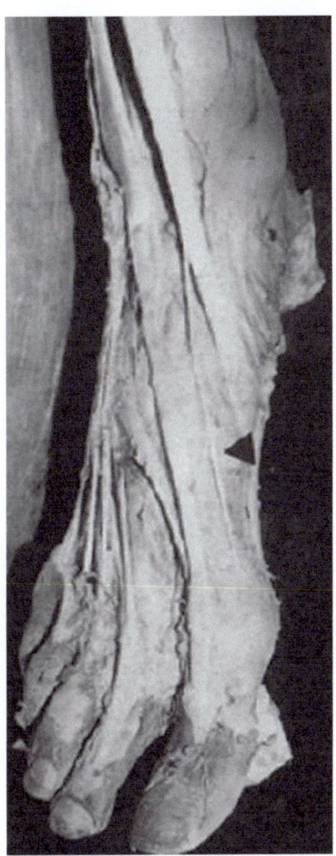

Relation of the Sural Nerve

Proximally, it lies posterior to the peroneus longus. According to Lawrene and Bolti from cadaveric specimens located 7 cm proximal to the distal tip of the fibula, it lies 26 mm posterior. This is less at the level of the tip of the malleolus at 14 mm, as well as 14 mm distal. At this point, it bifurcates distally (Figs. 1.20 and 1.21) [2].

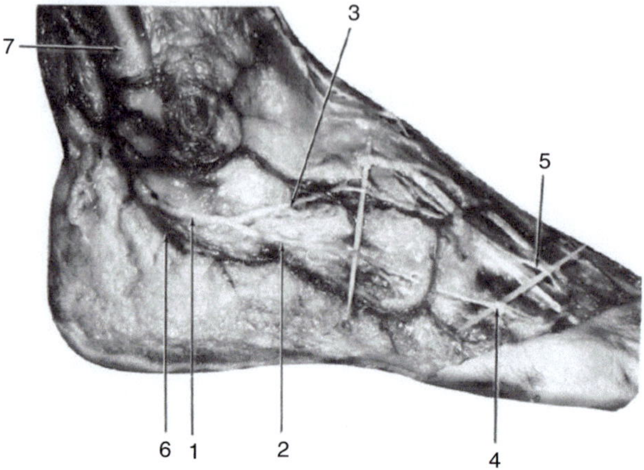

Fig. 1.20 Lateral aspect of the right foot and ankle. (1. sural nerve dividing into lateral branch (2) forming dorsolateral cutaneous nerve (4) and medial branch (3) uniting with intermediate dorsal cutaneous nerve (5) of superficial peroneal nerve; 6. shorter saphenous vein; 7. peronei tendons.) (From: Sarrafian SK (2011) Anatomy of the Foot and Ankle: Descriptive Topographic, Functional. J.B. Lippincott, Philadelphia. P. 385)

Fig. 1.21 Sural nerve. Four lateral calcaneal branches (small arrows), an anastomotic branch (large arrow), distal bifurcation (distal arrow). (From: Sarrafian [23], P. 387)

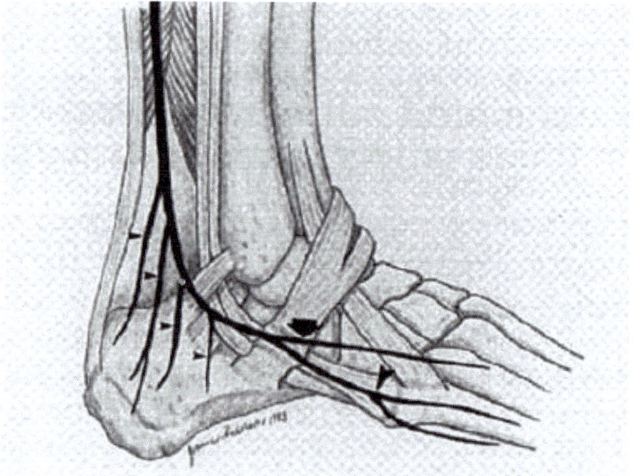

Blood Supply

Sobel et al. looked at the vascularity of the peroneus in a series of 12 specimens and determined there were three zones for each tendon, zone A, zone B, and zone C. Zone A included the regions from the musculotendinous junction to the proximal aspect of the fibular groove. Zone B is the portion of the tendon that traverses the fibular groove. Zone C is comprised of the tendon from the fibular groove to the bony attachment. Proximally, the tendons are provided blood supply from muscular branches of the posterior peroneus artery. In the study, they found that along the length of the peroneus longus, there was a rich vinculum supplied from the lateral periphery. The brevis tendon had a similar network of vinculum, except it was more prominent in zones A and C and less robust in zone B. In spite of this, in the ten specimens where both brevis and longus tendons were present, no hypovasulcar area was found [21].

Petersen et al. also studied the blood supply of the peroneus tendons in a two-part study. One utilized injection techniques of ten fresh cadaveric legs and the other looked at 20 peroneus brevis and longus tendons with bony attachments immuno-histochemically [22].

In the injection portion of the study, there was found to be a relatively avascular zone at the level of the fibular groove. They found the longitudinally oriented blood supply was interrupted in this region for an average length of 40 mm (29–55 mm).

The peroneus longus tendon was found to have avascular regions as well. The first was at the level of the turn around the distal fibula and another was found at the bend around the peroneus trochlea of the calcaneus. The first avascular zone was found along the anterior aspect of the tendon and spanned an average of 52 mm (38–63 mm). The second zone at the level of the cuboid bend was found to span an average of 25 mm (18–31 mm) [22].

The immunohistochemical portion of the study looked specifically at the presence of laminin, a basic component of a blood vessel's basement membrane. When looking at the peroneus brevis, there was a lack of laminin present at the level of the retromalleolar groove. The peroneus longus similarly showed a lack of evidence of laminin at the retromalleolar groove. The longus also showed a region, with a void of laminin at the bend it takes around the cuboid on the lateral aspect of the foot (Fig. 1.22) [22].

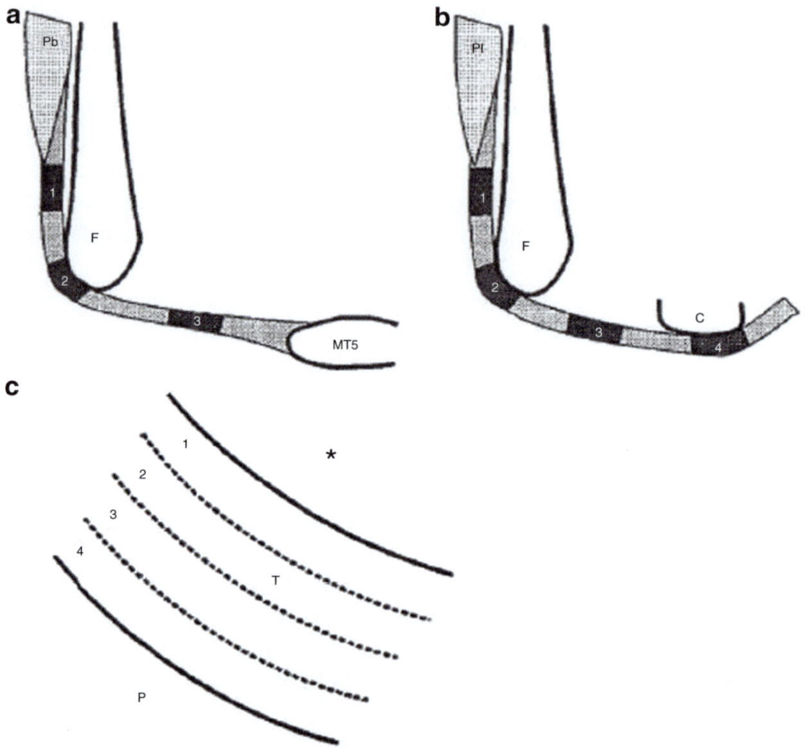

Fig. 1.22 (**a**) Location of three segments (dark marked) obtained from the peroneus brevis tendon for immunohistochemical proof of laminin. Segment 2 came from the region where the peroneus brevis wraps around the lateral malleolus. The segments measured 2 cm. (**b**) Location of biopsies (dark marked) from the peroneus longus tendon for immunohistochemical investigations. (PL peroneus longus muscle.) From each tendon, four segments (length 2 cm) were obtained. (**c**) Presence of positive immunoreactions in different quarters of the tendon. (1. anterior quarter adjacent to the gliding surface; 2 and 3. middle quarters; 4. peripheral quarters; (∗) location of the bony pulley, P peritendinum, T tendon.) (From: Sarrafian [23], P. 368)

Osteology

The lateral malleolus has a lateral, medial, and posterior surface. It has a pyramidal type shape. The peroneus brevis occupies the posterior surface. It twists with the fibular corpus. Edwards studied 178 dry fibula and found that 82% had a sulcus or concavity, 11% were flat and the remaining 7% were convex (Fig. 1.23) [2].

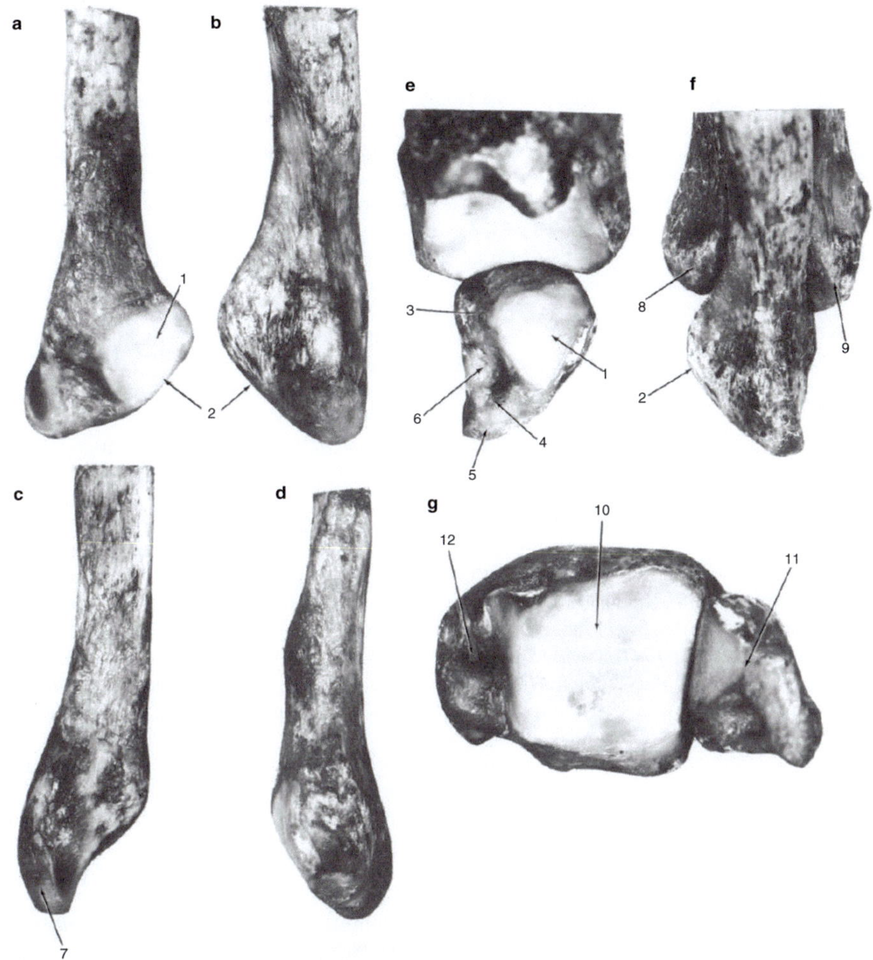

Fig. 1.23 (**a**) Medial view of left fibula. (**b**) Lateral view of fibula. (**c**) Posterior view of fibula. (**d**) Anterior view of fibula. (**e**) Medial view of tibia-lateral malleolus. (**f**) Lateral view of distal fibula–tibia. (**g**) Inferior view of distal tibia–fibula. (1. articular surface; 2. anterior border; 3. posterosuperior tubercle; 4. insertion tubercle of posterior talofibular ligament; 5. tip of lateral malleolus; 6. digital fossa; 7. gliding surface for peronei tendon; 8. anterior tibial tubercle; 9. posterior tibial tubercle; 10. tibial plafond; 11. lateral malleolus; 12. medial malleolus.) (From: Sarrafian [23], P. 43)

References

1. Kelikian AS, Sarrafian SK, Sarrafian SK. Sarrafian's anatomy of the foot and ankle: descriptive, topographical, functional. 3rd ed. Philadelphia: Wolters Kluwer Health/Lippincott Williams & Wilkins; 2011.
2. Edwards ME. The relations of the peroneal tendons to the fibula, calcaneus, and cuboideum. Am J Anat. 1928;42(1):213–53.
3. Ozbag D, Gumusalan Y, Uzel M, Cetinus E. Morphometrical features of the human malleolar groove. Foot Ankle Int. 2008;29(1):77–81.
4. Parsons FG, Keith A. Seventh report of the Committee of Collective Investigation of the Anatomical Society of Great Britain and Ireland, 1896-97. J Anat Physiol. 1897;32(Pt 1):164–86.
5. Köhler A, Zimmer EA, Wilk SP. Borderlands of the normal and early pathologic in skeletal roentgenology. 3d American ed. New York: Grune & Stratton; 1968.
6. Brandes CB, Smith RW. Characterization of patients with primary peroneus longus tendinopathy: a review of twenty-two cases. Foot Ankle Int. 2000;21(6):462–8.
7. Picou R. Bulletins de la Société anatomique de Paris. 1894.; http://gallica.bnf.fr/ark:/12148/bpt6k6413780t.
8. LeDouble A-F. Traité des variations du système musculaire de l'homme : et de leur signification au point de vue de l'anthropologie zoologique. T. 2 T. 2. Paris: Reinwald; 1897.
9. Patil V, Frisch NC, Ebraheim NA. Anatomical variations in the insertion of the peroneus (fibularis) longus tendon. Foot Ankle Int. 2007;28(11):1179–82.
10. Der RR. variable Streckapparat der kleinen Zehe. Konkurrierende Muskelgruppen im Wettbewerb um die Streckfunktion an dem in Rückbildung begriffenen fünften Strahl der unteren Extremität. Gegenbaurs Morphol Jahrb. 1981;127(2):188–209.
11. Testut L, Duval M. Les anomalies musculaires chez l'homme expliquées par l'anatomie comparée. Leur importance en anthropologie ... Précédé d'une préface par ... M. Duval. Paris; 1884. p. xv. 844.
12. Wood J. Variations in human myology observed during the winter session of 1867–68 at King's College, London. London: Royal Society of London; 1868.
13. Bareither DJ, Schuberth JM, Evoy PJ, Thomas GJ. Peroneus digiti minimi. Anat Anz. 1984;155(1–5):11–5.
14. Otto AW. Seltene Beobachtungen zur Anatomie, Physiologie und Pathologie gehörig. Wilibald August Holäufer: Breslau; 1816.
15. Gruber WL. Monographie über das Corpusculum triticeum und über die accidentelle Musculatur der Ligamenta hyo-thyreoidea lateralia. Nebst einem Anhange: mit Bemerkungen über die "Musculi thyreoidei marginales inferiores" - Gruber. St.-Pétersbourg: Eggers; 1876.
16. Hecker P. Étude sur le péronier du tarse (variations des péroniers latéraux). Strasbourg: [publisher not identified]; 1924.
17. Sobel M, Levy ME, Bohne WH. Congenital variations of the peroneus quartus muscle: an anatomic study. Foot Ankle. 1990;11(2):81–9.
18. Sönmez M, Kosar, Çimen M. The supernumerary peroneal muscles: case report and review of the literature. Foot Ankle Surg Foot Ankle Surg. 2000;6(2):125–9.
19. Zammit J, Singh D. The peroneus quartus muscle. Anatomy and clinical relevance. J Bone Joint Surg. British volume. 2003;85(8):1134–7.
20. Saupe N, Mengiardi B, Pfirrmann CW, Vienne P, Seifert B, Zanetti M. Anatomic variants associated with peroneal tendon disorders: MR imaging findings in volunteers with asymptomatic ankles. Radiology. 2007;242(2):509–17.
21. Sobel M, Geppert MJ, Hannafin JA, Bohne WH, Arnoczky SP. Microvascular anatomy of the peroneal tendons. Foot Ankle. 1992;13(8):469–72.
22. Petersen W, Bobka T, Stein V, Tillmann B. Blood supply of the peroneal tendons: injection and immunohistochemical studies of cadaver tendons. Acta Orthop Scand. 2000;71(2):168–74.
23. Sarrafian SK. Anatomy of the Foot and Ankle: Descriptive Topographic, Functional. Philadelphia: J.B. Lippincott; 2011.

Biomechanics of the Peroneal Tendons

2

Oliver Morgan, Jinsup Song, Rajshree Hillstrom, Mark Sobel, and Howard J. Hillstrom

Background

Purpose of the Peroneal Tendon

The foot-ankle complex is a structure that comprises 28 bones, 33 joints, and 112 ligaments, which are controlled by 13 extrinsic and 21 intrinsic muscles. One of its more understudied extrinsic structures are the peroneals, including the peroneus longus and brevis. The primary purpose of the peroneal tendon is to evert the hindfoot [1] and secondarily contribute to plantarflexion (Fig. 2.1). The peroneus longus combines these motions to keep the first metatarsal head purchased to the ground.

The peroneal tendon originates in the lateral compartment of the leg and travels around the lateral malleolus posteriorly and inferiorly [2] (Fig. 2.2a). The peroneus brevis tendon inserts into the base of the fifth metatarsal (Fig. 2.2a), while the peroneus longus tendon curves around the cuboid obliquely crosses the sole of the foot

O. Morgan (✉)
Faculty of Science and Engineering, Anglia Ruskin University, Chelmsford, Essex, UK
e-mail: oliver.morgan@anglia.ac.uk

J. Song
School of Podiatric Medicine, Temple University, Philadelphia, PA, USA
e-mail: jsong@temple.edu

R. Hillstrom
Tandon School of Engineering, New York University, New York, NY, USA
e-mail: rajshree.hillstrom@nyu.edu

M. Sobel
Private Practice, New York, NY, USA
e-mail: msobelmd@comcast.net

H. J. Hillstrom
Hospital for Special Surgery, New York, NY, USA
e-mail: hillstromh@hss.edu

© Springer Nature Switzerland AG 2020
M. Sobel (ed.), *The Peroneal Tendons*,
https://doi.org/10.1007/978-3-030-46646-6_2

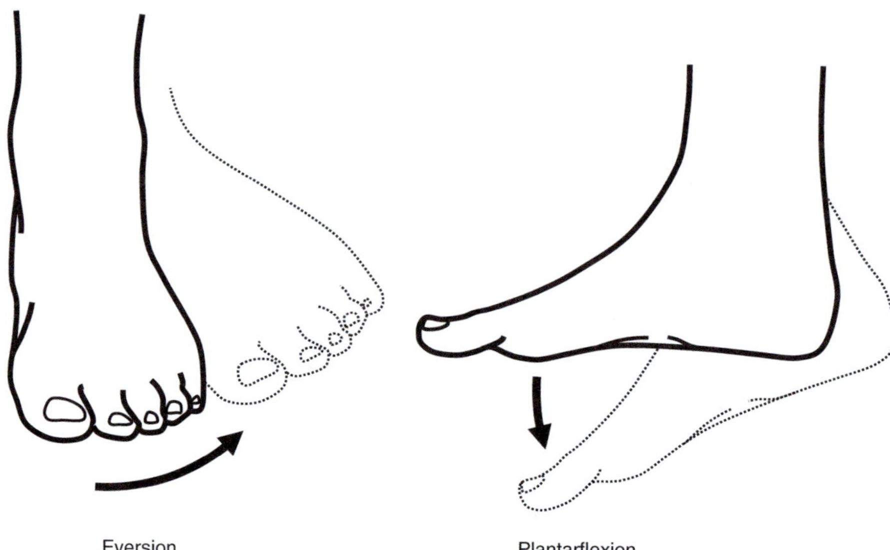

Fig. 2.1 The peroneal tendons and muscles elicit eversion and plantarflexion of the foot

Fig. 2.2 (**a**) The peroneus longus and peroneus brevis travel along the lateral compartment of the leg behind the lateral malleolus. (**b**) Insertion of the peroneus longus into the base of the first metatarsal and medial cuneiform

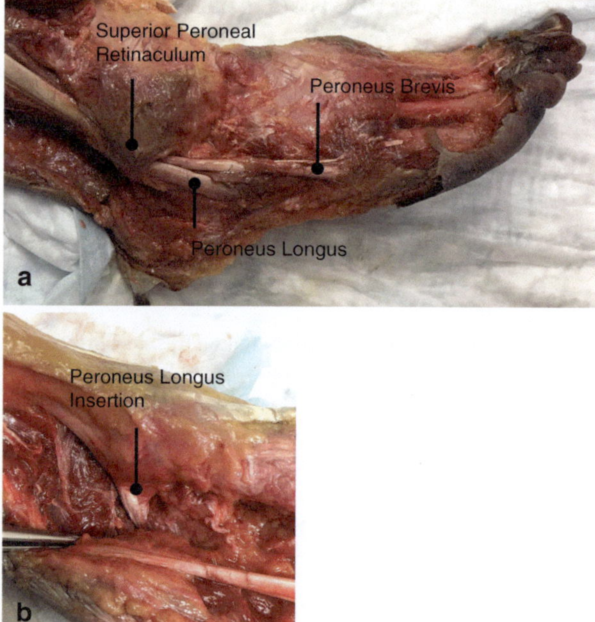

and inserts into the plantar-lateral aspect of the first metatarsal base and the medial cuneiform (Fig. 2.2b). The peroneal nerve innervates both the peroneus brevis and peroneus longus muscles. In healthy individuals, the musculotendinous junctions are located proximal to the superior peroneal retinaculum. The peroneus brevis and peroneus longus tendons pass through the common peroneal synovial sheath (~4 cm proximal to the lateral malleolus). The tendon sheath is stabilized by the posterior surface of the distal fibula (retromalleolar sulcus). This sulcus can vary in depth and width, which can contribute to dislocation and chronic subluxation of the peroneal tendons.

Clinical Presentation

The peroneus longus and brevis work to stabilize the foot when undergoing a forceful inversion and have been implicated in the lateral ankle ligament injury mechanism. Typically referred to as an ankle sprain, it is a common musculoskeletal injury that may be elicited by inversion or eversion. Such an injury may be self-treated with rest, ice, and elevation. The athletic trainer, physical therapist, podiatric physician, emergency room physician, sports medicine, or foot and ankle orthopedist may be consulted during the process of evaluation and treatment, especially if a complication is suspected. Both high and low arches have been implicated with lateral ankle ligament sprain risks. Ankle sprains have an incidence rate of 2.15 per 1000 (23,000/day) in the United States with an estimated annual cost of $2 billion [3].

Lateral ankle ligament injuries (anterior tibiofibular ligament (ATFL) and calcaneofibular ligament (CFL)) are often accompanied with peroneal tendinopathy. Rapid inversion and plantarflexion are known to potentially damage the lateral ankle ligaments, superior peroneal retinaculum, and peroneal tendons. Patients with chronic ruptures of the peroneal tendons typically present with a planus foot structure, difficulty everting the hindfoot, swelling, lateral pain, and functional instability with limited plantarflexion of the first ray and dorsiflexion of the ankle. In addition, the cavus foot structure has also been implicated in chronic rupture of the peroneal tendon. Untreated prior injury, chronic inflammatory changes, or tendon tension/friction have been implicated in chronic rupture of the peroneal tendons [4]. In a cadaveric model, Geppert et al. sectioned the lateral ankle ligaments to simulate ankle instability, demonstrating a concomitant increase in optical displacement of metal beads within the superior peroneal retinaculum [5]. This structure functions to restrain the peroneal tendons, and hence, when damaged from lateral ankle instability or sprain, the peroneal tendons are at risk.

Anatomical Variants

The tendons pass anteriorly to the peroneal tubercle of the calcaneus, which when hypertrophied can be associated with stenosis, inflammation, and attrition of tendons [2]. The os peroneum, an oval accessory bone within the peroneus longus tendon, maybe ossified in 20% of feet. In 13%–22% of ankles, an accessory muscle, the peroneus quartus, may also be present in the lateral aspect of the leg. In response to a discrepancy regarding the identification and location of the peroneal tubercle, Ruiz et al. developed a reliable method to measure the location of this osteologic landmark [6]. The results re-established the correct anatomical presentation of the retrotrochlear eminence and the peroneal tubercle along the lateral surface of the calcaneus.

One may divide the lateral calcaneal surface into thirds. The peroneal tubercle separates the peroneus longus and brevis tendons and is located in the middle third. Hypertrophy, or enlargement, of the peroneal tubercle could limit normal gliding motion of the peroneus longus tendon during movement. This friction could increase shear stress between the tubercle and tendons promoting tenosynovitis and ultimately lead to a tear. Tearing of the peroneus longus tendon at the level of the peroneal tubercle is uncommon [7]. Sobel et al. studied the lateral peroneal tendon of 124 cadaveric legs and found the accessory muscle, the peroneus quartus, present in 21.7% of the specimens [8]. Furthermore, 63% distally inserted into the peroneal tubercle.

It should also be noted that the peroneus longus tendon has two avascular zones: lateral malleolar region and cuboid. These zones correspond to the most frequent locations of peroneal tendinopathies. Etiology of the hypertrophied peroneal tubercle has been controversial and included occurrence of the peroneus quartus, peroneus longus tenosynovitis, peroneus longus rupture, osteochondroma, pes planus, and pes cavus [7]. The increased size of the peroneal tubercle imposes a larger moment arm about which the peroneus longus creates a pronatory moment to the subject's hindfoot. Loss, or limitation, of first-ray plantarflexion has also been observed with peroneal tendon dysfunction.

Peroneal Tendon Morphometry

A variety of tools have been employed to assess the morphometry of the peroneal tendons and associated muscles including dissection, plain film radiography, ultrasound, CT, tenography, and MRI. The tendon is comprised of a highly organized and dense array of collagen that presents challenges to most morphometric approaches. Jerban et al. used ultrashort echo time (UTE) magnetic resonance imaging (MRI) to form a biomarker of very short T2 values in conjunction with static tensile loads to assess the structure of tendons [9]. Six human peroneal tendons were evaluated at the following static tensile loads: 3 at 15 N (group A) and 3 at 15 N, followed by 30 N (Group B). Mean T2 values (relaxation time of transverse magnetization) were significantly reduced for group A and further reduced, albeit not significantly, for group B. These results suggest that UTE T2 values may be a biomarker for peroneal tendon biomechanics (load vs. deformation), although more research on larger sample sizes is required for confirmation.

The peroneal longus and brevis tendons transfer the loads both eccentrically and concentrically. Since tendinopathies may include stenoses with tendon sheaths, tensile and frictional loading across the peroneal tubercle, and the presence of other anatomical variants, proper evaluation of this system must include all load-bearing components. For example, pronatory runners with recurrent overuse injuries were found to have 12% smaller peroneal muscles compared with asymptomatic controls [10]. This symptomatic group also exhibited larger peak forefoot abduction;

however, no difference in rearfoot motion was observed. The overarching finding of this study was that larger peroneal muscles protected runners with pronated feet [11, 12].

A thinner peroneus longus may have difficulty locking the first metatarsal against the medial cuneiform, hence leaving the athlete with greater susceptibility to injury. Muscle geometry may also be affected by overall foot structure; subjects with pes planus exhibited a significantly smaller cross-sectional area (14.7%) of the peroneal muscles than those with a normal arch alignment [12].

The Peroneal Tendons Role in Foot Structure

Feet are often categorized into three general structures: Planus (a low arch with an everted calcaneus and/or varus forefoot); rectus (a moderate arch with the posterior calcaneal bisection close to perpendicular with the ground); and cavus (a high arch with an inverted calcaneus and/or valgus forefoot) [13]. These structural references describe different configurations of the medial longitudinal arch and identify common morphological and structural variations among the general population. It is accepted that foot structure and function are related to one another and that functional variations exist between these three distinct classifications [14–16].

Kokubo et al. examined the influence of the posterior tibialis and peroneus longus on stiffness of the foot's medial longitudinal arch [17]. They hypothesized that foot shock absorption and arch stiffness would be affected by force transmitted through each tendon. The posterior tibialis was shown to have more effect on arch stiffness than the peroneus longus, indicating the peroneal tendon does not function to maintain the medial longitudinal arch. However, loading of this tendon was shown to improve first metatarsocuneiform joint sagittal plane subluxation (reduced translation) and intermetatarsal angle (reduced abduction) [18]. This suggests that the peroneus longus interacts with the orientation of the first ray under weightbearing load.

From a structural perspective, the peroneus longus provides passive and active contributions to stabilizing and "locking" the first metatarsal against the medial cuneiform (Fig. 2.3). Torsion of the first metatarsal was suggested by Johnson and Christensen to tighten the midfoot ligaments, stabilize the medial column, and maintain integrity of the transverse arch [19]. Bohne et al. demonstrated a significant increase in medial displacement of the transverse arch after transecting the peroneus longus [20]. Conceptually, the peroneus longus may help the first ray to resist excessive motion by drawing it into plantarflexion due to the tendon's line of action across the lateral ankle.

The peroneus longus assists the windlass mechanism [21] by enhancing dorsiflexion of the first metatarsophalangeal joint [19, 22] (Fig. 2.4). The magnitude and direction of the peroneal force illustrates its role upon everting the hindfoot, plantarflexing the forefoot, and keeping the first ray purchased to the ground. During midstance, the rectus foot with a normally functioning peroneus longus will establish equilibrium with the plantar fascia and flexor hallucis longus tissues. In

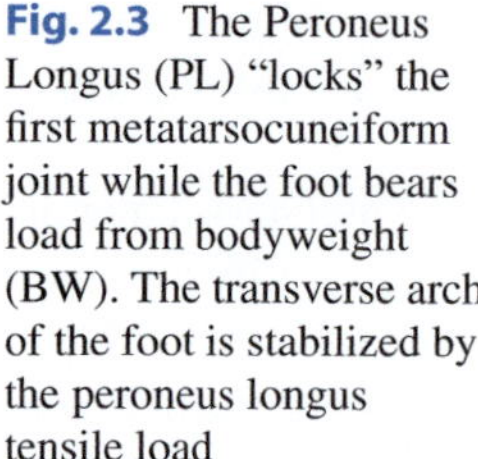

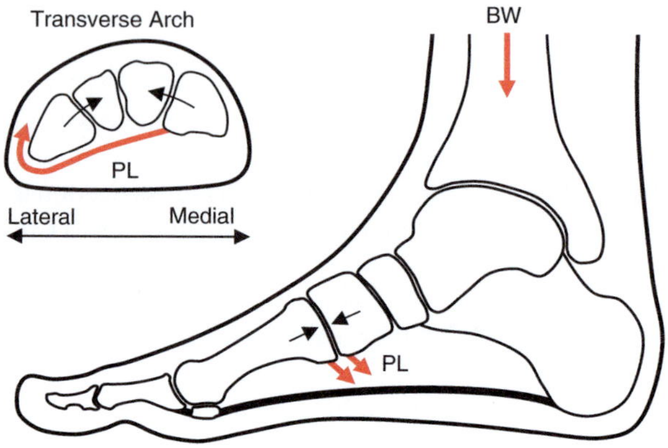

Fig. 2.3 The Peroneus Longus (PL) "locks" the first metatarsocuneiform joint while the foot bears load from bodyweight (BW). The transverse arch of the foot is stabilized by the peroneus longus tensile load

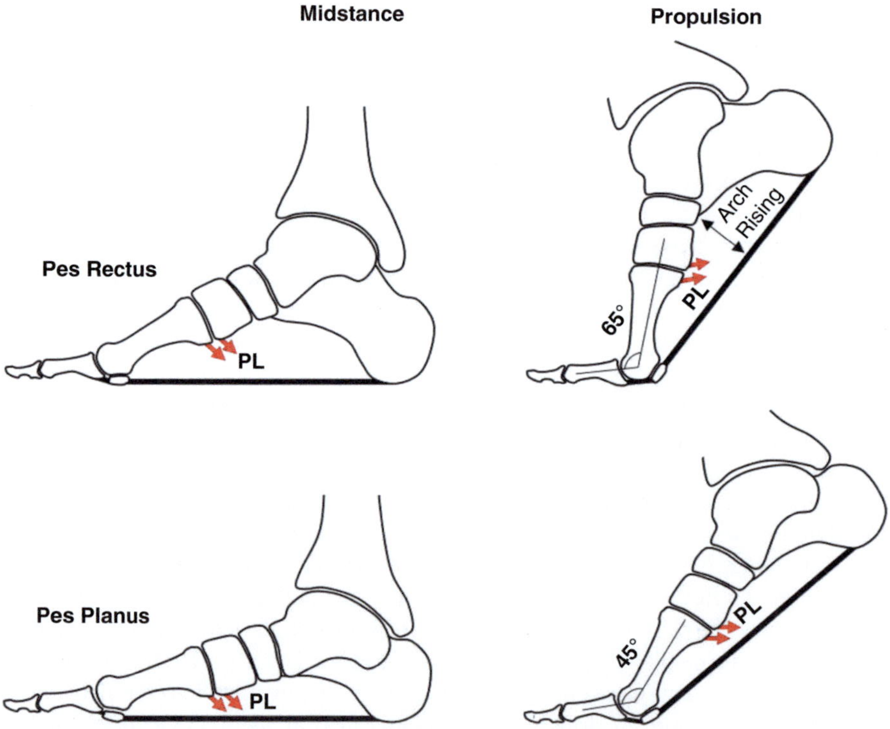

Fig. 2.4 Effect of the peroneus longus on the windlass mechanism for planus and rectus feet. During midstance, the rectus foot, with a normally functioning peroneus longus, will establish equilibrium with the plantar fascia and flexor hallucis longus tissues. In propulsion, all the residual elasticity of the plantar soft tissues is used to elongate these structures enabling 65° dorsiflexion of the first metatarsophalangeal joint. For the planus foot during midstance, the arch is lower with a reduced mechanical advantage from the peroneus longus leaving the plantar soft tissues in a nearly maximally elongated position. During propulsion, the windlass mechanism has less available range, limiting first metatarsophalangeal joint dorsiflexion to ≤45°

propulsion, all the residual elasticity of the plantar soft tissues is used to elongate these structures enabling 65° dorsiflexion of the first metatarsophalangeal joint. For the planus foot during midstance, the arch is lower with a reduced mechanical advantage from the peroneus longus, leaving the plantar soft tissues in a nearly maximally elongated position. During propulsion, the windlass mechanism has less available range, limiting first metatarsophalangeal joint dorsiflexion to ≤45°. The translational and rotational movements of the first metatarsophalangeal joint interact as part of the windlass mechanism, which may be modulated by peroneus longus function.

The Peroneal Tendon's Role in Foot Function

The peroneal muscles exert 63% of the total work required to evert the hindfoot and 4% of the total work required for plantarflexing the ankle. These muscles balance the forces from the tibialis posterior, flexor hallucis longus, and flexor digitorum longus tendons during single limb support. They contract eccentrically from 12% of the gait cycle until foot flat at midstance. Once the heel begins to rise in propulsion, the peroneal muscles contract concentrically, enhancing flexibility of the first metatarsophalangeal joint and the transfer of load from forefoot to rearfoot [2, 22].

Plantar Pressures

In an ideal rectus foot, the peroneus longus can evert the hindfoot and plantarflex the first ray to purchase the ground and bear load through the first metatarsal head. Peak plantar pressures are typically highest beneath the first metatarsal head followed by the second and lesser rays [16]. In the flexible planus foot, where the first ray is hypermobile, the first metatarsal head may not be able to remain purchased to the ground and share in forefoot loading. In fact, the second metatarsal head may demonstrate higher plantar pressures as hypermobility of the first ray ensues [23, 24]. As described in a study of 61 asymptomatic feet, the peak pressures (Fig. 2.5) beneath the first metatarsal head decreased while those beneath the second metatarsal head increased in planus ($n = 22$) compared to rectus ($n = 27$) feet [16]. Paradoxically to this effect of hypermobility, the center of pressure (origin of the ground reaction force vector) is reduced in concavity in the planus versus rectus foot as evidenced by the lower center of pressure excursion index (CPEI) [14–16].

Although this suggests that hypermobility of the first ray may be responsible for the transfer of load between the first and second metatarsal heads, no investigator has examined the potential relationships between plantar pressure, foot structure, first-ray mobility, and peroneal tendon function. Of the limited work performed in this area, Olson et al. found the peroneus longus to be the primary muscle for increasing plantar pressures beneath the first metatarsal head. In patients with clawed hallux deformity, ulceration beneath the first metatarsal head may occur due to increased overpull of the peroneus longus [25].

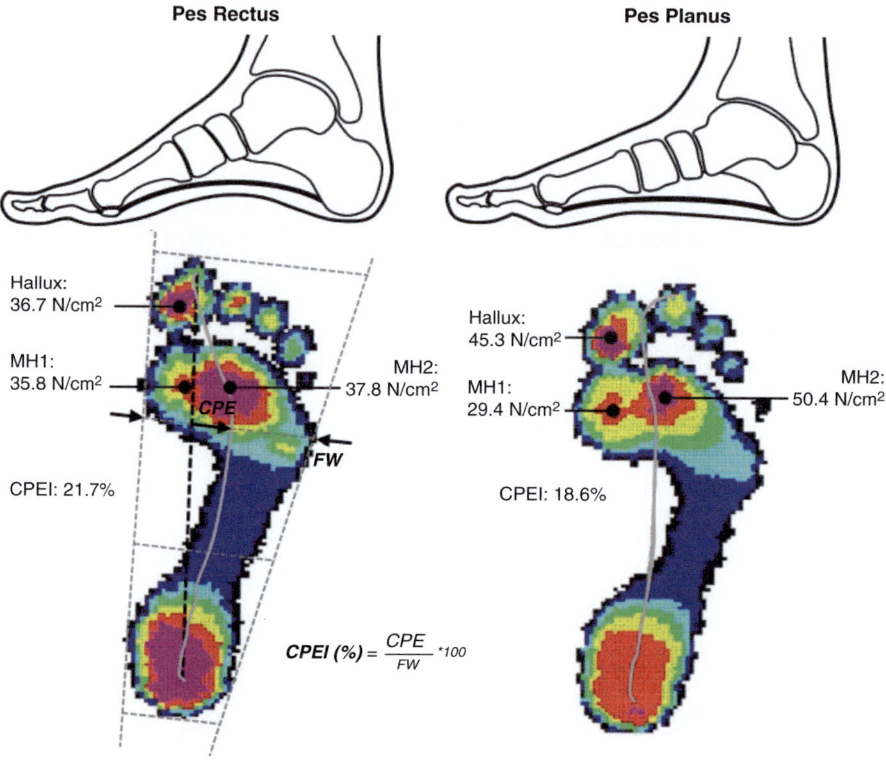

$$CPEI\,(\%) = \frac{CPE}{FW}\,{}^{*}100$$

Fig. 2.5 The rectus and planus foot types exhibit different biomechanical functions. The planus plantar pressure distribution demonstrates lateral transfer of forefoot load from the first to the second metatarsal, resulting from greater mobility of the first ray in the presence of a more medially oriented center of pressure. (*MH1* first metatarsal head, *MH2* second metatarsal head. *FW* foot width, *CPE* center of pressure excursion, *CPEI* center of pressure excursion index)

Vlahovic et al. reported a case in which a male with peroneal neuropathy-induced drop foot was evaluated with gait analysis [26]. The patient was tested 3 years post open reduction and internal fixation of a proximal fibular fracture and a distal, spiral, oblique tibial fracture of the right leg. The peroneal nerve innervates the tibialis anterior, extensor digitorum longus and extensor hallucis longus (dorsiflexors and digital extensors), peroneus longus and brevis (evertors and plantarflexors), and biceps femoris (knee flexor) muscles. Since the common peroneal nerve was damaged, the patient lost their ability to dorsiflex and evert the foot and extend the digits. A significant foot drop imposed initial contact at the lateral plantar forefoot as opposed to heel strike. The maximum plantar pressure throughout stance phase plot resulted in a "reverse check mark" center-of-pressure pattern (Fig. 2.6). Kinematically, there were increased transverse-plane rotations of the foot, and excessive knee and hip flexions in the sagittal plane. The excessive knee and hip flexions were compensation mechanisms to assist with floor clearance in the

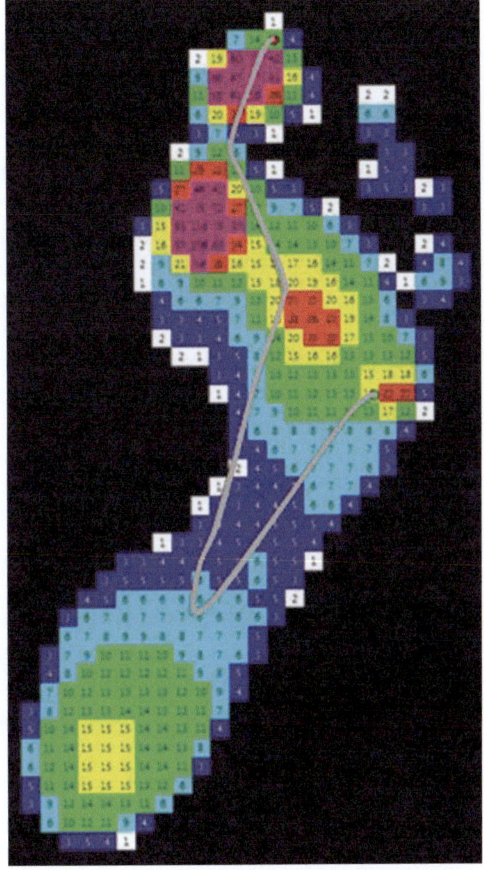

Fig. 2.6 Maximum pressure throughout stance phase for a patient with peroneal neuropathy induced flatfoot. The center of pressure excursion exhibits an irregular pattern as the foot moves through stance

presence of drop foot. For this patient, loss of the evertors (peroneus longus and brevis) was not as devastating as loss of the dorsiflexors and digital extenders (tibialis anterior, extensor hallucis longus, and extensor digitorum brevis).

Kinematics

Hypermobility of the first ray has been implicated in numerous disorders of the forefoot. The most prominent of these are hallux valgus [27] and functional hallux limitus [28]. While many potential causes of first ray hypermobility have been rejected due to a lack of convincing evidence, the peroneus longus' role and its relationship to first ray function has been the subject of numerous investigations. Duchenne suggested that without the peroneus longus to counteract the tibialis anterior, the first ray would gradually elevate resulting in a planus arch alignment [29]. This early research also found that contracture of the peroneus longus caused the arch to form a cavus-like appearance and the transverse arch to decrease foot splay. Although these early observations were in contrast to the modern understanding of the peroneals' interactions with foot structure, Duchenne correctly identified the need for balanced peroneus longus, tibialis anterior, and tibialis posterior activity in normal foot function.

Johnson and Christensen have also shown the importance of the peroneus longus on forefoot stability in vitro [19]. In a study of seven fresh frozen cadavers, they simulated static loads from bodyweight. Increased force in the peroneus longus caused the first metatarsal to evert and plantarflex, the first ray to lower, and the medial column to exhibit torsion while enhancing the transverse arch. Increasing tensile load in the peroneus longus caused a mean difference in first metatarsal motion of $8.1° \pm 3.1°$ in the frontal plane and $3.8° \pm 0.5°$ in the sagittal plane. Similarly, frontal plane motion of the medial cuneiform exhibited a mean increase of $7.4° \pm 2.6°$. Medial cuneiform motion in the sagittal ($3° \pm 0.6°$) and transverse ($2.1° \pm 1.8°$) planes also increased due to peroneus longus loading. No significant differences in arch height were observed. Lapidus arthrodesis may be performed to stabilize the metatarsocuneiform joint, restore peroneus longus function, and improve first-ray kinematics to mimic normal weightbearing activity [30].

Kinetics

Hintermann et al. determined displacements and moment arms of the peroneus longus and brevis during flexion-extension of the foot in a cadaver study [31]. The peroneal tendon was found to be one of the strongest evertors while the foot was in extension, but strength diminished as the foot was flexed. Loss of the peroneals' eversion function in deeper flexion is relevant to understanding the injury mechanism of lateral ankle sprains. These injuries occurred more frequently while the foot was in flexion. The reduced eversion capability of the peroneal tendons during flexion may reduce their ability to stabilize the ankle, indicating a potential mechanical pathway for ankle injury. Passive stabilization of the ankle from the peroneal tendon was demonstrated in a cadaveric study by Ziai et al. who found that transecting the peroneus longus caused a reduction in torque of 18% (0.9 Nm) compared to the intact tendon [32]. Transection of the peroneus brevis was not found to make a difference and was considered to play an ancillary role in passive instability of the ankle. Loss of peroneal tendon function/strength is one cause of lateral ankle instability, potentially increasing the risk for sprain.

Hunt and Smith examined rearfoot and forefoot kinematics, ankle joint moments, and EMG (tibialis anterior, peroneal, soleus, and medial and lateral gastrocnemius) between normal and planus feet during level walking [33]. The forefoot was less adducted at toe-off, and the total transverse plane range of motion was decreased in the planus group. Peak plantarflexory moment at push off and the inverting moment at foot flat were also greater in the planus group. Mean stance phase EMG was higher in the tibialis anterior and lower in the peroneals, soleus, and gastrocnemius muscles for the planus group. Interpretation of this study is complicated since it is not clear how many pronated, neutral, and supinated feet were included in the "normal" group. Still, the peroneus longus and brevis from a group of pronated individuals with a history of musculoskeletal symptoms demonstrated reduced magnitude in EMG compared with the normal (asymptomatic) group. This suggests that peroneus longus and brevis EMG are sensitive to foot structure and/or the presence of symptoms.

Electromyography

Denyer et al. studied if pronated or supinated foot structures contribute to neuromuscular deficits [3]. The reaction time between a simulated inversion sprain (30° inversion and a 20° plantarflexion tilt) and the EMG response was measured for the peroneus longus, gluteus medius, and tibialis anterior. Thirty healthy subjects were stratified into one of three groups based on the navicular drop test: pronated ($\geq$10 mm), neutral (5–9 mm), and supinated ($\leq$4 mm). The peroneus longus had a significantly slower reaction time for pronated (49.7 ms ± 9.5 ms) and supinated feet (47.2 ms ± 5.8 ms) compared to neutral (39.6 ms ± 5.1 ms). There were no differences in reaction time for the gluteus medius and tibialis anterior across foot structure.

Root et al. were some of the earliest researchers to theorize that the peroneus longus played a stabilizing role in forefoot kinematics during gait [34]. The authors suggested that pronation of the planus foot may reduce the mechanical advantage of the peroneus longus during gait. In lieu of proving the stabilizing role of the peroneus longus in vivo, Murley and Menz demonstrated a reduction in peroneus longus activation in flat feet compared to controls with subsequent compensation of the tibialis posterior [35]. The planus group exhibited a mean decrease in peak EMG amplitude of 12.8% during the contact phase of gait and 13.7% during midstance compared to the normal arched group (Fig. 2.7) [35].

In contrast to Duchenne's early theory that loss of peroneus longus function would cause compensation in the tibialis anterior, Murley and Menz did not find a significant difference in tibialis anterior EMG activity between flat and normal arched subjects during gait. However, they did observe a mean 26.5% increase in peak tibialis posterior EMG amplitude. Flat-arched feet may be utilizing the tibialis posterior as a compensation for the diminished capacity of the peroneus longus. These functional differences between foot types may reflect an adaptation in the peroneus longus to avoid further overloading of the first ray. Alternatively, Murley and Menz hypothesized that flat-arched feet may be more laterally unstable, therefore requiring less peroneus longus activity. These findings contrasted with an

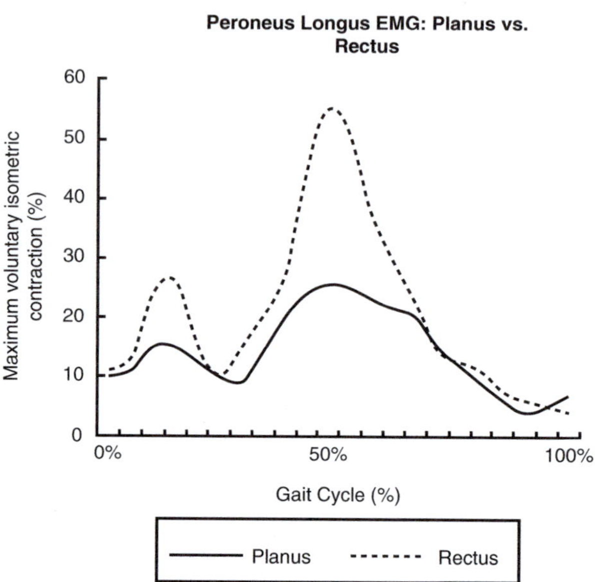

Fig. 2.7 Average EMG amplitude curves for peroneus longus activation in individuals with planus and rectus foot types. Adapted from Murley et al., 2009. J Foot Ankle Surg

earlier study by Gray and Basmajian, who found the peroneus longus to be more active in planus versus rectus individuals [36].

Introduction of a foot and ankle orthotic to realign the arch in pes planus individuals significantly increased peroneus longus activity ranging from 16% to 21% [37]. This finding, that foot orthoses increase peroneus longus amplitude, is consistent with prior research [38, 39]. Artificial heightening of the arch appears to balance the supinator muscles and help stabilize the medial forefoot while secondarily assisting in plantarflexion of the first ray.

Mitchell et al. studied the effect of ankle sprain mechanisms on peroneus longus and peroneus brevis reaction times [40]. Ankles presenting with instability were significantly slower in firing their peroneal tendons compared to controls. In this two-part series, the authors also investigated the relationship between postural sway and reaction time of the peroneal muscles [41]. A positive correlation was observed between the peroneal muscle's reaction time and lateral-medial sway. Both the peroneus longus and peroneus brevis had poor reaction times in unstable ankles. Foot eversion may predominantly be a defense mechanism against ankle sprain. In the presence of repeated lateral ankle ligament injuries, the peroneal muscles may be delayed in receiving afferent signaling from the inverting muscle spindles and Golgi tendon organs, hence resulting in an overall response time that is too slow for protecting against ankle sprains.

Contact Mechanics

Potthast et al. measured the magnitude and distribution of intra-articular joint contact pressures resulting from varying the extrinsic tendon loads of five cadaveric feet [42]. Increasing load in the peroneal tendons led to higher joint stress in the lateral ankle compartment. Peroneal tendon influence on lateral ankle compartment contact mechanics was also predicted by Morles-Orcajo et al. in a finite element modelling study of the foot [43]. Three-dimensional geometries of the ligaments, cartilages, bones, and the muscle-tendon system were reconstructed to develop a dynamic model. Similar to experimental observations, the peroneal tendon produced an eversion and abduction about the foot, increasing plantar pressures beneath the sesamoids. The tibialis anterior was also found to invert the foot and relieve pressure beneath the first ray, corroborating Duchenne's early theory that loss of peroneus longus function could result in gradual elevation of the first metatarsal.

Clinical Biomechanics of the Peroneal Tendon

Peroneal Tendon Rupture

Wagner et al. analyzed the mechanical strength of the peroneal tendon after a tear [44]. They disputed the conventionally accepted 50% rule proposed by Heckman et al. that primary repair and tubularization are necessary for tears involving <50% of the tendon [45], and tenodesis for tears involving >50% of the tendon. In their study, Wagner et al. artificially induced a tear of 66% of the peroneal tendon and performed cyclic loading and load-to-failure tests on cadaver specimens. Mean failure load of the peroneus brevis tendon was 416 N, while the peroneus longus tendon was 723 N. The peroneus longus and brevis muscles produce ~217 N of muscular force during gait [46]. The clinical relevance of this research for patients unresponsive to conservative care is to provide guidance as to when surgical repair of the tendon is necessary. In contrast to the 50% rule, the authors found that patients with a peroneal tendon tear of up to 66% were not at risk of spontaneous rupture and therefore not in need of tenodesis. Nevertheless, this research should be interpreted with caution. Since the authors only loaded the tendon statically, its dynamic functions during gait were not replicated. The changing orientation of the tendon during different flexion-extension and eversion-inversion positions may also contribute to risk of tendon failure.

Tendon Transfer

When the peroneal tendon becomes irreparably torn, the surgeon may perform a tendon transfer (a segmental resection with tenodesis to the peroneus longus tendon, autograft, or allograft) [47]. There is limited biomechanical research on peroneal tendon reconstruction. Pellegrini et al. loaded cadaveric feet in a custom-built jig to simulate normal weightbearing in midstance. Tenodesis was found to elicit greater tension than the uninjured peroneal tendon (range, 101%–120%), while allograft more closely emulated uninjured tensile load (range, 94%–101%). From the perspective of matching in vivo properties, the allograft procedure is preferred.

Peroneal tendinopathy is a condition characterized by structural changes of the peroneal tendon in response to excessive load and overuse. Immobilization, medication, and physical therapy are typically utilized as treatments. Surgical interventions for peroneal tendinopathy and concomitant rupture of the peroneus longus and brevis include end-to-end repair, allograft reconstruction, and reconstruction of the peroneal sheath. Since chronic peroneal dysfunction is associated with minimal excursion of the muscle-tendon complex, scarring, and atrophy of the muscle belly, this may be contraindicated to allograft reconstruction. An alternative to these is a tendon transfer of the flexor hallucis longus or flexor digitorum longus to the lateral forefoot, typically the fifth metatarsal. A similar excursion distance and work percentage of the flexor digitorum longus has been found for the peroneus brevis tendon, supporting its use in this case [48]. In contrast, Seybold et al. performed an in vitro investigation of lateral flexor hallucis longus and flexor digitorum longus transfers with respect to tendon length, diameter, and proximity to the posterior neurovascular bundle. They found the flexor hallucis longus provided superior length with which to secure the graft, offering a larger tendon diameter for transfer, and less need for additional posteromedial incision, without increasing muscle bulk within the peroneal groove. It was suggested that the use of flexor digitorum longus transfer may compress the tibial nerve and cause neuritic symptoms [49]. An in vivo study of five patients demonstrated no significant differences in the peak force loss, average power loss, and average velocity of the peroneal tendon, following flexor digitorum longus versus flexor hallucis longus lateral transfer [50].

Peroneal Groove Deepening

Recurrent dislocation of the peroneal tendon usually results from trauma. The superior peroneal retinaculum can detach with recurrent instability if unmanaged. If the distal fibula, which abuts the peroneal tendon, is flat or convex, this could impose excessive stress on the peroneal tendon and promote dislocation. Kollias and Ferkel recommended reducing the contact stress by surgically forming a retromalleolar groove, a concave interface to the peroneal tendon, within the distal fibula [51]. By recessing the posterior wall of the fibula, the peroneal tendon exhibits better tracking and lower intratendinous pressures, which improves pain and function. Peroneal groove deepening reduced pressure between the tendon-groove articulations at different foot orientations [52]. This procedure can potentially reduce the rate of peroneal tendon dislocation, as well as improve patient outcomes.

Gaps in Knowledge

Several gaps in knowledge from the literature should be noted:

- Epidemiological studies.
  - Large cohorts with healthy and diseased peroneal muscle-tendon systems to explore outcomes across BMI, sex, and foot type in vivo.

- In vitro studies.
  - Structural properties of peroneal muscle-tendon systems in response to controlled loading (e.g., digital image correlation, Bose tensiometer, material testing machines, high fidelity cadaveric simulators).
  - Treatment prediction with high fidelity cadaveric simulators.
- In vivo studies.
  - Structural properties of healthy and pathologic peroneal tendons (e.g., shear wave elastography, advanced 3D imaging (weightbearing CT, UTE MRI, and ultrasound)).
  - Comprehensive structural assessment (arch height index (AHI), arch height flexibility (AHF), malleolar valgus index (MVI), first-ray mobility and position, 2D radiographic parameters, 3D imaging (e.g., weightbearing CT, MRI), foot posture index (FPI)).
  - Comprehensive functional assessment during activities of daily living using multi-segment foot kinematics (e.g., marker-based motion capture, stereo radiography), hindfoot kinetics, intrinsic and extrinsic muscle EMG.
- In silico studies.
  - Prediction of forefoot contact forces (musculoskeletal modeling) and first metatarsophalangeal and first metatarsocuneiform joint stress (finite element models).
  - Subject-specific treatment planning with 3D-imaging-based musculoskeletal and finite element models in vivo.

Summary

The biomechanical interactions between the peroneal tendons and the foot are complex and not yet fully understood. An enlarged peroneal tubercle can increase the foot's pronatory moment arm and be subjected to tensile and shear stresses at the tubercle–tendon interface, which may be causative of tendinopathies and ruptures. Size of the peroneal tendon is a risk factor for lateral ankle instability, ankle sprain, and recurrent overuse injury. Peroneal function is also sensitive to foot type. Planus individuals experience reduced function of the peroneus longus, which may increase first-ray mobility and produce a concomitant limitation of first metatarsophalangeal joint dorsiflexion during gait. In contrast, realignment of the foot's medial longitudinal arch from an orthotic can elicit improved function of the peroneus longus. Loading of the peroneal tendon has been shown to increase lateral compartment stress within the ankle. Furthermore, a computational model of the foot confirmed experimental findings that the peroneal tendon produced eversion and abduction about the foot while increasing plantar pressures beneath the sesamoids. A tear of up to 66% of the peroneal tendon may not impose a risk of spontaneous rupture or require tenodesis, in contrast with the conventionally accepted 50% rule. Allograft of the tendon can provide better functional results than tenodesis. Peroneal groove deepening improves tendon-groove articulation and pressures, where recurrent dislocation of the tendon occurs. There are many gaps in knowledge including the foot-type sensitive roles of the peroneal muscle-tendon system, which could benefit from additional epidemiological, in vitro, in vivo, and in silico studies.

Acknowledgments We would like to thank Rogerio Bitar MD for his expert cadaveric dissection (Fig. 2.2a, b).

References

1. Kumar Y, Alian A, Ahlawat S, Wukich DK, Chhabra A. Peroneal tendon pathology: pre- and post-operative high-resolution US and MR imaging. Eur J Radiol. 2017;92:132–44.
2. Clarke HD, Kitaoka HB, Ehman RL. Peroneal tendon injuries. Foot Ankle Int. 1998;19:280–8.
3. Denyer JR, Hewitt NLA, Mitchell ACS. Foot structure and muscle reaction time to a simulated ankle sprain. J Athl Train. 2013;48:326–30.
4. Hamid KS, Amendola A. Chronic rupture of the peroneal tendons. Foot and Ankle Clinics of Northern America. 2017;22:843–50.
5. Geppert MJ, Sobel M, Bohne WHO. Lateral ankle instability as a cause of superior peroneal retinacular laxity: an anatomic and biomechanical study of cadaveric feet. Foot Ankle Int. 1993;14:330–4.
6. Ruiz JR, Christman RA, Hillstrom HJ. William J. Stickel Silver Award. Anatomical considerations of the peroneal tubercle. J Am Podiatr Med Assoc. 1993;83:563–75.
7. Palmanovich E, Laver L, Brin YS, Kotz E, Hetsroni I, Mann G, et al. Peroneus longus tear and its relation to the peroneal tubercle: a review of the literature. Muscle Ligaments Tendons J. 2012;1:153–60.
8. Sobel M, Levy ME, Bohne WHO. Congenital variations of the peroneus quartus muscle: an anatomic study. Foot Ankle Int. 1990;11:81–9.
9. Jerban S, Nazaran A, Cheng X, Carl M, Szeverenyi N, Du J, et al. Ultrashort echo time T2* values decrease in tendons with application of static tensile loads. J Biomech. 2017;61:160–7.
10. Zhang X, Pauel R, Deschamps K, Jonkers I, Vanwanseele B. Differences in foot muscle morphology and foot kinematics between symptomatic and asymptomatic pronated feet. Scand J Med Sci Sports. 2019;[Epub ahead of print].
11. Zhang X, Aeles J, Vanwanseele B. Comparison of foot muscle morphology and foot kinematics between recreational runners with normal feet and with asymptomatic over-pronated feet. Gait Posture. 2017;54:290–4.
12. Angin S, Crofts G, Mickle KJ, Nester CJ. Ultrasound evaluation of foot muscles and plantar fascia in pes planus. Gait Posture. 2014;40:48–52.
13. Ledoux WR, Shofer JB, Ahroni JH, Smith DG, Sangeorzan BJ, Boyko EJ. Biomechanical differences among pes cavus, neutrally aligned, and pes planus feet in subjects with diabetes. Foot Ankle Int. 2003;24:846–60.
14. Song J, Hillstrom HJ, Secord D, Levitt J. Foot type biomechanics. Comparisons of planus and rectus foot types. J Am Podiatr Med Assoc. 1996;1:16–23.
15. Ledoux WR, Hillstrom HJ. The distributed plantar vertical force of neutrally aligned and pes planus feet. Gait Posture. 2002;15:1–9.
16. Hillstrom HJ, Song J, Kraszewski AP, Hafer JF, Mootanah R, Dufour AB, et al. Foot type biomechanics part 1: structure and function of the asymptomatic foot. Gait Posture. 2013;37:445–51.
17. Kokubo T, Hashimoto T, Nagura T, Nakamura T, Suda Y, Matsumoto H, et al. Effect of the posterior tibial and peroneal longus on the mechanical properties of the foot arch. Foot Ankle Int. 2012;33:320–5.
18. Dullaert K, Hagen J, Klos K, Gueorguiev B, Lenz M, Richards RG, et al. The influence of the peroneus longus muscle on the foot under axial loading: a CT evaluated dynamic cadaver model study. Clin Biomech. 2016;34:7–11.

19. Johnson CH, Christensen JC. Biomechanics of the first ray part I. the effects of peroneus longus function: a three-dimensional kinematic study on a cadaver model. J Foot Ankle Surg. 1999;38:313–21.
20. Bohne WHO, Lee KT, Peterson MGE. Action of the peroneus longus tendon on the first metatarsal against metatarsus primus varus forces. Foot Ankle Int. 1997;18:510–2.
21. Hicks HJ. The mechanics of the foot II. The plantar aponeurosis and the arch. J Anat. 1954;88:25–30.
22. Roukis TS, Scherer PR, Anderson CF. Position of the first ray and motion of the first metatarsophalangeal joint. J Am Podiatr Med Assoc. 1996;86:538–46.
23. King DM, Toolan BC. Associated deformities and hypermobility in hallux valgus: an investigation with weightbearing radiographs. Foot Ankle Int. 2004;25:251–5.
24. Cooper AJ, Clifford PF, Parikh VK, Steinmentz ND, Mizel MS. Instability of the first metatarsal-cuneiform joint: diagnosis and discussion of an independent pain generator in the foot. Foot Ankle Int. 2009;30:928–58.
25. Olson SL, Ledoux WR, Ching RP, Sangeorzan BJ. Muscular imbalances resulting in a clawed hallux. Foot Ankle Int. 2003;6:477–85.
26. Vlahovic TC, Ribeiro CE, Lamm BM, Denmark JA, Walters RG, Talbert T, et al. A case of peroneal neuropathy-induced footdrop. Correlated and compensatory lower-extremity function. J Am Podiatr Med Assoc. 2000;90:411–20.
27. Min BC, Chung CY, Park MS, Choi Y, Koo S, Jang S, et al. Dynamic first tarsometatarsal instability during gait evaluated by pedobarographic examination in patients with hallux valgus. Foot Ankle Int. 2019;[Epub ahead of print].
28. Dannanberg HJ. Gait style as an etiology to chronic postural pain. Part I. functional hallux limitus. J Am Podiatr Med Assoc. 1993;83:433–41.
29. Duchenne GB. Physiologie de mouvements: translated and edited to physiology of motion. Bailliere, Paris: Saunders WB; 1949. p. 205–439.
30. Bierman RA, Christensen JC, Johnson CH. Biomechanics of the first ray. Part III. Consequences of Lapidus arthrodesis on peroneus longus function: a three-dimensional kinematic analysis in a cadaver model. J Foot Ankle Surg. 2001;40:125–31.
31. Hintermann B, Nigg BM, Sommer C. Foot movement and tendon excursion: an in vitro study. Foot Ankle Int. 1994;15:386–95.
32. Ziai P, Benca E, von Skrbensky G, Graf A, Wenzel F, Basad E, et al. The role of the peroneal tendons in passive stabilisation of the ankle joint: an in vitro study. Knee Surg Sports Traumatol Arthrosc. 2013;21:1404–8.
33. Hunt AE, Smith RM. Mechanics and control of the flat versus normal foot during the stance phase of walking. Clin Biomech. 2004;19:391–7.
34. Root ML, Orien WP, Weed JH. Normal and abnormal function of the foot. Clin Biomech. 1997;2:46–5.
35. Murley GS, Menz HB, Landorf KB. Foot posture influences the electromyographic activity of selected lower limb muscles during gait. J Foot Ankle Res. 2009;26:35.
36. Gray EG, Basmajian JV. Electromyography and cinematography of leg and foot ("normal" and flat) during walking. Anat Rec. 1968;161:1–15.
37. Murley GS, Landorf KB, Menz HB. Do foot orthoses change lower limb muscle activity in flat-arched feet in a pattern observed in normal-arched feet? Clin Biomech. 2010;25:72–736.
38. Ludwig O, Kelm J, Fröhlich M. The influence of insoles with a peroneal pressure point on the electromyographic activity of tibialis anterior and peroneus longus during gait. J Foot Ankle Res. 2016;9:33.
39. Mündermann A, Wakeling JM, Nigg BM, Humble RN, Stefanyshyn DJ. Foot orthoses affect frequency components of muscle activity in the lower extremity. Gait Posture. 2006;23:295–302.
40. Mitchell A, Dyson R, Hale T, Abraham C. Biomechanics of ankle instability. Part 1: Reaction time to simulated ankle sprain. Med Sci Sports Exerc. 2008a;40:1515–21.
41. Mitchell A, Dyson R, Hale T, Abraham C. Biomechanics of ankle instability. Part 2: Postural sway-reaction time relationship. Med Sci Sports Exerc. 2008;40:1522–8.

42. Potthast W, Lersch C, Segesser B, Koebke J, Bruggemann G-P. Intraarticular pressure distribution in the talocrural joint is related to lower leg muscle forces. Clin Biomech. 2008;23:632–9.
43. Morales-Orcajo E, Souza TR, Bayod J, de Las Cases EB. Non-linear finite element model to assess the effect of tendon forces on the foot-ankle complex. Med Eng Phys. 2017;49:71–8.
44. Wagner E, Wagner P, Radkievich R, Palma F, Guzmán-Venegas R. Biomechanical cadaveric evaluation of partial acute peroneal tendon tears. Foot Ankle Int. 2018;39:741–5.
45. Heckman DS, Sudheer R, David P, Wapner KL, Parekh SD. Operative treatment for peroneal tendon disorders. J Bone Joint Surg. 2008;90:404–18.
46. Jeng C, Thawait G, Kwon J. Relative strengths of the calf muscles based on MRI volume measurements. Foot Ankle Int. 2012;33:394–9.
47. Pellegrini MJ, Glissons RR, Matsumoto T, Schiff A, Lavar L, Easley ME, et al. Effectiveness of allograft reconstruction vs tenodesis for irreplaceable peroneus brevis tears: a cadaveric model. Foot Ankle Int. 2016;37:803–8.
48. Sherman TI, Koury K, Orapin J, Schon LC. Lateral transfer of the flexor digitorum longus for peroneal tendinopathy. Foot Ankle Int. 2019;40:1012–7.
49. Seybold JD, Campbell JT, Jeng CL, Myerson MS. Anatomic comparison of latera transfer of the long flexors for concomitant peroneal tears. Foot Ankle Int. 2013;34:1718–23.
50. Seybold JD, Campbell JT, Jeng CL, Short KW, Myerson MS. Outcome of lateral transfer of FHL or FDL for concomitant peroneal tendon tears. Foot Ankle Int. 2016;37:576–81.
51. Koallis SL, Ferkel RD. Fibular grooving for recurrent peroneal tendon subluxation. Am J Sports Med. 1997;25:329–35.
52. Title CI, Jung H-G, Park BG, Schon LC. The peroneal groove deepening procedure: a biomechanical study of pressure reduction. Foot Ankle Int. 2005;26:442–8.

Congenital Variations of the Peroneal Tendons

3

Jay M. Sobel and Mark Sobel

Peroneus Quartus Tendon

The presence of an anomalous peroneus quartus tendon within the fibular groove has been reported to contribute to chronic lateral ankle pain. The incidence of this tendon was reported to be present in 13% of dissections by Hecker in 1923 [1]. In 1990, Sobel et al. looked at the variations of the peroneus quartus in 124 cadaver legs from 65 human cadavers and found the peroneus quartus muscle to be present in 27 legs (21.7% of specimens). Although the origins, insertions, and size of the peroneus quartus varied, the most common anatomical variation, found in 17 legs (63% of specimens with peroneus quartus present), showed that the peroneus quartus took origin from the muscular portion of the peroneus brevis in the lower one-third of the leg and inserted onto the peroneal tubercle of the calcaneus, causing hypertrophy to the bony location, which is palpable to the examining physician (Fig. 3.1) [2].

Sobel's findings on the origins and insertions of the peroneus quartus are as follows [1]:

I. Peroneus quartus takes origin from the muscular portion of the peroneus brevis in the lower one-third of the leg and inserts on the peroneal tubercle of the calcaneus (Fig. 3.2): 63%.

Electronic Supplementary Material The online version of this chapter (https://doi.org/10.1007/978-3-030-46646-6_3) contains supplementary material, which is available to authorized users.

J. M. Sobel (✉)
Icahn School of Medicine at Mount Sinai, Biomedical Sciences, New York, NY, USA

M. Sobel
Lenox Hill Hospital – Northwell Health, Orthopaedic Surgery, New York, NY, USA
e-mail: msobelmd@comcast.net

© Springer Nature Switzerland AG 2020
M. Sobel (ed.), *The Peroneal Tendons*,
https://doi.org/10.1007/978-3-030-46646-6_3

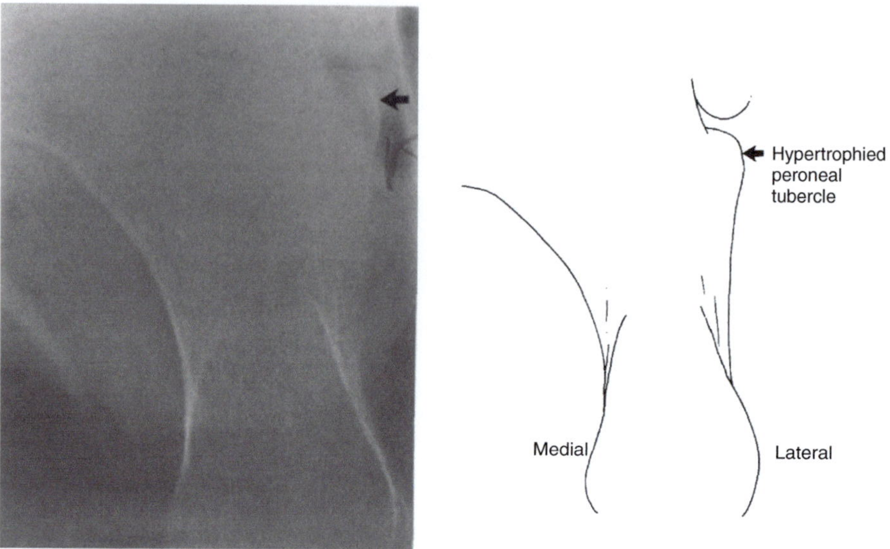

Fig. 3.1 Hypertrophied lateral process of the calcaneus, which is a common insertion site for the peroneus quartus. (From Sobel et al. [2])

   II. Peroneus quartus takes origin from the peroneus brevis and inserts into the peroneus longus just distal to the retromalleolar groove (Fig. 3.3): 3.7%.

  III. Peroneus quartus takes origin from the muscular portion of the peroneus brevis and inserts back into the peroneus brevis just distal to the fibular groove (Fig. 3.4): 3.7%.

  IV. Peroneus quartus takes origin from the peroneus brevis. The tendon divides into two tendinous slips that insert separately on the dorsum of the base and the head of the fifth metatarsal (Fig. 3.5): 7.4%.

   V. Peroneus quartus originates high in the leg from the peroneus longus and inserts into the peroneal tubercle of the calcaneus, or courses under the tendon of the peroneus longus and inserts into the peroneal tubercle of the calcaneus (Fig. 3.6a–d): 7.4%.

  VI. Peroneus quartus originates high in the leg from the peroneus longus and inserts back into the peroneus longus tendon just distal to the fibular groove (Fig. 3.7): 3.7%.

 VII. Peroneus quartus originates from the peroneus brevis and inserts into the lateral retinaculum: 11.1%.

VIII. Peroneus quartus originates from the peroneus longus and inserts into the peroneus brevis: 3.7%.

Of interest was the presence of peroneus brevis attrition (splits or tears), as depicted in Fig. 3.8 below, which was found in 18% of the peroneus brevis tendons in the fibular groove when the peroneus quartus was present

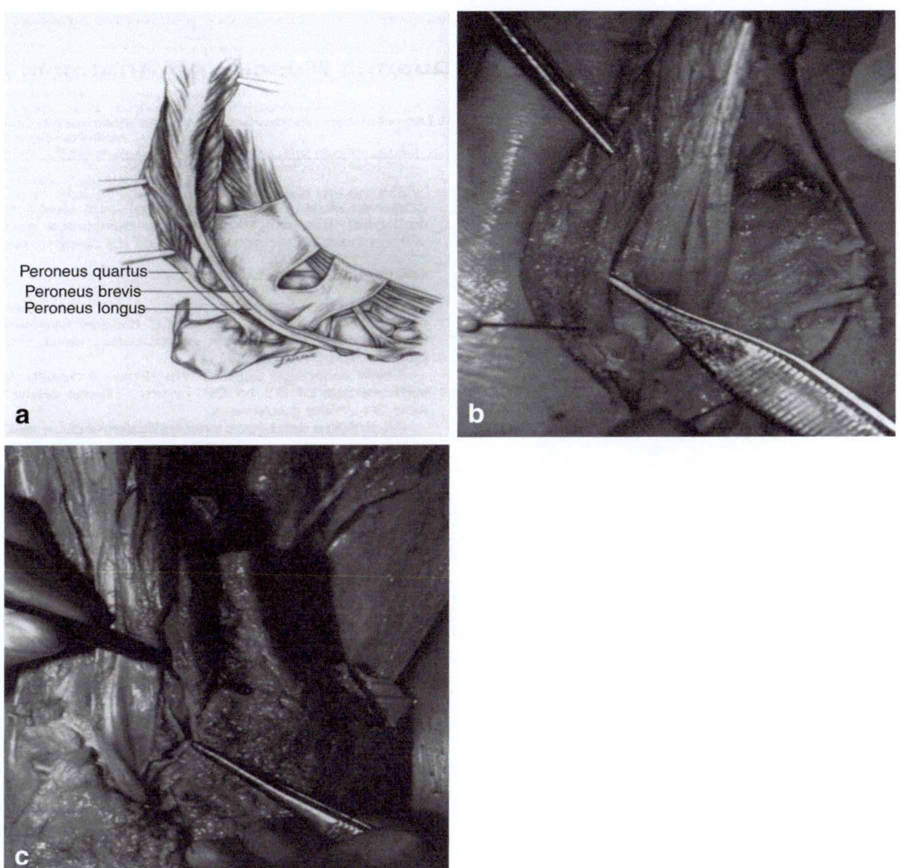

Fig. 3.2 (**a**) Illustration and (**b**, **c**) Cadaveric dissections. The peroneus quartus takes origin from the lower one-third portion of the peroneus brevis and inserts into the peroneal tubercle of the calcaneus. Hypertrophy of the peroneal tubercle is evident. (From Sobel et al. [2])

This anatomical finding may have clinical significance in that the peroneus quartus may produce overcrowding within the fibular groove and subsequent laxity of the superior peroneal retinaculum, allowing for partial subluxation of the peroneus brevis tendon over the sharp posterior ridge of the distal fibula resulting in splitting or tearing of the peroneus brevis tendon [3].

Since our original publications on the anatomy of the peroneus quartus tendon and its association with peroneus brevis splits or tears, there have been a number of case reports and other clinical and radiological studies calling attention to this clinical entity [2, 3].

We have summarized these findings below:

Donley reported a case of chronic ankle pain in a 15-year-old athlete caused by the presence of a peroneus quartus. There was no evidence of subluxation upon

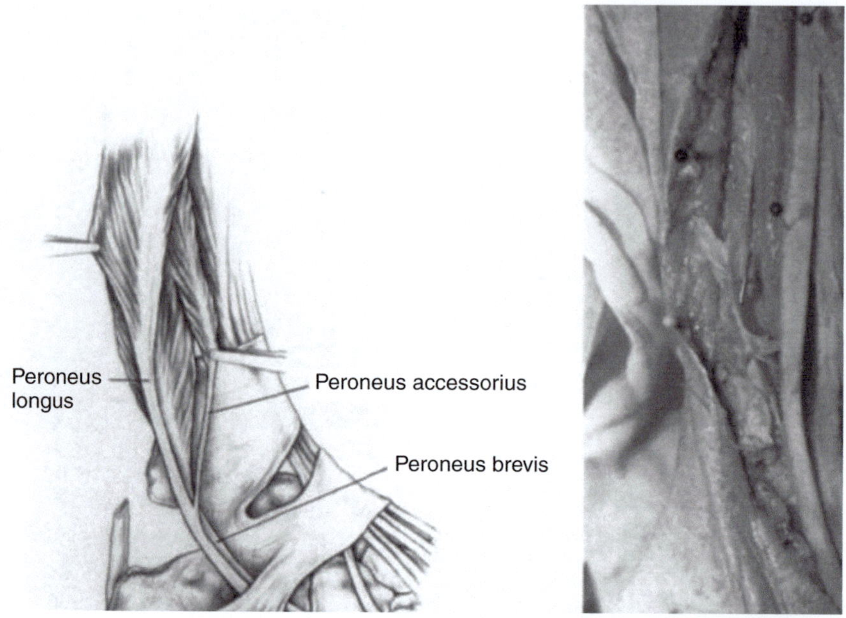

Fig. 3.3 The peroneus quartus takes origin from the peroneus brevis and inserts into the peroneus longus just distal to the fibular groove. (From Sobel et al. [2])

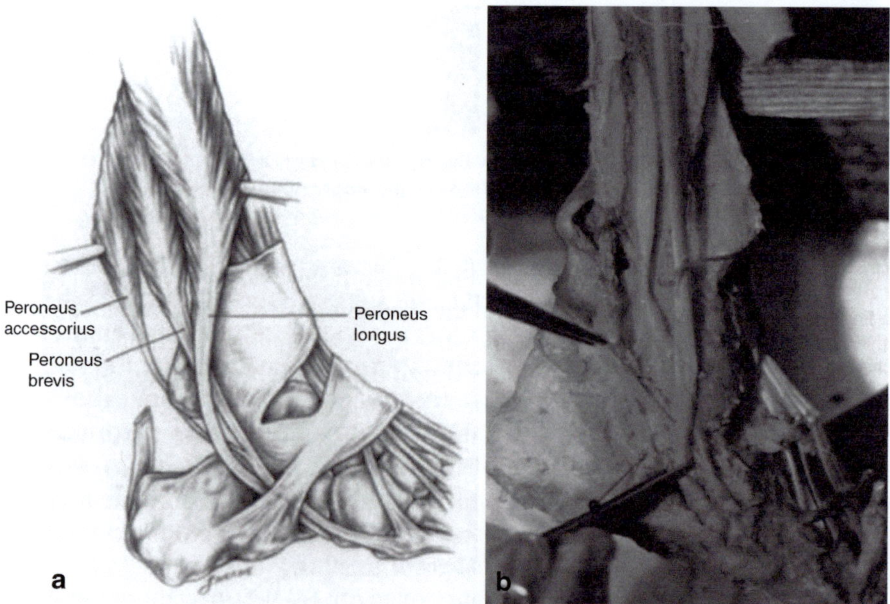

Fig. 3.4 Peroneus quartus takes origin from the muscular portion of the peroneus brevis and inserts back into the peroneus brevis just distal to the fibular groove. (From Sobel et al. [2])

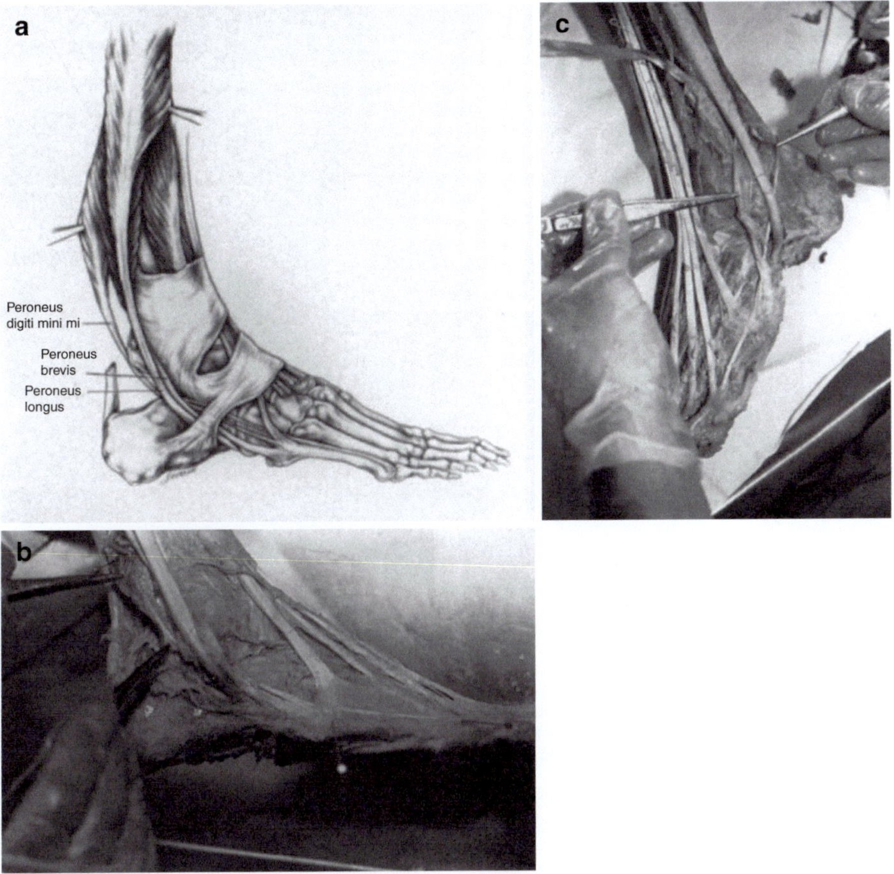

Fig. 3.5 The peroneus quartus takes origin from the peroneus brevis, and the tendinous portion splits into two tendons. One slip inserts dorsally at the base of the fifth metatarsal, and the long slip inserts into the dorsum of the head of the fifth metatarsal. (From Sobel et al. [2])

normal examination. MRI imaging disclosed a peroneus quartus in which the prominent muscle belly extended distally beneath the superior peroneal retinaculum [4]. In their cadaver study, Zammit and Singh dissected 102 cadaver legs and reported a peroneus quartus tendon to be present in 6.6% of their dissections. They showed the peroneus quartus muscle to be associated with a longitudinal tear in the peroneus brevis tendon, a prominent retrotrochlear eminence, and a thin and lax superior peroneal retinaculum [5]. In their research study on the prevalence of the peroneus quartus muscle, Bilgili and colleagues dissected 115 cadaver legs and found the peroneus quartus muscle to be present in six of the legs (5.2%). In five of the six legs, the peroneus quartus originated from the peroneus brevis muscle, while one originated from the distal fibula. The muscle most commonly inserted into the peroneal tubercle of the calcaneus. The authors found a strong relationship between degeneration of the peroneus brevis and existence of the peroneus quartus (p:0.03)

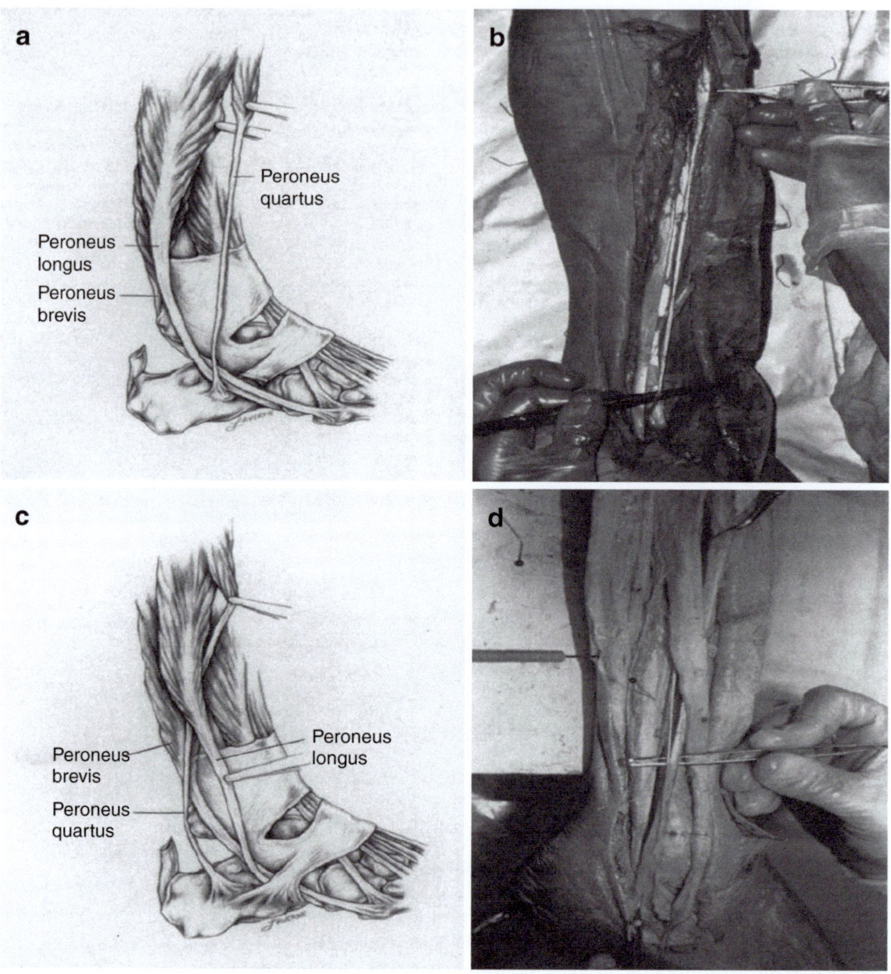

Fig. 3.6 (**a**, **b**) The peroneus quartus takes origin high in the leg from the peroneus longus and inserts into the peroneal tubercle of the calcaneus. Hypertrophy of the peroneal tubercle is evident. (From Sobel et al. [2]). (**c**, **d**) The peroneus quartus takes origin high in the leg from the peroneus longus, runs under the tendon of the peroneus longus, and inserts into the peroneal tubercle of the calcaneus. (From Sobel et al. [2])

[6]. Yammine performed a systematic review and meta-analysis of data from 46 studies and 3928 legs and found a prevalence of 10.2% for peroneus quartus. Of the seven studies reporting its origin, the peroneus quartus muscle most commonly originated from the peroneus brevis muscle. Of the ten studies reporting its insertion, the peroneus quartus most commonly inserted onto the retrotrochlear eminence of the calcaneus [7]. Athavale et al. dissected the superior peroneal tunnel in 58 embalmed lower limbs and reported that muscle fibers of the peroneus brevis muscle were the most frequent additional contents followed by an aberrant muscle,

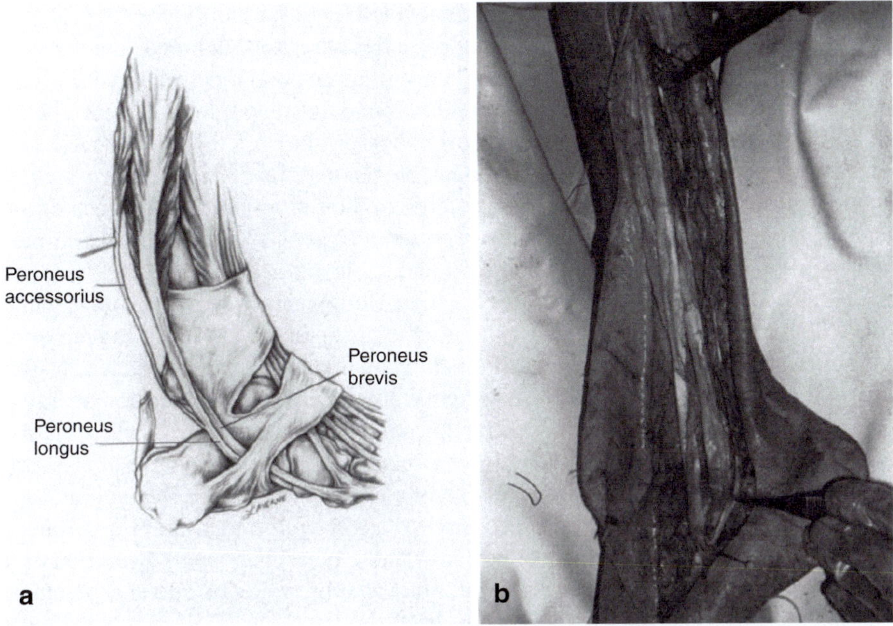

Fig. 3.7 The peroneus quartus takes origin high in the leg from the peroneus longus and inserts back into the peroneus longus just distal to the fibular groove. (From Sobel et al. [2])

Fig. 3.8 This illustration depicts the longitudinal tear in the peroneus brevis tendon, and the splaying out, as well as fraying of the tendon. The proximity of the tear in the tendon to the fibular groove is evident. (From Sobel et al. [2])

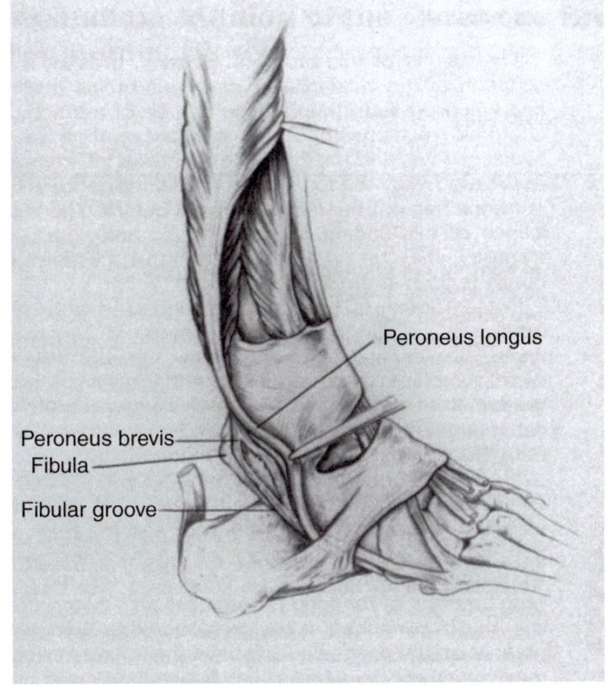

termed the peroneus quartus. Other variants noted by the authors were the presence of a split tear of the peroneus brevis tendon, a double peroneus longus tendon, and an accessory peroneal nerve [8]. A year later, Athavale conducted a cadaveric study on the prevalence of the peroneus quartus and found the muscle to be present in 21% of his 92 dissections. The peroneus quartus took origin from the lower lateral surface of the fibula, the base of the peroneus brevis, and the posterior intermuscular septum in all of his specimens, and inserted into the retrotrochlear eminence of the calcaneus [9]. Habashy et al. recently reported a case of a teenaged boy who presented with sharp right lateral ankle pain and subluxation of the peroneal tendons upon ankle eversion. He had a history of non-Hodgkin lymphoma and a palpable distal fibular osteochondroma. One year after excision of the exostosis and repair of the superior peroneal retinaculum (SPR), the pain recurred. Imaging showed a split tear of the peroneus brevis tendon. At surgery, a peroneus quartus muscle was found and excised, and the peroneus brevis tendon was repaired. At 1-year follow-up, the patient's symptoms were resolved [10]. Chinzei et al. reported a case of bilateral ankle pain and crepitation caused by a peroneus quartus muscle. The authors suggest that foot and ankle surgeons use MRI to assist with diagnosis of a peroneus quartus when patients present with posterior ankle pain [11]. Upon dissection of a 45-year-old male cadaver, Sonmez et al. noted the presence of bilateral peroneus quartus muscles. The muscle took origin from the lateral malleolus and tendinous portion of the peroneus brevis, and inserted into the peroneal trochlea of the calcaneus [12]. Moroney and Borton reported a case in which a 37-year-old soldier with chronic left posterolateral ankle pain 2 years after an inversion ankle injury. MRI scan showed inflammatory changes in both the peroneus longus tendon and an accessory muscle posterior to the peroneus brevis tendon. Surgical examination revealed two accessory muscles with large muscle bellies located in the retromalleolar groove. They called this a previously unreported variant: the peroneus quintus [13]. Prakash et al. conducted a cadaver study of the peroneal muscles in 70 specimens in the Indian population and found a peroneus quartus muscle in three of their dissections (4.3%). After observing the lateral compartment of each leg, they noted that 20 of the specimens (28.6%) had split or tear lesions of the peroneus brevis muscle. When compared to reports of peroneus quartus prevalence from 6.6% to 21.9% in American populations, the authors concluded that the presence of the peroneus quartus muscle in this Indian population was relatively low [14]. Saupe et al. looked at the anatomical variants associated with peroneal tendon disorders using MR imaging in 65 volunteers with asymptomatic ankles. They found a peroneus quartus muscle in 11 (17%) ankles and a peroneal tubercle in 36 (55%) ankles. Of these 36 ankles, 90% of all tubercles were 4.6 mm or smaller with a median height of 2.9 mm. "The retromalleolar groove was concave in 18 (28%), flat in 28 (43%), convex in 12 (18%), and irregular in 7 (11%) of the volunteers." The height of the retrotrochlear eminence was found to be significantly different ($P = 0.04$) between men and women with a median of 3.4 mm and 2.5 mm, respectively. Additionally, the authors found the peroneus brevis musculotendinous junction to be located between 27 mm proximal to and 24 mm distal to the fibular tip [15]. Chepuri et al. correlated the sonographic and MRI appearance of the peroneus quartus tendon in

32 patients over a four-year period. They found a peroneus quartus tendon in seven patients (six taking origin from the peroneus brevis muscle and seven inserting into the calcaneus). The authors noted a hyperechoic muscular portion and a hyperechoic/fibrillar tendinous portion of each peroneus quartus. The location of the peroneus quartus musculotendinous junction varied between patients, and accordingly, the sonographic appearance of the peroneus quartus muscle near the distal fibula ranged from completely muscle to completely tendon. Based on this finding, the authors concluded that sonographic appearance of the peroneus quartus muscle shows variations, and pinpointing these variations will allow for accurate diagnosis of a peroneus quartus muscle, and differentiation from adjacent tendon abnormality [16]. Cheung et al. performed a retrospective review of 136 consecutive MRI imaging studies and found the prevalence of the peroneus quartus to be 10% (14 of 136 cases). The peroneus quartus (muscle and tendon) descended medial and posterior to the peroneal tendons. Variability in the insertion site included the calcaneus, peroneus longus tendon, peroneus brevis tendon, and the cuboid bone. In 11 of 14 cases, the retrotrochlear eminence of the calcaneus was the insertion site. Compared to the group without the peroneus quartus muscle, the authors found the height of the retrotrochlear eminence to be significantly taller ($P < 0.01$) in the group with the peroneus quartus muscle [17]. Sammarco and Brainard reported a case of a 20-year-old female collegiate high jumper who described a continuous ache in her ankle at rest and a shooting pain with tightness along the outside of the ankle when jumping. MRI revealed a longitudinal mass posterolateral to the ankle behind the peroneal tendons consistent with muscle tissue. At surgery, an anomalous tendon was found to arise from the peroneus brevis muscle and the posterior interosseous membrane and insert into the trochlear process of the calcaneus. This accessory muscle and tendon was removed and at 14 weeks post-op, she successfully returned to normal competition and remained asymptomatic 2 years after this operation [18]. Martinelli and Bernobi reported a case of a 28-year-old amateur sportsman with complaints of pain and swelling in the right lateral retroperoneal region. The patient had sustained a twisting injury one year earlier, and no improvement was seen when treated with normal immobilization and rehabilitation procedures. MRI demonstrated post-traumatic peritendonitis. At surgery, a peroneus quartus muscle was discovered. This variant originated from the peroneus brevis muscle and abutted the peroneal tendons. A fasciotomy was performed and a 1-year post-op MRI demonstrated the presence of a normal peroneus quartus muscle. The patients symptoms were eliminated definitively [19]. Nascimento et al. evaluated 211 MRI scans on the ankle and hind foot. They found a peroneus quartus muscle to be present in 7.62% (16 ankles) of the examinations [20]. Kulshreshtha et al. reported on a patient with symptomatic dislocated peroneal tendons in combination with tear of the anterior talofibular ligament. The authors described a reconstruction of the lateral ankle ligaments using an accessory peroneus quartus muscle. There is an association of chronic lateral ankle instability with peroneal tendon injuries, which may include subluxation or tears of the peroneus brevis tendon and/or the presence a peroneus quartus tendon or low-lying peroneus brevis muscle belly either of which can create an encroachment phenomenon within the fibular groove and stretching out of the SPR. The fact that

there is a parallel relationship between the calcaneofibular ligament (CFL) and the SPR may link injuries to these two structures [21–23]. Upon routine dissection of a 75-year-old male cadaver leg, Gumasalan and Ozbag reported on an accessory muscle that originated from the lateral surface of the fibula and posterior intermuscular septum. They reported the origin to be 7.5 cm proximal to the distal tip of the fibula and described its fusiform-shaped muscle belly to be 4 cm long, 7 mm wide, and 3 mm thick. The muscle converged into a 5.8 cm tendon posterior to the peroneus longus and peroneus brevis and inserted onto the retrotrochlear eminence of the calcaneus. The authors named this muscle the "musculus fibulocalcaneus externum," which we call the peroneus quartus [24]. Regan and Hughston reported on a patient with chronic ankle "sprain" secondary to an anomalous peroneal tendon. The patient was a 51-year-old female who injured her right ankle while skiing. After 11 months of lateral ankle pain, the patient was reported to have tenderness to palpation and a sensation of fullness over the peroneal tendons posterior to the lateral malleolus. At surgery, she was found to have a trifurcation of the peroneus brevis tendon, and the smaller two of the three divisions of the anomalous tendon were excised. At 1-year follow-up, her symptoms had markedly improved [25]. Mick and Lynch reported a case of a patient who had recurrent peroneal tendon dislocation after 6 weeks of immobilization in a short leg cast. Originally, the authors had planned to use a Jones repair, but identified a peroneus quartus accessory muscle during the procedure. They decided to reconstruct the peroneal retinaculum with the peroneus quartus. With the authors' procedure, the superior peroneal retinaculum and a portion of the inferior peroneal retinaculum were reconstructed by anterior transfer of the peroneus quartus. After 5 weeks of immobilization in a short-leg cast, the patient returned to normal activity with no dislocation of the peroneal tendons [26]. White et al. reported a case of chronic ankle pain associated with a peroneus accessorius in a 40-year-old woman who had a 1-year history of swelling and severe pain in the right ankle following a varus strain of the joint. Examination revealed physical findings of tenderness over the course of the peroneal tendons in the ankle region and a palpable thickening at the peroneal sheath. Two years following the onset of symptoms, exploratory surgery was performed, which revealed an anatomic variation, the peroneus accessorius. The authors reported that the peroneus accessorius "originated from the peroneus brevis and continued as a small tendon which passed medial to the common peroneal sheath at the level of the lateral malleolus. The tendon then emerged at the distal end of the sheath and attached to the tendon of the peroneus longus just before the latter passed under the sole of the foot." After the structure, along with its muscle belly, was dissected free and excised, the peroneal tendon sheath was reconstructed. At two years follow-up, she was pain-free and symptom-free [27]. Taljanovic et al. reported on the use of high-resolution ultrasound and MR imaging of the peroneal tendons. They provided MRI and ultrasound examples of cases depicting the whole spectrum of peroneal tendon injuries including the peroneus quartus muscle [28]. Öznur et al. reported a case in which chronic persistent lateral ankle pain was caused by a peroneus quartus. The authors summarized that the presence of a peroneus quartus muscle should be considered in the differential diagnosis of chronic lateral ankle pain [29].

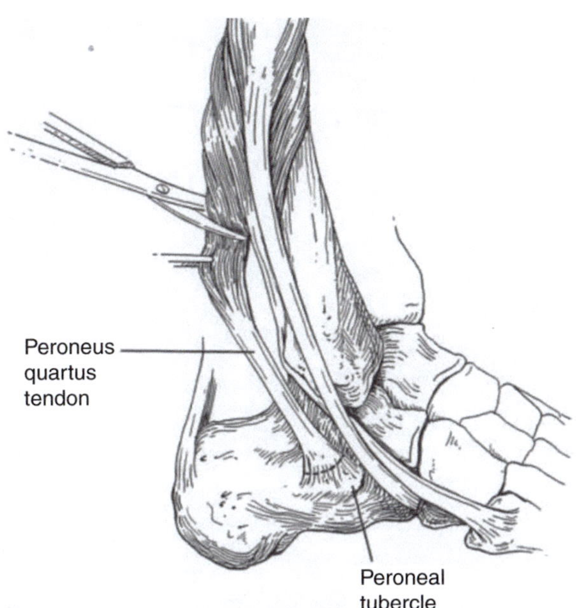

Fig. 3.9 This illustration depicts the surgical removal of the peroneus quartus tendon. (From Sobel and Mizel [30])

In summary, the presentation of chronic lateral ankle pain and chronic lateral ankle instability may be associated with an accessory peroneus quartus muscle and a good history and physical examination are imperative. MRI or high-resolution ultrasound has been found to be helpful in the diagnosis and surgical planning. Surgical removal of the peroneus quartus (Fig. 3.9) and superior peroneal retinaculum reconstruction is usually curative.

Anomalous Low-Lying Peroneus Brevis Muscle Belly Within the Fibular Groove

As previously discussed, the presence of an anomalous peroneus quartus can contribute to chronic lateral ankle pain, as well as peroneus brevis attrition. In addition to this etiology, a low-lying peroneus brevis muscle belly is a variation that can predispose the peroneus brevis tendon to tears, consequently leading to chronic lateral ankle pain (Figs. 3.10, 3.11, and 3.12). The mechanism by which this congenital variation can lead to peroneal tendon disorders includes an encroachment phenomenon within the fibular groove, stretching out of the superior peroneal retinaculum, longitudinal tearing of the peroneus brevis tendon, subluxation of the peroneal tendons, and peroneal tenosynovitis [31].

MRI studies have reported that 10–25% of patients with a peroneus brevis tear often have an anomalous low-lying muscle belly. In this case, the muscle tissue extends beyond the retromalleolar groove rather than converging into tendon above the distal fibula. This irregularity produces increased muscle mass in the

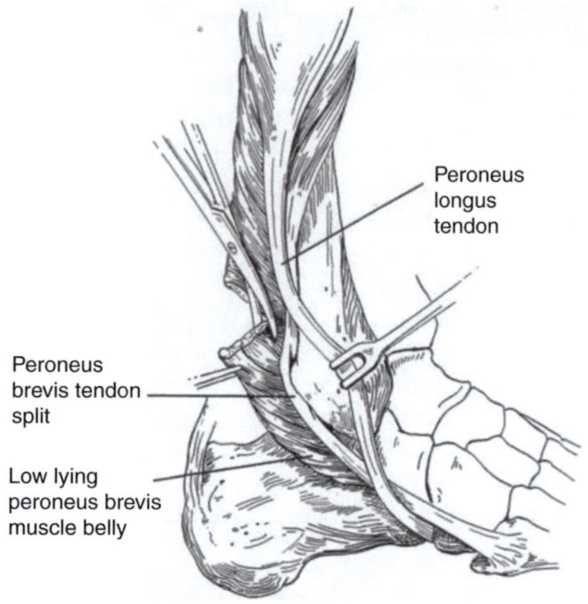

Fig. 3.10 This illustration depicts the presence of an anomalous low-lying peroneus muscle belly within the fibular groove. (From Sobel and Mizel [32])

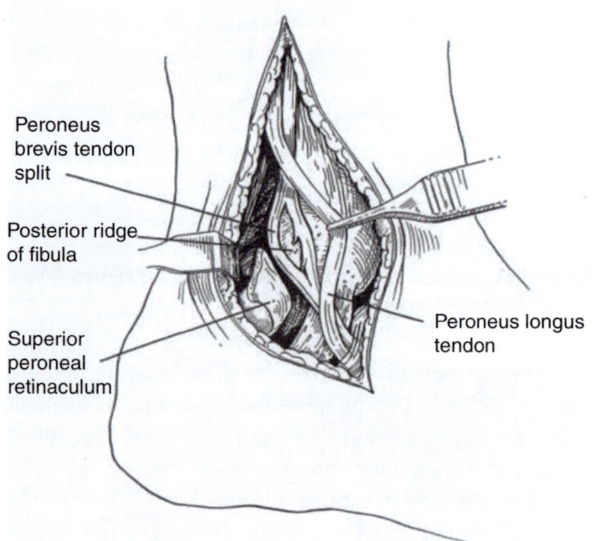

Fig. 3.11 This illustration depicts the relationship between the superior peroneal retinaculum, the posterior ridge of the fibula, and the split peroneus brevis tendon. (From Sobel and Mizel [32])

retromalleolar groove, which, in effect, generates an overcrowding phenomenon within the fibular groove, leading to peroneal tendon injury [34].

In 1992, Sobel et al. reported on a case of peroneal tendon subluxation as a result of an extension of the peroneus brevis muscle belly into the fibular groove. In this case, a 30-year-old woman, competitive athlete since childhood, presented with a 4-year history of chronic pain in the lateral aspect of the right ankle and instability

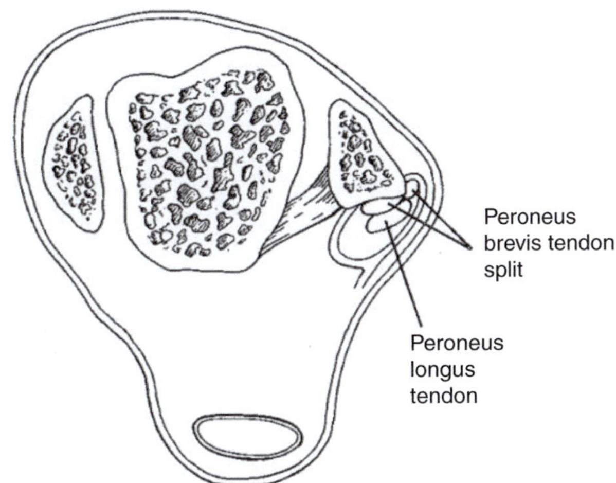

Fig. 3.12 This illustration displays the cross-sectional relationship of the split peroneus brevis tendon to the posterior ridge of the fibula. Please note that while the posterior half of the split peroneus brevis tendon remains within the fibular groove, the anterior half subluxates out over the sharp ridge of the fibula. (From Sobel and Mizel [33])

after an initial twisting injury while playing tennis. During routine examination, swelling was noted in the peroneal sheath at the fibular groove, and active dorsiflexion and eversion of the ankle caused the peroneal tendons to subluxate out from behind the lateral malleolus, causing pain through the entire distal course of the tendons. Upon surgical exploration, a posterior osteoperiosteal flap was raised from the lateral aspect of the fibula revealing an abnormally low-lying peroneus brevis muscle belly in the fibular groove (Fig. 3.13a, b) [31].

They noted an overpacking phenomenon within the fibular groove, a thick and inflamed tenosynovium around the peroneal tendons, and a partial thickness 1-cm longitudinal tear in the peroneus brevis tendon centered on the posterior ridge of the fibula (Fig. 3.14) [31].

The peroneal tendons fell back into their anatomic position after a synovectomy of the peroneal tendons and excision of peroneus brevis muscle approximately 3 cm proximal to the fibular groove. One year following the procedure, the patient reported no symptoms of pain or instability about the ankle, and there was no evidence of subluxation of the peroneal tendons [31].

Dombek et al. conducted a three-year retrospective review on the nature of peroneal tendon injury. In their study, 40 patients underwent surgery for chronic pain along the peroneal tendons. Using medical records and MRI, the authors identified that 88% of their cases involved peroneus brevis tendon tear, 33% low-lying peroneus brevis muscle belly, and 20% tendon subluxation [35].

In their cadaveric study, Geller et al. dissected 30 human specimens to measure the length of the musculotendinous junction (MTJ) between the tip of the fibula and peroneal tubercle. In four of their cases, they discovered degenerative longitudinal tear of the peroneus brevis tendon. In addition, "the MTJ was significantly more distal and the tendon was thicker in torn versus untorn specimens ($P < 0.05$)." Based on their findings, they proposed that the longitudinal location of the peroneus brevis MTJ as well as the width of the tendon may influence the development of degenerative peroneus brevis tears [36].

Fig. 3.13 (**a**) A fibular osteoperiosteal flap raised to expose the peroneal tendons. (**b**) An anomalous low-lying peroneus brevis muscle belly extending into the fibular groove. (From Sobel et al. [31])

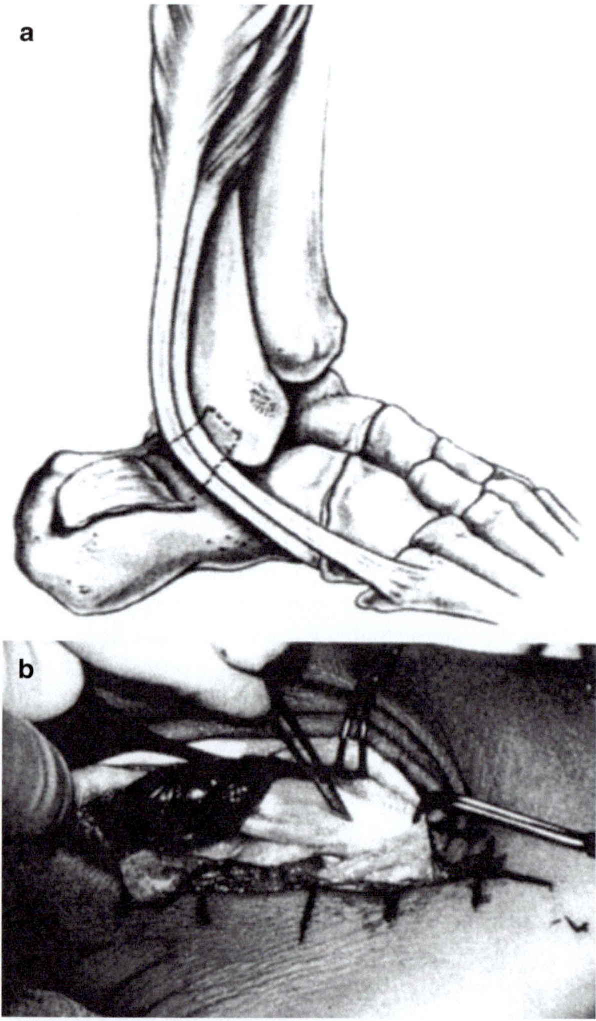

Fig. 3.14 Longitudinal tear in the peroneus brevis tendon. (From Sobel et al. [31])

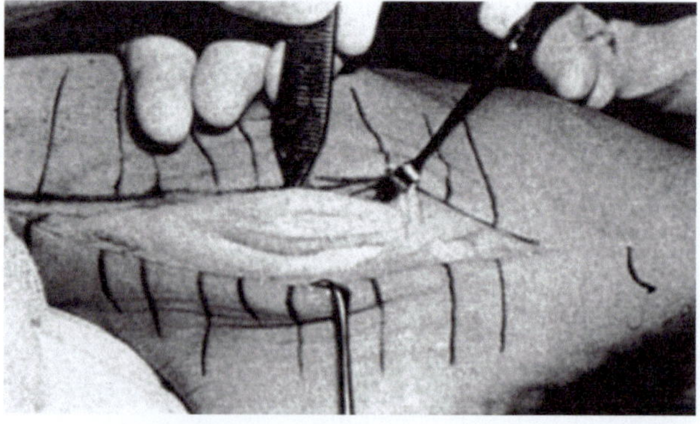

Over a 5-year period, Mirmiran et al. conducted a retrospective study evaluating the MRI and intraoperative findings of 50 consecutive patients undergoing a primary peroneal tendon surgery. Additionally, they used these data to compare the pathologic differences in patients with a low-lying peroneus brevis muscle belly to those without. The authors found no statistically significant association between the presence of a low-lying muscle belly and peroneus brevis tendon subluxation, but noted that nine out of their ten patients with an intraoperatively observed tendon subluxation had a concomitant low-lying muscle belly [37].

Highlander et al. conducted a case-control study comparing the MRI features of patients with symptomatic peroneal tendon pathology versus an asymptomatic control group. The presence of a low-lying peroneus muscle belly extending beyond the fibular groove was discovered in 87% of the patients with symptomatic peroneal tendon pathology and only 53.8% of controls ($P = 0.022$). Interestingly, the authors noted ankle instability and osteochondral defect of the talus or tibial plafond to be the most common diagnosis associated with peroneal tendon injury pathology. After discovering a low-lying peroneus brevis muscle belly to be a common anatomic variant in controls, the authors concluded that this variation, when combined with lateral ankle instability, can become a source of pain secondary to overcrowding [38]. Freccero et al. conducted a similar study on the MRI findings of patients with a surgically confirmed peroneus brevis tear. Specific attention was focused on the distance between the musculotendinous junction of the peroneus brevis tendon and the distal tip of the fibula. Their findings revealed an average distance of 33.1 cm between the MTJ and distal tip of the fibula. This distance was significantly lower than that of patients who were surgically inspected but did not have a confirmed tear ($P < 0.05$). These findings, when compared to controls, confirmed that the presence of a more distal insertion of the peroneus brevis muscle belly results in peroneus brevis tears [39].

These findings were contradicted by Unlu et al., who found that an increase, rather than a decrease, in distance from the MTJ of the peroneus brevis to the distal tip of the fibula increased the probability of peroneus brevis tendon tear. After examination of 115 fresh cadaver legs, they found 15 cases of peroneus brevis tendon tear. Interestingly, there were no cases of low-lying muscle belly reported in this study. The authors concluded that proximal, rather than distal, extension of the peroneus brevis MTJ may lead to peroneus brevis tear [40]. This phenomenon was further investigated by Housley et al., who studied the prevalence of longitudinal peroneus brevis tears in specimens with a proximal peroneus brevis insertion. After measuring the peroneus brevis tendon in 24 cadaveric legs and assessing for full thickness longitudinal tears, the authors found that a more proximal peroneus brevis muscle belly insertion was associated with longitudinal tears in the peroneus brevis tendon. Their findings suggest that a more proximal MTJ increases the likelihood of peroneal tendon subluxation or tears by reducing the stabilizing effect of the muscle belly against the posterolateral surface of the fibula [41].

Hammerschlag and Goldner reported on a case of peroneal tendon subluxation produced by an anomalous bifid peroneus brevis. In this case, the authors described the presence of a surgically discovered bifid peroneus brevis leading to chronic tendon subluxation. Once found, the duplicated tendon was resected, and the superior peroneal retinaculum was reinforced to fully relieve the patient's symptoms [42].

In summary, either the presence of a peroneus quartus or a low-lying peroneus brevis muscle belly within the fibular groove can produce an overcrowding or encroachment phenomenon, which, over time, can stretch out the SPR. The resulting incompetence of the SPR then allows partial subluxation of the peroneus brevis tendon over the sharp posterior ridge of the distal fibula and subsequent splitting or tearing of the peroneus brevis tendon. The peroneus longus tendon acts like a wedge in between the splayed out peroneus brevis tendon and the bony tunnel.

Variations of the Superior Peroneal Retinaculum

The superior peroneal retinaculum (SPR) is noted to be the primary restraint to subluxation and/or dislocation of the peroneal tendons as they pass posterior to the distal fibula (Fig. 3.15) [22]. Several anatomical variations of the SPR have been discovered [43]. The most common variation is that of a single band originating from the posterior ridge of the fibula and inserting onto the lateral wall of the calcaneus [22, 43].

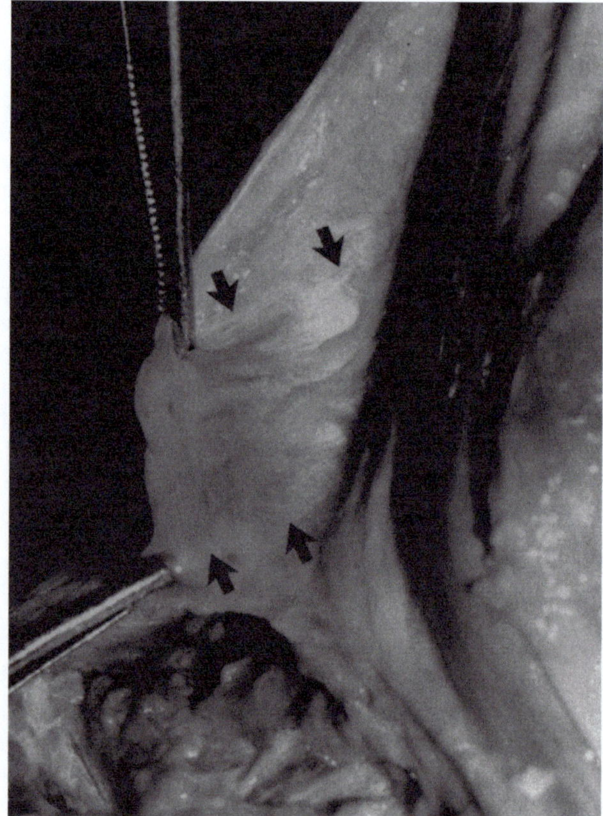

Fig. 3.15 This photograph depicts the inside of the peroneal sheath. The superior and inferior extents of the SPR, centered on the posterior ridge of the fibula, are depicted by the arrows. (From Davis et al. [22])

To better understand the anatomy of the SPR, as well as its role in peroneal tendon pathology, Davis et al. conducted a study that defined several variations of its form. In all of their specimens, the SPR had a common origin on the posterolateral ridge of the fibula. Interestingly, they found the width of the origin to be determined by the insertional variation present [22].

The authors reported five distinctly different insertional variations for the SPR [22]:

I. Type 1 SPR was the most common variation, seen in 47% of their specimens. The origin had an average width of 17.2 mm (5–18 mm). This variation had two bands that split after leaving the posterior ridge of the distal fibula. The superior band ran posterior and inserted into the anterior Achilles sheath. The inferior band inserted in the lateral wall of the calcaneus, parallel and just lateral/posterior to the insertion of the calcaneofibular ligament (CFL). The average width of the superior and inferior bands was determined to be 9.9 mm (5–18 mm) and 9.0 mm (range 4–15 mm), respectively. Please note that the parallel relationship to the CFL and the SPR may explain the coexistence of chronic lateral ankle instability and peroneal tendon subluxation/injury (Fig. 3.16a–c).
II. Type 2 SPR was the second most common variation seen in 17% of specimens. The retinacula originated from the fibula then split into two bands, both of which inserted into the calcaneus (Fig. 3.17).
III. Type 3 SPR, seen in 13% of specimens, had a single wider band inserting into the Achilles sheath (Fig. 3.18).
IV. Type 4 SPR, seen in 13% of specimens had a single wider band inserting broadly into the lateral wall of the calcaneus (Fig. 3.19).
V. Type 5 SPR, seen in 10% of specimens had a superior band inserting into the pretendinous fascia of the Achilles and an inferior band inserting into the lateral wall of the calcaneus (Fig. 3.20).

Examination of each lateral ankle revealed peroneus brevis attritional changes (tears) in specimens containing at least one insertion of the SPR on the calcaneus. Specimens with only an Achilles insertion of the SPR showed no sign of peroneal tendon abnormality. In all of their dissections, at least one of the two bands ran parallel to the CFL, placing the SPR at risk for concurrent injury following a severe inversion ankle sprain.

In their study, Davis and colleagues confirmed that the anatomy of the SPR varies in its width, thickness, and insertional patterns [22]. When diagnosing peroneal tendon pathology and lateral ankle injury, it is important to fully understand the anatomy of the lateral ankle structures, as well as the importance of the SPR as a primary restraint to peroneal tendon subluxation [22, 23].

Acute injury to the SPR had classically been thought to be caused by a dorsiflexion eversion movement of the ankle coupled with a forceful reflex contraction of the peroneal tendons [22, 23, 31, 44]. However, this mechanism does not characterize the cause of chronic lateral ankle injury, which usually follows an inversion injury to the ankle. To further investigate this injury complex in relation to incompetency

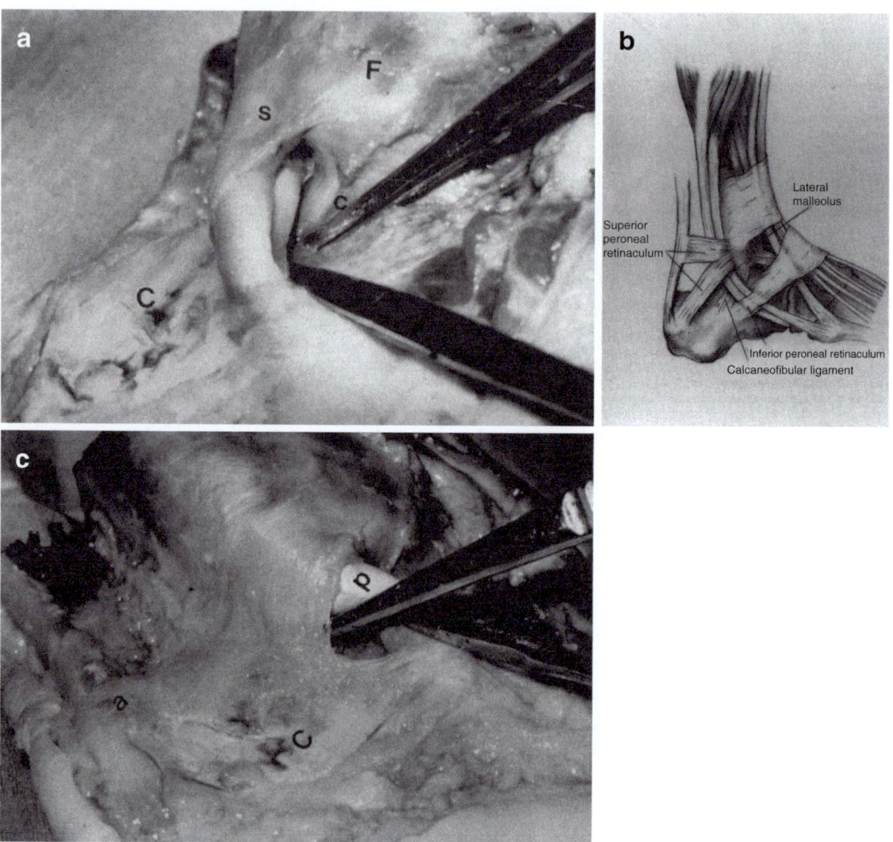

Fig. 3.16 (**a**) Photograph depicting the parallel relationship of the calcaneal band of the SPR and the CFL. (C calcaneus, F fibula, c CFL, s SPR). (**b**) Type 1 SPR illustration depicting the parallel relationship of the calcaneal band of the SPR and the CFL. (**c**) Photograph showing how type 1 SPR had a superior band inserting into the Achilles sheath and an inferior band inserting into the lateral wall of the calcaneus. (C calcaneus, a Achilles tendon, p peroneal tendons). (From Davis et al. [22])

of the SPR, subluxing peroneal tendons, and peroneus brevis tears, Geppert et al. constructed a cadaveric model of ankle instability by serial sectioning of the lateral ankle ligaments under applied mechanical inversion stress. As shown in Fig. 3.21, visual strain on the SPR was noted to increase with increasing degrees of lateral ankle instability, suggesting that the SPR serves as a secondary restraint to ankle inversion stress, and that the forces that result in chronic lateral ankle instability can also injure or attenuate the SPR [3, 23, 44]. This study confirmed that the SPR is in fact a secondary restraint to lateral ankle instability. In addition, the parallel alignment of the calcaneal band of the SPR to the CFL suggests that forces that injure the CFL would also affect the SPR, which, in effect, could account for coexistent pathology of the lateral ankle ligaments, specifically the anterior

Fig. 3.17 An illustration of type 2 SPR (arrows) showing two separate bands inserting into the calcaneus. (From Davis et al. [22])

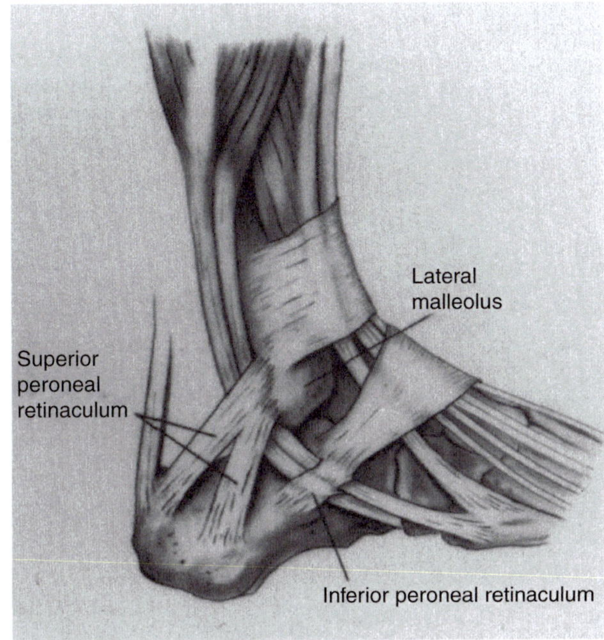

Fig. 3.18 An illustration of type 3 SPR showing a single wider band inserting into the Achilles sheath. (From Davis et al. [22])

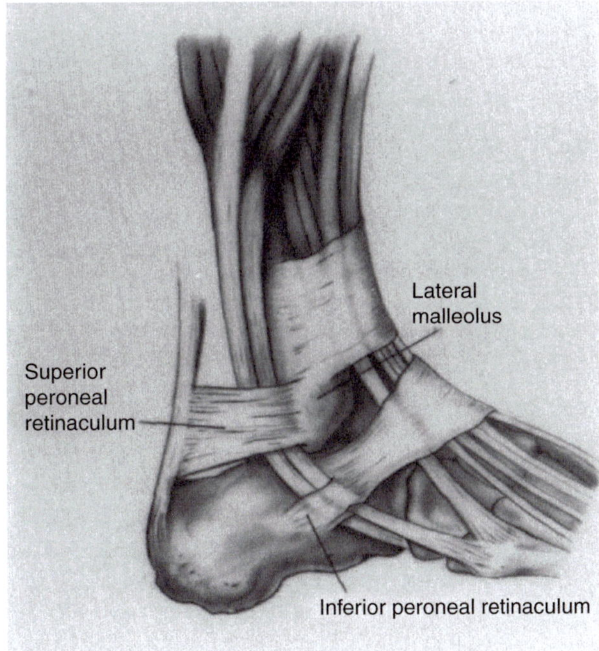

Fig. 3.19 An illustration of type 4 SPR showing a single wider band inserting into the calcaneus. (From Davis et al. [22])

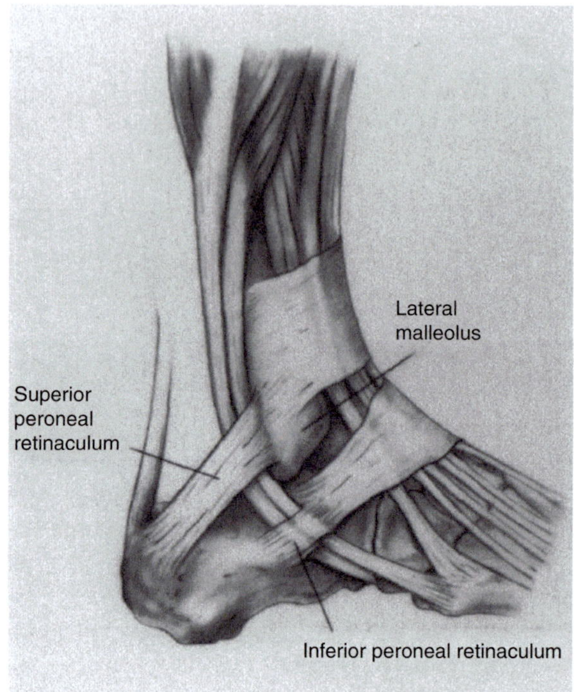

Fig. 3.20 An illustration of type 5 SPR showing a superior band inserting into the pretendinous fascia of the Achilles and an inferior band inserting into the lateral wall of the calcaneus. (From Davis et al. [22])

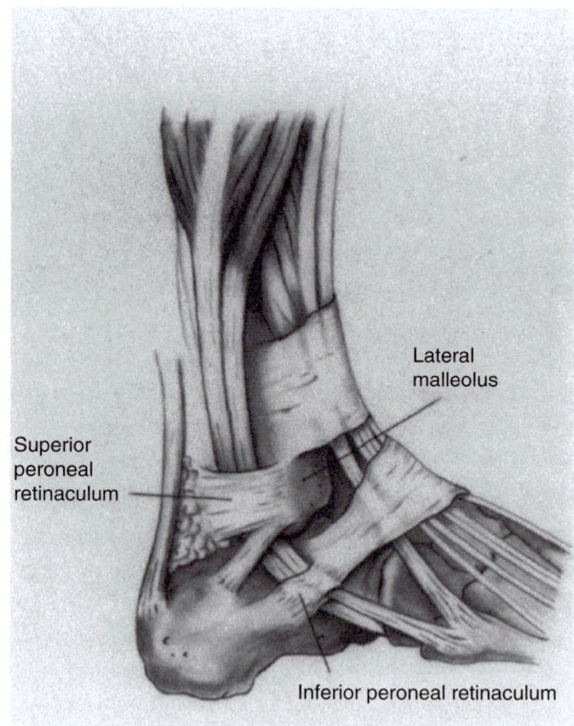

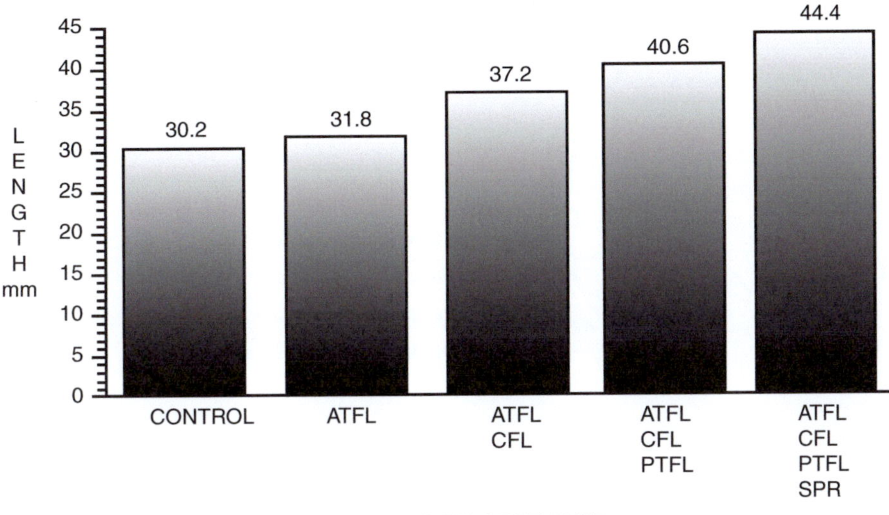

Fig. 3.21 This graph indicates increasing levels of instability to inversion stress with each ligament sectioned. Cutting the ATFL alone did not result in an increased instability to varus stress. The SPR contributes to lateral stability, and its sectioning yielded an increased intermetallic distance after all the lateral ligaments had been released [23]. (From Geppert et al. [23])

talofibular ligament (ATFL), CFL, SPR, and subsequently the peroneal tendons [22, 23].

Eckart and Davis described three grades of acute tears of the SPR, which were later classified into four grades by Oden. Oden's classification of injury to the SPR is as follows (Fig. 3.22) [45]:

- Type I: Elevation or stripping off of the periosteal attachment of the SPR to the lateral malleolus at the level of the fibular groove. The stripped-off periosteum and SPR form a pouch-like configuration lateral to the distal fibula into which the peroneal tendons can dislocate.
- Type II: Tear of the SPR at its attachment to the distal fibula.
- Type III: Distal fibular avulsion fracture at the attachment of the retinaculum to the lateral malleolus.
- Type IV: Tear of the retinaculum at its posterior attachment.

Rosenberg et al. demonstrated that axial MRI images are probably the best method for assessing SPR injury and allows direct visualization of any disruption [45, 46]. It is useful to be familiar with the typical MR imaging features of Oden's four types of SPR injuries. Imaging studies by Rosenberg et al. and Wang et al. thoroughly explain these MRI appearances, as well as the imaging features of diseases of the peroneal tendons, including tenosynovitis, rupture, and dislocation [45, 46].

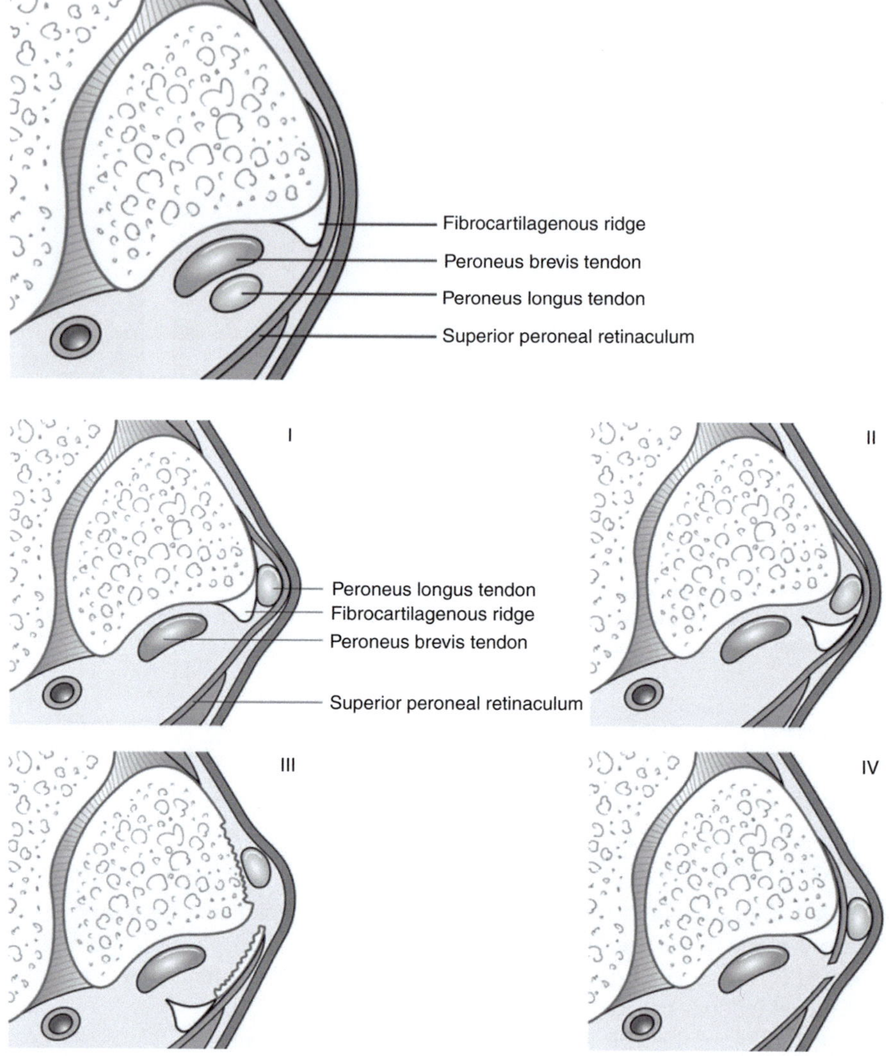

Fig. 3.22 The normal anatomy of the peroneus longus and peroneus brevis tendons contained within the retromalleolar groove, followed by Oden's classification of SPR injuries as described in the previous paragraph. (From Hamilton and Robinson [74])

In summary, the SPR is the primary restraint to peroneal tendon subluxation and has a variety of insertional variations. The parallel relationship of the SPR to the CFL is illustrated, and the SPR is a secondary restraint to inversion stress of the ankle. This parallel relationship of the CFL and SPR may help to explain the coexistence of peroneal tendon injury and chronic lateral ankle instability.

Morphologic Variations in the Retromalleolar Fibular Groove

In 1928, Edwards [47] conducted a cadaveric study and found the presence of a substantial concave groove on the posterior aspect of the fibula in 82% of specimens. He also noted a flat or convex groove in 11% and 7% of individuals, respectively, both of which can result in lateral subluxation/dislocation and longitudinal tears of the peroneal tendons. The depth and width of the groove vary from 2 to 4 mm and 5 to 10 mm, respectively, and the groove itself is accentuated by an osseous ridge that is covered by a fibrocartilaginous cap, adding an additional 2–4 mm to the depth of the sulcus. The SPR has no strong attachment to the ridge itself but rather blends in with the periosteum on the lateral surface of the fibula. Associated with the sharp posterior edge of the fibula is a dense fibrocartilaginous ridge that effectively deepens the groove, which has been shown to contribute to the stability of the tendons behind the fibula [47]. Tearing of the peroneus brevis tendon is often noted in this location. Most commonly, a shallow (congenital convex) groove or a sharp posterior ridge of the fibula may contribute or predispose one to peroneal tendon injury [3].

In Sobel et al.'s cadaveric work, they discovered that the presence of a sharp posterior ridge, as opposed to a rounded or flat posterior ridge, enhances the ability of the fibula to split the peroneus brevis tendon [3]. Peroneus brevis tendon tears are often noted as a result of dynamic mechanical insult within the fibular groove. A sharp edge at the fibrocartilaginous posterior ridge of the distal fibula where the SPR inserts may contribute to the tearing of the peroneus brevis tendon, as the anterior half of the splayed out peroneus brevis tendon subluxates out of the fibular groove under pressure from the peroneus longus tendon and splits over the sharp posterior ridge of the distal fibula [3]. Figures 3.23, 3.24, 3.25, and 3.26 illustrate the pull of the peroneus longus with eversion of the foot and resultant compression of the peroneus brevis by the peroneus longus at the fibular groove leading to peroneus brevis tears.

Kumai et al. [48] looked at the histological structure of the retromalleolar fibular groove in ten cadaveric specimens and noted that the contour and thickness of the groove differed significantly in its proximal and distal parts. Distally, the fibula is convex, and the shape of the groove is determined by the thick periosteal cushion of fibrocartilage covering the fibular surface. Proximally, the shape of the groove is determined by the fibula itself, and the periosteum is thin and fibrous. The authors concluded that the restriction of a thick periosteal fibrocartilage to the distal end suggests that it serves to promote stress dissipation by adapting the shape of the malleolar groove to that of the tendons within it [48]. However, by restricting the periosteum to the distal end, the tendons can be sliced longitudinally by the sharp posterior ridge created from periosteal fibrocartilage when the SPR becomes torn or incompetent, increasing the risk of damage to subluxated peroneal tendons. The

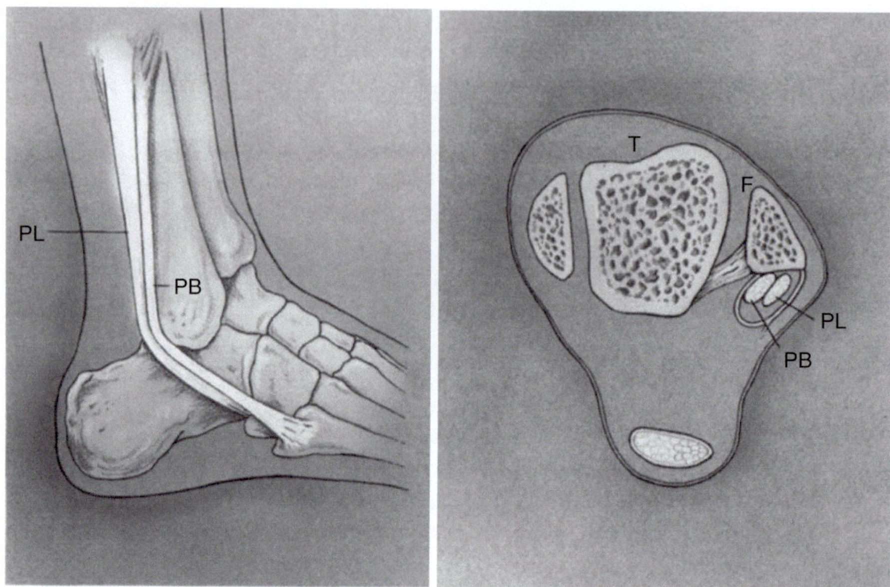

Fig. 3.23 The photograph (left) and cross section of the ankle at the level of the fibular groove (right) demonstrate the relationship between the peroneus brevis, peroneus longus, and posterior edge of the fibula, with no pull on the peroneus longus and the foot in neutral alignment. (From Sobel et al. [3])

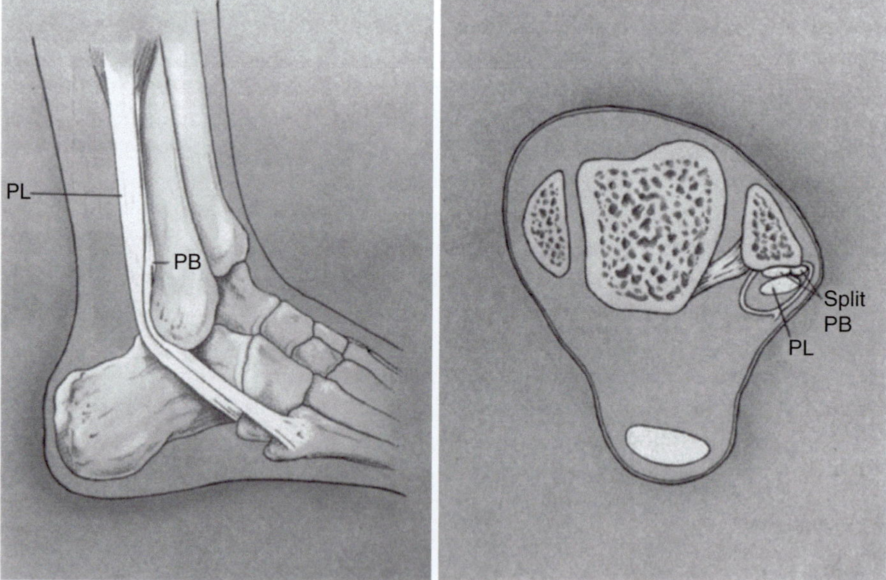

Fig. 3.24 The photograph (left) and cross section of the ankle at the level of the fibular groove (right) demonstrate the relationship between the peroneus longus and peroneus brevis, with moderate pull on the peroneus longus and moderate eversion of the foot. (From Sobel et al. [3])

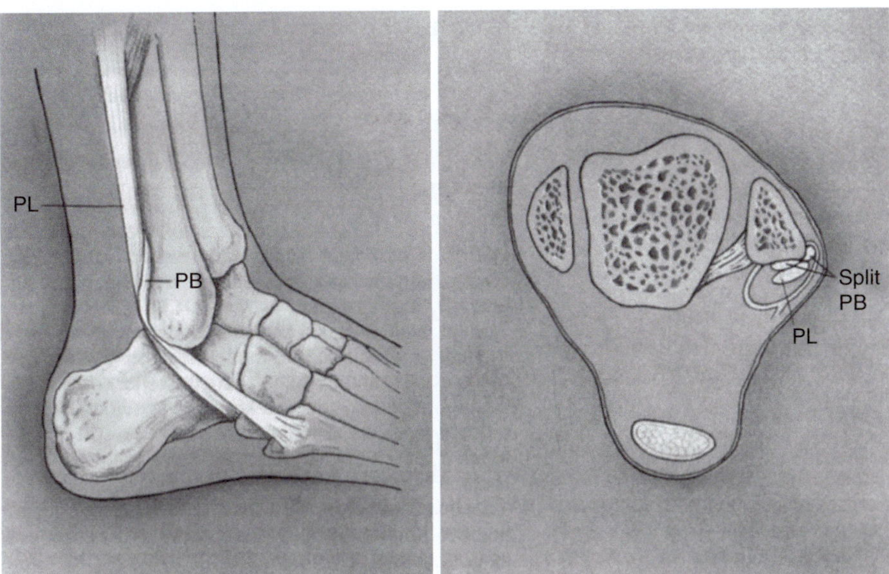

Fig. 3.25 The photograph (left) and cross section of the ankle at the level of the fibular groove (right) show the relationship between the peroneus longus and peroneus brevis, with maximal pull on the peroneus longus and maximal eversion of the foot. (From Sobel et al. [3])

medial periosteum was formed by both the posterior and inferior tibiofibular ligaments.

Athavale et al. looked at the anatomy of the superior peroneal tunnel in 58 cadaver limbs, as well as the contour of the retromalleolar groove is 60 dry fibulas [8]. The authors noted a spacious tunnel with its roof formed by the superior peroneal retinaculum. The floor of the tunnel had an osseous component formed by the retromalleolar groove of the fibula, and a nonosseous component formed by the lower portion of the posterior intermuscular septum of the leg [8]. Additional contents found within the fibular tunnel were the muscular tissue of the peroneus brevis muscle and an anomalous peroneus quartus tendon. Other findings included the presence of a split peroneus brevis tendon, a double peroneus longus tendon, and an accessory peroneal nerve. Their study of dry fibulas confirmed a constantly concave shape of the retromalleolar groove [8].

In summary, if a peroneus brevis tear is found upon exploration, debridement of the tendon edges and repair of the tear, in addition to tubularization of the tendon and reefing of the superior peroneal retinaculum, seem warranted. In addition, when present, the sharp posterior ridge of the fibula can be removed as well. Both these remove a possible insult to the tendon and create an excellent bony bed for the SPR advancement and repair.

Lateral Wall of the Calcaneus; Enlarged Peroneal Tubercle Variation

After coursing below the retromalleolar groove, the peroneus longus and peroneus brevis tendons separate into two distinctly separate synovial sheaths and traverse the lateral wall of the calcaneus. This surface may have two bony projections: the peroneal tubercle and the retrotrochlear eminence [49].

The peroneal tubercle is located at the junction of the anterior and middle one-third of the lateral wall of the calcaneus and separates the peroneus longus and peroneus brevis as they split into two distinct tendon sheaths [50, 51]. It also fixes the pulley of both tendons [51]. The peroneus brevis runs superior to the tubercle and later inserts onto the surface of the fifth metatarsal base, while the peroneus longus passes inferior to the tubercle and continues into the cuboid tunnel where the os peroneum articulates with the cuboid [50]. The retrotrochlear eminence is located posterior to the peroneal tubercle and tendons. Edwards reported this eminence to be present in 98% of individuals [47]. In their cadaveric study, Zammit and Singh [5] reported the retrotrochlear eminence to be most frequent insertion site for the peroneus quartus tendon. This often leads to hypertrophy of the bony location [46].

In 1928, Edwards examined 150 human heel bones and found the peroneal tubercle to be prominent and well developed in 24% of the specimens [47]. Hyer et al. studied 114 cadaveric calcaneus specimens and found the peroneal tubercle to be prominent in 29.1%, flat in 42.7%, and concave in 27.2% of specimens [52]. Hofmeister et al. studied the peroneal tubercle in 35 specimens and found that the average length was 10.3 mm, width 5.6 mm, height 4.0 mm, and average distance to the calcaneocuboid joint was 17.2 mm. The incidence of hypertrophy of the peroneal tubercle was 3% [53].

The presence of an enlarged or gigantic peroneal tubercle on the lateral aspect of the calcaneus can entrap the peroneus longus tendon and/or the os peroneum during tendon excursion [49]. Enlargement of the peroneal tubercle could be congenital, present as an acquired deformity, or caused by the insertion of an anomalous peroneus quartus tendon [2, 54]. This variation could interfere with the normal gliding motion of the peroneus longus tendon, leading to tenosynovitis and eventually to a tear of the tendon. Wang et al. also noted that an adventitial bursa can develop over the peroneal tubercle, which can be symptomatic when inflamed [46]. The acquired form has been associated most often with flat, cavus, or paralytic feet [54, 55]. Pierson and Inglis described a case in which an enlarged peroneal tubercle was associated with the formation of a bony tunnel over the peroneus longus tendon. The patient presented with a large osseous prominence along the lateral wall of the calcaneus, which was very tender to palpation. They also noted the presence of an enlarged os peroneum. The pain, clicking, and symptoms of unsteadiness

Fig. 3.26 Radiographically (A), an enlarged peroneal tubercle (arrow) is identified on the lateral aspect of the calcaneus, on the axial view of the calcaneus. An intraoperative photograph with the tendons retracted demonstrates a gigantic peroneal tubercle on the lateral wall of the calcaneus responsible for obstruction of os peroneum and peroneus longus tendon excursion [49].
(From Sobel et al. [49])

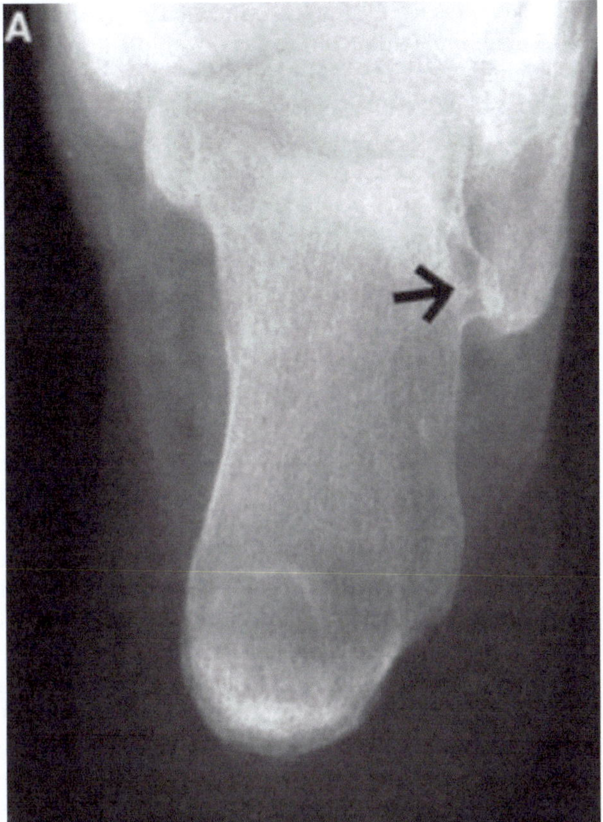
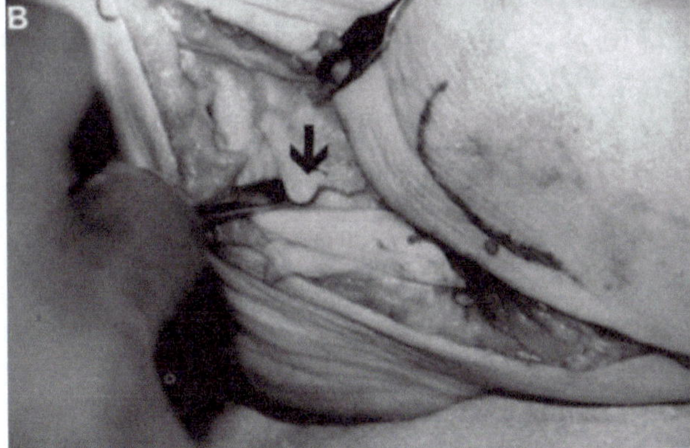

completely resolved after excision of the hypertrophied tubercle [56]. In 1994, Sobel et al. reported on ten patients with plantar lateral foot pain whose symptoms and findings demonstrated painful os peroneum syndrome. The majority of these cases presented with an enlarged or multipartite os peroneum. One patient demonstrated a gigantic peroneal tubercle on the lateral wall of the calcaneus responsible for obstruction of the os peroneum and peroneus longus tendon excursion [49]. Sugimoto et al. described three patients with peroneal tenosynovitis due to enlarged peroneal tubercles. All three patients were treated surgically with resection of the enlarged peroneal tubercle with good results [51]. Bruce et al. reported three patients with stenosing tenosynovitis of the peroneus longus tendon associated with a markedly enlarged peroneal tubercle. In one case, a bony tunnel enveloped the peroneus longus tendon in the absence of an os peroneum. In the other two patients, an os peroneum was present [57]. Lui reported on a case in which an enlarged peroneal tubercle was removed endoscopically. The endoscopic resection was performed through zone 2 peroneus longus tendoscopy, keeping the procedure at the level of the peroneal tubercle and peroneus longus [58]. Chen et al. described six patients with painful hypertrophy of the peroneal tubercle. X-ray and CT scanning revealed a bony prominence at the lateral calcaneal cortex and stenosing tenosynovitis at the peroneal tubercle in all patients. The symptoms were treated by synovectomy and peroneal tubercle resection with good results. The authors concluded that a hypertrophic peroneal tubercle creates a stenotic tunnel, which triggers a painful peroneal longus tenosynovitis [59]. Burman described stenosing tenovaginitis of the peroneal tendons in conjunction with a painful enlarged peroneal tubercle [60]. Brandes and Smith reported on 22 patients with primary peroneus longus tendon injury. Of the patients with partial tears, 89% involved the region of the lateral calcaneal process. The authors determined that the zone of the peroneus longus tendon from the inferior peroneal retinaculum to the cuboid notch is a high-stress area, responsible for the majority of peroneus longus tears [61]. Palmanovich et al. published a review of the literature on peroneus longus tear and its relation to the peroneal tubercle. The authors clarified the anatomy, biomechanics of the tendon, and the clinical features of tear of the peroneus longus tendon on the lateral surface of the calcaneus due to an enlarged peroneal tubercle [54]. Dutton et al. looked at the prevalence of painful peroneal tubercles in the pediatric population. During the study period, 2689 children were seen for foot and ankle pain. Of the 367 patients who underwent CT scan during their treatment, 57% had a measurable peroneal tubercle, and in 44% of patients, the peroneal tubercle was 3 mm or greater. Only three patients were found to have clinical symptoms and ultimately underwent surgical excision with successful relief of symptoms. The authors noted that hypertrophy of the peroneal tubercle is less likely to be associated with peroneal tendinopathy and tears in the pediatric population [62]. Taki et al. reported a case of bilateral stenosing tenosynovitis of the peroneus longus tendon associated with hypertrophied peroneal tubercle in an 11-year-old junior soccer player. MRI of each foot demonstrated that the peroneus longus tendon was pushed inferiorly by the hypertrophic peroneal tubercle, and the tendon sharply changed its course at the inferior border of the tubercle [63].

Watson et al. recently reported on 11 patients treated surgically for stenosing peroneal tenosynovitis. After discovering normal MRI findings in this population of patients, the authors concluded that ultrasound-guided anesthetic injection of the peroneal sheath to confirm diagnosis is paramount for the success of the surgical outcome. In this series, distal peroneal tenolysis was performed after independently opening the longus and brevis sheaths and excising any residual sheathing. The peroneal tendons were inspected to ensure that there were no peroneal tendon tears. The authors noted that an area of stenosis could be visualized by a dimpling of the tendon. In the event of a low-lying peroneus brevis muscle belly or thickened area of synovium, the muscle or synovial space was debrided. In the instance of an enlarged peroneal tubercle, the tubercle was removed, and the remainder of the calcaneal bone was smoothed. The authors reported significant improvement in all 11 patients that underwent surgery [64].

In summary, the presence of an enlarged peroneal tubercle along the lateral wall of the calcaneus can contribute to peroneus longus stenosing tenosynovitis. Surgical excision of the enlarged peroneal tubercle and tenosynovectomy of the peroneal tendons is usually curative.

Cuboid Tunnel: Incidence and Variations of the Os Peroneum in the Peroneus Longus Tendon

At the level of the cuboid tunnel, an osseous or fibrocartilaginous sesamoid is present in the fibers of the peroneus longus tendon (Fig. 3.27) [65]. This sesamoid, named the os peroneum or sesamum peroneum, is frequently round but may be divided into several portions as it glides along the anterior slope of the plantar surface of the cuboid at the cuboid tunnel [49, 65]. Sarrafian [65] reported that "the os peroneum is always present in an ossified, cartilaginous, or fibrocartilaginous stage. It may remain a fibrocartilaginous nucleus for life." Rarely, the os peroneum is found in the retromalleolar or calcaneal portions of the peroneus longus tendon. When present, the os peroneum is fully ossified in 20% of individuals, not fully ossified in 75%, and radiographically apparent in 5% [65]. Edwards [47] identified a groove on the lateral surface of the calcaneus for the peroneus longus tendon next to the peroneal tubercle in 128 of 150 bones (85%).

In 1994, Sobel et al. reported that painful os peroneum syndrome (POPS) was a spectrum of conditions responsible for plantar lateral foot pain and included one or more of the following: (1) an acute os peroneum fracture or a diastasis of a multipartite os peroneum, either of which may result in a discontinuity of the peroneus longus tendon; (2) chronic (healing or healed) os peroneum fracture or diastasis of a multipartite os peroneum with callus formation, either of which results in a stenosing peroneus longus tenosynovitis; (3) attrition or partial rupture of the peroneus longus tendon proximal or distal to the os peroneum; (4) frank rupture of the peroneus longus tendon with discontinuity proximal or distal to the os peroneum; and/or (5) the presence of a gigantic peroneal tubercle on the lateral aspect of the

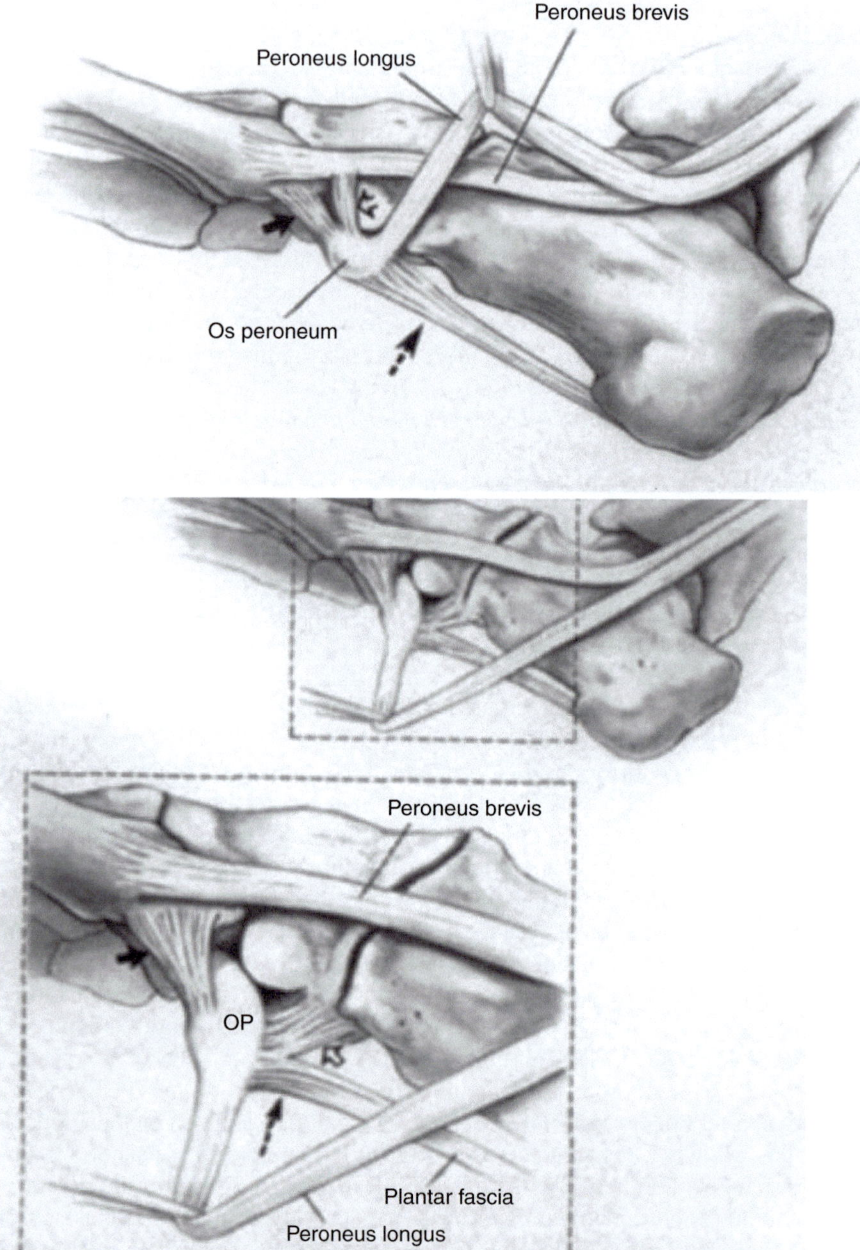

Fig. 3.27 Illustration demonstrating the four soft tissue attachments of the os peroneum sesamoid complex: (1) the plantar fascial band (dashed black arrow), (2) the fifth metatarsal band (short solid black arrow), which extends from the os peroneum (OP) to the base of the fifth metatarsal, (3) the band to peroneus brevis tendon (hollow black arrow on top), and (4) the cuboid band (hollow black arrow on bottom). (From Sobel et al. [49])

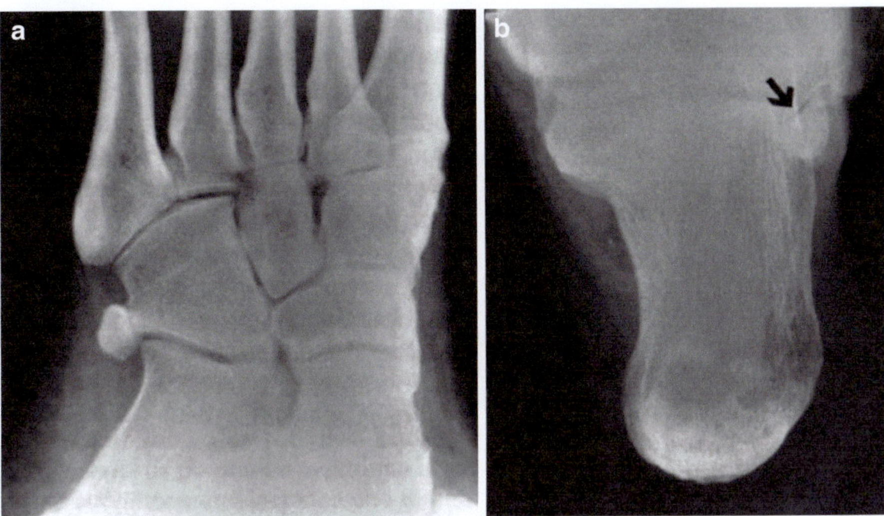

Fig. 3.28 Oblique view (**a**) of the foot and axial view of the calcaneus (**b**) demonstrate a large solitary os peroneum articulating with the posterior lateral surface of the cuboid (arrow). (From Sobel et al. [49])

calcaneus, which entraps the peroneus longus tendon and/or the os peroneum during tendon excursion [49].

Clinical diagnosis of painful os peroneum syndrome can be facilitated by the single stance heel rise and varus inversion stress test, as well as by resisted plantar flexion of the first ray, which can localize tenderness along the distal course of the peroneus longus tendon at the cuboid tunnel. Radiographic diagnosis should include an oblique radiograph of the foot for visualization of the os peroneum and, if indicated, other imaging studies (Figs. 3.28 and 3.29).

Recommended treatment ranges from conservative cast immobilization to surgical approaches including (1) excision of the os peroneum and repair of the peroneus longus tendon, and (2) excision of the os peroneum and degenerated peroneus longus tendon with tenodesis of the remaining remnant of the peroneus longus to the peroneus brevis tendon [49]. In the case where both tendons are gone, then autograft or allograft reconstruction or single-stage flexor digitorum longus transfer, or flexor hallucis longus tendon transfer are options [66–70]. Alternatively, as popularized by Wapner, the flexor hallucis longus can been used in a staged procedure after Hunter rod placement [67].

Barton et al. [70] reported on two patients with lateral instability of the hindfoot due to chronic transverse tears of both the peroneus longus and brevis tendons. Examination of each patient showed loss of continuity of the peroneal tendon with weakness of eversion of the hindfoot. Neither patient had an os peroneum. Surgical reconstruction was done by transfer of flexor digitorum longus (FDL) to peroneus brevis when end-to-end repair was not possible. Both patients had excellent function when reviewed after eight and six years, respectively, with no symptoms [70].

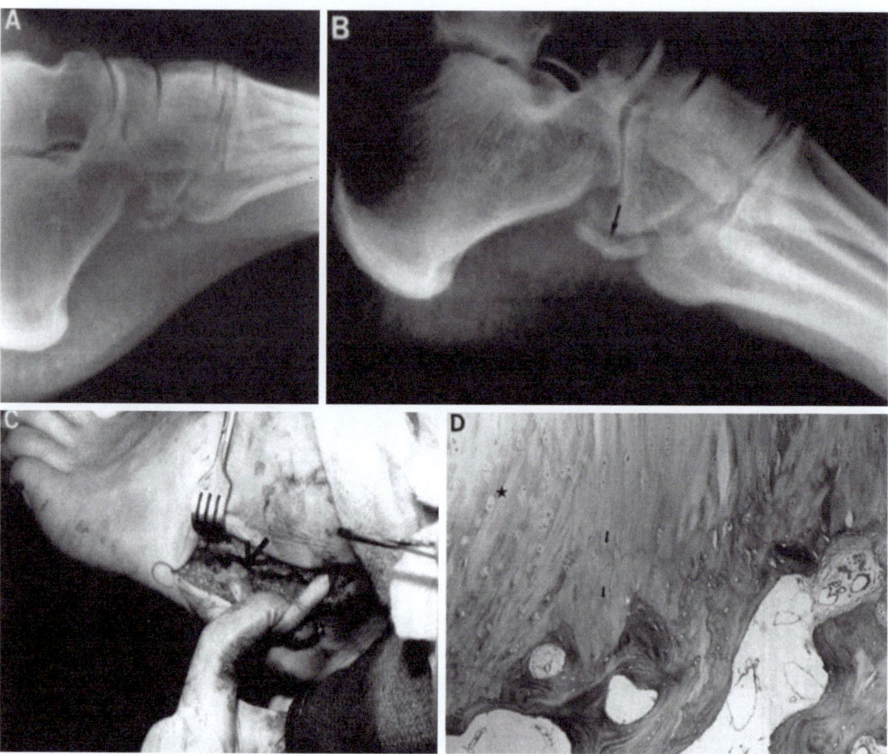

Fig. 3.29 (**a**) Lateral view of the left foot demonstrates a multipartite os peroneum articulating with the cuboid. Each of the fragments has a smooth corticated border. There is 2 mm of diastasis between the main fragments. (**b**) Lateral view demonstrates that the previously identified multipartite sesamoid has remodeled and coalesced to form a large elongated os peroneum. A faint vertically oriented radiolucency, suggesting partition, through the mid-portion is present (arrow). (**c**) Intraoperative photograph with the peroneus longus tendon retracted demonstrates the articular facet of the os peroneum (arrow) in the cuboid tunnel. (**d**) Photomicrograph from the edge of the os peroneum shows lamellar bone of the os peroneum and the degenerative cartilaginous metaplasia (star) at the insertion of the tendon with progression and duplication of the tidemark (arrows) as it extends into the tendon, which is indicative of a degenerative enthesopathy (hematoxylin and eosin, ×20 objective). (From Sobel et al. [49])

Although the CT showed a normal appearance of the FDL in both patients, the peroneal muscles looked abnormal. The authors concluded that transfer of the FDL provides a reliable solution to lateral hindfoot instability resulting from loss of function of both peronei [69]. Blitz and Nemes [71] reported a case of bilateral peroneus longus tendon rupture through a bipartite os peroneum. The patient had a cavovarus foot, which, when combined with an inversion force, has been a suggested mechanism of os peroneum injury [71]. In both feet, a peroneus longus to peroneus brevis tendon transfer was performed in conjunction with a partial excision of the fractured os peroneum. In a five-year retrospective review, Stockton and Brodsky [72] reported on 12 patients surgically treated for complex irreparable tears of the peroneus longus tendon with associated pathology of the os peroneum. In eight patients, the peroneus longus tendon tear was associated with a fracture of the os peroneum. In the remaining four patients, tear of the peroneus longus was associated with an enlarged and entrapped os peroneum preventing tendon excursion at the cuboid tunnel. At surgery, the peroneus longus tendon was found to be enlarged, fibrotic, and adhered to the surrounding tissues [72]. All of the patients had a viable peroneus brevis tendon and were successfully treated with excision of the os peroneum, debridement, and tenodesis of the peroneus longus to the peroneus brevis. Concomitant partial tears of the peroneus brevis tendon were found in 9 of the 12 patients, which were treated with debridement and suture repair. Between 1985 and 1996, Brandes and Smith reported on 22 patients with primary peroneus longus tendinopathy. 82% of the patients had a cavovarus hindfoot position. All six of the complete tears occurred at the cuboid notch. Seven of the cases (33%) had associated involvement of the peroneus brevis tendon [61]. Smith et al. showed that minimally displaced fracture of the os peroneum can be treated nonoperatively allowing a high-level athlete to return pain-free through restriction of weight bearing activities and physical therapy [73].

In summary, POPS is a spectrum of disease processes of the peroneus longus tendon and os peroneum, which is present at the lateral wall of the calcaneus and especially the cuboid tunnel which causes plantar lateral hindfoot pain. Awareness of these conditions together with proper history and physical examination can guide the most appropriate diagnostic studies for each condition and prevent delayed or missed diagnosis of this entity.

Bibliography

1. Hecker P. Study on the peroneus of the tarsus. Anat Rec. 1923;26:79–82.
2. Sobel M, Levy ME, Bohne WHO. Congenital variations of the peroneus quartus muscle: an anatomic study. Foot Ankle. 1990;11:81–9.
3. Sobel M, Geppert MJ, Olson EJ, Bohne WHO, Arnoczky SP. The dynamics of peroneus brevis tendon splits: a proposed mechanism, technique of diagnosis, and classification of injury. Foot Ankle. 1992;13:413–22.
4. Donley BG, Leyes M. Peroneus quartus muscle. Am J Sports Med. 2001;29:373–5.
5. Zammit J, Singh D. The peroneus quartus muscle. Anatomy and clinical relevance. J Bone Joint Surg Br. 2003;85-B:1134–7.
6. Bilgili MG, Kaynak G, Botanlıoğlu H, Basaran SH, Ercin E, Baca E, Uzun I. Peroneus quartus: prevalence and clinical importance. Arch Orthop Trauma Surg. 2014;134:481–7.
7. Yammine K. The accessory peroneal (fibular) muscles: peroneus quartus and peroneus digitiquinti. A systematic review and meta-analysis. Surg Radiol Anat. 2015;37:617–27.
8. Athavale SA, Vangara SV. Anatomy of the superior peroneal tunnel. J Bone Joint Surg. 2011;93(6):564–71.
9. Athavale SA, Gupta V, Kotgirwar S, Singh V. The peroneus quartus muscle: clinical correlation with evolutionary importance. Anat Sci Int. 2012;87:106–10.
10. Habashy A, Cook B, Sumarriva G, Treuting R. Peroneus quartus muscle. Am J Orthop. 2017;46:E419–22.

11. Chinzei N, Kanzaki N, Takakura Y, Takakura Y, Toda A, Fujishiro T, Hayashi S, Hashimoto S, Kuroda R, Kurosaka M. Surgical management of the peroneus quartus muscle for bilateral ankle pain. J Am Podiatr Med Assoc. 2015;105:85–91.
12. Sönmez M, Kosar ÇM. The supernumerary peroneal muscles: case report and review of the literature. Foot Ankle Surg. 2000;6:125–9.
13. Moroney P, Borton D. Multiple accessory peroneal muscles: a cause of chronic lateral ankle pain. Foot Ankle Int. 2004;25:322–4.
14. Prakash NC, Singh DK, Rajini T, Venkatiah J, Singh G. Anatomical variations of peroneal muscles. J Am Podiatr Med Assoc. 2011;101:505–8.
15. Saupe N, Mengiardi B, Pfirrmann CWA, Vienne P, Seifert B, Zanetti M. Anatomic variants associated with peroneal tendon disorders: MR imaging findings in volunteers with asymptomatic ankles. Radiology. 2007;242:509–17.
16. Chepuri NB, Jacobson JA, Fessell DP, Hayes CW. Sonographic appearance of the peroneus quartus muscle: correlation with MR imaging appearance in seven patients. Radiology. 2001;218:415–9.
17. Cheung YY, Rosenberg ZS, Ramsinghani R, Beltran J, Jahss MH. Peroneus quartus muscle: MR imaging features. Radiology. 1997;202:745–50.
18. Sammarco GJ, Brainard BJ. A symptomatic anomalous peroneus brevis in a high-jumper. A case report. J Bone Joint Surg Am. 1991;73:131–3.
19. Martinelli B, Bernobi S. Peroneus quartus muscle and ankle pain. Foot Ankle Surg. 2002;8:223–5.
20. Nascimento SRR, Costa RW, Ruiz CR, Wafae N. Analysis on the incidence of the fibularis quartus muscle using magnetic resonance imaging. Anat Res Int. 2012;2012:1–6.
21. Kulshreshtha R, Kadri S, Rajan DT. A case of unusual combination of injuries around the lateral malleolus. Foot. 2006;16:51–3.
22. Davis WH, Sobel M, Deland J, Bohne WH, Patel MB. The superior peroneal retinaculum: an anatomic study. Foot Ankle Int. 1994;15:271–5.
23. Geppert MJ, Sobel M, Bohne WH. Lateral ankle instability as a cause of superior peroneal retinacular laxity: an anatomic and biomechanical study of cadaveric feet. Foot Ankle. 1993;14:330–4.
24. Gumusalan Y, Ozbag D. A variation of fibularis quartus muscles: musculus fibulocalcaneusexternum. Clin Anat. 2007;20:998–9.
25. Regan TP, Hughston JC. Chronic ankle "sprain" secondary to anomalous peroneal tendon. Clin Orthop Relat Res. 1977;123:52–4. https://doi.org/10.1097/00003086-197703000-00020.
26. Mick CA, Lynch F. Reconstruction of the peroneal retinaculum using the peroneus quartus. A case report. J Bone Joint Surg. 1987;69:296–7.
27. White AA, Johnson D, Griswold DM. Chronic ankle pain associated with the peroneus accessorius. Clin Orthop Relat Res. 1974;103:53–5.
28. Taljanovic MS, Alcala JN, Gimber LH, Rieke JD, Chilvers MM, Latt LD. High-resolution US and MR imaging of peroneal tendon injuries. Radiographics. 2015;35(1):179–99.
29. Öznur A, Arik A, Alanay A. Peroneus quartus muscle as a rare cause of the chronic lateral ankle pain. Foot Ankle Surg. 2002;8(3):227–30.
30. Sobel M, Mizel MS. Peroneal tendon injury. In: Pfeffer GB, Frey CC, editors. Current practice in foot and ankle surgery. New York: McGraw-Hill, Health Professions Division; 1993. p. 33.
31. Sobel M, Bohne WHO, Obrien SJ. Peroneal tendon subluxation in a case of anomalous peroneus brevis muscle. Acta Orthop Scand. 1992;63:682–4.
32. Sobel M, Mizel MS. Peroneal tendon injury. In: Pfeffer GB, Frey CC, editors. Current practice in foot and ankle surgery. New York: McGraw-Hill, Health Professions Division; 1993. p. 34.
33. Sobel M, Mizel MS. Peroneal tendon injury. In: Pfeffer GB, Frey CC, editors. Current practice in foot and ankle surgery. New York: McGraw-Hill, Health Professions Division; 1993. p. 35.
34. Amini B. Low-lying peroneus brevis muscle belly [Internet Blog]. Roentgen ray reader 2011. Accessed 5 Nov 2018. Available from: http://roentgenrayreader.blogspot.com/2011/11/low-lying-peroneus-brevis-muscle-belly.html.

35. Dombek MF, Lamm BM, Saltrick K, Mendicino RW, Catanzariti AR. Peroneal tendon tears: a retrospective review. J Foot Ankle Surg. 2003;42:250–8.
36. Geller J, Lin S, Cordas D, Vieira P. Relationship of a low-lying muscle belly to tears of the peroneus brevis tendon. Am J Orthop (Belle Mead NJ). 2003;32:541–4.
37. Mirmiran R, Squire C, Wassell D. The prevalence and role of a low-lying peroneus brevis muscle belly in patients with peroneal tendon pathologic features: a potential source of tendon subluxation. J Foot Ankle Surg. 2015;54:872–5.
38. Highlander P, Pearson KT, Burns P. Magnetic resonance imaging analysis of peroneal tendon pathology associated with low-lying peroneus brevis muscle belly. Foot Ankle Spec. 2015;8:347–53.
39. Freccero DM, Berkowitz MJ. The relationship between tears of the peroneus brevis tendon and the distal extent of its muscle belly: an MRI study. Foot Ankle Int. 2006;27:236–9.
40. Unlu MC, Bilgili M, Akgun I, Kaynak G, Ogut T, Uzun I. Abnormal proximal musculotendinous junction of the peroneus brevis muscle as a cause of peroneus brevis tendon tears: a cadaveric study. J Foot Ankle Surg. 2010;49:537–40.
41. Housley SN, Lewis JE, Thompson DL, Warren G. A proximal fibularis brevis muscle is associated with longitudinal split tendons: a cadaveric study. J Foot Ankle Surg. 2017;56:34–6.
42. Hammerschlag WA, Goldner JL. Chronic peroneal tendon subluxation produced by an anomalous peroneus brevis: case report and literature review. Foot Ankle. 1989;10:45–7.
43. Sobel M, Mizel MS. Peroneal tendon injury. In: Pfeffer GB, Frey CC, editors. Current practice in foot and ankle surgery. New York: McGraw-Hill, Health Professions Division; 1993. p. 32.
44. Sobel M, Mizel MS. Peroneal tendon injury. In: Pfeffer GB, Frey CC, editors. Current practice in foot and ankle surgery. New York: McGraw-Hill, Health Professions Division; 1993. p. 30–3.
45. Rosenberg ZS, Bencardino J, Astion D, Schweitzer ME, Rokito A, Sheskier S. MRI features of chronic injuries of the superior peroneal retinaculum. Am J Roentgenol. 2003;181:1551–7.
46. Wang X-T, Rosenberg ZS, Mechlin MB, Schweitzer ME. Normal variants and diseases of the peroneal tendons and superior peroneal retinaculum: MR imaging features. Radiographics. 2005;25:587–602.
47. Edwards ME. The relations of the peroneal tendons to the fibula, calcaneus, and cuboideum. Am J Anat. 1928;42:213–53.
48. Kumai T, Benjamin M. The histological structure of the malleolar groove of the fibula in man: its direct bearing on the displacement of peroneal tendons and their surgical repair. J Anat. 2003;203:257–62.
49. Sobel M, Pavlov H, Geppert MJ, Thompson FM, Dicarlo EF, Davis WH. Painful Os peroneum syndrome: a spectrum of conditions responsible for plantar lateral foot pain. Foot Ankle Int. 1994;15:112–24.
50. Davda K, Malhotra K, O'Donnell P, Singh D, Cullen N. Peroneal tendon disorders. EFORT Open Rev. 2017;2:281–92.
51. Sugimoto K, Takakura Y, Okahashi K, Tanaka Y, Ohshima M, Kasanami R. Enlarged peroneal tubercle with peroneus longus tenosynovitis. J Orthop Sci. 2009;14:330–5.
52. Hyer CF, Dawson JM, Philbin TM, Berlet GC, Lee TH. The peroneal tubercle: description, classification, and relevance to peroneus longus tendon pathology. Foot Ankle Int. 2005;26:947–50.
53. Hofmeister E, Juliano P, Lippert F. The anatomical configuration and clinical implications of the peroneal tubercle. Foot. 1996;6:138–42.
54. Palmanovich E, Laver L, Brin YS, Kotz E, Hetsroni I, Mann G, Nyska M. Peroneus longus tear and its relation to the peroneal tubercle: a review of the literature. Muscles Ligaments Tendons J. 2011;4:153–60.
55. Dr-P A Peroneal Tendon Complex Injury And Rehabilitation. In: 986 Dr Pributs Blog. https://www.drpribut.com/wordpress/2017/10/peroneal-tendon-complex-injury-and-rehabilitation/. Accessed 24 Oct 2018.

56. Pierson JL, Inglis AE. Stenosing tenosynovitis of the peroneus longus tendon associated with hypertrophy of the peroneal tubercle and an os peroneum. A case report. J Bone Joint Surg Am. 1992;74:440–2.
57. Bruce WD, Christofersen MR, Phillips DL. Stenosing tenosynovitis and impingement of the peroneal tendons associated with hypertrophy of the peroneal tubercle. Foot Ankle Int. 1999;20:464–7.
58. Lui TH. Endoscopic resection of the peroneal tubercle. J Foot Ankle Surg. 2012;51:813–5.
59. Chen YJ, Hsu RW, Huang TJ. Hypertrophic peroneal tubercle with stenosing tenosynovitis: the results of surgical treatment. Changgeng Yi Xue Za Zhi. 1998;21:442–6.
60. Burman M. Stenosing tendovaginitis of the foot and ankle: studies with special reference to the stenosing tendovaginitis of the peroneal tendons at the peroneal tubercle. AMA Arch Surg. 1953;67:686.
61. Brandes CB, Smith RW. Characterization of patients with primary peroneus longus tendinopathy: a review of twenty-two cases. Foot Ankle Int. 2000;21:462–8.
62. Dutton P, Edmonds EW, Lark RK, Mubarak SJ. Prevalence of painful peroneal tubercles in the pediatric population. J Foot Ankle Surg. 2012;51:599–603.
63. Taki K, Yamazaki S, Majima T, Ohura H, Minami A. Bilateral stenosing tenosynovitis of the peroneus longus tendon associated with hypertrophied peroneal tubercle in a junior soccer player: a case report. Foot Ankle Int. 2007;28:129–32.
64. Watson GI, Karnovsky SC, Levine DS, Drakos MC. Surgical treatment for stenosing peroneal tenosynovitis. Foot Ankle Int. 2018;40:282–6.
65. Sarrafian SK. Anatomy of the foot and ankle: descriptive, topographic, functional. Philadelphia: J.B. Lippincott; 2011.
66. Mook WR, Parekh SG, Nunley JA. Allograft reconstruction of peroneal tendons. Foot Ankle Int. 2013;34:1212–20.
67. Wapner KL, Taras JS, Lin SS, Chao W. Staged reconstruction for chronic rupture of both peroneal tendons using hunter rod and flexor hallucis longus tendon transfer: a long-term follow up study. Foot Ankle Int. 2006;27:591–7.
68. Jockel JR, Brodsky KW. Single-stage flexor tendon transfer for the treatment of severe concomitant peroneus longus and brevis tendon tears. Foot Ankle Int. 2013;34:666–72.
69. Seybold JD, Campbell JT, Jeng CL, Short KW, Myerson MS. Outcome of lateral transfer of the FHL or FDL for concomitant peroneal tendon tears. Foot Ankle Int. 2016;37:576–81.
70. Barton DC, Lucas P, Jomha NM, Cross MJ, Slater K. Operative reconstruction after transverse rupture of the tendons of both peroneus longus and brevis: surgical reconstruction by transfer of the flexor digitorum longus tendon. J Bone Joint Surg Br. 1998;80:781–4.
71. Blitz NM, Nemes KK. Bilateral peroneus longus tendon rupture through a bipartite os peroneum. J Foot Ankle Surg. 2007;46(4):270–7.
72. Stockton KG, Brodsky JW. Peroneus longus tears associated with pathology of the os peroneum. Foot Ankle Int. 2014;35:346–52.
73. Smith JT, Johnson AH, Heckman JD. Nonoperative treatment of an osperoneum fracture in a high-level athlete: a case report. Clin Orthop Relat Res. 2011;469:1498–501.
74. Hamilton P, Robinson AHN. Peroneal tendon disorders. In: Bentley G. (eds) Eur Surg Orthop Traumatol. Springer, Berlin, Heidelberg. 2014:3637–57.

History and Physical Examination in Peroneal Tendon Injury

Mark J. Geppert

The ankle region, including bones, ligaments, and tendons, constitutes one of the most commonly affected sites in sports and traumatic injuries accounting for up to 20% of all sports injuries [1]. Though not as common as ankle sprains, peroneal tendon injury or pathology is not rare, with increasing attention to this condition being reported in the last few decades [2–9]. Unfortunately, peroneal tendon injury can be missed because of the difficulty in differentiating peroneal tendon injury from lateral ankle injury in the setting of acute ankle trauma [10]. Additionally, the majority of ankle injuries are labeled "ankle sprains" and are first evaluated by parents, coaches, trainers, family practitioners, and emergency room personnel. The ankle "sprain" that fails to improve will eventually seek an orthopedic surgeon or foot and ankle specialist, and a significant percentage of these ankle sprain failures will be found to have a peroneal tendon condition. Peroneal tendon problems can also present with no revealed history of injury or trauma. Peroneal tendon injury or pathology can be organized into peroneal tendonitis, tendinopathy, tears, ruptures, acute subluxation, acute dislocation, chronic subluxation, and chronic dislocation. These conditions represent a spectrum of pathology with either no antecedent event or trauma, or with an acute event potentially leading to a chronic condition unless an accurate and timely diagnosis is made and appropriate interventions initiated [11].

The key to an accurate diagnosis of peroneal tendon pathology can be revealed by taking a detailed history and then performing a directed physical examination. The physician mentally hypothesizes potential pathology before touching the patient or body part and is directed in his or her thought process by listening to the patient and determining precisely where the patient complains of pain.

M. J. Geppert (✉)
Department of Orthopedic Surgery, Wentworth Health Partners Seacoast
Orthopedics & Sports Medicine, at Wentworth-Douglass Hospital, Dover, NH, USA
e-mail: mgeppert@sosmed.org

© Springer Nature Switzerland AG 2020
M. Sobel (ed.), *The Peroneal Tendons*,
https://doi.org/10.1007/978-3-030-46646-6_4

Past Medical History and Family History

Before examining the ankle and before asking for a history of specific ankle complaints, the past medical history is reviewed to exclude systemic conditions that are associated with peroneal tendon pathology. Lyme disease and gout have been diagnosed in the author's experience after initial presentation of peroneal tendon complaints. Rheumatoid arthritis, psoriasis, hyperparathyroidism, diabetic neuropathy, and seronegative conditions are similarly associated [12]. Bilateral atraumatic tendon or joint complaints may suggest an undiagnosed systemic condition which should be investigated. Fluoroquinolone use has a well-documented negative affect on Achilles tendons leading to rupture [13], but fluoroquinolones have not, to the author's knowledge, been reported in peroneal tendon pathology.

The astute physician tries to exclude pre-existing medical conditions associated with ankle problems and potential tendon pathology. The past medical history includes a history of prior surgery, fracture, or injury to the foot and ankle as surgical fixation of a fibula fracture can commonly lead to peroneal tendon complaints. Prior fractures of the lateral process of the talus can result in peroneal tendonitis. Calcaneus fractures can lead to a broadened heel and peroneal impingement, or operative fixation of calcanei can lead to peroneal symptoms secondary to impinging hardware.

Ankle pain or injury is so common a complaint that before focusing on a specific peroneal tendon pathology other conditions or injuries can be rapidly excluded on an anatomic basis. Location of pain is the most important element in the history-taking process. Anterior, medial, posteromedial, and direct posterior ankle pain is rarely associated with peroneal tendon pathology. Anterior symptoms may reveal anterior tibialis tendonitis, rupture, or anterior ankle impingement. Medial ankle pain can indicate deltoid injury or posterior tibial tendonitis (PTT). Initial symptoms of PTT are predominately medial with late secondary lateral peroneal symptoms due to fibular impingement in stage 3 [14] and stage 4 [15] PTT dysfunction. Pain just anterior to the posterior process on the medial aspect of the ankle can indicate flexor hallucis longus tendonitis or "dancer's tendonitis" [16].

The differential diagnosis of direct posterior ankle pain is extensive and most commonly affects the Achilles tendon. Visible swelling in the Achilles hypovascular zone, 4 cm proximal to its insertion, may indicate chronic Achilles tendinosis. Crepitus within the Achilles reveals tendonitis whereas a palpable gap or ecchymosis can indicate a rupture. The classic Thompson test with lack of plantarflexion of the Achilles confirms a rupture. Insertional Achilles tendonitis is evident in the middle-aged individual with exquisite palpation tenderness at the insertion whereas tenderness on the anterior distal Achilles can indicate retrocalcaneal bursitis. Inferior calcaneal pain at the tuberosity is the most common site of tenderness in a calcaneal stress fracture, whereas pain slightly inferior to this in an 8- to 12-year-old child may indicate Sever's disease or calcaneal apophysitis. Soft tissue masses in the lateral hindfoot may mimic peroneal tendon pathology but actually can represent ganglions arising from degenerative tibiotalar or subtalar arthritis (Fig. 4.1).

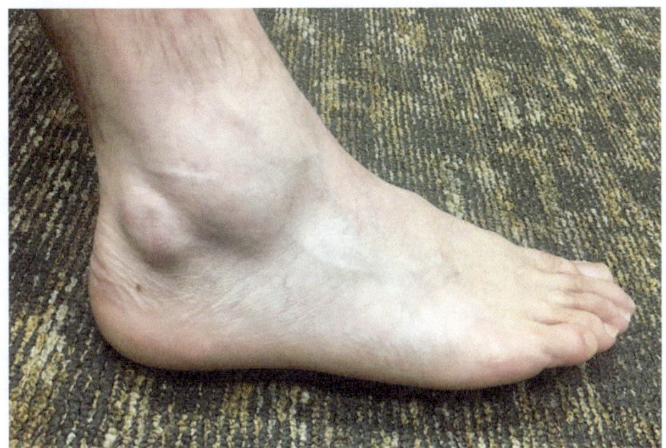

Fig. 4.1 Photograph of a ganglion arising from degenerative posterior facet arthrosis. Note the circular appearance of the mass

Direct posterior tenderness in the talar region may indicate a talar compression syndrome, posterior impingement syndrome, or lateral talus process fracture. An os trigonum is present in approximately 5% of normal foot radiographs [17] and is in close proximity to the peroneal tendons. Passive plantarflexion accompanied by posterior pain is a classic finding in posterior impingement syndrome whereas pain to posterolateral palpation likely indicates peroneal tendon pathology.

It is fairly straightforward to accurately exclude peroneal tendon injury on an anatomic basis of anterior, medial, and direct posterior ankle or tendon pain. Peroneal tendon injury manifests as pain in the anterolateral, lateral, and posterolateral ankle region. Fortunately, the bones, tendons, and ligaments of the ankle region are superficial and these structures can be visualized and/or palpated by the experienced physician (Figs. 4.2 and 4.3).

Anatomy

Though the regional anatomy of the peroneal tendons is described in detail in Chapter One, a brief review is required as focal tenderness at very specific anatomic regions can reveal likely distinct peroneal tendon pathologies. The peroneus longus (PL) tendon originates from the proximal lateral aspect of the tibia and the fibula to insert on the inferior and lateral aspect of the medial cuneiform and first metatarsal. The function of the longus is to plantar flex the ankle and evert the foot and to plantar flex the first metatarsal. The peroneus brevis (PB) originates in the middle of the lateral portion of the fibula and plantar flexes the ankle and everts the foot with its insertion into the base of the fifth metatarsal. Both tendons are innervated by the superficial peroneal nerve.

The PL becomes tendinous a few centimeters proximal to the tip of the fibula whereas the PB muscular portion can extend a few centimeters distal to the fibula. This distal extension of PB muscle is thought to potentially contribute to overcrowding of the peroneal tendons within their retinacular attachments with resultant attenuation of the superior peroneal retinaculum (SPR) and subsequent pathology [18].

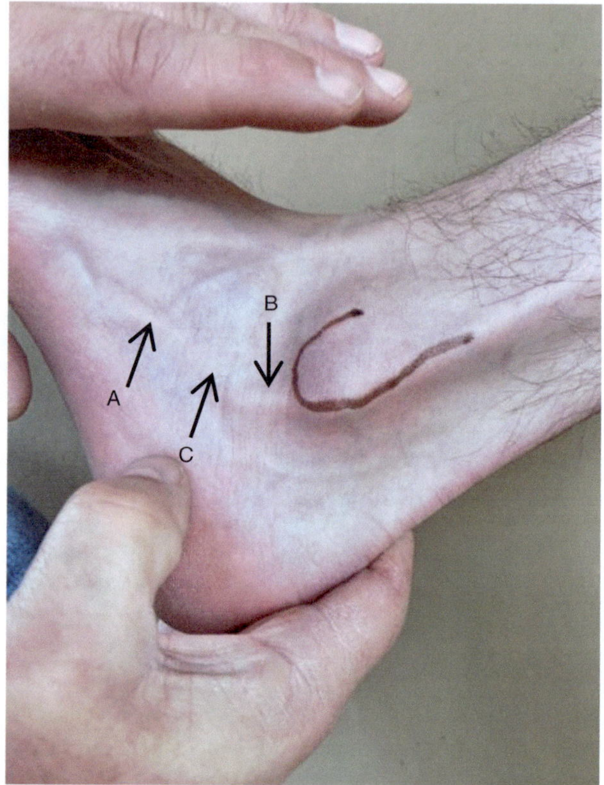

Fig. 4.2 Note the distal peroneus brevis tendon inserting into the base of the fifth metatarsal (A). The peroneus longus tendon can be seen at the posterior aspect of the fibula and distal to the fibula (B). Separation of the longus and brevis is noted at the peroneal tubercle (C)

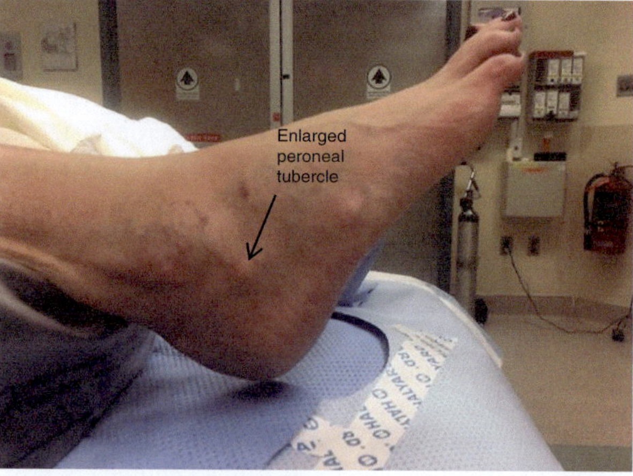

Fig. 4.3 Easily visible enlarged peroneal tubercle

An extra peroneal tendon, the peroneus quartus has been found in 22% of anatomic dissections [19]. This normal tendon can be mistaken for a peroneal tendon tear on imaging studies and can also contribute to overcrowding at the SPR.

The PL rides posterolateral to the brevis and is restrained behind the fibula by the highly variable SPR. At the tip of the fibula, the PL turns sharply toward the peroneal tubercle (PT) where it is restrained by the inferior peroneal retinaculum (IPR). The PT was found to be present in 90% of 114 calcaneal dissections and enlarged in 29% [20]. An enlarged peroneal tubercle has been associated with stenosing tenosynovitis [21] and peroneal tendon tears. Distal to the PT, the longus encompasses the os peroneum present as a calcified structure in approximately 5–20% of specimens in radiographic and anatomic studies [22] and then turns sharply and medially toward the cuboid tunnel. Comprising the fourth layer of plantar foot musculature, the PL inserts on the plantar lateral aspect of the medial cuneiform and first metatarsal.

The PB lies beneath the PL above the fibula with both tendons restrained by the highly variable SPR and held beneath the sharp posterior ridge of the distal fibula. Injury to the SPR or anatomic variation of a flattened, convex, or irregular posterior fibula [23] can lead to incompetence of the SPR and attendant subluxation, tendonitis, and peroneal tendon tears. Inferior to the tip of the fibula, the PB is superior to the PL and is restrained above the PT by the inferior peroneal retinaculum (IPR). It travels directly to its broad insertion at the base of the fifth metatarsal. Understanding this normal anatomy is a key to define zones of injury to help identify suspected peroneal tendon pathology revealed by palpation tenderness during the physical examination. The foot is amenable to visualization and palpable detection of topographic landmarks (Fig. 4.4).

Recent biochemical and histologic studies have helped define the pathologic process that differentiates tendonitis and tendinosis [13]. Tendonitis is an acute inflammatory process that is largely reversible and accompanied by peripheral tendon damage. Because it is of acute onset, its diagnosis should be detected within the history and is generally associated with a change in usual activity. It can arise from intense overtraining, lack of rest, and excessive acute strain on normal tendons. A history of a mild prior injury in the recent past, major change in training regimen or shoe wear, or altered surface environment increases the risk of tendon pathology. Tendonitis is seen much less frequently in a young athlete compared to adults

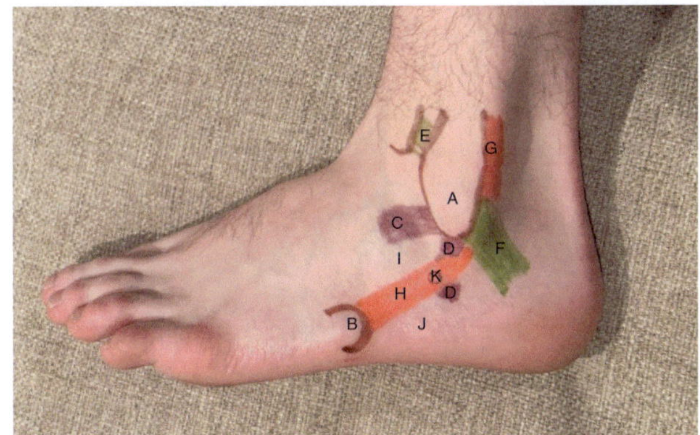

Fig. 4.4 Normal foot: (A) distal fibula, (B) fifth metatarsal, (C) anterior talofibular ligament, (D) calcaneofibular ligament, (E) anterior inferior tibiofibular ligament, (F) superior peroneal retinaculum, (G) posterior ridge of fibula and peroneus longus tendon, (H) peroneus brevis tendon, (I) sinus tarsi, (J) cuboid tunnel, (K) peroneal tubercle

because the apophysis or tendon site attachment to the bone is weaker than the tendon itself and is more susceptible to injury.

Tendinosis is an irreversible process of intrinsic tendon damage resulting in histopathologic change to the tendon. It is found as a result of chronic stress, aging, and faulty repair. Healing from tendon injury is dependent upon adequate vascularity. Studies have identified zones of hypovascularity in both peroneal tendons that correlate with usual sites of peroneal tendon pathology. Peterson [24] detected hypovascularity of both peroneal tendons as they turn distally at the tip of the fibula towards the peroneal tubercle. A second zone of hypovascularity of the longus is near the cuboid tunnel as it turns medially toward the bottom of the foot.

Widespread orthopedic awareness of peroneal tendon pathology lags behind the familiar "too many toes sign" of posterior tibial tendonitis (PTT) because PTT pathology has been reported earlier and more extensively in the orthopedic literature. A multitude of peroneal tendon basic science articles, case series, and operative techniques have appeared in the last three decades [12, 25–29]. As familiarity with peroneal tendon pathology increases, the frequency of its diagnosis will increase and "failed" ankle sprains will likely decrease.

Trauma

If there is a history of significant trauma, swelling, focal tenderness, or inability to bear weight, screening radiographs to exclude fracture should be taken, as it is unfair to the patient to manipulate, palpate, and perform range of motion or strength testing if a fracture is present. It is helpful to place a small metallic marker at the point of maximal tenderness prior to obtaining X-rays, as markers may correlate with an enlarged peroneal tubercle, os peroneum, or other structures.

Anteroposterior standing foot films (if tolerated) can reveal fractures at the base of the fifth metatarsal, cuboid fractures, chopart joint avulsion fractures, Lis Franc injury, and navicular fractures. Oblique foot films can reveal an avulsion fracture of the anterior process of the calcaneus, calcaneonavicular tarsal coalition, or the presence of an os peroneum.

Lateral standing foot X-rays can reveal fractures of chopart joint, talus, or calcaneus. A break in the lateral talo-metatarsal angle from $0°$ can indicate a pes cavus ($>0°$) or pes planus (angle $<0°$). An increased calcaneal pitch ($>30°$) suggests a cavus foot.

Mortise and oblique radiographs of the ankle can reveal fibular fractures, an os subfibulare, avulsion fibular fractures, lateral process of talus fractures, talus fractures, and osteochondral injury or osteochondritis dessicans. The orthopedist is the one physician who should not miss a fracture evident on easily obtainable plain radiographs.

History of the Onset of Peroneal Symptoms

Acute peroneal tendon symptoms associated with tendonitis, tear, rupture, or dislocation is generally identified by an event recognized by the patient. The clinician needs to elicit the mechanism of injury which can be associated with specific peroneal tendon pathology. Was the ankle loaded in a weight-bearing position? What was the position of the foot and the direction of force? Was there impact or a torsional mechanism of injury? Was there a popping sensation or any sound associated with the injury? Can the patient point to the location of pain, and can the patient reproduce the pathology by a specific motion or maneuver? Though the clinician may be seeing a patient with "new" ankle or peroneal problems, careful questioning can reveal this to be a progression of symptoms from a remote injury. The persistence and worsening of symptoms may indicate a chronic peroneal pathology.

Other important elements in the history-taking process include questions regarding onset, duration, course, ameliorating and exacerbating factors, quality, and intensity of pain [30]. Stress fracture pain usually worsens with activity and if severe, may also occur with rest. Conversely, tendinopathy generally improves with a warm up, yet worsens following a run [30]. A significant increase in exercise intensity or running mileage indicates a training error with greater than 20 miles per week correlated with a significant increased risk of injury [31].

Over-Reliance on Imaging Studies

All of this background information regarding medical associations with tendon pathology, anatomy, blood supply, acute and chronic conditions, and exclusion of nonperoneal tendon pathology based on the location of pain allows the astute physician to formulate a differential diagnosis and test this through a detailed physical examination. This includes inspection, palpation, manipulation, strength assessment, and special tests with a directed and knowledgeable physical examination to reveal or exclude peroneal tendon pathology suggested in the history. This focused examination on the anterolateral, lateral, and posterolateral ankle region from origin to insertion of the peroneal tendons with attention to topographical anatomy helps to accurately diagnose peroneal tendon pathology. Ancillary tests such as X-rays, high-resolution ultrasounds, and MRIs should confirm a suspected diagnosis, and are ideally ordered by the treating specialist. A significant percentage of positive MRI findings of peroneal tendon pathology in asymptomatic volunteers has been reported [32, 33]. In one study, the positive predictive value, accuracy rate, and interobserver reliability of MRI were relatively low indicating that thorough physical examination should be performed in combination with MRI scanning for a definitive diagnosis of peroneal tendinopathy [34]. Peroneal tendon tears are often incidental findings on MRI [35]. Conversely, MRI studies that were reported normal have also missed operatively confirmed peroneal tendon tears [36].

Multiple practitioners can order ancillary tests that may reveal clinically insignificant findings and result in inappropriate intervention. For example, the author treated a patient whose primary care physician had ordered an ankle MRI which revealed a small tear of the peroneus brevis tendon. The initial foot and ankle subspecialist performed a PB repair but the lateral "ankle pain" persisted. Careful physical examination noted pain distal and anterior to the peroneal tendons. A missed nonunited anterior process of the calcaneus fracture was diagnosed and excised with complete symptom resolution. Findings from sophisticated imaging techniques should not drive the management of reported pathology, and the tests themselves should be ordered by physicians capable of diagnosing and directing appropriate therapy or surgical treatment.

Physical Examination

Visual inspection is the initial step in physical diagnosis. At a minimum, the bare-footed leg must be visualized from the knees distally with either a gown or shorts allowing a more thorough examination. Barefooted gait should be witnessed from the front and rear of the patient, usually facilitated by walking down the hall, outside the examining room. Smooth reciprocating gait with equal stride length and lack of an antalgic limp serve as a sufficient screen. From the rear, the physician should observe heel inversion and supination of the foot during heel lift off. At heel strike, the heel should evert and the foot pronate to give a flat foot appearance at mid-stance.

While the patient has removed their shoes, the physician should examine the shoe-wear pattern with lateral heel-wear indicating supination [37]. Medial counter and medial sole-wear indicate pronation deformity [37]. While inspecting the shoes, ask about and look at any orthotic devices or history of devices. Whether the patient benefitted from or abandoned orthotics and who and why an orthotic trial was prescribed provides valuable information.

Comparison to the unaffected leg will often reveal differences that suggest peroneal tendon pathology (Fig. 4.5). Visual differences between the two legs are most

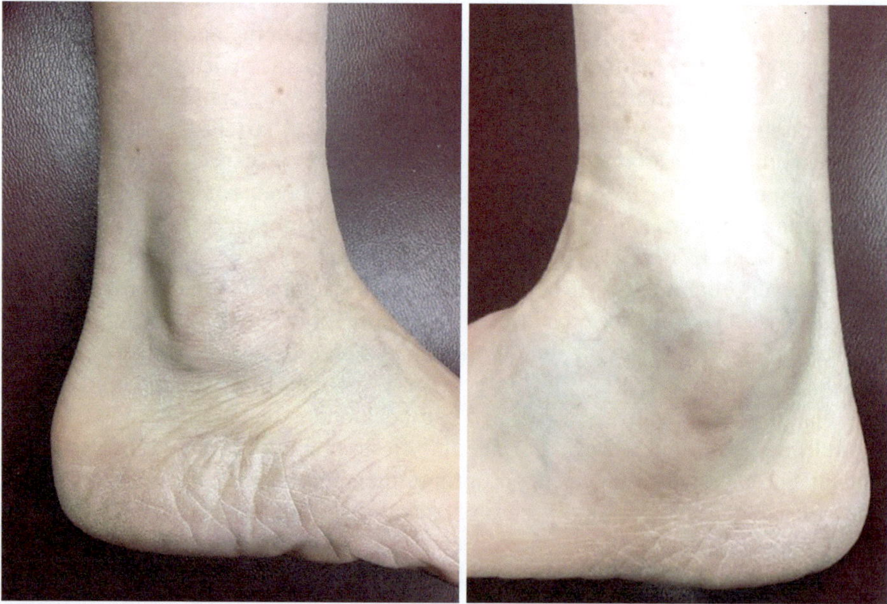

Fig. 4.5 Left: Photograph of normal leg with a visible concavity posterior to the fibula. Right: Obvious atraumatic posterior swelling with loss of normal fibula outline indicating likely chronic peroneal tendon pathology

significant in the absence of trauma or acute injury. Significant acute ankle injury may reveal a massively swollen ankle that hurts "everywhere" with the patient unable to differentiate posterior (peroneal) tenderness from anterior (ankle sprain) symptoms.

Visual examination includes inspection of the standing patient. From the front, visual inspection can reveal a subtle cavus foot with a visible or "peek-a-boo" [38] heel (Fig. 4.6, Left). Viewed from behind, detection of heel varus is a little more subtle due to a lack of anatomic landmarks, if one focuses on the heel. However, opposite of the familiar "too many toes" sign of the lateral toes in PTT, a cavus foot viewed from the rear will reveal a view of the big toe and an absence of the lesser toes (Fig. 4.6, Right). Because PTT is more often unilateral than pes cavus, this medial toe sign is not as evident as the unilateral "too many toes." Determination of subtle pes cavus is important, as peroneal tendon pathology is more frequently associated with pes cavus than a normal or flat foot [39, 40]. The cavus foot is then further evaluated with the familiar lateral Coleman block test to determine if the subtalar joint is supple and whether the varus is a forefoot- driven-hindfoot-varus [41]. This distinction has importance in treatment implications, which will be discussed in Chap. 22. Carefully inspect for differences between extremities from all angles. Visual inspection of differences may reveal a broadened heel of retrocalcaneal bursitis, hindfoot varus, and loss of anatomic landmarks with peroneal swelling. Visual inspection from the side viewing the inside weight bearing foot will, with experience, differentiate a pes planus, pes cavus, or normal arch.

The patient is then asked to rise on both toes keeping the knee straight. "Cheating" by forward flexion of the knee or limited heel inversion may indicate posterior tibialis weakness. Loss of heel inversion may also suggest a tarsal coalition, subtalar

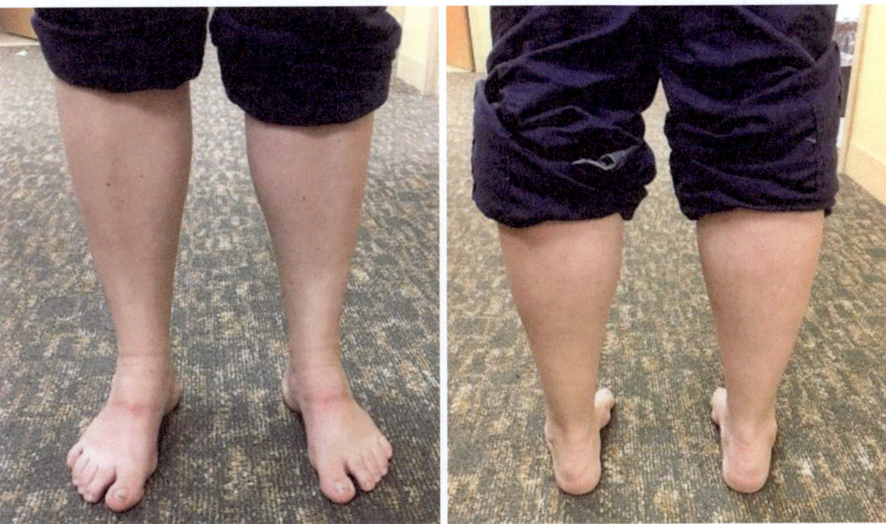

Fig. 4.6 Left: From the front, the "peek-a-boo" heel is visualized. Right: Standing view of a cavus foot from the rear, note the visibility of the great toe compared to the "too many toes" sign of posterior tibial tendon insufficiency

pathology, sinus tarsi syndrome, or peroneal spastic flatfoot. Once both feet are simultaneously tested, the patient is asked to perform ten single toe rises which may be required to unmask weakness.

The patient is then asked to take several steps on his heels and on his toes. More than once, in the author's experience, this maneuver has revealed a ruptured tibialis anterior tendon masquerading as an "ankle sprain." Weakness of toe or heel walking is also a rapid screen for lumbar pathology which can masquerade as peroneal tendon pathology. The standing patient then is asked to try to touch their toes with knees kept straight which is a rapid test for sciatic nerve tension.

The individual with toe or heel walk difficulty will need manual motor testing of the extensor hallucis longus, tibialis anterior, gastrocnemius, and knee and hip flexors and extensors. Assessment of patella and Achilles reflexes and a supine-positive straight leg raise test screen for spinal pathology. In the author's practice, a patient initially triaged as peroneal tendonitis actually suffered from a herniated lumbar disc with radiculitis presenting as posterolateral leg pain. The patient lacked point tenderness on palpation of the peroneals and had positive sciatic screening signs described above. The foot and ankle specialist must think outside his "box."

Tenderness to focused palpation of anatomic structures is the key step in physical examination of peroneal tendon injury. Pain within the peroneal tendons proximal to the SPR may indicate a referred pain from distal tendonitis if proximal referred spinal pathology has been excluded. Percussion tenderness at a region 15 cm proximal to the tip of the fibula may indicate a superficial peroneal nerve (SPN) neuritis or compression neuritis as the nerve exits the fascia. Both SPN and sural nerve neuropraxic injuries are associated with inversion ankle sprains and may be confused with peroneal tendon injury.

Boney tenderness proximal to the SPR may indicate a stress fracture, particularly in an elderly patient with an overuse history. The visual inspection of the standing individual with excess heel valgus can be associated with a chronic stress fracture 5–8 cm proximal to the tip of the fibula. This is particularly common in the extremely flatfooted, elderly, osteoporotic patient. Peroneal crowding due to an excessively everted calcaneus can result in subfibular impingement and peroneal tendonitis in Stage 3 or 4 PTT. Careful palpation of bone tenderness versus posterior soft tissue tenderness can differentiate between bone and tendon pathology.

Obvious and rare external traumatic injury may affect the proximal portion of the peroneal tendons, or they may be damaged by tibia/fibula fractures lacerating the muscle belly. Even a rare traumatic "thorn" penetrating injury has been reported as a cause of peroneal tendonitis [42].

Differentiating Ankle Sprains from Peroneal Tendon Injury

Twisting injuries of the ankle are one of the most common mechanisms of ankle injury and are most commonly regarded as sprains. Anterolateral pain over the anterior inferior distal fibula is regarded as a "low ankle sprain" and the mechanism is a plantarflexion and inversion strain. The anterior talofibular ligament (ATFL) is the most commonly injured of the three collateral ligaments of the ankle.

In the acute setting, global swelling and exquisite tenderness may prevent a complete physical examination. Tenderness slightly superior to this region indicates injury to the anteroinferior tibiofibular ligament (AITFL) classically sustained by an eversion injury. This "high ankle sprain" generally requires twice the time for recovery and has a similar mechanism of injury as the peroneal tendon. The difference is in the location of tenderness. Peroneal tendon injury is revealed by tenderness directly over the peroneal tendons propagating superiorly and posteriorly. Swelling of the peroneal sheath and focal peroneal tenderness suggests soft tissue injury. Palpation tenderness or injury of the posterior talofibular ligament (PTFL) is considered rare and is suggestive of peroneal tendon injury. Pain with compression of the tibia/fibula, several inches proximal to the ankle joint or pain with external foot rotation, helps differentiate peroneal tendon injury from a high ankle sprain.

The peroneal compression test [43] is a sensitive test that highly suggests peroneal tendon pathology and is performed with the patient seated and the knee bent 90° and the foot and ankle relaxed in an inverted and plantar flexed position. The examiner places their thumb over the posterior ridge of the fibula and compresses the peroneal tendons while the patient forcefully everts and dorsiflexes their ankle against resistance (Fig. 4.7). A positive test reproduces the pain and occasionally crepitus may be detected. Sometimes the anterior half of the peroneus brevis tendon

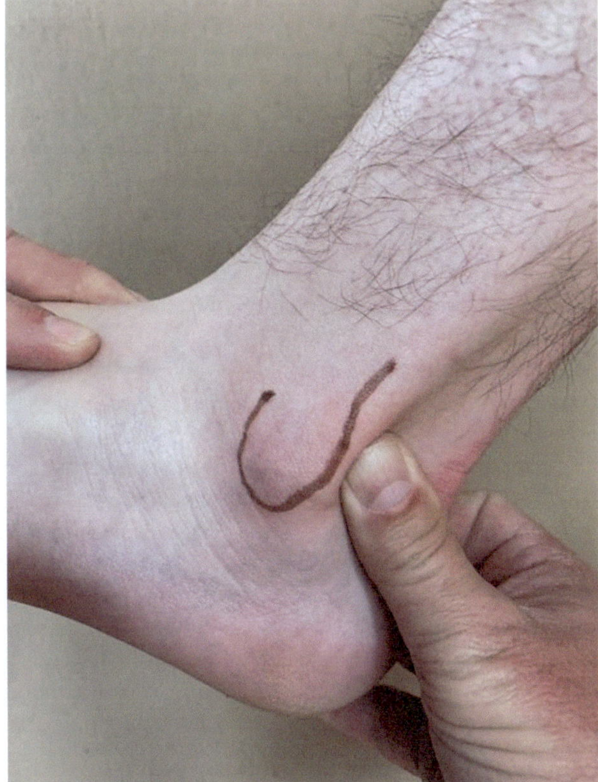

Fig. 4.7 Peroneal compression test performed with the thumb

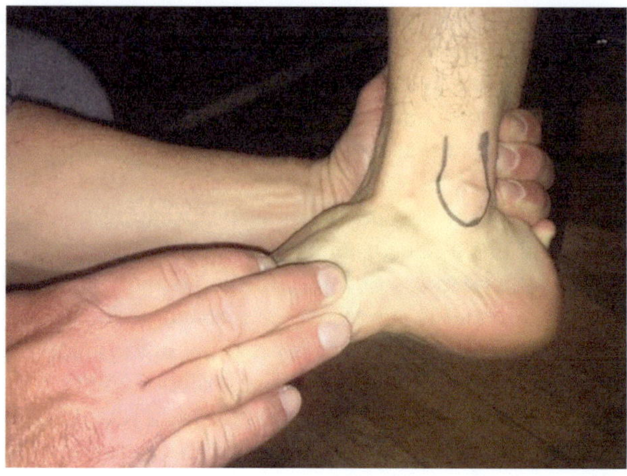

Fig. 4.8 Peroneal compression test performed with the second, third, and fourth fingers

may be noted to trigger, click, or jump over the posterior ridge of the fibula and the peroneal compression test can detect a subluxatable tendon. The patient may resist this and exhibit an "apprehension sign" during performance of the peroneal compression test. Alternatively, the examiner may place the second, third, and fourth fingers against the posterior fibula and resist the ankle eversion with the opposite hand (Fig. 4.8). Initially, the tendon is pressed against the fibula to detect tenderness. Then the examiner pushes the tendon anteriorly to attempt to recreate a partial tendon subluxation or dislocation.

The patient may report a snapping or visual tendon dislocation anterior to the fibula. Frank dislocation of the peroneal tendons acutely will oftentimes be accompanied by a radiographic "crescent sign" where the attached SPR avulses forwardly and is accompanied by a small rim of bone. The tendons will generally reduce posteriorly with eversion and can redislocate with forward pressure directed anteriorly from the posterior fibula. If acutely dislocated peroneal tendons have been reduced, it is generally too painful to reproduce acute dislocation in a clinical evaluation. A chronic subluxatable peroneal tendon, however, is much less painful, and can be reproduced with a peroneal compression test with particular attention to pushing the peroneal tendons anteriorly. The patient may also be able to demonstrate voluntary peroneal tendon subluxation or dislocation with plantar flexion and dorsiflexion of the ankle (Fig. 4.9).

Acute peroneal tendon dislocation is generally accompanied by significant force which should be revealed by a history of ankle injury. The fleck sign may or may not be evident on injury X-rays. Chronic ankle sprains may lead to incompetence of the SPR with its inability to effectively restrain the peroneal tendons. Biomechanical studies have demonstrated the contribution of the SPR to ankle stability [44]. Chronic lateral ankle instability leading to attenuation of the SPR can result in its incompetence, leading to partial tendon subluxation or frank dislocation. Once healing has occurred, an attenuated SPR may reveal a dislocatable peroneal tendon. The general orthopedist is familiar with the diagnosis of ankle instability and

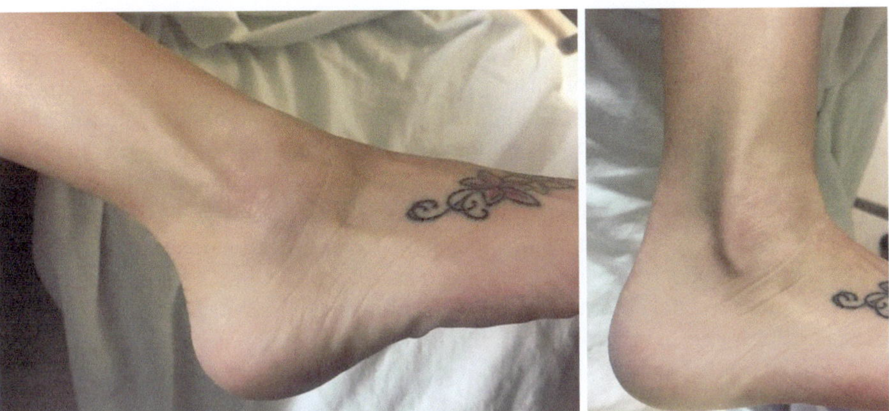

Fig. 4.9 Left: Plantarflexion of ankle with reduced peroneal tendons. Right: Dorsiflexion with voluntary subluxation/dislocation of peroneal tendons

performance of inversion and anterior drawer stress x-rays. When thinking of chronic lateral ankle instability, the orthopedist needs to remember potential peroneal tendon pathology due to the frequent coexistence of subluxation, SPR injury, peroneal tendon tears, and ankle ligament laxity [5, 45].

Incompetence of the SPR allows partial anterior subluxation of the anterior portion of the flattened PB resulting in its overriding the sharp fibrocartilaginous ridge of the posterior fibula. Reflex contraction of the PL will compress the PB and has been postulated as the mechanism of PB tendon tears [43]. Muscle weakness is not generally demonstrable, but compression over the fibula ridge will be painful. Comparison to the contralateral peroneal tendons will often reveal swelling. Both complete tendon dislocation and partial subluxation can reveal peroneal tendon tears. Earlier in the pathologic process, tenosynovitis, swelling, and flattening of the PB tendon are evidenced. It is relatively rare to find peroneus longus tears within the SPR sheath.

Frank dislocation of the peroneal tendons is generally associated with a significant eversion trauma, and the patient will often point to the displaced peroneal tendon. Restricted eversion of the foot will often be painful and will reveal the subluxed tendon. Comparison to the unaffected contralateral limb will make the diagnosis obvious. Patients may complain of a history of clicking or subjective feeling of tendon movement that may not be demonstrable upon physical exam. Difficulty in making a definitive diagnosis of subluxatable tendons may be clarified with an MRI, looking for incompetence of the SPR, avulsion from the posterior cartilaginous ridge, or at least fluid within the sheath on axial T2 images. Generally, within the SPR region, pathology of the PB tendon will be evident with longitudinal "tears in continuity" and splitting of the PB with anterior subluxation of its anterior portion.

Raikin and colleagues [46] have described two types of subluxation within the SPR sheath itself with patients describing a painful clicking or tendinous movement without anterior subluxation of the brevis or swelling of the peroneal sheath. The most common type revealed a posterolateral subluxation of the brevis over the peroneus longus accompanied by a click and termed this syndrome "intrasheath subluxation" [46]. Demonstration of this physical finding may be difficult to discern and may be accompanied by a "normal" MRI reading. Dynamic high-resolution ultrasound evaluation is required to reveal intrasheath subluxation but is highly operator-dependent and not readily available in all clinics. A presumptive diagnosis of intrasheath tendon subluxation requires an astute clinician and an experienced ultrasonographer for confirmation. This nuance of peroneal tendon pathology serves as a constant reminder that "the eye only sees what the mind knows" (William G. Hamilton, personal communication). The intrasheath peroneal subluxation of the PL and PB tendons in relation to one another without subluxation over the posterior ridge of the fibula has been confirmed under direct visualization with peroneal tendonoscopy [47].

In addition to a specific anatomic site of pain, a temporal element can suggest pathology. Acute ankle sprains, tendon dislocations, or ruptures are revealed by a history of trauma. Chronic lateral ankle instability or failure of recovery from a prior injury may indicate a chronic process. Peroneal tendon weakness is one of the most common causes of persistent pain post ankle sprain. With slow and incomplete recovery from a common ankle sprain, attention can be directed to potential peroneal tendon injury to explain persistent ankle complaints.

Location of Peroneal Tendon Tears

Brandes and Smith [39] defined three anatomic zones of peroneal tendon pathology of the peroneus longus (PL) tendon (Figs. 4.10 and 4.11). These zones are also useful to define zones of brevis pathology. Zone A is the region of the tip of the lateral malleolus and includes the SPR. Zone B is the region of the lateral calcaneal trochlear process or peroneal tubercle. Both tendons are coursing towards separate

Fig. 4.10 Photograph of foot. Zone A indicates the tip of the fibula, including the superior peroneal retinaculum. Zone B includes the peroneal tubercle and the inferior peroneal retinaculum. Zone C Region of cuboid notch where peroneus longus travels plantar to eventually insert on the base of the first metatarsal

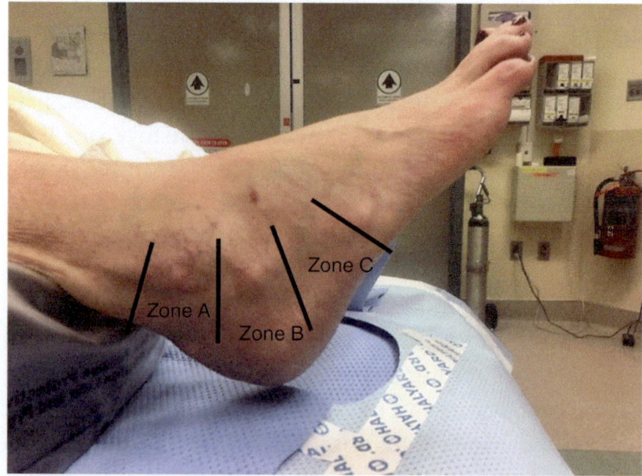

Fig. 4.11 Anatomic drawing of underlying structures present in the three zones of peroneal tendon pathology. Sobel, M. MIzel, M.S. Peroneal Tendon Injury. Chapter 2 In: Current Practice in Foot and Ankle Surgery Volume 1 Eds. Pfeffer, G.B. Frey, C.C. McGraw-Hill, Inc. Figure 2.1 page 32

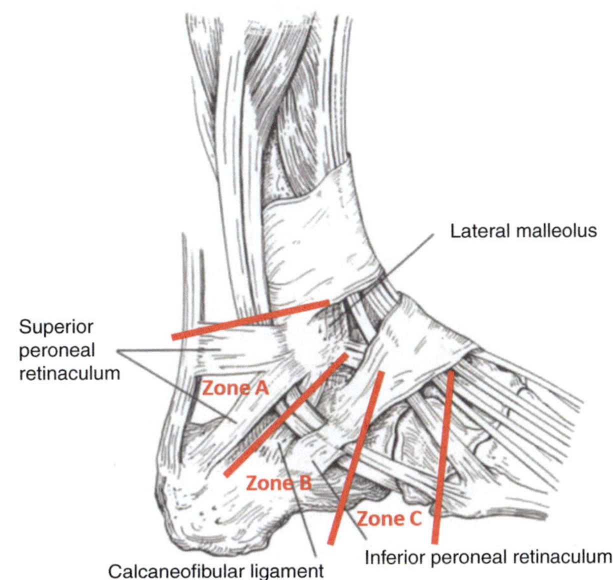

sheaths of the inferior peroneal retinaculum with the PL making a more acute turn around the tip of the fibula and correlates with Petersen's hypovascular region of the PB and PL [24]. Focal tenderness often correlates with an enlarged peroneal tubercle. A small metallic marker can be placed at the site of tenderness and readily obtainable lateral and axillary calcaneal radiographs can confirm an enlarged peroneal tubercle. Operative exploration will often reveal tendon swelling and an hourglass constriction proximal to the IPR indicates a stenosing tenosynovitis.

Distal to the PT, the brevis travels directly to its insertion at the base of the fifth metatarsal. This region is defined as Zone C. Tenderness here can indicate peroneal insertional tendonitis in the absence of a fracture easily excluded with routine radiographs. Pain in this region can indicate PL or PB pathology but the PB tenderness is slightly superior and extends to the base of the fifth metatarsal.

The PL encompasses the os peroneum (OP) which is always present [48] but not always calcified and therefore not always evident on routine oblique foot radiographs. The painful os peroneum syndrome (POPS) [22] has become a more commonly recognized explanation for pain between the PT and calcaneocuboid joint. Sometimes progressive elongation of a multipartite OP indicated on serial radiographs will confirm POPS. POPS is a popularized term that indicates an os peroneum fracture, diastasis or PL tendinosis, or rupture in zone C as subsequently described by Brandes and Smith [39]. POPS can present acutely with a complete PL rupture or diastasis of an os peroneum. More commonly, a chronic presentation is associated with attritional tears of the PL tendon, chronic diastasis, or nonhealing os peroneum fracture. Physical examination reveals pain with resisted plantarflexion of the first ray when the foot is placed in an inverted, supinated, and adducted position. Patients can also report a sensation of stepping on a pebble due to PL rupture or malalignment due to proximal migration of the os peroneum from its articulation with the cuboid facet.

These three zones are helpful in organizing peroneal tendon pathology by focal region of tenderness. Subluxation and dislocation of peroneal tendon tears occur with a positive peroneal compression test and demonstration of subluxation or dislocation in Zone A. PB tears are common in Zone A; PL tears are more commonly detected in Zone B and C. Stenosing tenosynovitis of both tendons occurs proximal to the PT in Zone B. An enlarged peroneal tubercle, particularly if tender, correlates with tears of both tendons and peroneal tenosynovitis. In Zone B, an enlarged PT can also envelope the PL causing tenosynovitis of the PL tendon [49]. Zone C is most frequently the region of PL pathology or POPS. Most peroneal tendon tears are tears in continuity with pain detected with palpation. Motor weakness is not always detectable though loss of eversion strength theoretically can reveal PB pathology and loss of plantar flexion strength of the first metatarsal indicating PL pathology. Though rare, a complete peroneal rupture of both tendons can occur with no demonstrable peroneal weakness, and most commonly occurs in Zone C, involving the PL tendon [39]. Pain rather than weakness will be usually detected with resistance testing, likely due to tears in continuity being far more frequent than complete ruptures.

Though most series report pathology of either the PL or PB, it appears most PB pathology occurs in zones A and B and is most frequently "tears in continuity." Complete rupture is rarer than tears in continuity and most frequently involves the PL in Zone C. Zone B has pathology of stenosing tenosynovitis, tears in continuity, and involves both PB and PL. Surgical case series and MRI findings indicate pathology is more common in the PB than the PL tendon [5]. Pain slightly dorsal to the peroneal tendons in Zone C, at the region of the cuboid tunnel, may also indicate a controversial condition termed "cuboid syndrome." This condition has been described more in the physical therapy, sports, and dance medical literature [50, 51]. It can be treated with manipulation and reduction maneuvers that have been reported to immediately relieve the symptoms. Some comprehensive foot and ankle textbooks do not include this diagnosis. Though the author is well aware of this condition, admittedly it (a patient with cuboid syndrome) may have seen the author yet escaped his diagnosis.

Tenderness at the sinus tarsi region slightly dorsal and distal to the peroneal tubercle can be due to sinus tarsi syndrome [52] and can be mistaken for peroneal tendon pathology. Spasm or rigidity of the peroneal tendons may be noted on physical exam by tight and tender peroneal tendons and a loss of heel inversion. The classic test for peroneal spastic flat foot is a quick inversion subtalar stress on the forefoot that can be performed after the peroneal compression test in a seated patient. Reflex beats of contraction, rigidity, or pain can indicate some form of subtalar pathology that could include tarsal coalition, subtalar instability, or sinus tarsi syndrome. Subtalar instability secondary to injury to the subtalar ligaments can be detected by stress views performed by a knowledgeable clinician, aware of these conditions.

Almost all primary care referrals in my practice have been for an "ankle sprain"; almost no one presented with a suspected diagnosis of subtalar instability, sinus tarsi syndrome, cuboid syndrome, or peroneal tendon injury. In these difficult cases, an MRI or high-resolution ultrasound can be a valuable adjunct to a competently performed and directed history and physical examination.

The responsibility of the clinician evaluating foot and ankle injury is to accurately diagnose conditions at the appropriate time in a cost-effective manner. Recognition of conditions that require urgent care should be addressed but not every complaint or injury require comprehensive radiographic, ultra sound or MRI study, nor does every condition require surgical treatment. Options for care and an appropriate list of conditions that could account for the symptoms (differential diagnosis) should be supplied to the patient to plot a course of expected clinical recovery. The most common complication of the treatment of peroneal tendon injuries is a failure to make the right diagnosis [53].

The treatment algorithms for peroneal tendonitis, tendinosis, tear, subluxation, dislocation, and rupture mandate an accurate diagnosis. The role of the foot and ankle specialist is to be aware of and to recognize potential pathologies when presented with a patient with these complaints so that an accurate diagnosis can be made. The clinician provides a diagnosis and outlines an appropriate course of treatment. The clinician also needs to recognize when certain suspected or diagnosed conditions require urgent and potential surgical intervention. The diagnosis of these conditions has been outlined. More detailed treatment algorithms are the subject of adjacent chapters.

References

1. Baumhauer JF, Nawoczenski DA, DiGiovanni BF, Flemister AS. Ankle pain and peroneal tendon pathology. Clin Sports Med. 2004;23:21–34.
2. Brodsky JW, Zide JR, Kane JM. Acute peroneal injury. Foot Ankle Clin. 2017;22:833–41.
3. Dombek MF, Lamm BM, Saltrick K, Mendicino RW, Catanzariti AR. Peroneal tendon tears: a retrospective review. J Foot Ankle Surg. 2003;42:250–8.
4. Heckman DS, Gluck GS, Parekh SG. Tendon disorders of the foot and ankle, part 1 peroneal tendon disorders. Am J Sports Med. 2009;37:614–25.
5. Roster B, Michelier P, Giza E. Peroneal tendon disorders. Clin Sports Med. 2015;34:625–41.
6. Sammarco GJ. Peroneal tendon injuries. Orthop Clin North Am. 1994;25:135–45.
7. Sammarco GJ, Mangone PG. Review article: diagnosis and treatment of peroneal tendon injuries. Foot Ankle Surg. 2000;6:197–205.
8. Slater HK. Acute peroneal tendon tears. Foot Ankle Clin. 2007;12:659–74.
9. Wukich DK, Tuason DA. Diagnosis and treatment of chronic ankle pain. Instr Course Lect. 2011;60:335–50.
10. Scanlan RL, Gehl RS. Peroneal tendon injuries. Clin Podiatr Med Surg. 2002;19:419–31.
11. Lau BC, Moore LK, Thuillier DU. Evaluation and management of lateral ankle pain following injury. JBJS Rev. 2018;6:1–10.
12. Selmani E, Gjata V, Gjika E. Current concepts review: peroneal tendon disorders. Foot Ankle Int. 2006;27:221–8.
13. Sharma P, Maffulli N. Current concepts review: tendon injury and tendinopathy: healing and repair. J Bone Joint Surg Am. 2005;87:187–202.

14. Johnson KA, Strom DE. Tibialis posterior tendon dysfunction. Clin Orthop Relat Res. 1989;239:196–206.
15. Myerson MS. Adult acquired flatfoot deformity: treatment of dysfunction of the posterior tibial tendon. J Bone Joint Surg Am. 1996;78:780–92.
16. Hamilton WG, Geppert MJ, Thompson FM. Pain in the posterior aspect of the ankle in dancers. Differential diagnosis and operative treatment. J Bone Joint Surg Am. 1996;78:1491–500.
17. Bizarro AH. On sesamoid and supernumerary bones of the limbs. J Anat. 1921;55:256–68.
18. Cerrato RA, Myerson MS. Peroneal tendon tears, surgical management and its complications. Foot Ankle Clin. 2009;14:299–312.
19. Sobel M, Levy ME, Bohne WH. Congenital variations of the peroneus quartus muscle: an anatomic study. Foot Ankle Int. 1990;11:81–9.
20. Hyer CF, Dawson JM, Philbin TM, Berlet GC, Lee TH. The peroneal tubercle: description, classification, and relevance to peroneus longus tendon pathology. Foot Ankle Int. 2005;26:947–50.
21. Bruce WD, Christoferson MR, Phillips DL. Stenosing tenosynovitis and impingement of the peroneal tendons associated with hypertrophy of the peroneal tubercle. Foot Ankle Int. 1999;20:464–7.
22. Sobel M, Pavlov H, Geppert MJ, Thompson FM, DiCarlo EF, Davis WH. Painful os peroneum syndrome: a spectrum of conditions responsible for plantar lateral foot pain. Foot Ankle Int. 1994;15:112–24.
23. Wang XT, Rosenberg ZS, Mechlin MB, Schweitzer ME. Normal variants and diseases of the peroneal tendons and superior peroneal retinaculum: MR imaging features. Radiographics. 2005;25:587–602.
24. Petersen W, Bobka T, Stein V, Tillmann B. Blood supply of the peroneal tendons: injection and immunohistochemical studies of cadaver tendons. Acta Orthop Scand. 2000;71:168–74.
25. Arbab D, Tingart M, Frank D, Abbara-Czardybon M, Waizy H, Wingenfeld C. Treatment of isolated peroneus longus tears and a review of the literature. Foot Ankle Spec. 2013;7:113–8.
26. Diaz GC, van Holsbeeck M, Jacobson JA. Longitudinal split of the peroneus longus and peroneus brevis tendons with disruption of the superior peroneal retinaculum. J Ultrasound Med. 1998;17:525–9.
27. Squires N, Myerson MS, Gamba C. Surgical treatment of peroneal tendon tears. Foot Ankle Clin. 2007;12:675–95.
28. Stockton KG, Brodsky JW. Peroneus longus tears associated with pathology of the os peroneum. Foot Ankle Int. 2014;35:346–52.
29. Wind WM, Rohrbacher BJ. Peroneus longus and brevis rupture in a collegiate athlete. Foot Ankle Int. 2001;22:140–3.
30. Plastaras CT, Rittenberg JD, Rittenberg KE, Press J, Akuthota V. Comprehensive functional evaluation of the injured runner. Phys Med Rehabil Clin N Am. 2005;16:623–49.
31. Macera CA. Lower extremity injuries in runners. Advances in prediction. Sports Med. 1992;13:50–7.
32. Saupe N, Mengiardi B, Pfirrmann CWA, Vienne P, Seifert B, Zanetti M. Anatomic variants associated with peroneal tendon disorders: MR imaging findings in volunteers with asymptomatic ankles. Radiology. 2007;242:509–17.
33. Galli MM, Protzman NM, Mandelker EM, Malhotra AD, Schwartz E, Brigido SA. An examination of anatomic variants and incidental peroneal tendon pathologic features: a comprehensive MRI review of asymptomatic lateral ankles. J Foot Ankle Surg. 2015;54:164–72.
34. Park HJ, Cha SD, Kim HS, Chung ST, Park NH, Yoo JH, et al. Reliability of MRI findings of peroneal tendinopathy in patients with lateral chronic ankle instability. Clin Orthop Surg. 2010;2:237–43.
35. Giza E, Mak W, Wong SE, Roper G, Campanelli V, Hunter JC. A clinical and radiological study of peroneal tendon pathology. Foot Ankle Spec. 2013;6:417–21.
36. Redfern D, Myerson M. The management of concomitant tears of the peroneus longus and brevis tendons. Foot Ankle Int. 2004;25:695–707.

37. Davis WH, Mann RA. Principle of the physical examination of the foot and ankle. In: Coughlin MJ, Mann RA, Saltzman CL, editors. Surgery of the foot and ankle. 8th ed. Philadelphia: Mosby; 2007. p. 45–70.
38. Manoli A II, Graham B. The subtle cavus foot, "the underpronator," a review. Foot Ankle Int. 2005;26:256–63.
39. Brandes CB, Smith RW. Characterization of patients with primary peroneus longus tendinopathy: a review of twenty-two cases. Foot Ankle Int. 2000;21:462–8.
40. Hodgkins CW, Kennedy JG, O'Loughlin PF. Tendon injuries in dance. Clin Sports Med. 2008;27:279–88.
41. Coleman SS, Chestnut WM. A simple test for hindfoot flexibility in the cavovarus foot. Clin Orthop Relat Res. 1977;123:60–2.
42. Yewlett A, Oakley J, Makwana N, Patel HJ. Retained blackthorn causing peroneal tendonitis: a case report. Foot Ankle Surg. 2009;15:205–6.
43. Sobel M, Geppert MJ, Olson EJ, Bohne WHO, Arnoczky SP. The dynamics of peroneus brevis tendon splits: a proposed mechanism, techniques of diagnosis, and classification of injury. Foot Ankle Int. 1992;13:413–22.
44. Geppert MJ, Sobel M, Bohne WHO. Lateral ankle instability as a cause of superior peroneal retinacular laxity: an anatomic and biomechanical study of cadaveric feet. Foot Ankle Int. 1993;14:330–4.
45. DiGiovanni BF, Fraga CJ, Cohen BE, Shereff MJ. Associated injuries found in chronic lateral ankle instability. Foot Ankle Int. 2000;21:809–15.
46. Raikin SM, Elias I, Nazarian LN. Intrasheath subluxation of the peroneal tendons. J Bone Joint Surg Am. 2008;90:992–9.
47. Vega J, Golano P, Batista JP, Malagelada F, Pellegrino A. Tendoscopic procedure associated with peroneal tendons. Tech Foot Ankle Surg. 2013;12:39–48.
48. Sarrafian SK. Osteology. In: Sarrafian SK, editor. Anatomy of the foot and ankle. Philadelphia: JB Lippincott; 1983. p. 35–106.
49. Pierson JL, Inglis AE. Stenosing tenosynovitis of the peroneus longus tendon associated with hypertrophy of the peroneal tubercle and an os peroneum. J Bone Joint Surg Am. 1992;74:440–2.
50. Jennings J, Davies GJ. Treatment of cuboid syndrome secondary to lateral ankle sprains: a case series. J Orthop Sports Phys Ther. 2005;35:409–15.
51. Marshall P, Hamilton WJ. Cuboid subluxation in ballet dancers. Am J Sports Med. 1992;20:169–75.
52. Frey C, Feder KS, DiGiovanni C. Arthroscopic evaluation of the subtalar joint: does sinus tarsi syndrome exist? Foot Ankle Int. 1999;20:185–91.
53. Molloy R, Tisdel C. Failed treatment of peroneal tendon injuries. Foot Ankle Clin. 2003;8:115–29.

High-Resolution Ultrasound and MRI Imaging of Peroneal Tendon Injuries

L. Daniel Latt, Gokhan Kuyumcu, and Mihra S. Taljanovic

Introduction

Common disorders of the peroneal tendons include peroneal tendonitis, peroneal tendon tears, and peroneal subluxation or dislocation. While the presence of a peroneal tendon disorder is often suspected from the history and physical examination, advanced imaging is usually required to arrive at a precise diagnosis. Both MRI and US have been used in the evaluation of peroneal tendon disorders. There are advantages and disadvantages to each, although neither has demonstrated clear superiority. Ultrasound (US), with its dynamic imaging capabilities, is the study of choice in the evaluation of peroneal tendon instability, particularly transient intrasheath subluxation. Whereas, MRI is the better imaging modality to diagnose bone marrow edema like changes, as these cannot be detected on ultrasound.

A number of studies have evaluated the sensitivity and specificity of MRI in detecting tears of the peroneus brevis and longus tendons by comparison with intraoperative findings (Table 5.1). The majority of these have found MRI to be highly specific, but to lack some sensitivity in diagnosis of peroneal tendon tears. In contrast, studies comparing US to intraoperative findings have concluded that US is 100% sensitive, and more than 80% specific.

Our study of 21 patients with retromalleolar pain comparing US to MRI to intraoperative findings found that MRI identified 13/13 peroneus brevis tears, whereas

L. D. Latt (✉)
Department of Orthopaedic Surgery, University of Arizona College of Medicine, Tucson, AZ, USA
e-mail: dlatt@ortho.arizona.edu

G. Kuyumcu · M. S. Taljanovic
Department of Medical Imaging, University of Arizona College of Medicine, Tucson, AZ, USA
e-mail: mihrat@radiology.arizona.edu

© Springer Nature Switzerland AG 2020
M. Sobel (ed.), *The Peroneal Tendons*,
https://doi.org/10.1007/978-3-030-46646-6_5

Table 5.1 Results of studies comparing MRI and US to intraoperative findings

Modality	Study	Comparison	Peroneal tendon tear (sens/spec)	PB tear (sens/spec)	PL tear (sens/spec)
MRI	Lamm et al. [1]	Intraop. finding		83%/75%	50%/99%
	Khoury et al. [2]	Intraop. finding	91%/50%[a]		
	Park et al. [3]	Intraop. finding		44%/99%	50%/96%
US	Waitches et al. [4]	Intraop. finding (PL/ PB/PT/ FDL)	100%/88%		
	Grant et al. [5]	Intraop. finding (PL/ PB)	100%/85%		

[a]Values calculated from data presented in paper

Table 5.2 Results of unpublished study comparing MRI and US to intraoperative findings of peroneal tendinopathy, PB tear, PL tear, and subluxation in 21 patients with retromalleolar pain

	Tendinopathy	PB tear	PL tear	Subluxation
Intraoperative examination	18	16	4	3
MRI	18	16	4	1
US	18	14	4	3

US only found 11/13 (90% sensitivity); however, US detected 3/3 subluxating tendons whereas MRI only detected 1/3 (Table 5.2). In other words, MRI and US were both highly accurate in the detection of tears, but US was far more sensitive in detection of subluxation – a finding that was not discussed elsewhere in the literature.

To summarize, in the evaluation of peroneal tendon disorders, MRI has the advantage of supplying information about a wide array of related conditions that cause chronic lateral ankle pain including chronic ankle instability, osteochondral lesion of the talus (OLT), syndesmotic, and lateral ankle ligament injuries [6]. Moreover, MR images can be used by the orthopedic surgeon for operative planning. In comparison, US has the advantages of the following: (1) being a less expensive, shorter examination, (2) being capable of interactive dynamic examination which can be guided by the patient's symptoms such as the location of pain, or during provocative maneuvers, (3) allows for easy comparison with the contralateral side [7, 8], and (4) is more sensitive for detecting peroneal instability.

Imaging Techniques

Radiographs

The evaluation of all patients with chronic ankle pain should include weight-bearing three-view radiographs of the ankle (anteroposterior, lateral, and mortice). In the setting of retromalleolar pain, these radiographs are particularly useful for the following: (1) evaluating hindfoot alignment, (2) detecting avulsion fractures (Fig. 5.1), and (3) detecting a fracture of the os peroneum. Weight-bearing three views of foot

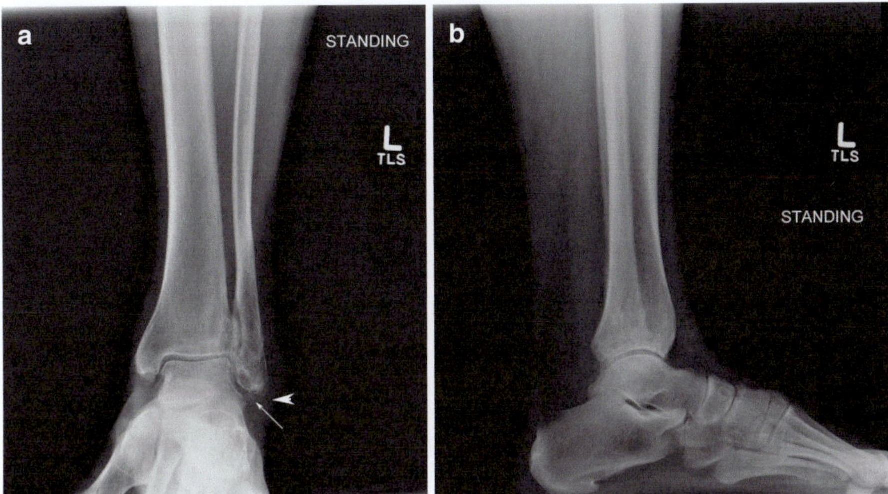

Fig. 5.1 Mortise (**a**) and lateral (**b**) standing radiographs of the left ankle. Mortise view shows soft tissue swelling overlying the lateral ankle (arrowhead) and small avulsion bone fragment (thin arrow) related to calcaneofibular ligament avulsion fracture

(anteroposterior, lateral, and oblique) should be obtained when varus or valgus hindfoot malalignment is suspected on clinical exam. Cavovarus malalignment (Fig. 5.2) causes lateral foot overload, is associated with peroneal tendon tears, and leads to protracted healing of lateral ankle ligaments and tendons. Cavovarus alignment is present in over 80% of patients undergoing surgery for peroneus longus tendon tears [9]. Similarly, planovalgus malalignment can cause narrowing of the inframalleolar space (subfibular impingement) leading to peroneal tendonitis and tendon tears. The standard weight-bearing radiographic views are usually sufficient, though a hindfoot alignment view [10] or long calcaneal alignment view may be useful to quantify the hindfoot varus.

MRI

Technique

MRI evaluation of the peroneal tendons is usually performed using a routine ankle protocol on a 1.5 T or 3.0 T machine [11, 12]. The ankle is placed in neutral inversion/eversion and approximately 20° of plantarflexion within a dedicated extremity coil (Fig. 5.3). The slight plantarflexion helps to separate the peroneal tendons within the common tendon sheath. Imaging sequences typically include both T1-weighted (anatomy) and T2-weighted or PD-weighted with fat saturation or STIR (fluid sensitive) in all three anatomic planes (axial, coronal, and sagittal relative to the distal tibia). The T1-weighted sequences are performed without fat saturation. A 3 mm slice thickness is used for all sequences except for sagittal STIR (4 mm slice thickness/0.5 mm gap). An additional three-dimensional gradient echo

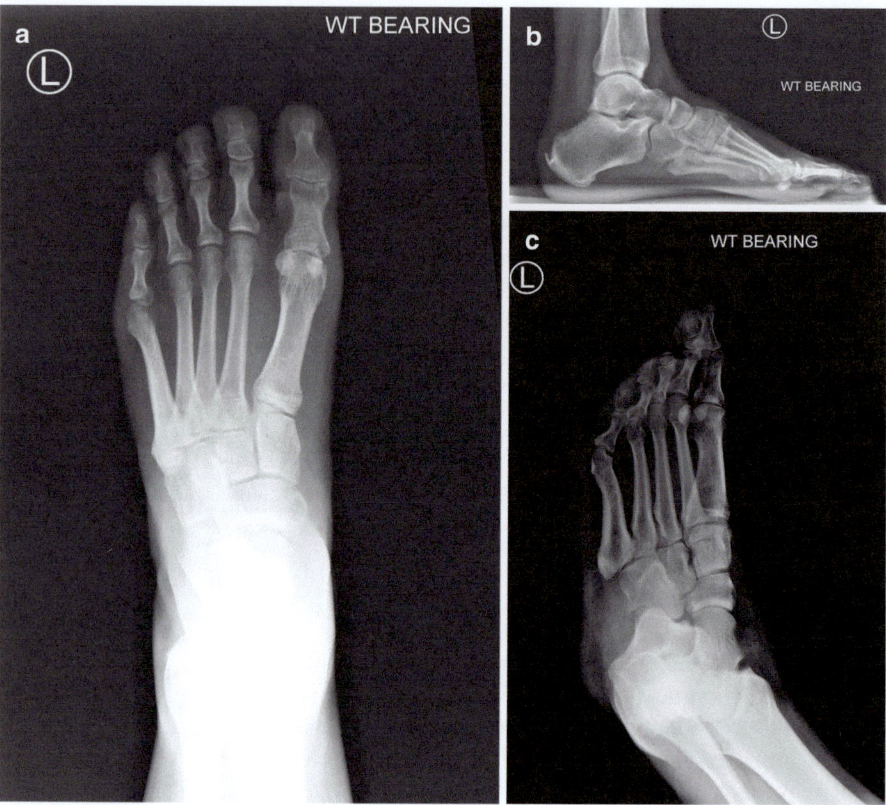

Fig. 5.2 Anteroposterior (**a**), lateral (**b**) and oblique (**c**) standing views of the left foot show cavovarus alignment of the left foot as evidenced by increased calcaneal pitch, sinus tarsi drive through sign, positive Meary's angle, and absent base of first and fifth metatarsal overlap on the lateral view as well as increase in parallelism between the talus and calcaneus and stacking of the tarsal bones on the anteroposterior view

sequence with submillimeter slice thickness (in our institution 0.7 mm) is often used to image the tibiotalar cartilage. Injuries to the peroneal tendons are usually well seen on the T1-weighted and fluid-sensitive sequences in three planes. However, injury to the distal portion of the PL on the plantar surface of the foot is sometimes better evaluated on additional sequences parallel and perpendicular to the long axis of the metatarsals.

Normal Findings and Pitfalls

Normal tendons have low signal intensity (black) on all MRI sequences (Fig. 5.4). Increased signal on all sequences indicates tendon disease that can be either tendinosis or tear. Fluid-sensitive sequences can help to identify the particular derangement. Signal heterogeneity and tendon thickening is typically associated with tendinosis while focal defects with associated increased signal are consistent with partial thickness tendon tears. Moreover, a collection of fluid around the tendon but within the sheath is characteristic of tenosynovitis. Signal heterogeneity and tendon

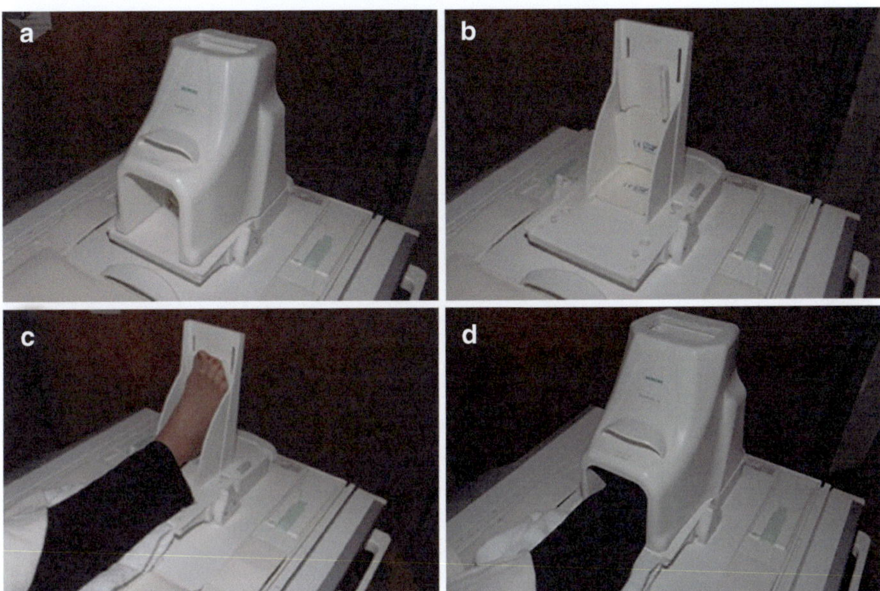

Fig. 5.3 Dedicated ankle extremity coil. The outer shell (**a**) and foot support (**b**) of a transmit–receive multichannel extremity coil for MRI. Ankle MRI is performed with the patient in the supine position and the ankle joint in the neutral position, with approximately 20° of plantar flexion (**c**). In the axial plane, the use of 20° of plantar flexion helps to separate the peroneal tendons in the common peroneal sheath. (**d**) The fully assembled ankle coil with patient in position

thickening is typically associated with tendinosis while focal defects with associated increased signal are consistent with partial thickness tendon tears. However, increased signal intensity can also be due to the magic angle effect whereby a structure oriented at 55° relative to the magnetic field has increased signal on T1-weighted (ET < 38 ms) sequences [13]. Plantarflexion of the ankle to 20° helps to minimize this effect. Furthermore, all findings made on T1-weighted sequences should be checked against the corresponding images on fluid-sensitive sequences to avoid misdiagnosis.

The configuration and shape of the tendons are also useful in determining the specific derangement. Within the retromalleolar groove, the normal PB has an oval, flat, or mildly crescentic appearance (fettuccini shaped) on axial sequences, whereas the PL has a more globular or circular cross-section (spaghetti shaped) [6, 12]. The slightly flattened cross-section of the PB should not be mistaken for a tear.

Ultrasound

Technique

In contrast to MRI in which routine imaging protocols are sufficient for the evaluation of the peroneal tendons, a specific protocol is required for the dynamic ultrasound evaluation of the peroneal tendons. The author's preferred technique is to use

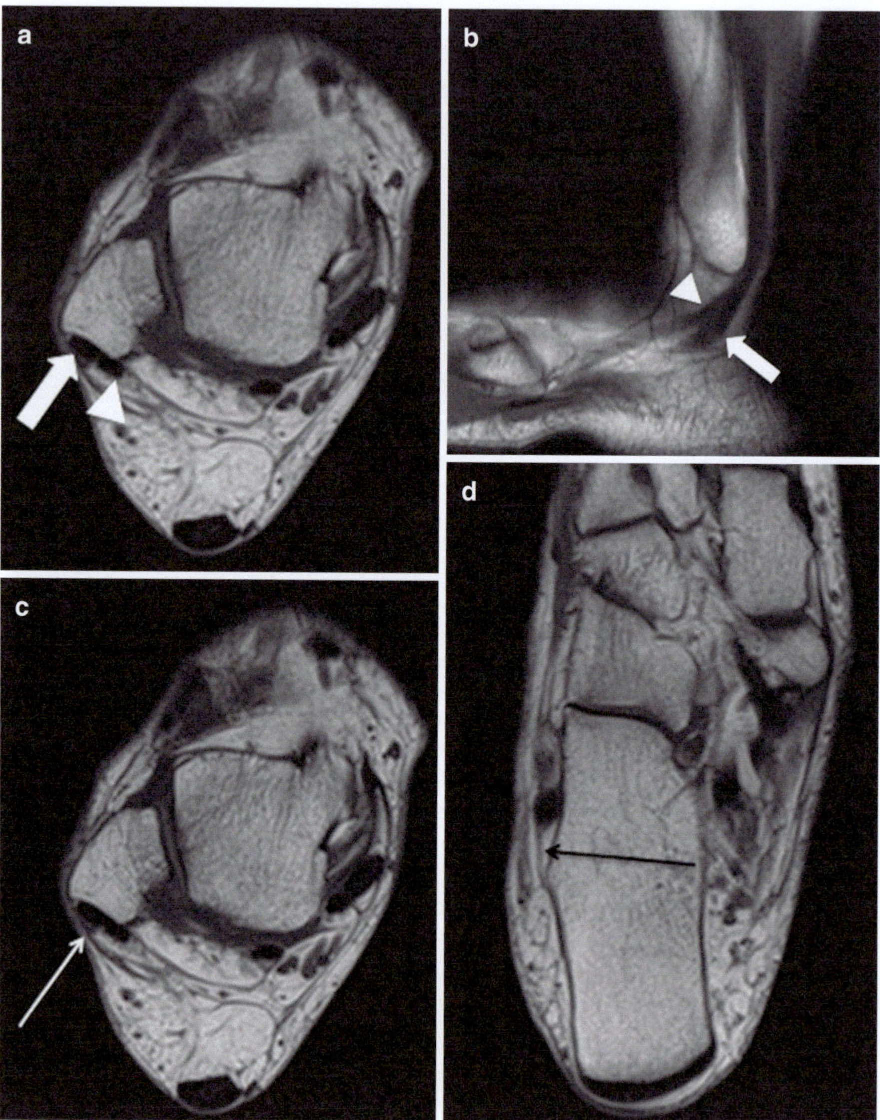

Fig. 5.4 Normal peroneal tendons, superior peroneal retinaculum (SPR) and inferior peroneal retinaculum (IPR): (**a**) Axial T1-weighted MR image shows the normal anatomy and positioning of the peroneal tendons. Peroneus longus (PL) tendon (white thick arrow) is situated anterior to the peroneus brevis (PB) tendon (white arrowhead) in the retromalleolar groove. The PB tendon is mildly flattened and crescentic and PL tendon is rounded. (**b**) T1-weighted sagittal MR image shows course of the PB tendon (white arrowhead) and attachment to the fifth metatarsal base. PL tendon course is also seen (white thick arrow). Note the homogenous hypointense signal through-out the PB and PL tendon course. (**c**) Axial T1-weighted MR image shows SPR (white thin arrow) overlying the peroneal tendons in the retromalleolar groove. (**d**) IPR (black thin arrow) is shown overlying both peroneal tendons at the hindfoot. (**e**) Axial T1-weighted MR image shows a normal concave retromalleolar groove (black arrow). (**f**) A shallow convex retromalleolar contour (white arrow) which is associated with an increased risk of peroneal tendon instability

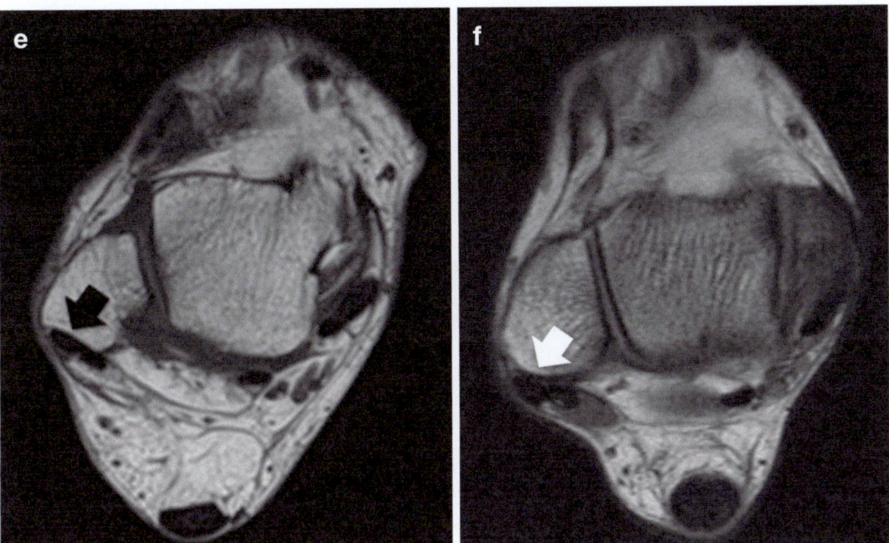

Fig. 5.4 (continued)

a high-resolution 8–18 MHz linear "hockey stick" probe with a small footprint. The patient is positioned in the supine position with the knee flexed approximately 45°–90° and the hip internally rotated to expose the lateral side of the ankle and foot. A large amount of gel is used especially around the curved surface of the lateral malleolus to avoid unnecessary pressure with the transducer which could displace the tendons. Imaging of the supramalleolar, retromalleolar, and inframalleolar portions of the PL and PB including the distal portion of their muscle bellies is performed in both the transverse (short-axis) and longitudinal (long-axis) planes. The examination begins proximally and proceeds distally. The tendons are imaged together until they take separate sheaths at the IPR, after which they are examined separately. The tendon sheaths are also examined for thickening, increased synovial fluid complexes, and hypervascularity using power Doppler or color Doppler imaging. The SPR is examined by orienting the transducer obliquely along its course. Dynamic examination of the SPR is performed to look for transient subluxation or dislocation of the peroneal tendons from within the sheath or intrasheath subluxation by having the patient perform resisted maximal dorsiflexion and eversion while the probe is oriented along the short axis of the tendons. The plantar portion of the PL is then imaged with the patient is prone position with the ankle plantar flexed to expose the plantar surface of the foot. The tendon is identified at its attachment at the base of the first metatarsal and followed on long and short axis views laterally and proximally until it reaches the cuboid tunnel.

Normal Findings and Pitfalls

The normal peroneal tendons appear hyperechoic and fibrillated on US [6, 7] (Fig. 5.5). They may appear hypoechoic due to anisotropy if the ultrasound transducer is not perpendicular to the examined tendon. This occurs commonly in the

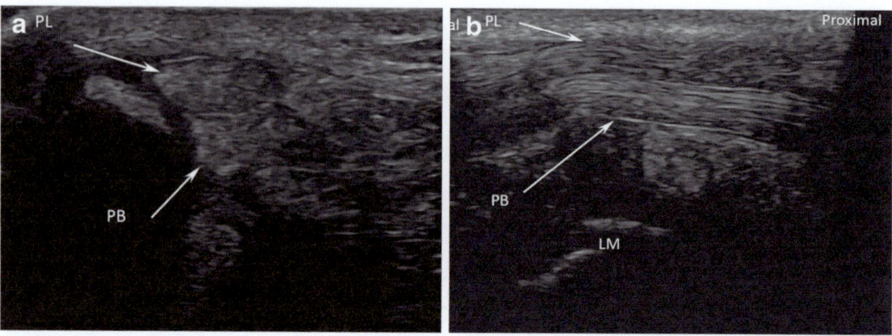

Fig. 5.5 US of normal peroneal tendons. Short-axis (**a**) and Long-axis (**b**) US images at the fibular retromalleolar groove show normal fibrillar texture and echogenicity of the PB and PL tendons

inframalleolar region where the probe must be tilted at the correct angle to follow each of the tendons [8]. The peroneal tendon sheaths are not normally seen on US unless they are distended by the presence of excess synovial fluid or synovial hypertrophy. The anterior portion of the SPR can be seen as a thin hyperechoic or hypoechoic band inserting onto the fibrocartilaginous ridge, whereas its posterior portion is difficult to visualize [7, 14]. The peroneal tubercle is seen protruding from the lateral aspect of the calcaneus with the overlying IPR which is often difficult to visualize. The os peroneum (when present) can be seen as a hyperechoic structure within the PL.

Functional Imaging

Shear wave elastography [15] is a recently developed technique which quantifies soft tissue stiffness (elasticity) in vivo and may eventually play a role in determining the prognosis for tendon and ligament disorders and thereby play a role in treatment decision making [16].

A shear wave is a secondary acoustic wave that is emitted by the linear US array prior to the imaging wave and is oriented perpendicular to the principal wave. The speed of propagation of the shear wave through the tissue is recorded. The shear modulus of the tissue can then be calculated from the shear velocity ($G = \mathrm{rho} \times c^2$) if the tissue density is known [15].

Shear wave imaging is now FDA-approved on most state-of-the-art US scanners (including those offered by Philips, GE Healthcare, Siemens Healthineers, Ultrasonix, and Supersonic Imagine) for diagnostic imaging of the musculoskeletal system. Despite its use in research studies of a number of musculoskeletal tissues, including Achilles tendon, patellar tendon, and supraspinatus tendon, it has not gained wide clinical acceptance for musculoskeletal examination, as normative values and its role have not been defined. SWE of the chronically injured peroneal tendons might help determine which tendons are capable of healing and which require repair, tenodesis, or allograft reconstruction.

Peroneal Tendinosis, Tendonitis, and Tenosynovitis

Peroneal tendonitis (tenosynovitis) occurs commonly as a result of inversion ankle injuries and is often concurrent with ankle sprains, osteochondral lesions of the talus and other hindfoot derangements [17]. The tendon is injured by the forceful reflexive activation of the peroneal muscles to prevent the complete inversion of the foot. Tenosynovitis can also result from repetitive stress, rheumatologic diseases, or infection [6, 7, 12]. Patients often present with swelling and tenderness along the tendon sheath. On MRI, the tendons appear thickened with increased or heterogenous intensity signal (Fig. 5.6). The normal tendon sheath contains a small amount

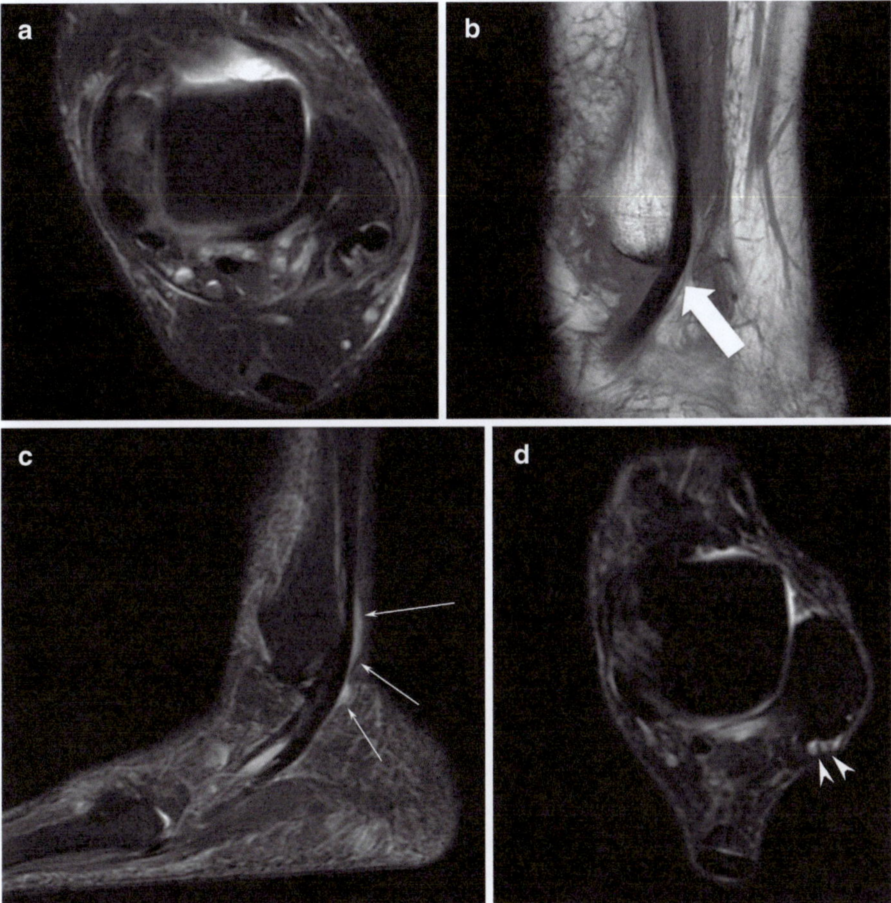

Fig. 5.6 Marked tendinosis of PB tendon without tear. (**a**) axial T2 Sagittal T1-weighted and (**b**) sagittal T1-axial T2-weighted fat-saturated MR images show marked thickening of the PB tendon (block arrow) without any tear or cleft consistent with tendinosis. Stenosing Tenosynovitis. (**c**) Sagittal STIR and (**d**) axial T2-weightedfat-saturated MR images show irregular distended peroneal tendon sheath with increased heterogeneous synovial fluid complex (thin arrows). In (**d**), note multiple linear low-signal-intensity bands (arrowheads) consistent with stenosing tenosynovitis

of tenosynovial fluid, up to 3 mm is considered normal [6, 18–20]. Edema may extend into the peritendious structures. The inflamed tenosynovium is best seen on fat-saturated contrast-enhanced T1 images. On US examination, the inflamed and thickened tendon, synovium, and peritendinous structures appear hypoechoic, whereas the synovial fluid appears anechoic. Power or color Doppler imaging can be used to show the increased vascularity of the inflamed synovium consistent with hyperemia.

In contrast, peroneal tendinosis is a noninflammatory degenerative process. It occurs in a number of settings that either decreases the space available for the peroneal tendons or chronically overloads the tendons. On MRI, the tendon appears thickened with increased signal intensity within the tendon substance on both T1 and T2 weighted sequences [6, 12, 18, 21, 22], whereas on US, the tendon appears hypoechoic and thickened, with no discrete tear [6] (Fig. 5.7). A decrease in the volume of the inframalleolar space can occur from subfibular impingement as in seen in patients with severe long-standing flatfoot when the lateral wall of the calcaneus comes to impinge on the distal fibula reducing the inframalleolar space available for the peroneal tendons. A relative decrease in the inframalleolar or retromalleolar space can be caused by a low-lying PB muscle belly or a peroneus quartus. Malunited calcaneus fracture also causes peroneal tendinosis as the blown out lateral wall decreases the retromalleolar and inframalleolar space. Chronic overload of the peroneal tendons can be caused by lateral ankle ligament instability, as the peroneal tendons must then assume the full role of stabilizing the ankle against inversion forces. This problem is commonly seen after an ankle sprain in patients with cavovarus alignment where the varus of the hindfoot puts all of the lateral ankle structures under constant load, including the peroneal tendons.

Stenosing tenosynovitis is a chronic condition which results from friction between the peroneal tendons and a narrowed inferior osseofibrous tunnel due to a hypertrophied peroneal tubercle and/or a thickened IPR [23, 24]. Long-standing compression of the tendons in the tunnel leads to tenosynovial fibrosis and synovial

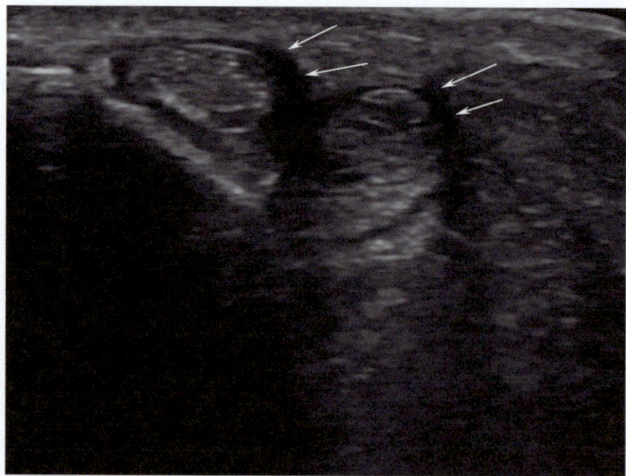

Fig. 5.7 Tendinosis and Tenosynovitis of PB and PL tendons. Short axis gray scale US image shows thickened heterogeneous peroneal tendons (thin white arrows) with increased surrounding hypoechoic synovial fluid complex in distended tendon sheath consistent with tendinosis and tenosynovitis

proliferation that limits tendon excursion. On MRI, the tendon fibrosis is seen as linear areas of intermediate or low signal intensity on all routine noncontrast sequences within the synovial fluid and tendon sheath which may contrast enhance. The absence of synovial fluid can be seen on the fluid-sensitive sequences [6, 12].

Peroneal Tendon Tears

Peroneal tendon tears should be suspected in any patient presenting with chronic lateral ankle pain located posterior or inferior to the tip of the lateral malleolus. They can occur as the result of either acute trauma (e.g., ankle sprain) or chronic degeneration. Tears are common (found in 11% of cadaveric specimens [25]), but fortunately, most are asymptomatic, thus they only require imaging investigation when symptoms persist after the acute injury has subsided. Tears usually occur as part of a complex injury (found in 30% of patients undergoing ankle instability surgery [26]) or in a malaligned hindfoot (cavovarus foot or planovalgus foot with subfibular impingement.

Peroneus brevis tears occur most commonly in the retromalleolar region where the PB is subjected to compression between the PL and the retromalleolar groove. There are a number of factors that predispose to tearing of the PB including the following: (1) shallow, convex, or irregular retromalleolar groove, (2) crowding due to low-lying PB muscle belly or (3) a peroneus quartus, and (4) subluxation or dislocation due to SPR tear [27]. In partial thickness tears, the PB is boomerang-shaped and envelops the PL, and this corresponds to the central thinning that occurs with tendon degeneration (Fig. 5.8). On MRI, the affected portion of the tendon has irregular intermediate signal intensity or hyperintensity. There is a corresponding hypoechoic internal echotexture with loss of normal fibrillation on US examination. Partial thickness longitudinal split tears are often associated with tendon thickening or thinning. In a thickened tendon, it is difficult to differentiate tendinopathy from partial thickness tear, whereas tendon thinning is almost always associated with partial thickness tearing [6, 7, 12].

Partial thickness longitudinal split tears usually involve the posterior portion of the PB. The fissuring of the tendon can progress anteriorly leading to a complete longitudinal split tear with the PL lying between two PB hemitendons (Fig. 5.9) [6, 7, 27]. The split tears always start in the retromalleolar region but may extend distally into the inframalleolar region where the tendon reconstitutes. On MRI, complete longitudinal split tears have a high or intermediate signal with discontinuity of the fibers [6, 12]. The hemitendons associated with these tears often have irregular borders. These tears are usually best visualized on axial and coronal MR images. On US, complete split tears appear hypoechoic or anechoic, with fluid at the tear site and discontinuity of the fibers. These tears can usually be seen on both short and long axis images at rest. Dynamic US examination in in ankle plantarflexion and subtalar eversion can help to bring out occult tears. Longitudinal split tears of the PB most often occur in conjunction with other lateral ankle soft tissue disorders including ATFL rupture (50%) and SPR tear. Complete tears (rupture) of the PB are

                                                                L. D. Latt et al.

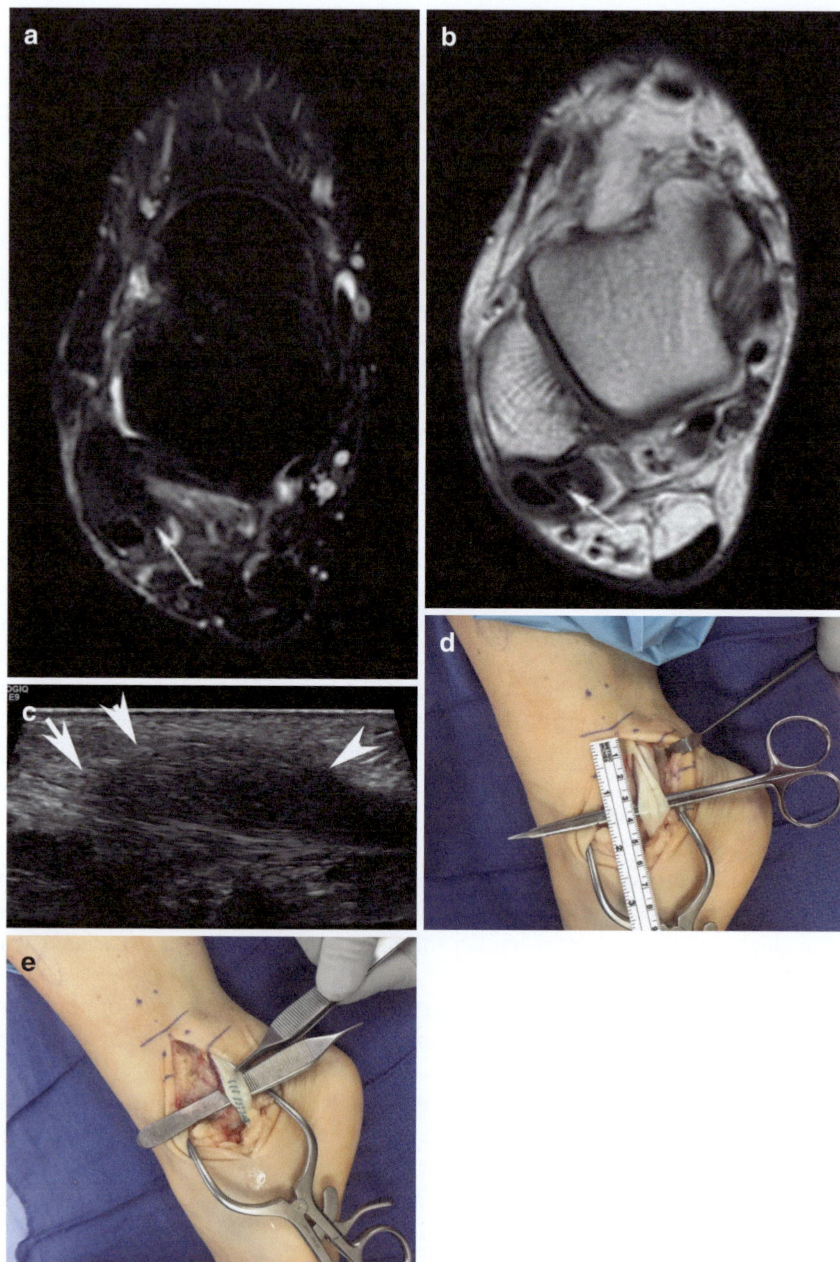

Fig. 5.8 Partial-thickness longitudinal PB tendon tear. (**a**) Axial fat-saturated T2-weighted and (**b**) axial T1-weighted MR images show an irregularity at the posterior aspect of the PB tendon with an associated intermediate- to high-signal-intensity cleft (arrow), consistent with a partial-thickness tear. (**c**) Long- axis US image shows irregularity and thickening of the PB tendon with partial loss of the normal fibrillar echotexture (arrowheads), consistent with a partial-thickness tear. (**d**) intraoperative photograph demonstrating the partial thickness tear and (**e**) following debridement of the tear and suture repair

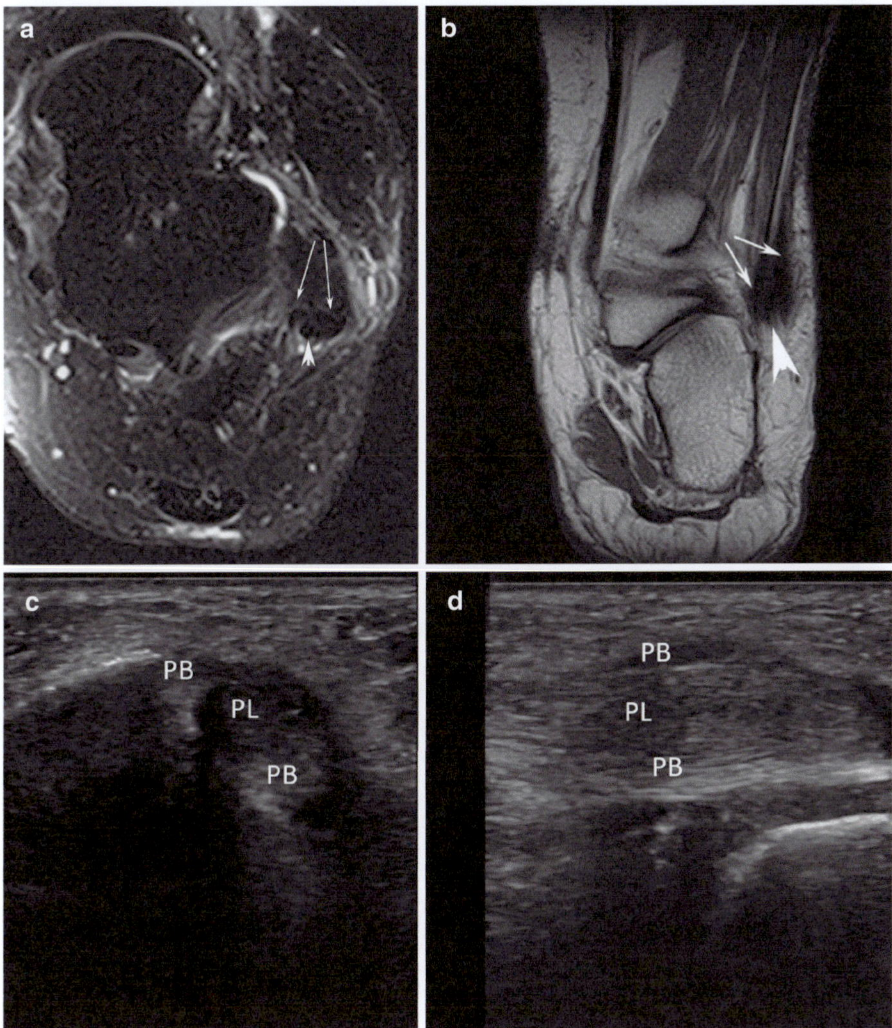

Fig. 5.9 Longitudinal split tear of PB tendon. (**a**) Axial fat-saturated T2-weighted and (**b**) coronal T1-weighted MR images show longitudinal split tear of the PB tendon at the level of retromalleolar groove with PL tendon (arrowhead) between two hemitendons of the PB (thin arrows). (**c**) Short axis and long axis (**d**) US images of the peroneal tendons at the retromalleolar groove show longitudinal split tear of the PB tendon with peroneus longus tendon between two PB hemitendons. Note heterogeneity and decreased echogenicity of the PB hemitendons and of the PL tendon consistent with pre-existing tendinosis. (**e**) Intraoperative photograph confirmed longitudinal split tear of the PB tendon

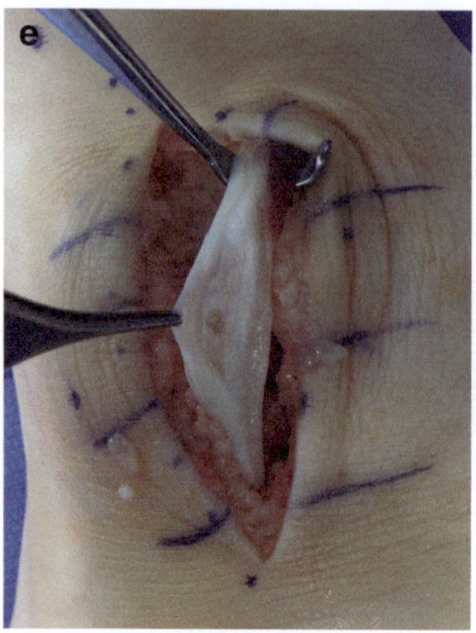

Fig. 5.9 (continued)

fortunately rare. Full-width tears or tendon ruptures show complete discontinuity of tendon fibers with variable amount of retraction (Fig. 5.10).

Peroneus longus tears are far less common than PB tears. Acute tears are more often caused by direct trauma or sporting injury. Chronic tears are commonly associated with cavovarus foot alignment [9] and hypertrophy of the peroneal tubercle [12]. PL tears can assume the same configurations as PB tears with partial and full-thickness longitudinal split tears and tendon ruptures. Longitudinal split tears commonly occur in the inframalleolar portion of the tendon in association with a hypertrophic peroneal tubercle, whereas acute tears most often occur at the cuboid tunnel where the tendon makes a 90-degree turn from the lateral to the plantar surface of the foot [9]. PL tears are often accompanied by tendinosis and tenosynovitis [20]. Other findings may include bone marrow edema in the hypertrophied peroneal tubercle and erosive changes in the cuboid [28].

Peroneal Instability

The superior peroneal retinaculum (SPR) stabilizes the peroneal tendons within the retromalleolar peroneal groove. Injury to the SPR, the fibrocartilaginous ridge (FCR) or the attachment on the SPR on the posterior fibula can lead to peroneal tendon instability (subluxation or dislocation). The initial injury often occurs with a sudden contraction of the peroneal muscles in an attempt to resist ankle inversion either during sporting activities [29, 30] or in patients with chronic ankle instability. Peroneal tendon subluxation and dislocation are common disorders with an estimated prevalence of 0.3–0.5% [31]. Factors which reduce the volume of the retromalleolar space (including low-lying PB muscle belly, peroneus quartus, and shallow retromalleolar groove), congenital absence of SPR, and ligamentous laxity all create a predisposition to peroneal instability [12]. SPR tears are classified according to their location of the tear [30]: Grade I tears (51% of cases) involve

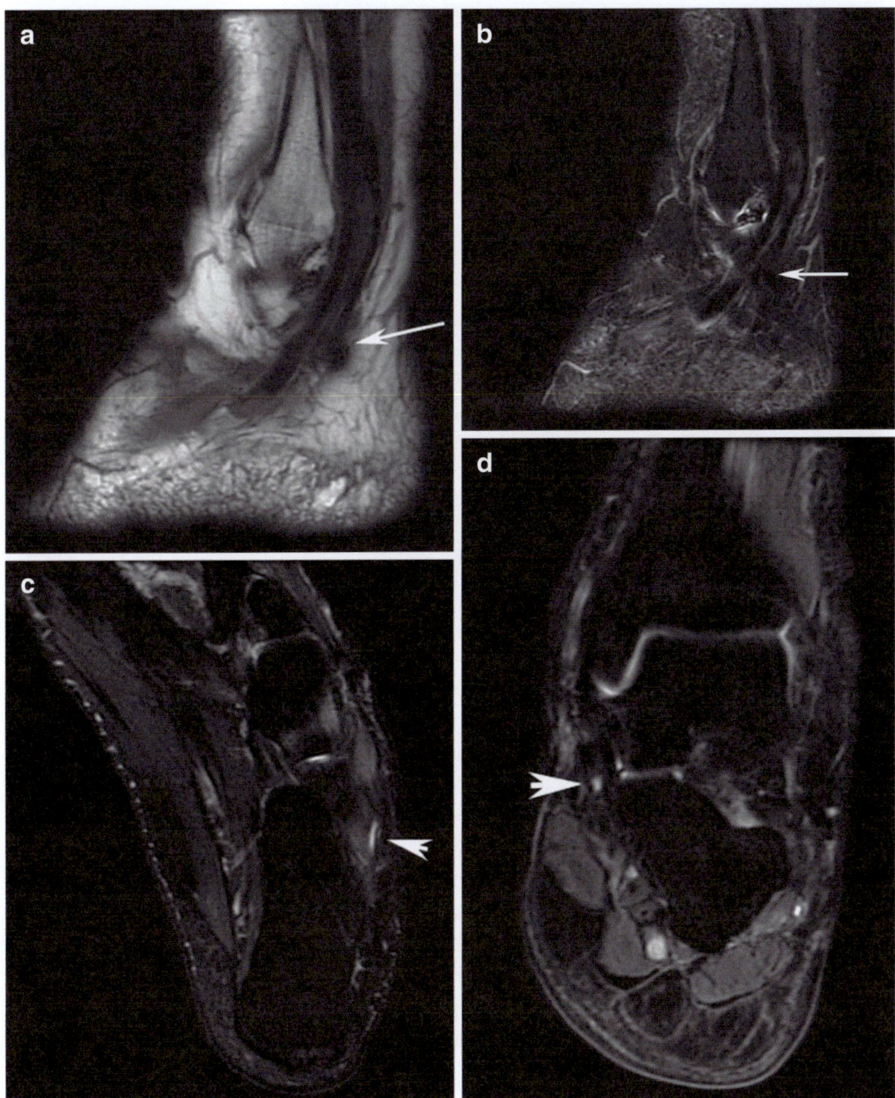

Fig. 5.10 Complete PB tendon tear with retraction. (**a**) Sagittal T1-weighted and (**b**) STIRMR images show thickening of the PB tendon. (**c**) Axial T2-weighted fat saturated and (**d**) coronal PD-weighted fat-saturated MR images show retraction of the ruptured PB tendon with fluid cleft and absence of the tendon below the lateral malleolus (arrowheads). (**e**) Intraoperative photograph confirms intact PL and completely torn PB tendons

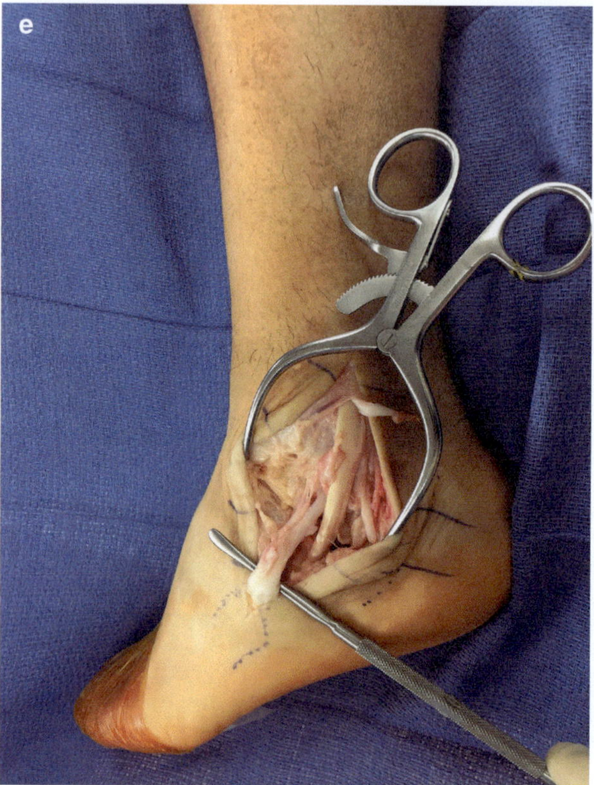

Fig. 5.10 (continued)

stripping of the SPR from the fibula, in grade II tears (33% of cases), the FCR is elevated along with the SPR, and in grade III injuries (13% of cases), a thin fragment of bone is avulsed along with the soft tissues [32]. A grade IV injury is one in which the SPR is torn from its posterior attachment allowing the tendons to lay outside the retinaculum [30].

The ability of imaging to detect peroneal tendon instability depends on the pattern of injury. Peroneal subluxation and dislocation are not seen on plain radiographs, but can sometimes be inferred from the presence of avulsion fragment(s) at the posterior fibula which correspond to an avulsion fracture of the fibular cortex adjacent to the peroneal groove, the so-called "fleck" sign in a type III SPR tear (Fig. 5.2).

On axial MRI, the normal SPR appears as a thin low signal intensity band on all sequences. The adjacent FCR appears as a meniscus like triangular structure that is also low in signal [14]. Whereas, the injured SPR appears thickened with high signal intensity in the surrounding soft tissues on all sequences. Bone marrow edema may be present as high signal intensity seen on the fluid sensitive sequences. Peroneal subluxation or dislocation can be seen on MRI when the displacement is present at rest (Fig. 5.11). MRI is highly sensitive for fixed subluxation or dislocation of the peroneal tendons, but may miss transient subluxation and dislocation that occur only with loading and dorsiflexion of the ankle.

On US, the normal SPR appears as a thin linear hypoechoic or hyperechoic band adjacent to the peroneal tendons [7]. In contrast, the injured SPR appears thickened, irregular, and hypoechoic, and often, increased vascularity can be seen on power or color Doppler evaluation.

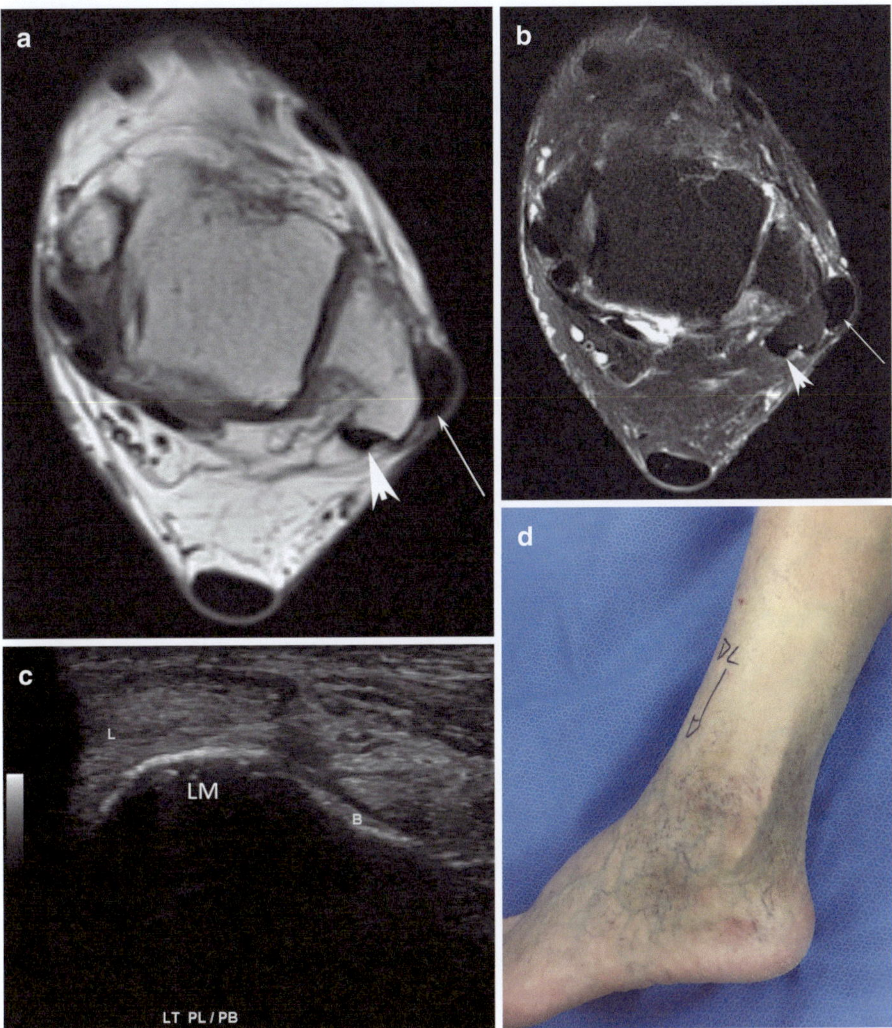

Fig. 5.11 Peroneal tendon subluxation, (**a**) axial T1-weighted and (**b**) T2-weighted fat saturated MR images show anterior dislocation of PL (long thin arrow) tendon, PB tendon (arrowhead) is seen in retromalleolar groove. Short axis US image shows PL tendon is anteriorly dislocated from the retromalleolar groove. Clinical images showing (**d**) anteriorly dislocated and (**e**) reduced peroneal tendons. (**f**) Intraoperative image showing dislocated peroneal tendons – note the synovialized lateral surface of the distal fibula resulting from the chronic subluxation

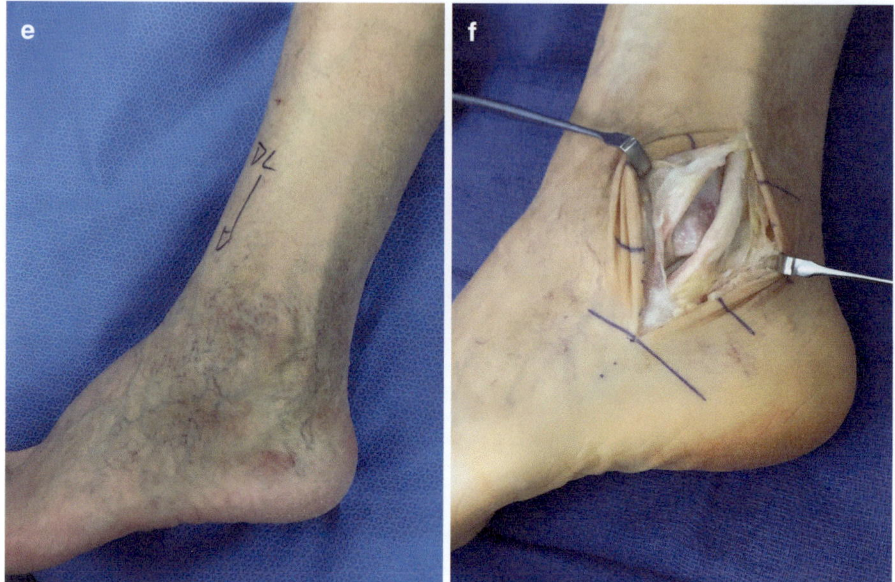

Fig. 5.11 (continued)

Ultrasound has the advantage of being able to be performed as a dynamic examination where the examiner can elicit symptoms or perform provocative maneuvers. In the case of peroneal subluxation or dislocation, this involves observing the position of the peroneal tendons in the fibular groove with transverse plane US during resisted dorsiflexion and eversion of the ankle [33–35] (Fig. 5.11).

Intrasheath subluxation of the peroneal tendons occurs when the SPR is intact, but the peroneal tunnel is enlarged, allowing the tendons to reverse their position behind the fibula during eversion and dorsiflexion of the hindfoot [35]. Patients who present with painful clicking but without apparent dislocation or subluxation should be evaluated with dynamic ultrasound, which demonstrates the reversal of the tendon positions.

Anatomic Variants

Os Peroneum

The os peroneum is a sesamoid bone which lies within the peroneus longus tendon at the cuboid groove. It can be either cartilaginous or ossified, ossified os peronei are found in 30% of feet [36]. It functions to enhance the moment arm of the peroneus longus [6, 7, 12]. On US it appears as a hyperechoic shadow within the PL. On MRI, an ossified os has the signal characteristics of normal bone marrow. Painful os peroneum syndrome (POPS) can occur with fracture of the os, diastasis of a multipartite os, PL tendinosis, tenosynovitis, or tendon tear (Fig. 5.12) [12, 37, 38]. The os peroneum

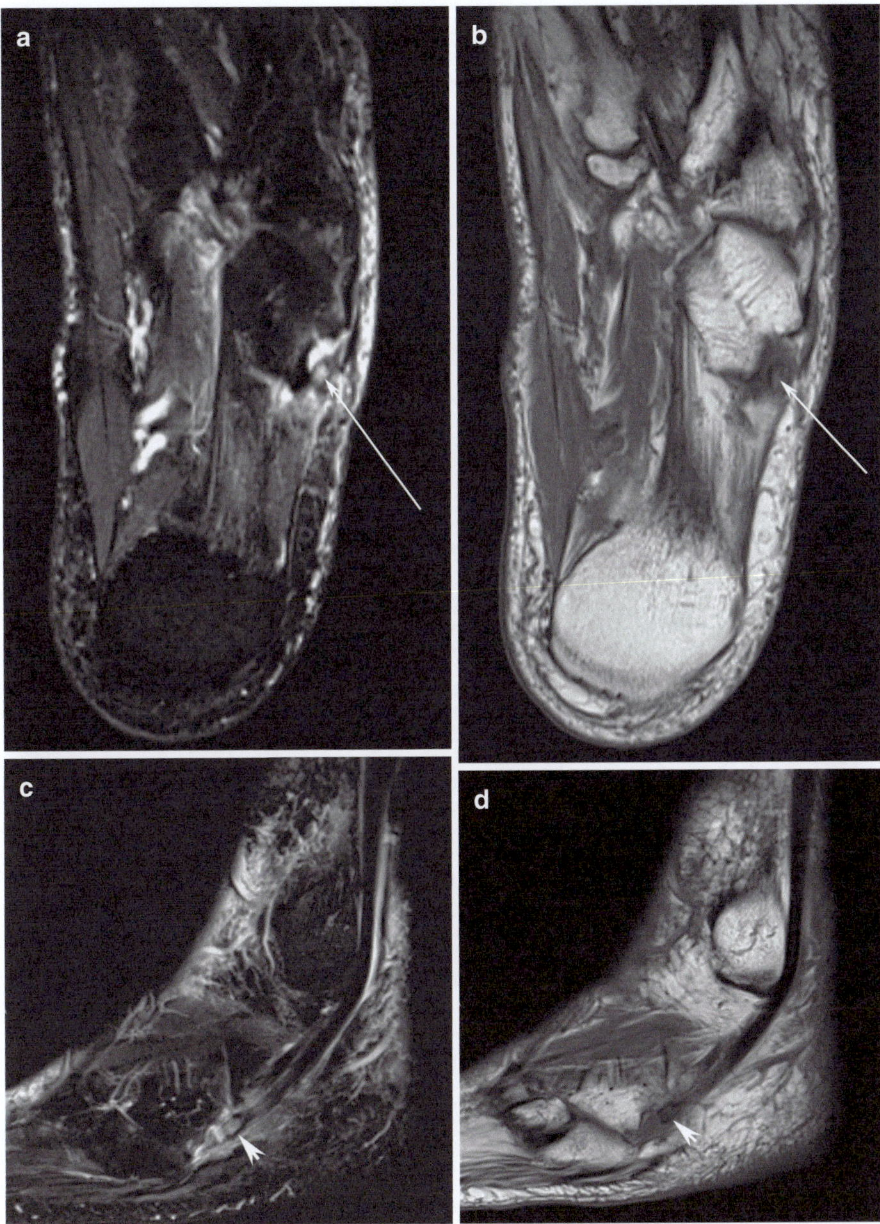

Fig. 5.12 Os peroneum syndrome secondary to bipartite os peroneum. Axial (**a**) T2-weighted fat saturated, (**b**) axial T1-weighted and sagittal (**c**) STIR and (**d**) T1-weighted MR images show bone marrow edema of the bipartite os peroneum consistent with clinical painful os peroneum syndrome (POPS)

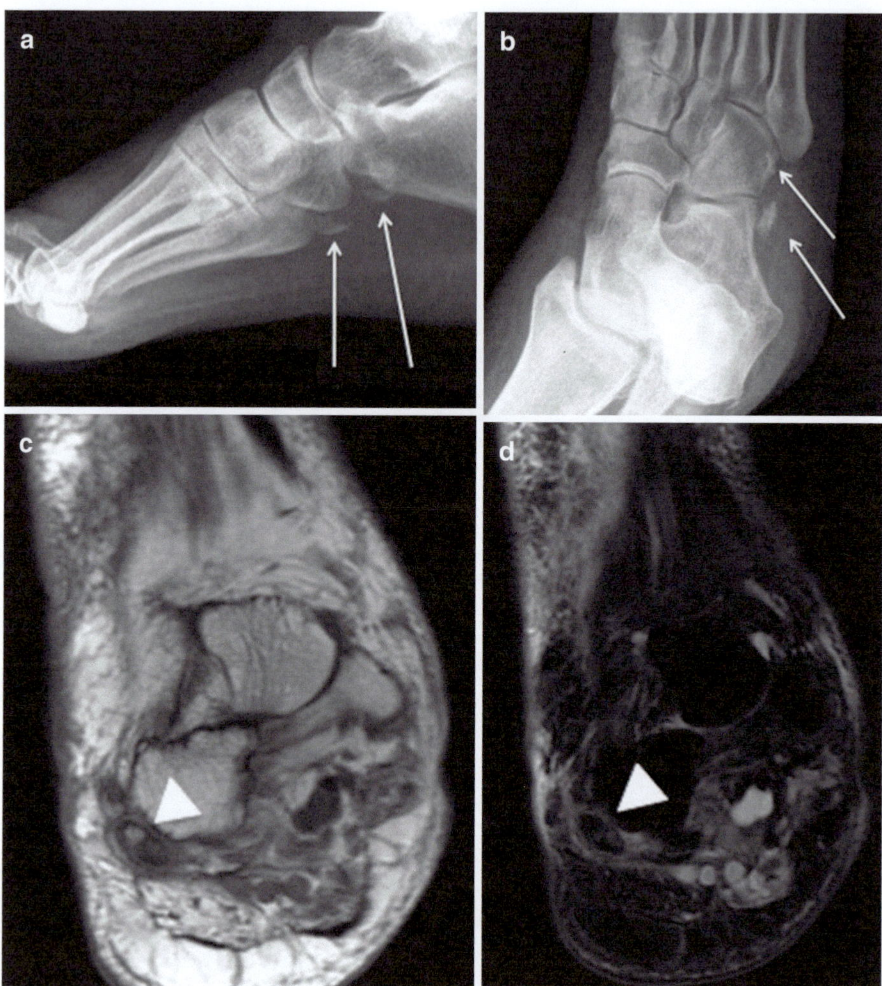

Fig. 5.13 Os peroneum fracture. (**a**) Lateral and (**b**) oblique radiographs show a fractured os peroneum (arrows) with a more than 6-mm distraction of the fracture fragments about the calcaneocuboid joint, a finding indicative of a PL tendon tear. (**c**) Coronal T1-weighted and (**d**) PD-weighted fat saturated MR images show fractured os peroneum (arrowhead) with associated PL tendon rupture

can be displaced in peroneus longus tears (displaced distally in proximal tears, and displaced proximally in distal tears). The displaced os peroneum in PL tendon tear or the displaced fragments in os peroneum fracture can be seen on XR (Fig. 5.13a and b).

Peroneus Quartus

The peroneus quartus is an accessory muscle that is present in 12–22% of individuals [39, 40]. It normally originates from the peroneus brevis. It most commonly inserts into a hypertrophied peroneal tubercle on the calcaneus, though it can also insert on other locations on the calcaneus, the PL, the PB, or the fifth metatarsal. It does not have a defined function. It occupies space within the peroneal groove and its presence is associated with a doubling of the risk of peroneal tendonitis and peroneal tendon tears [25]. On MRI, the peroneus quartus muscle shows intermediate signal intensity and its tendon shows low signal intensity on all sequences. On US, the peroneus quartus muscle belly appears hypoechoic with respect to its hyperechoic tendon [41] (Fig. 5.14).

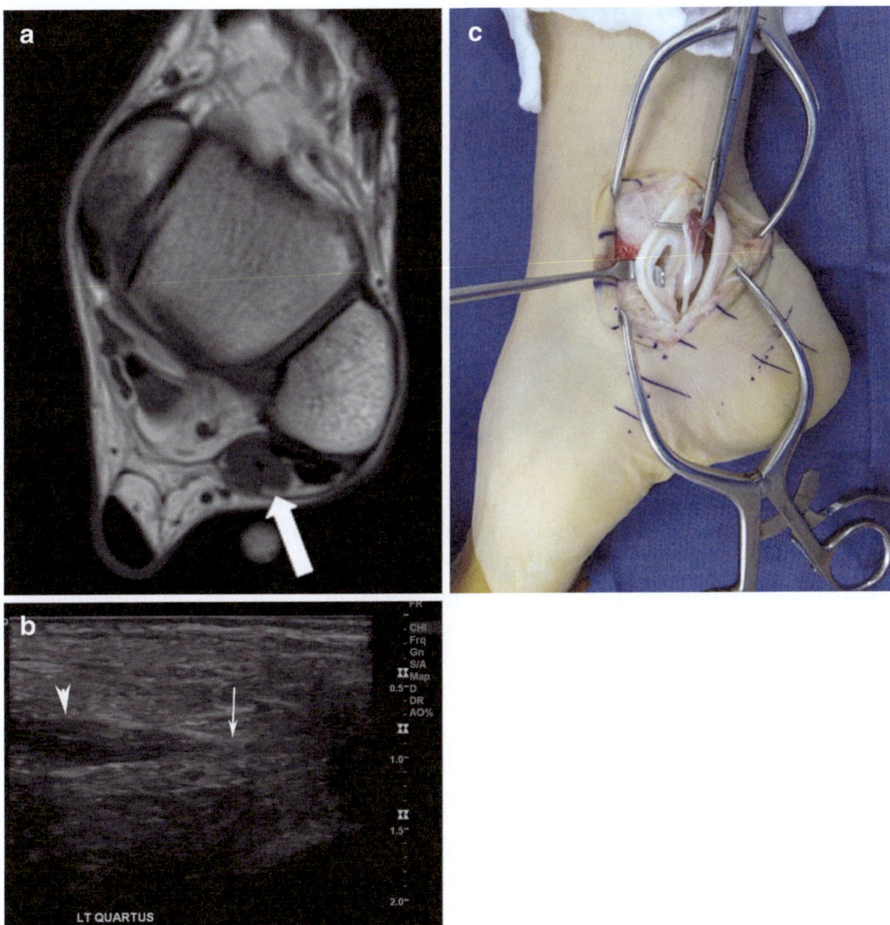

Fig. 5.14 Peroneus quartus muscle. (**a**) Axial T1-weighted MR image shows a small peroneus quartus muscle (white block arrow) posterior to PL and PB tendons causing crowding in the retromalleolar groove. (**b**) Long axis US image at the lateral malleolus shows a hypoechoic peroneus quartus muscle (arrowhead) with hyperechoic tendon (arrows) coursing distally. (**c**) Intraoperative image showing peroneus quartus muscle and tendon lying posterior to longitudinally split PB tendon

Low-Lying Peroneus Brevis Muscle Belly

The muscle belly of the peroneus brevis extends more distally than that of the peroneus longus. The distance between the PB muscle belly and the tip of the fibula is highly variable and depends on the angle of ankle flexion at the time of measurement. There is a lack of consensus as to how far distal the muscle belly normally extends. A number of studies have found the distal extent of the muscle belly occurring somewhere between 27 mm proximal to and 13 mm distal to the tip of the fibula with a median of 0 mm in normal individuals [19]. Thus, it is generally accepted that a muscle belly that extends more than 15 mm below the tip of the fibula is considered "low lying" [19]. The low-lying PB muscle belly can cause congestion within the peroneal groove and is associated with peroneal tendonitis and peroneal tendon tears [37, 42, 43] (Fig. 5.15).

A retrospective review of patients surgically treated for peroneal tendon symptoms found a lower lying muscle belly in patients with surgically confirmed tears (30.3 ± 9 mm above the tip) compared to those without tears(38.4 ± 8 mm above) and those without peroneal tendon symptoms(46.3 ± 11 mm) [44].

Hypertrophic Protuberances of the Lateral Calcaneus

The retrotrochlear eminence is a bony prominence located posterior to the peroneal tendons and is present in 98% of calcanei [12]. Hypertrophy is associated with the presence of a PQ. The peroneal tubercle is a bony prominence, which serves as the attachment site for the IPR and functions to provide a fulcrum for the PL as its course diverges from that of the PB. It is present in 90% of calcanei [45]. It is considered to be enlarged when it projects more than 5 mm past the lateral wall of the calcaneus (Fig. 5.16). A little over one-quarter of peroneal tubercles are enlarged with a concave shape [45]. The hypertrophied peroneal tubercle can irritate the PL or its sheath leading to tenosynovitis, partial or complete tendon tear, or bursitis [12, 23, 45].

Peroneal Groove Shape

The retromalleolar peroneal groove is variable in shape. The shape of the groove is best assessed on axial MR images taken 1 cm proximal to the level of the plafond. The groove is determined to have a concave shape when the posterior fibular surface has an anteriorly directed depression, a flat shape when there is no depression, and a convex shape when the central portion of the posterior cortex bulges posteriorly [46]. A concave fibular groove is found in 68% of cadaveric fibulae and a flat or convex groove in 32% [47]. The flat and convex groove are thought to be associated with an increased risk of peroneal tendon instability. However, the association of fibular groove shape with risk of dislocation has recently become the subject of

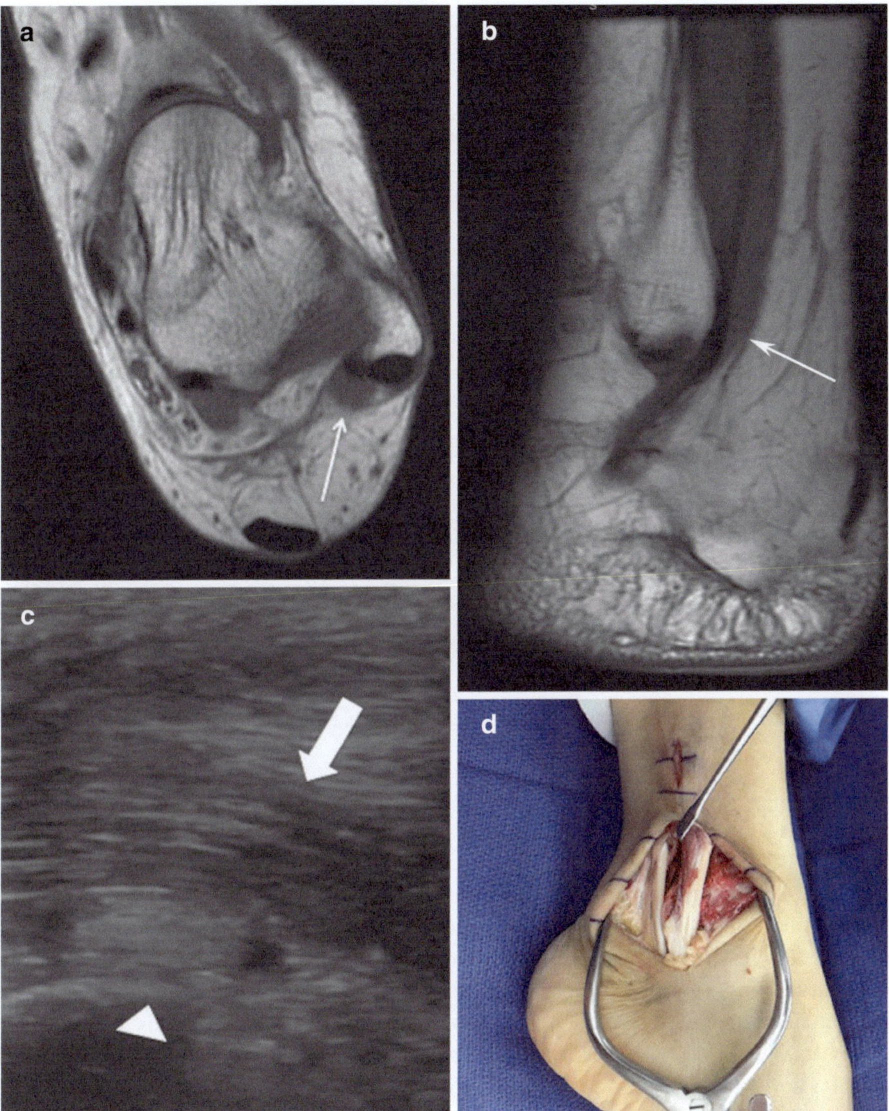

Fig. 5.15 Low-lying PB muscle belly. (**a**) Axial and (**b**) sagittal T1-weighted MR images show low-lying PB muscle belly (white thin arrows) extending below the lateral malleolus. (**c**) Long axis US image shows low-lying PB muscle belly (block arrow) extending below the lateral malleolus (white arrowhead). (**d**) Intraoperative image showing low-lying PB muscle belly

controversy, as recent studies have found no differences in morphology between patients with and without instability instead focusing on the fibrocartilaginous ridge as the primary stabilizer of the tendons [48].

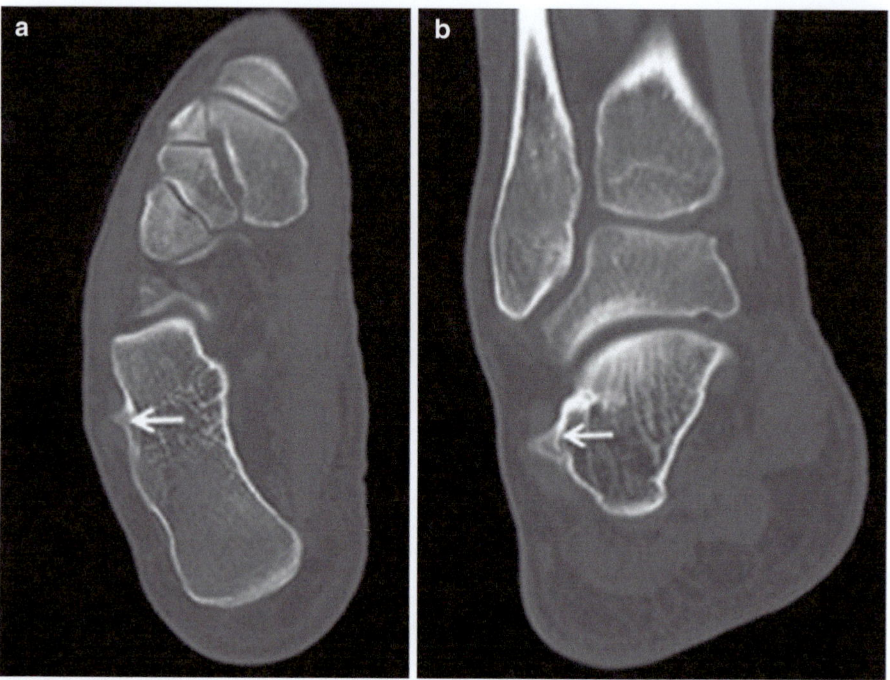

Fig. 5.16 (**a**) Axial and (**b**) coronal reformatted CT images show enlarged peroneal tubercle (arrow)

Summary

Imaging of patients with suspected peroneal tendon disorders should include weight-bearing radiographs of the ankle and foot, as they are useful for the detection of avulsion fractures, the presence of an os peroneum, and for the evaluation of cavovarus alignment. Advance imaging in the form of MRI or ultrasound imaging is often needed to differentiate between peroneal tendonitis (tendinosis and/or tenosynovitis), tears, and subluxation. MRI has the advantages of supplying information about a wide array of related and concomitant conditions and being useful for preoperative planning. In contrast, US is a less time-consuming and a less costly examination, which provides equivalent diagnostic accuracy for tears and is superior in the detection of tendon subluxation. Both modalities are capable of providing information about the presence the anatomic variants, including low-lying peroneus brevis muscle belly, os peroneum, peroneus quartus, and hypertrophied peroneal tubercle.

References

1. Lamm BM, Myers DT, Dombek M, Mendicino RW, Catanzariti AR, Saltrick K. Magnetic resonance imaging and surgical correlation of peroneus brevis tears. J Foot Ankle Surg. 2004;43(1):30–6. https://doi.org/10.1053/j.jfas.2003.11.002.
2. Khoury NJ, el-Khoury GY, Saltzman CL, Kathol MH. Peroneus longus and brevis tendon tears: MR imaging evaluation. Radiology. 1996;200(3):833–41.
3. Park HJ, Lee SY, Park NH, Rho MH, Chung EC, Kwag HJ. Accuracy of MR findings in characterizing peroneal tendons disorders in comparison with surgery. Acta Radiol. 2012;53(7):795–801. https://doi.org/10.1258/ar.2012.120184.
4. Waitches GM, Rockett M, Brage M, Sudakoff G. Ultrasonographic-surgical correlation of ankle tendon tears. J Ultrasound Med. 1998;17(4):249–56.
5. Grant TH, Kelikian AS, Jereb SE, McCarthy RJ. Ultrasound diagnosis of peroneal tendon tears. A surgical correlation. J Bone Joint Surg Am. 2005;87(8):1788–94. https://doi.org/10.2106/JBJS.D.02450.
6. Lee SJ, Jacobson JA, Kim SM, et al. Ultrasound and MRI of the peroneal tendons and associated pathology. Skelet Radiol. 2013;42(9):1191–200. https://doi.org/10.1007/s00256-013-1631-6.
7. Bianchi S, Delmi M, Molini L. Ultrasound of peroneal tendons. Semin Musculoskelet Radiol. 2010;14(3):292–306. https://doi.org/10.1055/s-0030-1254519.
8. Klauser AS, Peetrons P. Developments in musculoskeletal ultrasound and clinical applications. Skelet Radiol. 2010;39(11):1061–71. https://doi.org/10.1007/s00256-009-0782-y.
9. Brandes CB, Smith RW. Characterization of patients with primary peroneus longus tendinopathy: a review of twenty-two cases. Foot Ankle Int. 2000;21(6):462–8. https://doi.org/10.1177/107110070002100602.
10. Saltzman CL, el-Khoury GY. The hindfoot alignment view. [see comment]. Foot Ankle Int. 1995;16(9):572–6.
11. Schubert R. MRI of peroneal tendinopathies resulting from trauma or overuse. Br J Radiol. 2013;86(1021):20110750. https://doi.org/10.1259/bjr.20110750.
12. Wang XT, Rosenberg ZS, Mechlin MB, Schweitzer ME. Normal variants and diseases of the peroneal tendons and superior peroneal retinaculum: MR imaging features. Radiographics. 2005;25(3):587–602. https://doi.org/10.1148/rg.253045123.
13. Mengiardi B, Pfirrmann CW, Schottle PB, et al. Magic angle effect in MR imaging of ankle tendons: influence of foot positioning on prevalence and site in asymptomatic subjects and cadaveric tendons. Eur Radiol. 2006;16(10):2197–206. https://doi.org/10.1007/s00330-006-0164-y.
14. Demondion X, Canella C, Moraux A, Cohen M, Bry R, Cotten A. Retinacular disorders of the ankle and foot. Semin Musculoskelet Radiol. 2010;14(3):281–91. https://doi.org/10.1055/s-0030-1254518.
15. Taljanovic MS, Gimber LH, Becker GW, et al. Shear-wave elastography: basic physics and musculoskeletal applications. Radiographics. 2017;37(3):855–70. https://doi.org/10.1148/rg.2017160116.
16. Taljanovic MS, Melville DM, Klauser AS, et al. Advances in lower extremity ultrasound. Curr Radiol Rep. 2015;3(6):1–12.
17. DiGiovanni BF, Fraga CJ, Cohen BE, Shereff MJ. Associated injuries found in chronic lateral ankle instability. Foot Ankle Int. 2000;21(10):809–15.
18. Kijowski R, De Smet A, Mukharjee R. Magnetic resonance imaging findings in patients with peroneal tendinopathy and peroneal tenosynovitis. Skelet Radiol. 2007;36(2):105–14. https://doi.org/10.1007/s00256-006-0172-7.
19. Saupe N, Mengiardi B, Pfirrmann CW, Vienne P, Seifert B, Zanetti M. Anatomic variants associated with peroneal tendon disorders: MR imaging findings in volunteers with asymptomatic ankles. Radiology. 2007;242(2):509–17. https://doi.org/10.1148/radiol.2422051993.
20. Wang CC, Wang SJ, Lien SB, Lin LC. A new peroneal tendon rerouting method to treat recurrent dislocation of peroneal tendons. Am J Sports Med. 2009;37(3):552–7. https://doi.org/10.1177/0363546508325924.

21. Bencardino JT, Rosenberg ZS, Serrano LF. MR imaging features of diseases of the peroneal tendons. Magn Reson Imaging Clin N Am. 2001;9(3):493–505, x.
22. Mota J, Rosenberg ZS. Magnetic resonance imaging of the peroneal tendons. Top Magn Reson Imaging. 1998;9(5):273–85.
23. Bruce WD, Christofersen MR, Phillips DL. Stenosing tenosynovitis and impingement of the peroneal tendons associated with hypertrophy of the peroneal tubercle. Foot Ankle Int. 1999;20(7):464–7. https://doi.org/10.1177/107110079902000713.
24. Taki K, Yamazaki S, Majima T, Ohura H, Minami A. Bilateral stenosing tenosynovitis of the peroneus longus tendon associated with hypertrophied peroneal tubercle in a junior soccer player: a case report. Foot Ankle Int. 2007;28(1):129–32. https://doi.org/10.3113/FAI.2007.0022.
25. Sobel M, Bohne WH, Levy ME. Longitudinal attrition of the peroneus brevis tendon in the fibular groove: an anatomic study. Foot Ankle. 1990;11(3):124–8.
26. Squires N, Myerson MS, Gamba C. Surgical treatment of peroneal tendon tears. Foot Ankle Clin. 2007;12(4):675–95, vii. https://doi.org/10.1016/j.fcl.2007.08.002.
27. Sobel M, Geppert MJ, Olson EJ, Bohne WH, Arnoczky SP. The dynamics of peroneus brevis tendon splits: a proposed mechanism, technique of diagnosis, and classification of injury. Foot Ankle. 1992;13(7):413–22.
28. O'Donnell P, Saifuddin A. Cuboid oedema due to peroneus longus tendinopathy: a report of four cases. Skelet Radiol. 2005;34(7):381–8. https://doi.org/10.1007/s00256-005-0907-x.
29. Butler BW, Lanthier J, Wertheimer SJ. Subluxing peroneals: a review of the literature and case report. J Foot Ankle Surg. 1993;32(2):134–9.
30. Oden RR. Tendon injuries about the ankle resulting from skiing. Clin Orthop Relat Res. 1987;216:63–9.
31. Magnano GM, Occhi M, Di Stadio M, Toma P, Derchi LE. High-resolution US of non-traumatic recurrent dislocation of the peroneal tendons: a case report. Pediatr Radiol. 1998;28(6):476–7. https://doi.org/10.1007/s002470050388.
32. Eckert WR, Davis EA Jr. Acute rupture of the peroneal retinaculum. J Bone Joint Surg Am. 1976;58(5):670–2.
33. Neustadter J, Raikin SM, Nazarian LN. Dynamic sonographic evaluation of peroneal tendon subluxation. AJR Am J Roentgenol. 2004;183(4):985–8. https://doi.org/10.2214/ajr.183.4.1830985.
34. Raikin SM. Intrasheath subluxation of the peroneal tendons. Surgical technique. J Bone Joint Surg Am. 2009;91(Suppl 2 Pt 1):146–55. https://doi.org/10.2106/jbjs.h.01356.
35. Raikin SM, Elias I, Nazarian LN. Intrasheath subluxation of the peroneal tendons. J Bone Joint Surg Am. 2008;90(5):992–9. https://doi.org/10.2106/jbjs.g.00801.
36. Muehleman C, Williams J, Bareither ML. A radiologic and histologic study of the os peroneum: prevalence, morphology, and relationship to degenerative joint disease of the foot and ankle in a cadaveric sample. Clin Anat. 2009;22(6):747–54. https://doi.org/10.1002/ca.20830.
37. Bashir WA, Lewis S, Cullen N, Connell DA. Os peroneum friction syndrome complicated by sesamoid fatigue fracture: a new radiological diagnosis? Case report and literature review. Skelet Radiol. 2009;38(2):181–6. https://doi.org/10.1007/s00256-008-0588-3.
38. Sobel M, Pavlov H, Geppert MJ, Thompson FM, DiCarlo EF, Davis WH. Painful os peroneum syndrome: a spectrum of conditions responsible for plantar lateral foot pain. Foot Ankle Int. 1994;15(3):112–24. https://doi.org/10.1177/107110079401500306.
39. Cheung YY, Rosenberg ZS, Ramsinghani R, Beltran J, Jahss MH. Peroneus quartus muscle: MR imaging features. Radiology. 1997;202(3):745–50. https://doi.org/10.1148/radiology.202.3.9051029.
40. Sobel M, Levy ME, Bohne WH. Congenital variations of the peroneus quartus muscle: an anatomic study. Foot Ankle. 1990;11(2):81–9.
41. Griffith, James F. An introduction to musculoskeletal ultraound. In. Rotations in Radiology-Musculoskeletal Imaging Volume 2 Metabolic, Infectious, and Congenital Diseases; Internal Derangement of the Joints; and Arthrography and Ultrasound In: Mihra ST, Imran MO, Kevin BH, and Tyson SC, editors. Musculoskeletal imaging, rotations in radiology. New York:

Oxford University Press; 2019. p. 329–40. https://global.oup.com/academic/product/musculoskeletal-imaging-volume-2-9780190938178?lang=en&cc=us#.

42. Geller J, Lin S, Cordas D, Vieira P. Relationship of a low-lying muscle belly to tears of the peroneus brevis tendon. Am J Orthop (Belle Mead NJ). 2003;32(11):541–4.

43. Mirmiran R, Squire C, Wassell D. Prevalence and role of a low-lying peroneus brevis muscle belly in patients with peroneal tendon pathologic features: a potential source of tendon subluxation. J Foot Ankle Surg. 2015;54(5):872–5. https://doi.org/10.1053/j.jfas.2015.02.012.

44. Freccero DM, Berkowitz MJ. The relationship between tears of the peroneus brevis tendon and the distal extent of its muscle belly: an MRI study. Foot Ankle Int. 2006;27(4):236–9.

45. Hyer CF, Dawson JM, Philbin TM, Berlet GC, Lee TH. The peroneal tubercle: description, classification, and relevance to peroneus longus tendon pathology. Foot Ankle Int. 2005;26(11):947–50.

46. Rosenberg ZS, Bencardino J, Astion D, Schweitzer ME, Rokito A, Sheskier S. MRI features of chronic injuries of the superior peroneal retinaculum. AJR Am J Roentgenol. 2003;181(6):1551–7. https://doi.org/10.2214/ajr.181.6.1811551.

47. Ozbag D, Gumusalan Y, Uzel M, Cetinus E. Morphometrical features of the human malleolar groove. Foot Ankle Int. 2008;29(1):77–81. https://doi.org/10.3113/fai.2008.0077.

48. Adachi N, Fukuhara K, Kobayashi T, Nakasa T, Ochi M. Morphologic variations of the fibular malleolar groove with recurrent dislocation of the peroneal tendons. Foot Ankle Int. 2009;30(6):540–4. https://doi.org/10.3113/fai.2009.0540.

Conservative Treatment of Peroneal Tendon Injuries: Immobilization/Bracing/Orthotics

6

Glenn Garrison

Conservative treatment for peroneal tendon injuries may be desirable for a number of reasons. First, conservative treatment may delay or eliminate the need for surgical intervention, especially when the patient has a relatively mild condition. Many patients have a great deal of anxiety associated with foot and ankle pain, reduced function [1], loss of mobility, and even the stress associated with seeing their physician. The prospect of surgery and post-surgical immobilization/rehabilitation only serves to increase patient anxiety. Patients, as a result, often choose conservative, less invasive options as part of an initial treatment plan.

A second advantage of conservative care is that treatments may begin almost immediately and are generally less expensive options. Conversely, conservative care may take a longer period of time, sometimes months, to be fully effective. Additionally, the financial cost of surgical interventions may be prohibitive, especially for the uninsured or underinsured.

In some situations, application of an orthosis or some other splint will limit foot and/or ankle motion in much the same fashion as surgical interventions. The patient is afforded the opportunity to "live with the results" of surgery without having it completed. This "trial period" helps the patient and physician to make a more informed decision prior to surgery. Every orthotic intervention, however, has its own unique set of advantages and disadvantages that should be considered carefully with the patient prior to implementation. Some factors to consider are cost, fabrication/delivery timeline, length of treatment, cosmesis, patient commitment, and difficulty in adapting to device and lifestyle changes.

G. Garrison (✉)
Hospital for Special Surgery, New York, NY, USA
e-mail: garrisong@hss.edu

© Springer Nature Switzerland AG 2020
M. Sobel (ed.), *The Peroneal Tendons*,
https://doi.org/10.1007/978-3-030-46646-6_6

Ankle Walkers

The first step in conservative foot and ankle care is often immobilization of the foot and ankle. Traditionally, immobilization was achieved with the use of a plaster or fiberglass foot and ankle cast. Casts create superior immobilization; however, they are not removable by the patient or caregiver. This inability to remove the cast guarantees compliance but may also create skin care, skin inspection, and hygiene issues, and may be contraindicated in patients prone to volume changes or ulcerations.

A more contemporary method of immobilization is the application of a prefabricated off-the-shelf ankle walker orthosis. These devices are available from a wide variety of manufacturers under a multitude of trade names. These devices generally come in three different styles and two heights. The styles include pneumatic support, non-pneumatic support, and vacuum-system support. The different styles have common features including a fixed ankle, which does not allow plantar- or dorsiflexion and a rocker sole to help the patient transition from heel-strike to foot-flat to toe-off in the gait cycle. These devices are ordinarily designed for temporary use of up to 3 months. Should more long-term solutions be needed, a custom-made orthosis may be necessary.

The pneumatic ankle walker (Fig. 6.1) consists of a rigid plastic outer shell lined with pneumatic bladders. The amount of air in the pneumatic bladders is normally

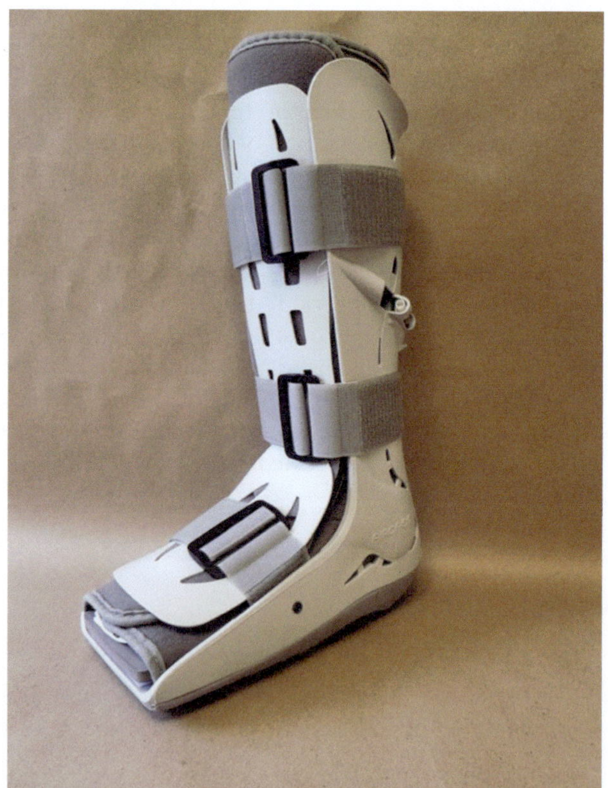

Fig. 6.1 Aircast "FP Walker." (Photo taken by Glenn Garrison)

adjustable as is the removable anterior shell which is adjusted with straps. The pneumatic bladders are designed to contour to the shape of the patient's leg and apply consistent total contact. The key, however, is not to over-inflate the bladders. Lower inflation pressure allows for more contact with the limb much like a flatter tire has more contact area with the road. By contrast, an over-inflated tire has less contact with the road. The overall tension of the orthotic support should be controlled by the outer straps. The advantages of pneumatic walkers are superior patient contact and consistent circumferential pressure. The disadvantage is limited ability to modify the shape/contour of the device to accommodate patients with very large or small shanks and wide feet and ankles.

Non-pneumatic ankle walkers (Fig. 6.2) are usually the least expensive option. They consist of a lightweight foam and cloth inner boot, which is attached to a rigid footplate with lateral moldable midline struts. The footplate has a rocker sole. The lateral struts may be contoured by a competent fitter to match the shape of the patient's leg. The advantage of this design is the ability to modify and adjust the device to fit almost any patient. The inner boot is breathable and therefore cooler to wear. Price is also an advantage. The disadvantage is the foam and cloth inner boot does not provide as much support as the plastic shells and pneumatic bladders of the pneumatic walker or vacuum bladder of the vacuum system.

Vacuum system ankle walker supports (Fig. 6.3) are the least commonly used devices. They consist of a rigid plastic frame lined with a plastic bead filled vacuum liner. The liner is very flexible and easily conforms to the shape of a patient's leg.

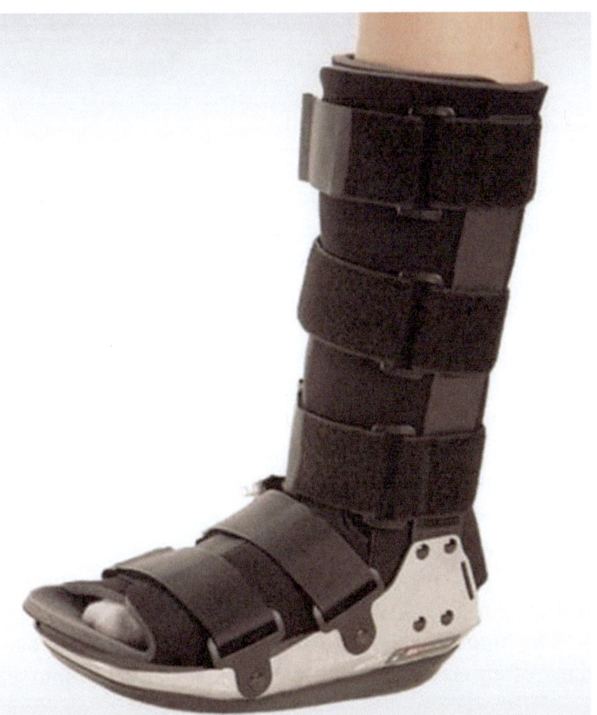

Fig. 6.2 Breg "J Walker Boot." (Online open source)

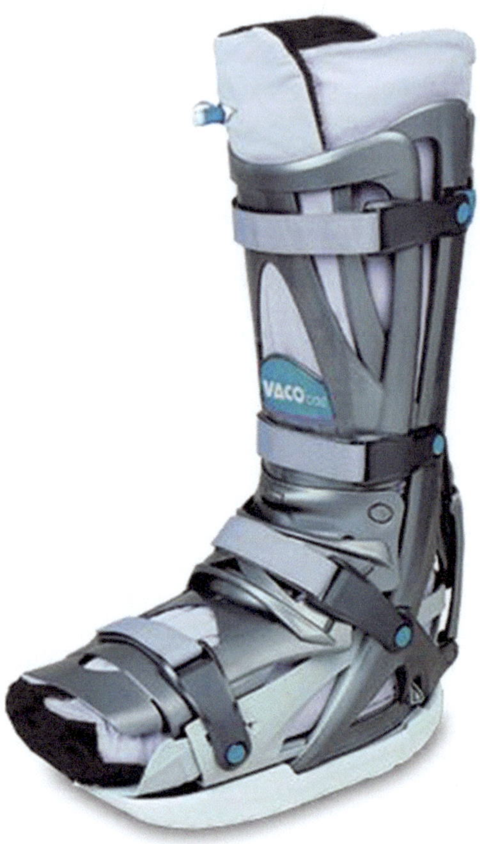

Fig. 6.3 VACOped "Achilles Injury/Fracture Orthosis Boot." (Online open source)

Once applied and straps adjusted for tension, air is expelled from the liner by the patient using a hand held expulsion pump. Once air is removed from the liner, the "beads," which once moved about freely in the liner, are locked rigidly into place. The once pliable liner becomes a rigid shell within the plastic frame which has conformed to the shape of the patient's leg and foot. This rigid shell offers superior support to the foot and ankle. This orthosis is available in a variety of designs which may be rigid or articulated at the ankle and may be adjusted or locked into a variety of positions in the sagittal plane. The liner will return to its soft, pliable, moldable condition with the release of negative pneumatic pressure. This is easily achieved by pulling out the valve collar and allowing air into the liner. This liner may be reshaped an unlimited number of times by evacuating air to create a vacuum and rigidity and allowing air back into the liner in order to make it pliable and easily reshaped. This device is very useful for patients who may have significant changes in limb volume from day to day or who have very thin or very large legs.

The biggest disadvantage of the vacuum system supports is the cost. These systems often cost much more than insurance reimbursement amounts and vendors,

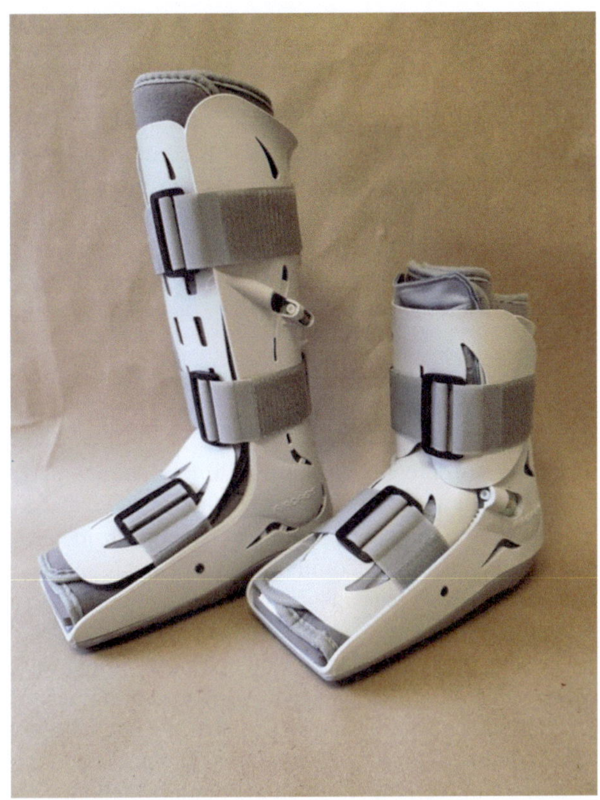

Fig. 6.4 Aircast "FP & SP Walkers." (Photo taken by Glenn Garrison)

therefore, do not offer this product as a patient option. Vendors who do dispense these devices often require patients to pay an "up charge" or "premium" for the device.

Most ankle walking orthoses are available in either a standard long length or shorter supra-malleolar height device (Fig. 6.4).

The standard-height ankle walker should extend from the plantar surface of the foot to just below the popliteal fossa when the patient is sitting and the knee bent to 90°. The full-length device incorporates the entire foot, ankle, and nearly the full length of the shank. It offers superior control of the foot and ankle in the sagittal plane. Control of the ankle in the frontal plane depends on the size relationship between the patient and the device, the design of the orthosis, and the quality of the fitting. It is difficult to control all varus/valgus movement in a prefabricated ankle walking orthosis. This length walker is preferable in patients with peroneal tendon injuries as the length of the device offers better control of the foot and ankle, limiting ankle movement, thereby offering more relief to muscles and long tendons.

As is common with most orthoses, the orthotist wants longer lever arms for better control with the least soft-tissue pressure. Patients, on the other hand, want the smallest, least-restrictive device possible. They prefer the supra-malleolar-height ankle walker which extends from the foot proximally to 2″–5″ above the malleoli.

These devices tend to be light and less obtrusive under clothing. While they may work well for stabilizing some mid and forefoot conditions, they generally do not provide the stabilization required for peroneal tendon injuries. The short lateral struts and the shorter general length do not effectively control the tibial shaft and ankle motion. Ankle movement will continue to stress the peroneal muscles and tendons and therefore not provide the desired relief.

Most ankle walking orthoses are sized according to the patient's foot length. The patient's toes should not extend beyond the length of the footplate to prevent possible trauma during ambulation. The toes should also be visible distally especially if there are circulation concerns with the lower extremity.

Foot Orthoses

The least restrictive devices for mild to moderate peroneal tendon injuries are foot orthoses. These devices may be prefabricated or custom-made to the shape of the patient's foot. They are designed to be worn inside an enclosed shoe that has ample room in the upper to accommodate the orthosis and the patient's foot. Many walking and athletic shoes have insoles that may be removed to allow more space for the foot orthosis.

Foot orthoses should be designed or modified to relieve pressure/stress on the peroneal tendons. This is done by incorporating a lateral heel wedge (Fig. 6.5) into the sole of the foot orthosis. The heel wedge may be supplemented with a lateral mid-foot post. These modifications will place the foot in a pronated position, which in turn should relieve stress on the peroneal tendons [2].

Patients who present with peroneal tendon injuries along with a cavovarus foot may require more in-depth foot orthosis modifications. Special attention may be required to relieve the metatarsal heads especially medially. Additional foot orthosis components such as medial arch pads, metatarsal pads, medially winged metatarsal pads, and wells for first metatarsal heads may be necessary to improve weight

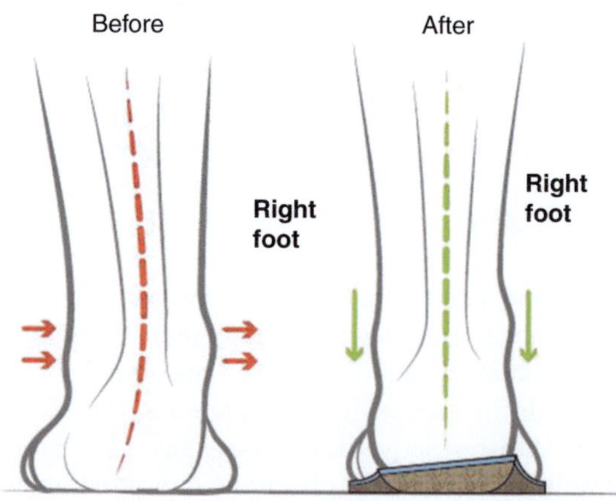

Fig. 6.5 Type 3: cavovarus/supination (high arch). (This drawing was copyrighted by Foot Scientific. Moore [4])

distribution and alleviate discomfort. These same foot orthosis components may be incorporated in custom ankle foot orthotic designs.

Prefabricated Ankle Foot Orthoses

There are commercially available prefabricated plastic Ankle Foot Orthoses (AFOs) (Fig. 6.6) that have been used for mild to moderate peroneal tendon injuries. As discussed, the goal of conservative care especially in moderate to severe cases is foot and ankle immobilization to allow the affected muscles and tendons to unload and rest during the acute phase of irritation. Prefabricated AFOs, by design, are plastic splints that generally fit over the shank and ankle and extend under the foot. Most of these devices are designed to control "foot drop" and provide some type of flexibility, particularly toward dorsiflexion, to allow the patient to roll smoothly over the affected foot during the gait cycle. These devices are generally too flexible to truly immobilize the foot and ankle. The few prefabricated devices that are rigid

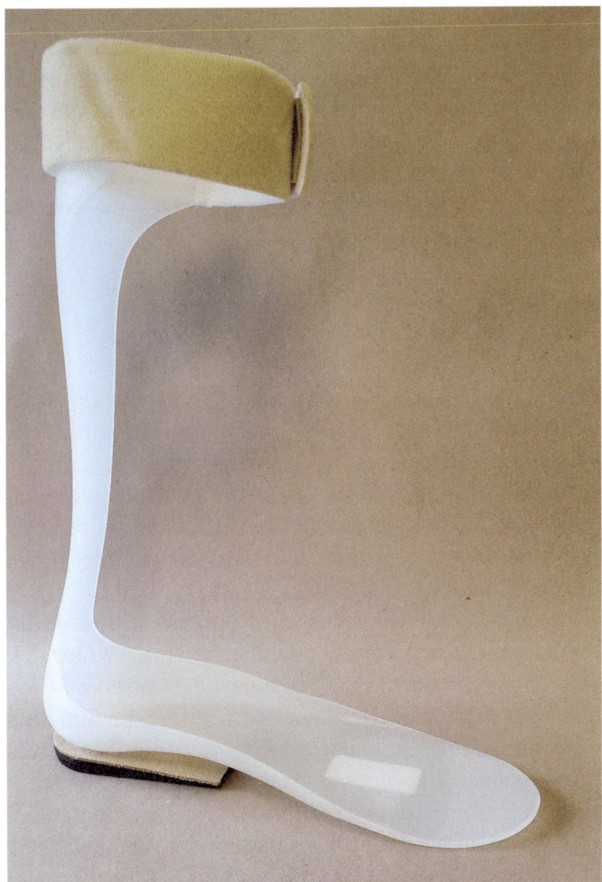

Fig. 6.6 "Pre Fab AFO." (photo taken by Glenn Garrison)

enough to immobilize the ankle in the sagittal plane often have a very generic shape in order to fit a large number of patients. The neutered design often does not provide sufficient control of the ankle and foot in the frontal plane to be effective in immobilizing the foot and ankle.

Custom Ankle Foot Orthoses

The most effective long-term control and immobilization of the foot and ankle is achieved with a custom-made AFO. These custom molded devices are made from either a casting or scanning of the patient's limb. From the cast or scan, an exact model of the limb is made for fabrication of the finished device. The model may be an actual model of plaster or some other rigid material or a virtual model reviewed on a computer screen or printout. The patient model is modified or manipulated to correct alignments, create reliefs for pressure-intolerant areas, or to increase corrective forces in pressure-tolerant areas. Once the model is corrected or rectified, a custom device is fabricated to its parameters. The orthosis is traditionally fabricated by thermo-molding plastic or molding leather to the patient model. With the advent of 3-D printing, AFOs may be printed to match the virtual design created from the patient scans. The efficacy of custom AFO design is dependent upon patient model rectification and fabrication, material selection, and design. There are a multitude of plastics, leathers, liners, padding, and strapping materials that may be employed in the fabrication process that may influence the control of the limb and comfort for the patient. Custom fabrication optimizes the component material selection and design/fitting processes.

Ankle Gauntlets

One of the oldest designs of ankle orthosis is a gauntlet which is a circumferential wrap around the lower shank and some portion of the foot. Gauntlets are still popular and are the foundation design for many devices. Many contemporary gauntlets are made of cloth, canvas, nylon, elastic, neoprene, and plastic. The rigidity of a gauntlet is heavily dependent on the materials used in fabrication, reinforcements provided to the design, the length of the gauntlet both proximally and distally, and the customization of the fit.

Recent gauntlet designs have combined the rigidity of custom-molded plastic AFOs with custom-molded leather gauntlet wraps. These custom hybrid designs, sometimes referred to as "Arizona-type" orthoses (Fig. 6.7), allow a large number of options for final trimlines and reinforcements. Some of the possible modifications include posting and/or wedging of the heels, relief windows at the heel, and limitless design choices as to rigidity and size of reinforcing plastic shells. Newer features include ankle gauntlets with articulating ankle joints.

For maximum control necessary for peroneal tendon relief, the custom ankle gauntlet should include a solid ankle plastic reinforcement design, extend distally to

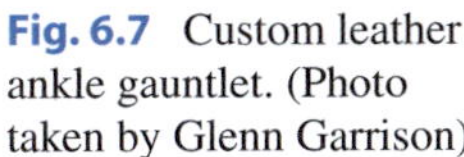

Fig. 6.7 Custom leather ankle gauntlet. (Photo taken by Glenn Garrison)

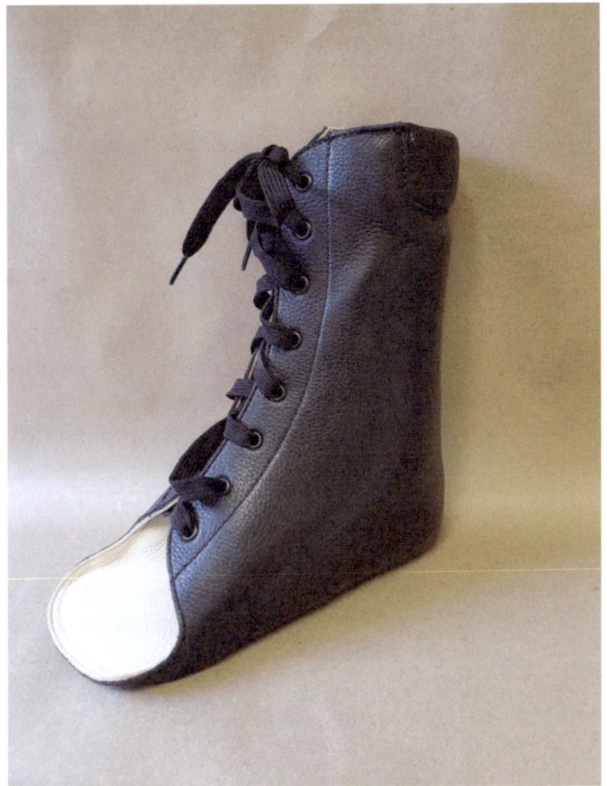

the metatarsal heads, and extend proximally at least 23 cm (9″) from the plantar surface. The proximal trim usually ends at or near the distal portion of the calf musculature and therefore does not increase bulk or restrict movement of the calf muscles. Careful attention should be paid to the casting or scanning technique to assure the ankle position (fabricated heel height) matches the shoe(s) to be used by the patient. Similarly, the foot and ankle should be positioned properly with the subtalar joint and forefoot in the desired position. Post-casting modifications to the model in the sagittal plane are fairly simple. Pronation-supination and adduction-abduction changes post-casting are extremely difficult to achieve.

The advantages of the custom ankle gauntlet include the following:

- The circumferential firm leather wrap provides excellent control of the ankle in all planes.
- The soft leather liner "feels" nice against the patient's skin, although the patient should always wear a sock between their leg and the leather gauntlet.
- The leather wrap will mold to the shape of the patient's limb over time, giving it a more contoured appearance and better control of the patient's limb.
- This device may be significantly shorter than a conventional plastic AFO.

- The outer leather may be any number of colors including natural leather, tan, black, white, brown, and beige. Other colors may be available depending on availability of leather from the fabricator.

The disadvantages of the custom ankle gauntlet include the following:

- Leather absorbs perspiration and is difficult to clean. Long-term use may lead to a deterioration of the leather surfaces and possible odor issues. This type of device may require routine maintenance for cleaning or rehabilitation/replacement of deteriorated leather.
- Arizona-type orthoses tend to be a bit thick and bulky as there are two layers of leather, a molded plastic shell, padding, and possible corrective pads. Sometimes patients require a size larger or wider shoe to accommodate the device.
- For maximum immobilization and control, the leather gauntlet works best if a lace closure is used anteriorly for donning purposes and to adjust tension. It may take a little time to lace up the orthosis when applying (this is similar to lacing up a boot or skate). It controls well but takes time to apply.
- Difficult to don independently if the patient has compromised hand function.
- Custom-fabricated device and may take 2–4 weeks to fabricate.
- Costly custom device. Utilizes recognized insurance billing codes.
- Orthosis wraps entirely around ankle and foot. Feels warm/hot to wear. Leg cannot "breathe."
- Limits foot and ankle motion.

As plastics technology advances, so does the range of materials available for orthotic fabrication. To offset some of the noted disadvantages of the custom leather ankle gauntlet, custom foot and ankle gauntlets are recently available fabricated entirely of plastic (Fig. 6.8). Instead of using leather as the primary gauntlet wrap, a very soft pliable plastic inner boot is used. This soft plastic liner is molded to the patient model and will gently control the position of the foot and ankle. A rigid plastic frame is then placed on the outside of the soft plastic inner boot. The plastic frame provides the same function as the custom-molded reinforcing plastic shells found within the traditional custom ankle gauntlet. Besides being made entirely of plastic, the two sections, soft plastic inner boot and rigid frame, are not normally attached to one another. This allows the patient the ability to don the molded inner boot first then apply the rigid frame.

The advantages of this new all-plastic design as compared to the custom leather ankle gauntlet are as follows:

- Plastic can be easily cleaned inside and out.
- Material does not deteriorate especially when exposed to moisture. Odors are not an issue.
- Less bulky, may not require larger footwear.
- Limits foot and ankle motion.
- Separate shells may be easier to don for some patients.
- Has a very high-tech appearance.

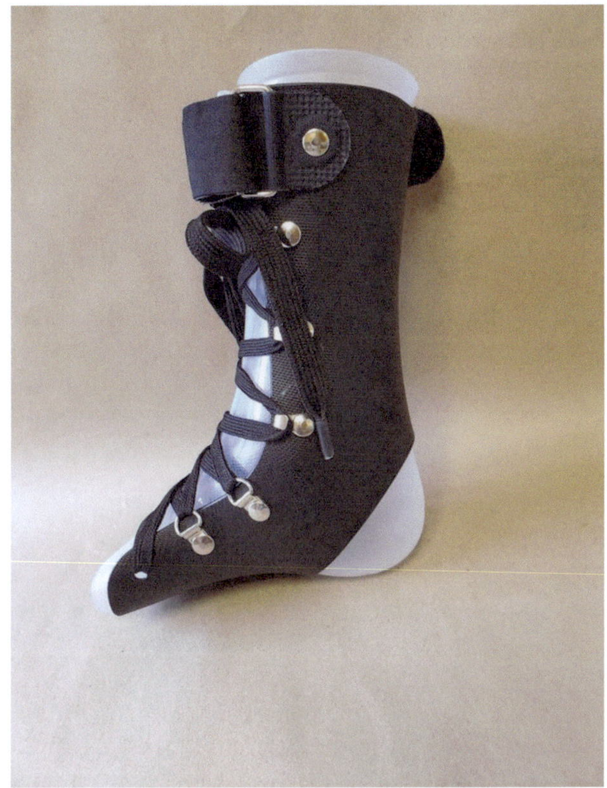

Fig. 6.8 Phoenix Ankle Stabilizer System, "PASS Rigid Orthosis." (Photo taken by Glenn Garrison)

There are some notable disadvantages to the all-plastic ankle gauntlet. The soft plastic inner shell is not as soft or conforming as leather. The touch and feel of leather are more desirable for some patients and the plastic still "feels" hard. These devices still require more time to don due to lacing the rigid frame across the anterior of the leg. The all-plastic ankle gauntlet generally is a slightly more expensive option.

There has been more acceptance of and requests for the all-plastic ankle gauntlet by athletes and other active patients. The ease of cleaning and more high-tech appearance have made it the device of choice for many patients.

Posterior Solid Ankle AFO – "Sobel Special"

A common device for immobilization of the foot and ankle is a custom-molded Posterior Solid Ankle AFO (Fig. 6.9). This orthosis is custom-molded to the patient model. It consists of a posterior shell for the shank that extends under the foot to the toes. There are numerous design features that vary from one practitioner to another according to the preferences of the providers.

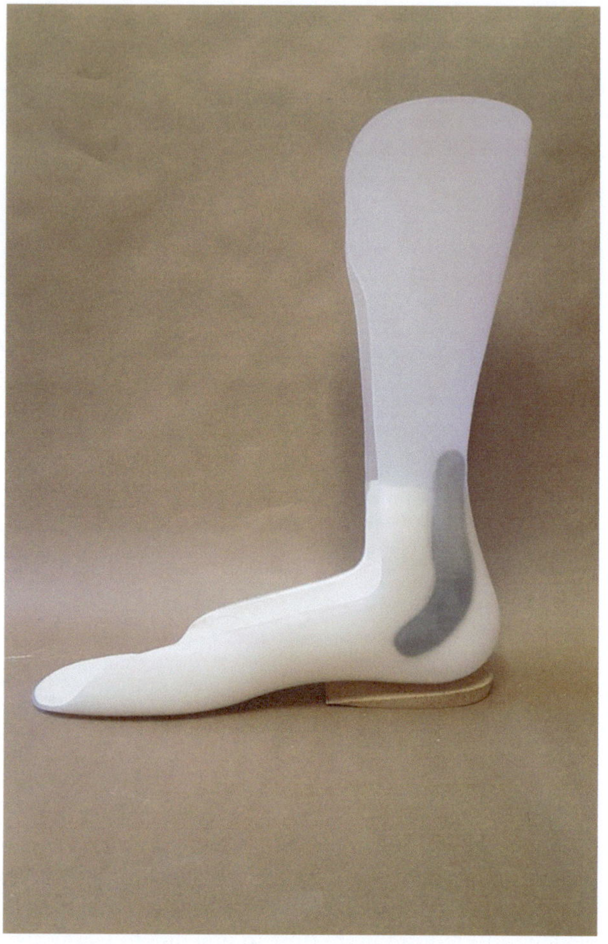

Fig. 6.9 Posterior Solid Ankle AFO. (Photo taken by Glenn Garrison)

Over years of practice, we have developed a specific design of custom-made Posterior Solid Ankle AFO to immobilize the foot and ankle for patients suffering from a variety of ailments including peroneal tendon injuries. The key to any device is the details of the design, fabrication, and fit. The communication between the physician and the orthotist is of paramount importance. Areas of particular interest and discussion include the diagnosis and specific needs of the patient, any extraordinary anatomic features of the patient, and any significant pertinent issues such as vocation, family support, household barriers, hobbies and/or recreational activities, fabrication time, and finally, resources to pay for device and services.

The Posterior Solid Ankle AFO design (Sobel Special) (Fig. 6.10) we use extends proximally posterior to 1–2 cm (1/2″) proximal to the apex of the gastrocnemius muscle belly. Proximal to that point, a well-molded AFO would begin to flare inward toward the tibia and may "dig" into the soft tissue during ambulation or when the patient sits down. Only in rare instances should the proximal edge of the AFO extend within 4–5 cm (1½–2″) of the fibular neck.

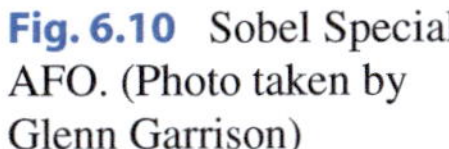

Fig. 6.10 Sobel Special AFO. (Photo taken by Glenn Garrison)

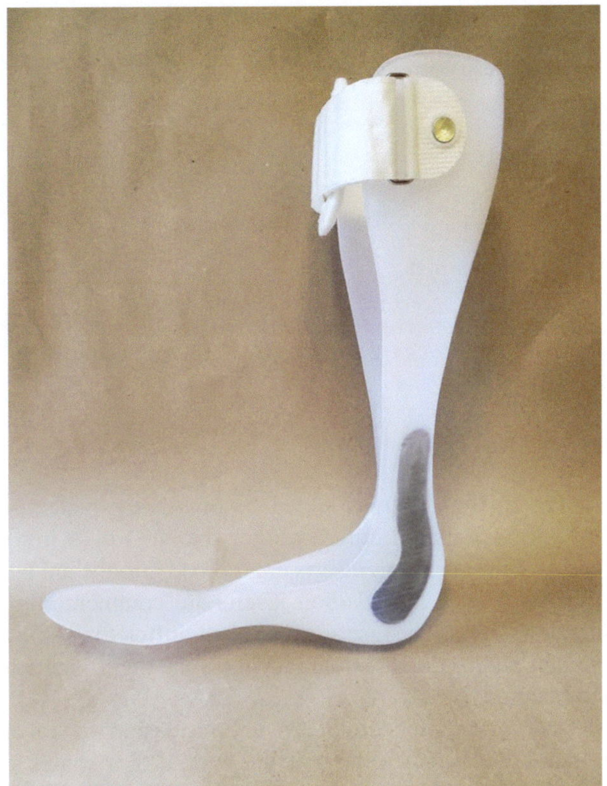

The sides of the AFO should extend forward roughly 4–5 cm (1½–2″) anterior of midline for the proximal 7–8 cm (3″) of length. This portion of the AFO serves as the anchor and transition point for the proximal anterior strap of the AFO. From this point distally, the lateral trimlines flare posteriorly to roughly 2–3 cm (1″) behind the midline of the shank, just behind the apex of the malleoli and anterior along the midline of the foot.

The lateral walls of the footplate should not be trimmed lower than the midline of the metatarsal shafts especially if the orthosis is to control forefoot abduction or adduction. Normally, the sidewalls are trimmed down toward the footplate just proximal to the metatarsal heads. Should there be a need to limit movement of the toes, the lateral trimlines may extend beyond the metatarsal heads. It should be noted that leaving the lateral trimlines higher, toward the dorsum of the foot, than midline of the metatarsal shafts may make donning of the footplate more difficult as the foot may not drop into the footplate. Additionally, higher lateral footplate walls will make shoe fitting more difficult because of the added foot width.

It is customary with our design to use a full plate. The length of the footplate is trimmed to clear the toes during the patient-fitting process. A full footplate eliminates the awkward transitions some patients feel should the footplate be trimmed proximal to the metatarsal heads or sulcus length. The full footplate also dampens if not eliminates toe movement particularly at push-off during the gait cycle.

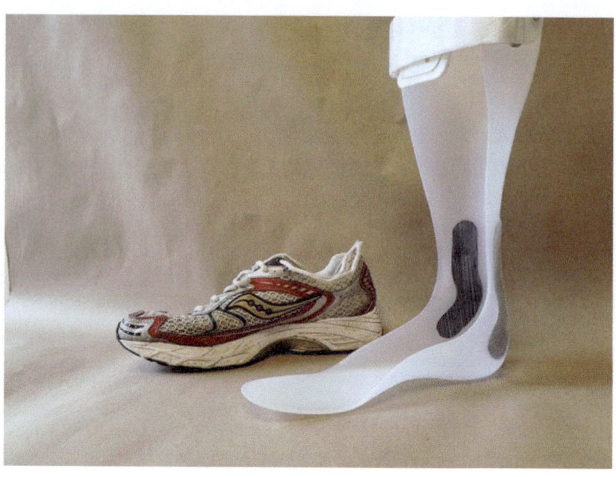

Fig. 6.11 Sobel Special AFO with shoe. (Photo taken by Glenn Garrison)

The custom AFO is molded out of slightly thicker polypropylene than would be used for a standard dorsiflexion-assist AFO (4–6 mm). To aid in immobilization, carbon reinforcement inserts are molded into the ankle area of the AFO during fabrication (Fig. 6.11). Carbon inserts are commercially available from a variety of manufacturers. The inserts themselves stiffen the ankle area of the AFO to eliminate plantar and/or dorsiflexion and stop splaying or spreading of the ankle area during ambulation.

A critical component of any orthotic design that involves the ankle and foot is the relationship between the patient's foot, orthosis, and footwear. The footwear must be large enough to accommodate the orthosis without crowding the foot or toes inside the shoe. There should be enough room in the toe box for the toes to wiggle if desired by the patient [3]. The throat of the upper should be large enough to allow the foot and orthosis combination to slide gently into the footwear. Blucher or surgical last shoes are preferable as these designs allow more room in the throat. The shoes should include lace closures which are easily adjustable and the lace stays should extend proximally to the end of the shank. The lace closures are a key component to keeping the patient's foot down and back into the orthosis, an important factor in foot and ankle immobilization.

An equally important relationship is the shape and contour of the plantar surface of the AFO compared to the shape and contour of the inside of the sole of the footwear (Fig. 6.12).

A lower wide heel in the shoe is most desirable. This heel provides a more stable base of support and smoother transition during the gait cycle. The foot and ankle should be cast and/or scanned in a position that matches the heel height of the shoe the patient will be using. Similarly, the patient model should be prepared with the shank vertical (tibia anterior tilt of 10°) while the foot is positioned with the same heel height of the patient's footwear. Should the patient use a shoe with a higher heel than built into the AFO, the net effect will be a dorsiflexed orthosis/shoe combination and the patient will feel like they are walking "downhill." They will also

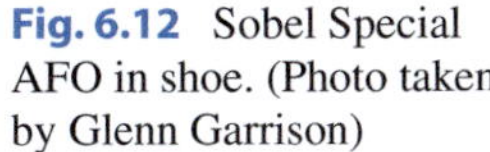

Fig. 6.12 Sobel Special AFO in shoe. (Photo taken by Glenn Garrison)

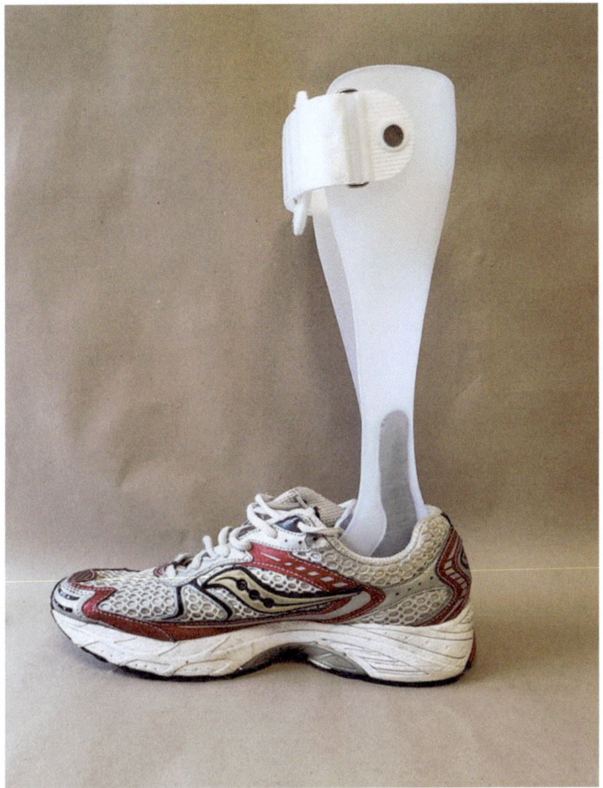

have difficulty keeping their knee straight, as the AFO will apply a flexion force to the knee. Conversely, should the patient use a shoe with a lower heel height than built into the AFO, the net effect will be a plantar-flexed orthosis/shoe combination and the patient will feel like they are walking "uphill." The patient will feel difficulty in bending their knee as the AFO will exert an extension force on their knee. Ample time should be spent when evaluating and measuring the patient to educate them on the importance of maintaining a consistent heel height while using a Posterior Solid Ankle AFO.

A second footwear consideration is the amount of toe spring built into the shoe. Toe spring is the amount of rise from the ball (metatarsal heads area) of the shoe to the end of the toe box. This is a form of forefoot rocker built into the shoe. Since the Posterior Solid Ankle AFO is designed to dampen or eliminate toe movement, it is imperative that the shape of the forefoot of the AFO and the amount of toe spring built into the AFO match the inside of the shoe (Fig. 6.13). If the AFO were made flat from the ball of the foot distally and not to match the shape of the shoe, there would be unnecessary and uncomfortable crowding of the foot and toes inside the shoe at the ball and inside the toe box. Additionally, there would not be enough forefoot rocker built into the AFO, which would add stress to the orthosis and force the patient's foot toward dorsiflexion during the heel-off to toe-off phase of gait.

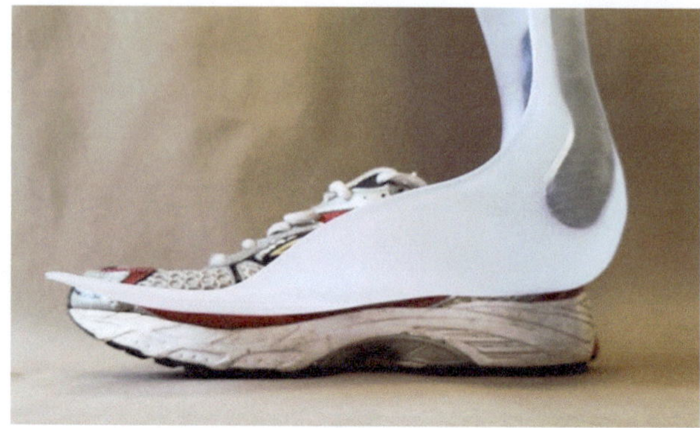

Fig. 6.13 Sobel Special AFO aligned with shoe. (Photo taken by Glenn Garrison)

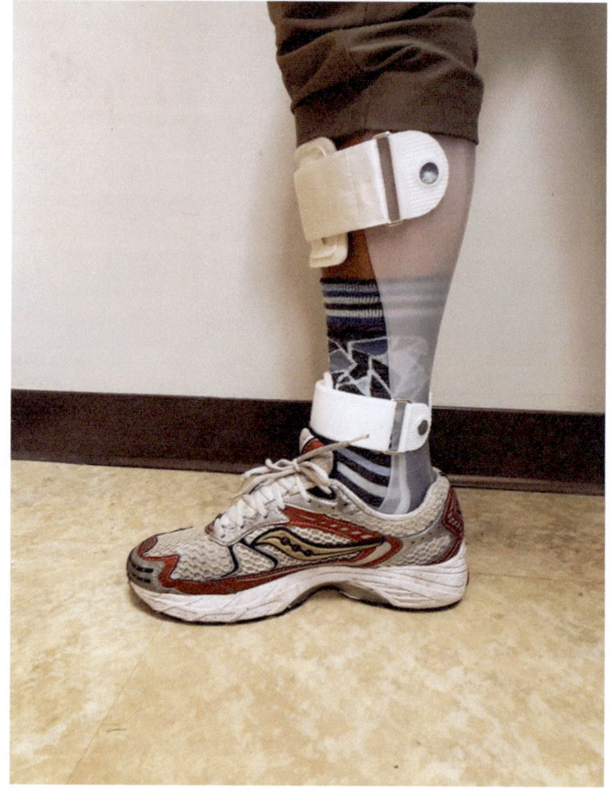

Fig. 6.14 Sobel Special AFO on patient. (Photo taken by Glenn Garrison)

Finally, the Posterior Solid Ankle AFO has an anterior proximal strap to hold the patient's shank back into the orthosis. This is normally a 5 cm (2″) wide strap with an additional pad to protect the tibial crest. A second strap may be incorporated into the design just proximal to the malleoli if the vamp closure of the footwear is not sufficient to keep the foot and ankle down and back into the orthosis (Fig. 6.14).

The advantages of the Posterior Solid Ankle AFO (Sobel Special) are as follows:

- Long orthotic lever arms provide superior immobilization of the foot and ankle.
- Contoured full-length footplate matches heel height of footwear and provides long forefoot rocker which eliminates dorsiflexion forces on foot and ankle.
- Slimmer design eliminates the need for larger/wider footwear.
- Orthosis is custom-shaped to provide frontal plane control without encapsulating the entire ankle and foot.
- Easier to don and doff, only two Velcro straps to adjust.
- Only posterior plastic, cooler orthosis to wear.
- Easy to clean and maintain.
- Maybe easily concealed under a sock.

The disadvantages of the Posterior Solid Ankle AFO (Sobel Special) are as follows:

- Long device which extends from high on calf to end of toes.
- Depends on footwear to hold patient properly in the device.
- Custom-fabricated device and may take 2–3 weeks to fabricate.
- Costly custom device. Utilizes recognized insurance billing codes.
- Limits foot and ankle motion.

The ease of use, cleaning, and maintenance, along with the effectiveness of this device, makes it increasingly popular for patients with moderate to severe peroneal tendon injuries.

Summary

Conservative treatment of peroneal tendon injuries requires effective, often long-term, positioning and possible immobilization of the ankle and foot. Ankle walkers may be used for immediate treatment of short duration but are not designed for long-term use. Ankle walkers are commercially available in pneumatic, non-pneumatic, and vacuum-system designs and function to eliminate motion in all planes. Foot orthoses may be used in mild to moderate cases and may be either prefabricated or custom-made. Foot orthoses should be modified with lateral heel wedges to position the foot in pronation relieving stress on the lateral peroneal tendons.

Moderate to severe cases of peroneal tendon injuries will require immobilization of the foot and ankle. While prefabricated ankle foot orthoses are available, most are designed to support "foot drop" and allow some ankle motion. The prefabricated AFOs that are rigid enough to immobilize the foot and ankle generally do not have the intimate contours necessary to control the foot and ankle in the frontal plane.

The most effective treatment for moderate to severe peroneal tendon injuries for the long term is a custom-made AFO. Custom-made devices are available in a few basic designs that may be customized to meet the individual needs of the patient. Arizona-type ankle gauntlets are shorter and completely enclose the lower shank, ankle, and foot. They may be fabricated of leather or a soft, flexible plastic reinforced with a rigid plastic support shell. Custom-made posterior solid ankle AFOs are longer, extending from the upper calf to the end of the foot. These orthoses cover only the posterior aspect of the leg and foot and are dependent on the patient's footwear to hold the foot properly in place.

Although custom orthotic devices tend to be expensive, they are considerably less expensive than surgical options and are usually eligible for insurance reimbursement. These devices may take several days to weeks to fabricate. Once properly fit to the patient, a custom device may be an effective tool for immobilizing the ankle and foot and relieving the peroneal tendons for several years. This less aggressive treatment plan gives the patient the opportunity to "heal" on their own, "see and feel" what may be the results of surgery, and buy the time necessary to make an informed surgical decision.

References

1. Nixon DC, Schafer KA, Cuswoth B, McCormick JJ, Johnson JE, Klein SE. Preoperative anxiety effect on patient-reported outcomes following foot and ankle surgery. Foot Ankle Int. 2019;40(9):1007–11. https://doi.org/10.1177/1071100719850806.
2. Anderson RB, Folmar E, Gans M, Sobel M. Peroneal tendon injury in the elite athlete. In: The peroneal tendons: a clinical guide to evaluation and management. New York: Springer; 2020.
3. Janisse DJ, Janisse E. Shoe modification and the use of orthoses in the treatment of foot and ankle pathology. J Am Acad Orthop Surg. 2008;16:152–8.
4. Moore G. Arches™ type 3 specialty orthotics [Internet]. Foot Scientific. Utah: Gary Moore; 2016 [cited 2019 Aug 26]. Available from https://www.footscientific.com/type-3-arches-orthotics/

Conservative Treatment of Peroneal Tendon Injuries: Rehabilitation

7

Eric Folmar and Michael Gans

Learning Objectives

On completion of this chapter, the reader will be able to:

1. Identify risk factors associated with peroneal tendon injuries, including abnormal biomechanics.
2. Explain the evaluative process used for identification of peroneal tendon injuries, including physical evaluation, functional evaluation, and use of outcome measures.
3. Formulate a comprehensive differential diagnosis for peroneal tendon injuries and associated disorders.
4. Describe the various types of peroneal tendon disorders and associated clinical presentations.
5. Describe evidence-based treatment strategies for the management of non-operative peroneal tendon injuries.
6. Apply knowledge of normal and pathological gait, assessment of impairment, and functional potential in the selection of appropriate supportive measures, including taping and bracing.

The original version of this chapter was revised. The correction to this chapter can be found at
https://doi.org/10.1007/978-3-030-46646-6_26

E. Folmar (✉)
Department of Physical Therapy, Movement & Rehabilitation Sciences,
Northeastern University, Boston, MA, USA
e-mail: e.folmar@northeastern.edu

M. Gans
PTSMC Orthopedic Residency Program, West Hartford, CT, USA

Physical Therapy and Sports Medicine Centers, Guilford, CT, USA

© Springer Nature Switzerland AG 2020, corrected publication 2020
M. Sobel (ed.), *The Peroneal Tendons*,
https://doi.org/10.1007/978-3-030-46646-6_7

Introduction

The peroneal longus and brevis muscles comprise the lateral compartment of the lower leg. Along with the extrinsic muscles of the anterior and deep compartments, they play a significant role in providing static and dynamic stability of the foot and ankle complex. The primary muscle function of the peroneal musculature is to evert the rear foot, with the peroneus longus additionally acting to plantar flex the first ray of the foot, providing stability against the ground [1]. The peroneal musculature serves to balance the actions of the tibialis posterior, tibialis anterior, and flexor halluces longus [1]. In particular, the peroneus longus and tibialis posterior function to control the subtalar and mid-tarsal joints during gait [2]. Tension through the tibialis posterior may increase stiffness of the foot, whereas tension through the peroneus longus serves to decrease tension in the foot [3]. Optimal balance and timing of tension created through activation of these muscles may serve to optimize foot biomechanics during gait. Imbalances and/or weakness in these muscles can negatively impact stability and lead to pain and recurrent ankle injury [4].

Effective clinical management of peroneal tendon injuries requires a detailed understanding of normal and pathological biomechanics, as well as the interaction of these biomechanics with the environment. Nonsurgical management of peroneal injuries requires the detailed evaluation of the nature of the tendon injury, associated pathomechanics, environmental stressors, and identification of concomitant injuries, such as ligamentous injuries and chronic ankle instability.

Peroneal tendon injuries are often the result of structural abnormalities and injuries that require alteration of the bony biomechanics and reconstruction of the tendons and ligaments involved. Effective management requires detailed examination and assessment of foot alignment and deformity. In particular, pathologies of the peroneal muscles are often found in individuals with chronic ankle instability and in those with cavovarus foot types. Repetitive activities or repeated sprains/inversion injuries are often associated with peroneal pathology.

Patient History

Most peroneal tendon injuries occur as a result of an ankle sprain. Persons who have had one ankle sprain are more likely to have a second ankle sprain [5–12]. In a prospective cohort study of high school soccer and basketball players, the risk of sustaining an ankle sprain was twice as high (risk ratio = 2.14) in those with a previous sprain [13]. Peroneal tendon injuries are more likely to occur with chronic ankle instability (CAI) resulting from repeated ankle sprains. In the case of an acute ankle sprain, our primary screening questions are used to determine who requires X-rays to rule out fracture. The Ottawa Ankle Rule (OAR) is a reliable and valid tool shown to be 100% sensitive for fractures, and to have the potential to allow physicians to safely reduce the number of radiographs ordered in patients with ankle injuries by one-third [14]. Since originally published, there have been 21 primary studies on the sensitivity and specificity of the OAR that range from 92% to 100% and from 16%

to 51%, respectively [15]. To improve the OAR specificity, other tools are proposed such as the Bernese ankle rules. Vibrating tuning fork test and ultrasound could be useful in patients with OAR positive to decrease the need for radiographs. X-rays are recommended to rule out fracture if the person is unable to bear weight for four steps, or has tenderness at any of the following places: the posterior aspects of the distal 5 cm of the fibular head, the medial malleolus, the navicular,; the base of the fifth metatarsal (see Fig. 7.1).

The mechanism of injury for the peroneal muscles usually involves an inversion sprain causing a tension to the peroneal tendons. Both peroneal muscles function to plantar flex and evert the foot, but peroneus longus muscle also causes plantarflexion of the first ray. This creates pain and difficulty with multiple phases of gait, but specifically with initial contact stabilizing an inverted foot as it accepts weight and

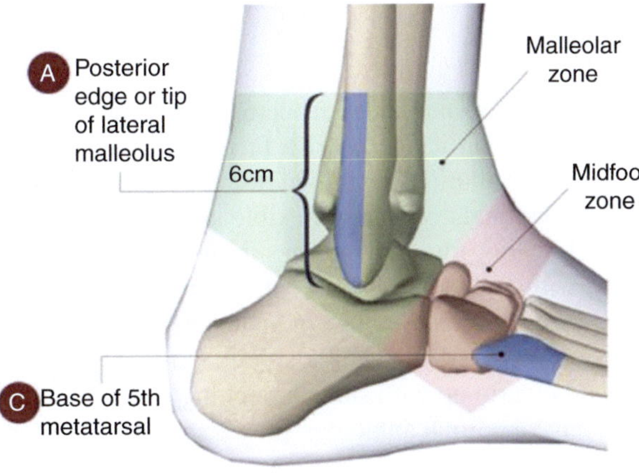

Fig. 7.1 Ottawa Ankle Rules for use in radiography in acute ankle injuries (http://www.theottawarules.ca/ankle_rules)

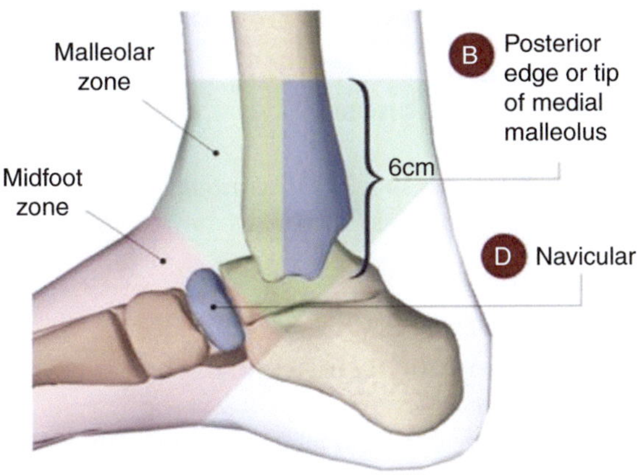

push-off when the ankle rapidly plantar flexes to propel forward. Peroneal muscles function in stabilizing the lateral ankle during all weight-bearing activities. Movements that involve twisting, bending, or uneven surfaces are usually aggravating. Other complaints including feelings of instability or "giving way" may help diagnose CAI. The patient with an acute subluxation may present with a history of a traumatic dorsiflexion or inversion episode during a cutting maneuver. They may report a forceful pop at the posterolateral ankle and will likely have pain at the lateral ankle. The patient may describe a feeling of instability on uneven surfaces, sometimes accompanied by a snapping or popping sensation about the lateral malleolus. With an inversion injury, the clinician should have a higher index of suspicion for peroneal tendon injury if pain is localized to the retrofibular groove, as an isolated posterior talofibular ligament injury is uncommon [16].

Risk Factors

There is no substantial evidence to support physical characteristics such as gender, age, height, and weight as risk factors for ankle sprain [17]. There are risk factors related to limitations in the ankle range of motion, specifically ankle dorsiflexion [18]. Individuals with an inflexible ankle (average dorsiflexion of 34° measured in weight-bearing) were five times more likely to suffer an ankle sprain compared to those with an average dorsiflexion range of motion of 45° [19]. Clinicians should recognize the increased risk of acute lateral ankle sprain in individuals who (1) have a history of a previous ankle sprain, (2) do not use an external support, (3) do not properly warm up with static stretching and dynamic movement before activity, (4) do not have normal ankle dorsiflexion range of motion, and (5) do not participate in a balance/proprioceptive prevention program when there is a history of a previous injury [17]. Clinicians should also be aware of the increased risk for developing ankle instability in patients who (1) have an increased talar curvature, (2) are not using an external support, or (3) did not perform balance or proprioception exercises following an acute lateral ankle sprain [17].

Differential Diagnosis

A thorough history should differentiate between peroneal tendonitis/tendinopathy, os peroneum syndrome, peroneus brevis and longus tears, and peroneal tendon subluxation.

Peroneal Tendonitis/Tendinopathy

Tendonitis of the peroneal tendons is typically related to overuse. Symptoms most commonly incurred are pain with contraction or excessive use of the peroneal muscles, inflammation, and tenderness. Tendinopathy is an encompassing term utilized to describe painful conditions that affect tendons in response to abnormal stresses or overuse. In contrast to tendonitis, which implies pain secondary to inflammation, tendinopathy is more reflective of the histopathologic changes that occur due to abnormal stresses over a period of time. Some of these changes included have led to these conditions being regarded as degenerative in nature, including vascular hyperplasia, increase in cellularity, and a consistent absence of inflammatory cells. Tendon thickening, tearing, pain, and minimal inflammation are associated, impacting the mechanical function of the tendon [20]. Tendinopathy of the peroneal brevis is often associated with pain along the peroneal muscles, whereas peroneus longus symptoms may be found distal to the separation of the two tendons and along the course of the longus tendon around the cuboid and under the foot.

Tendon Splits/Tears

Split peroneal tendon injuries typically involved the peroneus brevis at the level of the fibular groove behind the lateral malleolus. At this point, the longus tendon lies over the brevis tendon. The primary cause of longitudinal splitting is mechanical stress [21, 22]. A typical patient history includes description of an inversion ankle injury. Often the superior peroneal retinaculum is injured, creating instability of the tendon within the groove. This leads to the tendon riding over the ridge of the fibular groove, creating physical wearing of the tendon. These tears typically are degenerative in nature as this mechanical wearing occurs over a period of time (see Fig. 7.2).

Os Peroneum

The os peroneum is a round or oval-shaped ossicle located distally near the cuboid within the peroneus longus tendon. Painful os peroneum syndrome (POPS), described by Sobel et al., encompasses a spectrum of conditions that can cause pain in the lateral aspect of the foot [23]. A fracture or bipartite ossicle is most typical

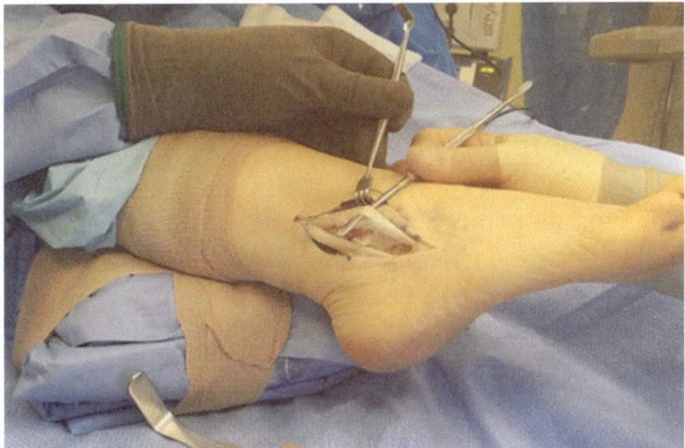

Fig. 7.2 Split peroneal tendon – longitudinal tear of the peroneus brevis is noted with instrument passing through a tear to identify injury https://www.faant.com/blog/surgical-repair-of-peroneal-tendon-tear.cfm

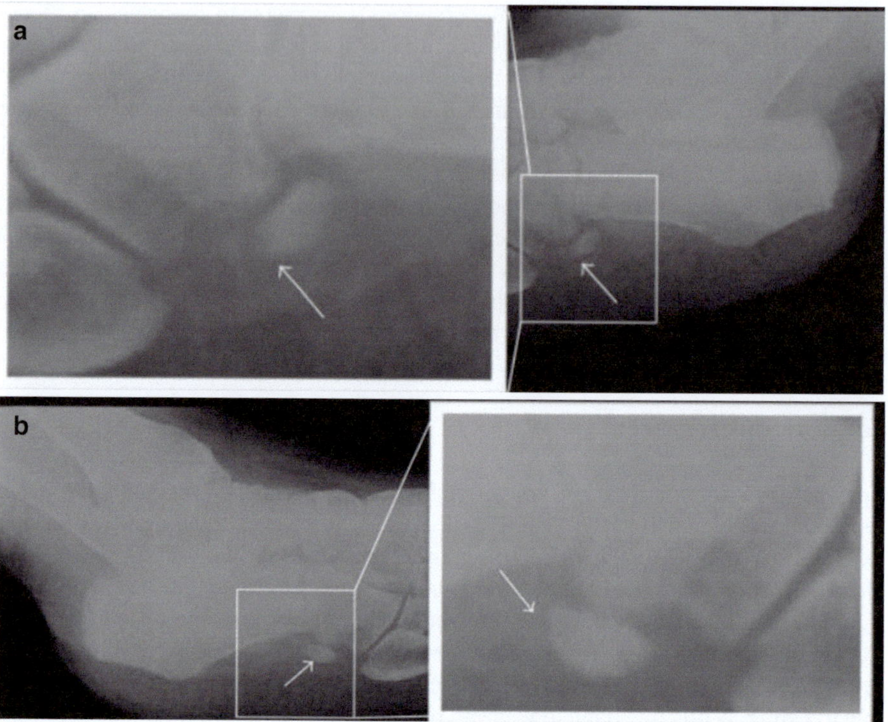

Fig. 7.3 (**a**) Right foot: complaint side, showing an irregular and fragmented os peroneum with heterogeneous density (arrow). (**b**) Left foot: comparative contralateral side, showing a regular and complete os peroneum with regular contours and homogeneous density (Chagas-Neto et al. [87])

and may cause discontinuity of the peroneus longus tendon. Chronic fracture resulting in callus formation and stenosis of the tendon, attrition or rupture (partial or full), or an enlarged peroneal tubercle can all be characteristic of this condition. Radiography is key to diagnosis (see Fig. 7.3). Clinical presentation may demonstrate acute or chronic pain, though acute conditions are much less common. Pain is typically distal to the fibula along the peroneus longus tendon, with notable discomfort with a heel rise and associated plantar flexion of the first ray [23].

Peroneal Tendon Subluxation/Dislocation

The superior peroneal retinaculum is the primary structure responsible for maintaining the peroneal tendons in the fibular groove. Injuries causing subluxation/dislocation of the tendons (see Fig. 7.4) can be acute or chronic in nature. Acute injuries often involve forced dorsiflexion of the ankle, causing a strong contraction of the peroneal muscles to counter the movement. Chronic injuries often occur as the result of repetitive strain in extreme positions, such as in ballet. Acute injuries are subject to recurrence with conservative management, typically requiring surgical intervention to prevent recurrence. Peroneal subluxation often presents with

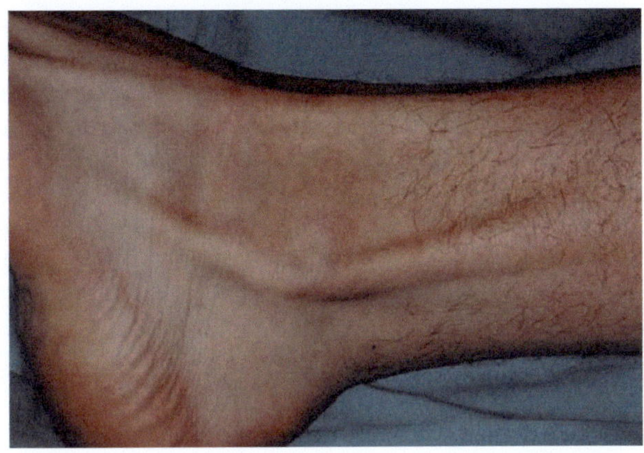

Fig. 7.4 Subluxation of the peroneal tendons in a plantar-flexed ankle position (Oliva et al. [88])

simultaneous splitting/tearing of the peroneal tendon, as the tendon subluxes over the sharp ridge of the fibular groove.

Physical Exam

Outcome Measures

Self-reported outcome measures are an excellent way to gather more information about the patient's overall condition. As recommended by current clinical practice guidelines for Ankle Stability and Movement Coordination Impairments: Lateral Ankle Sprains, clinicians should incorporate validated functional outcome measures, such as the Foot and Ankle Ability Measure (FAAM) and the Lower Extremity Functional Scale (LEFS), as part of a standard clinical examination [17]. These should be utilized before and after interventions intended to alleviate the impairments of body function and structure, activity limitations, and participation restrictions associated with ankle sprain and instability.

The FAAM is a region-specific instrument designed to assess activity limitations and participation restrictions for individuals with general musculoskeletal foot and ankle disorders [24]. This includes those who sustained an ankle sprain. It consists of the 21-item activities of daily living (ADL) and separately scored 8-item sports subscales. The FAAM has strong evidence for content validity, construct validity, test–retest reliability, and responsiveness with general musculoskeletal foot and ankle disorders [25]. There is also evidence for validity in those with chronic ankle instability. Test–retest ICCs and minimal detectable change values at 95% confidence (MDC95) were 0.89 and 5.7 for the ADL subscale and 0.87 and 12.5 for the sports subscale. The minimal clinically important difference was reported to be 8 and 9 points over a 4-week time frame for the ADL and sports subscales, respectively. The FAAM is an updated version of the Foot and Ankle Disability Index (FADI). The FADI contains five additional items, four about pain, and one about sleep, which were removed after factor and item response theory analyses [25].

The LEFS was created to be a broad region-specific measure appropriate for individuals with musculoskeletal disorders of the hip, knee, ankle, or foot [26]. The LEFS consists of 20 items that assess activity limitations and participation restrictions. The test–retest reliability was $r = 0.87$, with an MDC90 of 9.4 over a 1-week interval with subjects who sustained an acute ankle sprain. A significant difference between changes in scores over a 1-week period was noted when comparing those 6 or more days to those less than 6 days of post-ankle sprain. In a group of subjects with hip, knee, ankle, and foot pathologies, the minimal clinically important difference was reported to be 9 points over a 4-week interval [26].

Foot Posture and Gait Assessment

The Foot Posture Index (FPI 6) is a highly reliable and valid way to assess static foot positioning [27, 28]. The FPI 6 includes six static foot posture assessments ranking each on a scale of −2 to +2. Negative scores indicate supinated positions and positive scores indicate pronated foot positions (see Fig. 7.5a, b). Patients

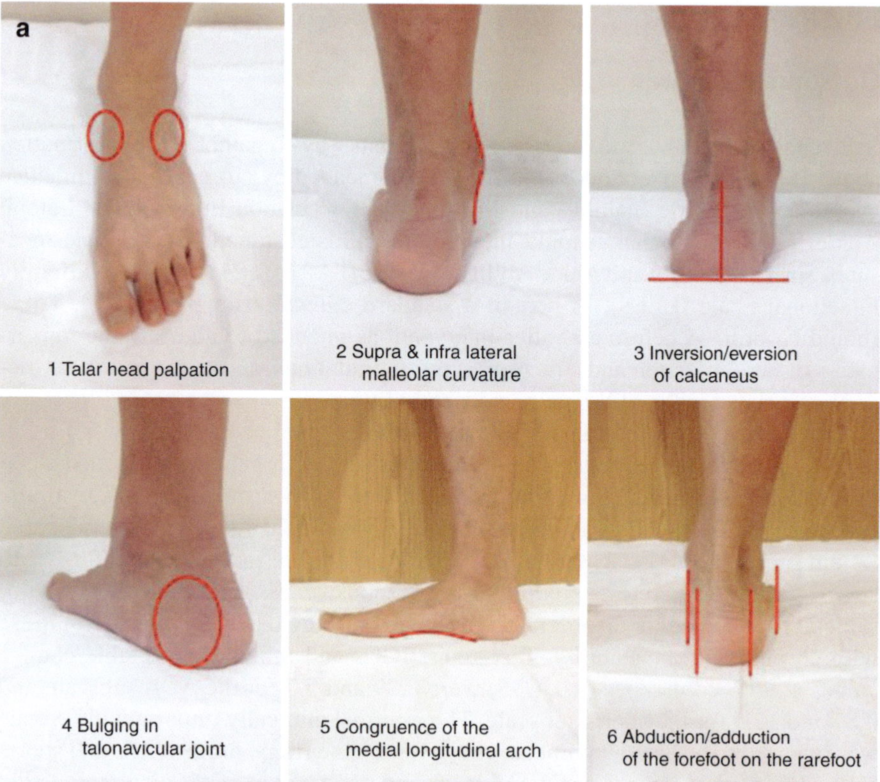

Fig. 7.5 Foot posture index (FPI 6): (**a**) six items of the FPI; (1) Talar head palpation, (2) supra and infra lateral malleolar curvature, (3) inversion/eversion of calcaneus, (4) bulging in talonavicular joint, (5) congruence of the medial longitudinal arch, (6) abduction/adduction of the forefoot on the rarefoot and (**b**) scoring of the FPI (Lee et al. [89])

b

	-2	-1	0	1	2
Talar head palpation	Talar head palpable on lateral side/but not on medial side	Talar head palpable on lateral side/ slightly palpable on medial side	Talar head equally palpable on lateral and medial side	Talar head slightly palpable on lateral side/palpable on medial side	Talar head not palpable on lateral side/but palpable on medial side
Supra and infra lateral malleolar curvature	Curve below the malleolus either straight or convex	Curve below the malleolus concave, but flatter/more than the curve above the malleolus	Both infra and supra malleolar curves roughly equal	Curve below the malleolus more concave than curve above malleolus	Curve below the malleolus markedly more concave than curve above malleolus
Calcaneal frontal plane position	More than an estimated 5° inverted (varus)	Between vertical and an estimated 5° inverted (varus)	Vertical	Between vertical and an estimated 5° everted (valgus)	More than an estimated 5° everted (valgus)
Prominence in the region of the talonavicular joint (TN)	Area of TNJ markedly concave	Area of TNJ slightly, but definitely concave	Area of TNJ flat	Area of TNJ bulging slightly	Area of TNJ bulging markedly
Congruence of the medial longitudinal arch	Arch high and acutely angled towards the posterior end of the medial arch	Arch moderately high and slightly acute posteriorly	Arch height normal and concerntrically curved	Arch lowered with some flattening in the central portion	Arch very low with severe flattening in the central portion-arch making ground contact
Abduction/adduction of the forefoot on the rarefoot	No lateral tose visible. Medial tose clearly visible	Medial tose clearly more visible than lateral	Medial and lateral tose equality visible	Lateral tose clearly more visible than medial	No medial lose visible. Lateral tose clearly visible

Fig. 7.5 (continued)

who exhibit low foot posture scores (0 to −5) are defined as supinators [29–31]. Supination includes excessive rear foot inversion. Alterations in gait kinematics, particularly excessive inverted rear foot positions at initial contact, may predispose someone to ankle sprains. Individuals with chronic ankle instability in particular have been shown to have a tendency to ambulate in an overly inverted ankle position [32, 33].

Measuring ROM

Ankle range of motion measurements lack reliability [34]. Ankle subtalar joint motions have questionable interrater reliability and only moderate intrarater reliability [35]. Non-weight-bearing goniometric measure of ankle dorsiflexion is done with the knee extended to 0° and flexed to 45°. Measures with the knee extended are intended to be descriptive of gastrocnemius flexibility, whereas those with the knee flexed are thought to reveal soleus flexibility. These measures can be done in standing as well. This is an important measure as it looks at the ability of the tibia to advance over the ankle in loaded positons. Loss of weight-bearing dorsiflexion ROM has been linked to biomechanical changes lending to a higher risk ankle sprain, as well as other pathologies of the kinetic chain (see Fig. 7.6).

Strength Testing

Often clinicians rely on manual muscle testing procedures (as outline by multiple texts) as the primary method of assess muscle function. Access to and cost of more expensive devices can be prohibitive in the clinical setting. Isokinetic tests of ankle inversion and eversion strength for healthy adults are highly reliable with the Biodex

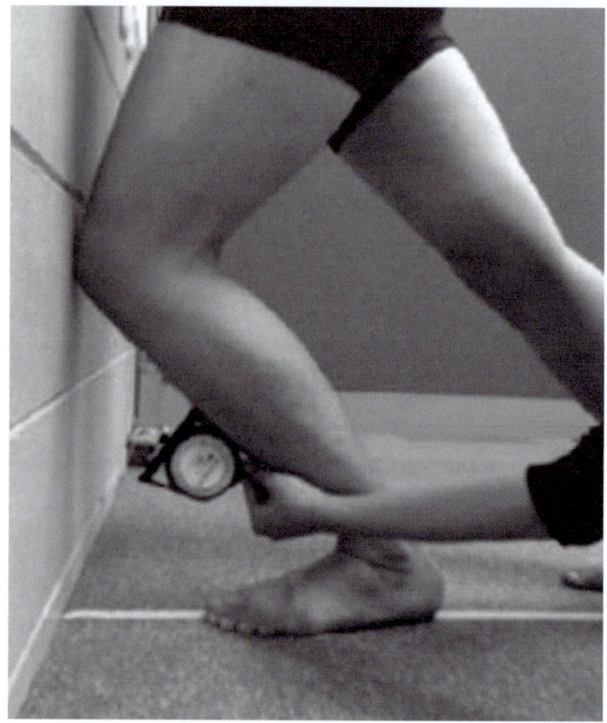

Fig. 7.6 Weight-bearing ankle dorsiflexion range of motion measurement (weight-bearing lunge test) (Kang et al. [90])

dynamometer [36]. The test–retest reliability and interrater reliability of handheld dynamometric measures were found to be good to excellent for ankle dorsiflexion, inversion, and eversion [37–40].

Special Tests

Ligamentous stability should be assessed. Peroneal subluxation is tested by flexing the knee and having the patient actively plantar flex and dorsiflex the ankle with resisted eversion. The test yields positive results when the peroneal tendons can be felt or seen to subluxate anterior to the lateral malleolus. Intrasheath subluxation should be suspected if the tendons are noted to translate relative to one another without truly subluxating anterior to the lateral malleolus. The peroneal compression test can be used to evaluate for peroneus brevis tendonitis; to perform this test, the foot is everted and dorsiflexed while manual pressure is placed against the fibular groove. Pain elicited with this maneuver is considered a positive result of test [23] (see Fig. 7.7).

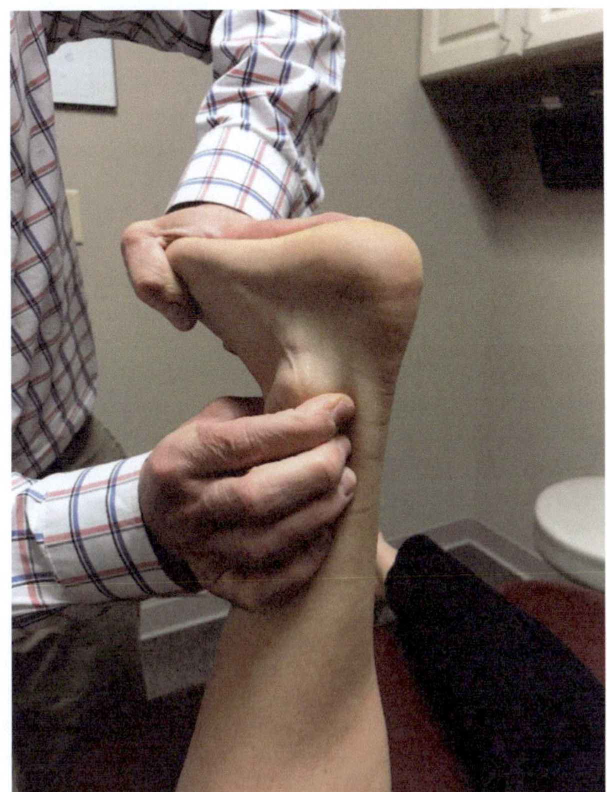

Fig. 7.7 The peroneal compression test

Functional Testing

Functional testing serves many purposes in the clinical and research settings. Often these tests are used to establish baseline levels of function, are markers to indicate progress, and can serve as thresholds for return to activity or sport. Though not specific to pathology, these tests serve a broad population and can serve very useful in determining the level of dysfunction.

The simple balance test is performed by having an individual stand on one leg for 1 minute with eyes open and 1 minute with eyes closed. Each surface contact with the contralateral leg was counted a "touch" or failure point. Alternately, the time the individual is able to maintain balance up to 60 seconds has also been described as the single-limb balance test (SLBT) [41]. Performances on the simple balance test and SLBT were different between individuals with and without unstable ankles, as well as between injured and uninjured ankles in individuals with ankle instability [41–44]. Average single-limb balance times for individuals between 20 and 49 years of age ranged between 29.7 and 30.0 seconds with eyes open and between 24.2 and 28.8 seconds with eyes closed. The average times decreased to between 14.2 and 29.4 seconds with eyes open and between 4.3 and 21.0 seconds with eyes closed for those between the ages of 50 and 79 years [45].

The Balance Error Scoring System (BESS) is a measurement of impairment of function and proprioception and consists of counting the number of deviations from a standardized stance position. The test positions to maintain balance are double limb, single limb, and tandem stances on both firm and foam surfaces and the "errors" in a 20-second time period for each of the six conditions. The stance position requires the individuals to stand with their hands on iliac crests, head in neutral, and eyes closed. An "error" is counted when the individual (1) opens their eyes; (2) steps, stumbles, or falls out of test position; (3) removes hands from their hips; (4) moves into more than 30° of hip flexion or abduction; (5) lifts the toes or heels; or (6) remains out of the test position for more than 5 seconds. Normative data: average total BESS scores ranged from 11 to 13 "errors" for those between the ages of 20 and 54 years and 15–21 "errors" for those between the ages of 55 and 69 years ($n = 589$) [46]. Minimum detectable change is 7–9 points [47] (see Fig. 7.8).

The Star Excursion Balance Test (SEBT) and the Y-balance test require the patient to maintain balance on one lower extremity while reaching as far as possible with the other extremity (see Fig. 7.9). The SEBT reach is in eight different directions while the Y Balance test reach is only for the anterior, posterolateral, and posteromedial directions [48]. The SEBT layout consists of eight lines from a center point arranged at 45° angles. The lines can be labeled according to their position in a counterclockwise direction as follows: anterior, anterolateral, lateral, posterolateral, posterior, posteromedial, medial, and anteromedial. The Y Balance test uses a platform reaching in only the anterior, posterolateral, and

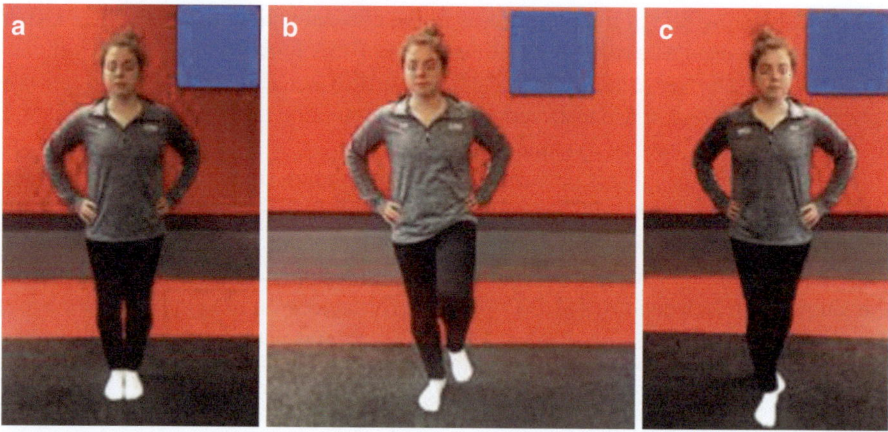

Fig. 7.8 Balance Error Scoring System (BESS) and scoring: (**a**) double leg, firm surface; (**b**) single leg, firm surface; (**c**) tandem stance, firm surface; (**d**) double leg, soft surface; (**e**) single leg, soft surface; (**f**) tandem stance, soft surface

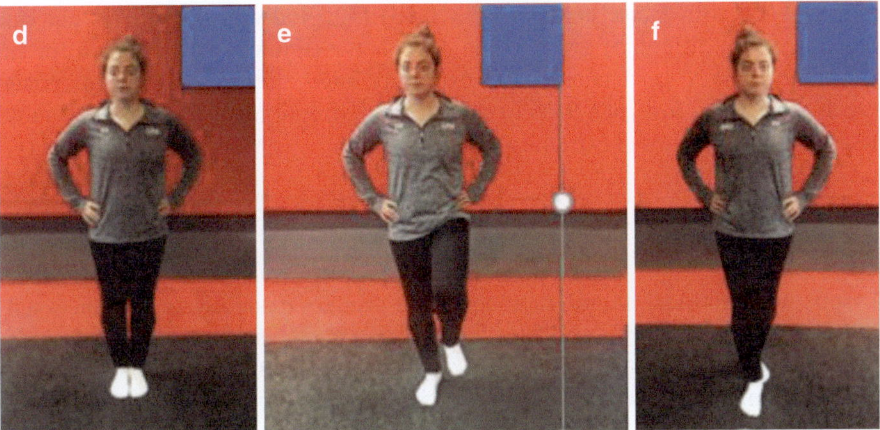

Fig. 7.8 (continued)

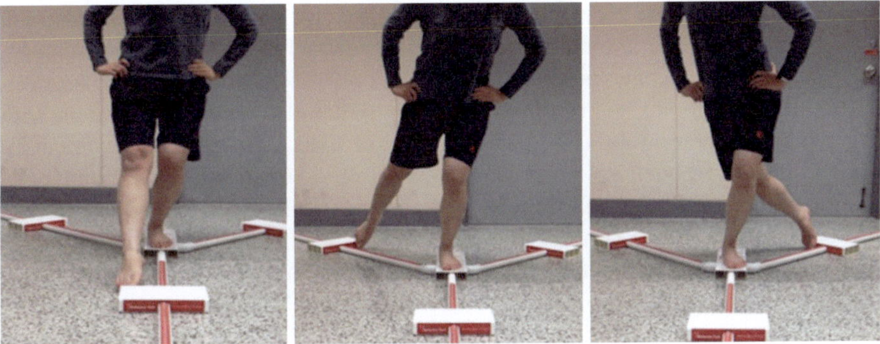

Fig. 7.9 The "Y" Balance Test (Lee et al. [91])

posteromedial directions. The test consists of having the subject stand with the lower extremity being tested in the center while the maximum reach distance of the contralateral lower extremity achieved along each of the direction lines is measured. Subjects are not allowed to move the support foot and should keep their hands on their hips. The test consists of six practice and three test trials in each of the eight directions. Reach distances can be normalized by dividing excursion distance by lower extremity length [49]. The SEBT and Y balance tests have good inter- and intrarater reliability and validity [49, 50]. Individuals with ankle instability had decreased reach distances compared to their uninvolved side and compared to healthy individuals [51–53]. Decreased anterior and posteromedial reach distances on the involved side were predictive of ankle instability [54]. Anteromedial, medial, and posteromedial directions were found to represent the best directions to discriminate those with ankle instability from healthy individuals [52]. The posteromedial direction had the highest correlation to overall SEBT performance with factor analysis ($\alpha = 0.96$) [52]. Individuals with an anterior reach distance difference greater than 4 cm between lower extremities were 2.5 times more likely to sustain a lower extremity injury. Females with a composite reach distance of less than 94% of their lower extremity length were 6.5% more likely to sustain a lower extremity injury [48].

Intervention

In a pathoanatomical model, there are three primary categories of peroneal tendon lesions: (1) tendinitis and tenosynovitis, (2) tendon subluxation and dislocation, and (3) tendon tears and ruptures. There are various models of tendon pathology in the literature that can generally be categorized based upon the primary feature of the pathology, including collagen disruption, inflammation, and tendon cell response, among others [55]. Regardless, gearing interventions toward the appropriate tendon pathology stage is of the utmost importance. The continuum model, proposed by Cook and Purdham, proposes interventions based upon the stages of pathology being either in a reactive tendinopathy/early tendon dysrepair versus late tendon dysrepair/degeneration [56]. In the reactive stage, pharmacological management focuses on reduction of inflammation and minimization of tenocyte upregulation. Physical rehab includes load management, with assessment to determine and alter the harmful load, as well as adjustment of intensities and frequencies accordingly [56]. In the late, degenerative phases of tendon pathology, the primary focus is to stimulate cellular activity and increase protein production to potentially facilitate restructuring and repair, though literature suggests this may not actually occur. Pharmacological interventions may include options such as prolotherapy, whereas physical management may include eccentric training and friction therapy among others. Pain may have an influence anywhere within these stages. Pain management will also be integral to moving through the continuum with the ultimate goal of improving tendon load capacity and overall function.

Tendons are tissues responsible for transferring forces from muscle to bone. It is important to recognize that rest is detrimental in the long term to tendons. To maintain tendon health, normal, physiologic loads are necessary to maintain homeostasis of the tendon tissue and ultimately prevent increased degradation of the extracellular matrix [57]. Mechanotransduction is a process in which cells turn mechanical stimulus into electrochemical activity. Tendons respond to normal and abnormal mechanical stresses, including the direction, frequency, magnitude, and duration of these stresses. Tendons are exposed to tensile, compressive, and shear forces. Exposing these tissues to external forces at the appropriate point within the pathological process (exercise, manual therapy, etc.) and normalizing the forces during function provide an optimal environment for tendon healing.

Conservative Management of Specific Peroneal Tendon Pathologies

Peroneal Tendonitis/Tenosynovitis

Patients with peroneal tendinitis respond well to conservative treatment including NSAIDs, lateral heel wedges, and possibly a period of immobilization when symptoms are severe [58]. Physical therapy intervention is also recommended. Physical therapy should follow an impairment-based approach and include stretching and strengthening activities, use of tools such as a biomechanical ankle platform system (BAPS) board, manual therapy to improve ankle dorsiflexion and eversion, and balance/proprioceptive activities. Additional physical agents such as electrical stimulation, ultrasound, and low-level laser therapy may be indicated as well.

Peroneal Tendinopathy

Due to the chronic, degenerative nature of peroneal tendinopathy, an antiinflammatory approach to management of this condition is not recommended. NSAIDs and corticosteroids have not demonstrated long-term effectiveness in managing this condition, though short pain relief may be achieved. Physical therapy management may require the use of highly specific therapeutic exercise programs. Eccentric strengthening and mixed concentric–eccentric strengthening programs have been advocated in the treatment on Achilles tendinopathy and lateral epicondylitis. Other modalities such as low-level laser, ultrasound, deep friction massage, iontophoresis, and phonophoresis have been documented. Low-level laser and therapeutic ultrasound have demonstrated mixed results in effectiveness during clinical trials. Deep friction massage has demonstrated minimal benefit. Iontophoresis and phonophoresis involve the use of anti-inflammatory medications, again with minimal benefits demonstrated.

Painful Os Peroneum Syndrome (POPS)

Patients with POPS are initially treated with conservative modalities. This includes NSAIDs, lateral heel wedges, physical therapy, and possibly a period of immobilization if painful tenderness is present. Physical therapy should include stretching and strengthening activities, proprioceptive training, and other modalities employed by the therapist, including massage therapy and modalities as indicated. If a period of immobilization is required, a short leg weight-bearing cast or CAM boot may be initiated to control inflammation. Once the pain subsides, patients start with physical therapy.

Peroneal Tendon Dislocation

Nonoperative treatment may be attempted for acute peroneal tendon dislocations; however, it is associated with a high rate of recurrence, particularly in athletes who subject the peroneal tendons to high stresses. Conservative management may involve immobilization in a short leg cast with the foot in neutral to slight inversion to allow the superior peroneal retinaculum to heal to the posterolateral aspect of the fibula [1].

Peroneal Tendon Tears

Patients with peroneal tendon tears can be initially treated with conservative modalities. This includes NSAIDs, lateral heel wedges, physical therapy, and possibly a period of immobilization if there is painful tenderness or edema. Physical therapy should include stretching and strengthening activities, use of a BAPS board, and other modalities employed by the therapist, including massage therapy, ultrasound, and electrical stimulation as indicated. If a period of immobilization is required, a short leg weight-bearing cast or CAM boot may be initiated to control inflammation. Once the pain subsides, patients start with physical therapy.

Conservative treatment of peroneal tendon tears includes NSAIDs, physical therapy, activity modification, and immobilization in a brace or short leg walking cast. However, symptoms frequently persist despite nonoperative management, especially in the setting of chronic ankle laxity, chronic peroneal tendon subluxation, or hindfoot varus deformity [59, 60].

Rehabilitation Strategies

Modalities

There are a variety of therapeutic modalities available to the practitioner. Selection of the appropriate modality is based upon the therapeutic outcome that is desired and the timing of the use of the modality. Therapeutic ultrasound has been a modality of choice for many years. Generally, the literature has not shown benefit of utilizing therapeutic ultrasound in addition to exercise programs and to low-level laser. Low-level laser therapy has demonstrated some potential in accelerating healing, though the level of clinical research is low. Therapeutic ultrasound and low-level laser therapy may have more benefit in the management of pain at various stages of the healing process. Utilizing them in isolation is not recommended, but rather should be done as an adjunct to physical management strategies.

Manual Therapy

Manual therapy procedures, such as joint mobilizations, manipulations, and mobilization with movement techniques, are utilized to improve ankle ROM and proprioception in patients suffering from peroneal injuries, ankle sprains, and other ankle pathologies.

Joint mobilizations are recommended to improve ankle mobility and have been shown to improve pain, range of motion, and function in inversion ankle sprains [61–64]. Methods to improve ankle dorsiflexion include talar thrust distraction manipulation, talocrural posterior talar glides, and weight-bearing mobilization with movement. Talar thrust distractions are a perfect technique to be used in peroneal tendon injuries because the ankle is placed in slight eversion prior to the thrust, reducing stress on the tendons. The technique is performed in supine, ideally with the patient's lower leg stabilized to the table. The therapist overlaps their hands and their fifth digits are placed over the anterior talus. The ankle is placed into slight dorsiflexion and eversion and a high velocity, low amplitude thrust longitudinally is performed. This can be performed multiple times in varying degrees of dorsiflexion if needed, but even one manipulation can create a cavitation or "pop" that creates relaxation in the surrounding musculature, decreases pain, and improves range of motion (see Fig. 7.10).

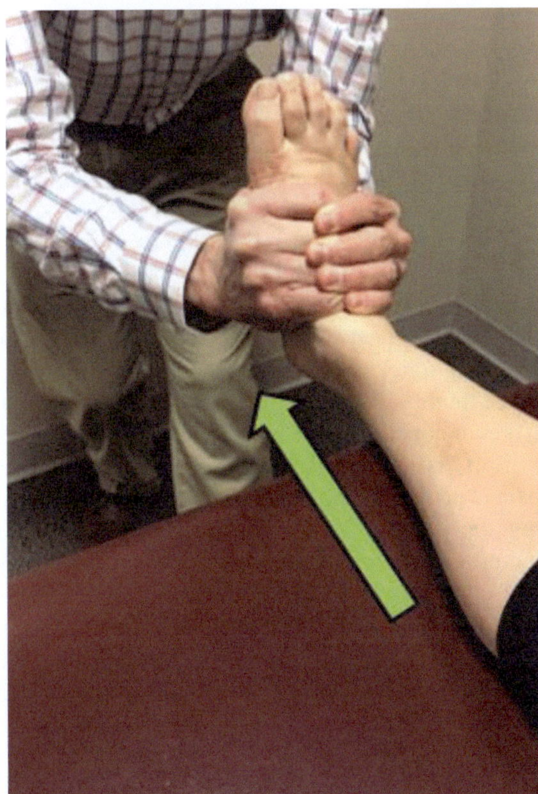

Fig. 7.10 Talar thrust distraction

When performing posterior talar joint mobilizations, it is important to take into account the total arc of motion between dorsiflexion and plantarflexion. The open packed position of the ankle is slight plantarflexion and is the preferred position for posterior talar mobilizations, but if the patient is already lacking dorsiflexion, the ankle might need to be placed in further PF. A clinical indication that this is required is a patient feeling "pinching" in the anterior ankle during the technique. When performing mobilization, it is important to stabilize the posterior distal tibia with the table or a bolster and your hand while performing the posteriorly directed force at the talus with the mobilizing hand. Using your leg on the plantar surface of the foot can help stabilize the foot plantar flexion angle while the hand performs the mobilization.

Mobilization with movement (MWM) was originally described by Brian Mulligan in 1995. A therapist applies a passive glide mobilization to a joint (usually an accessory motion) and sustains it while the client performs a physical task involving the limbs. The mobilization with movement can be performed in a supine, non-weight-bearing position or in a weight-bearing position. The recommended position for weight-bearing is with the patient's foot on a chair or table. The practitioner places a belt or strap on the distal tibia and stabilizes the foot on the table with their hands. Then to mobilize the belt is used to provide a posterior to anterior force on the tibia while the patient moves the knee over the toes. It is important that the belt stays perpendicular to the tibia to create even pressure on the posterior leg and to prevent pinching.

Subtalar joint mobilizations can be used to help improve ankle eversion and reduce the need for lateral heel wedges or taping.The preferred position side-lying is with the patient on the involved side. The practitioner stabilizes the forefoot in a dorsiflexed and everted position and the mobilizing hand is placed on the calcaneus, mobilizing into eversion (see Fig. 7.11).

Cuboid Whip: The cuboid whip can improve joint mobility and improve pronation. The technique is performed in prone with the lower leg in a 45-degree knee flexion foot off the table. The practitioner grasps the midfoot overlapping thumbs on the plantar aspect of the cuboid. The thrust is performed by moving the foot and lower leg quickly toward the knee extension, which rapidly plantar flexes the ankle as the thumbs provide the plantar to dorsal thrust to the cuboid as shown in Fig. 7.12. It is common to use the supination correction taping technique after this manipulation.

Soft Tissue Mobilization can be used to improve flexibility, reduce swelling and pain in peroneal tendon injuries, and ankle sprains. There is weak evidence supporting the efficacy of Instrument Assisted Soft Tissue Mobilization(IASTM) for increasing lower extremity joint ROM for a short period of time [65]. There is minimal evidence to support the use of soft tissue mobilization to promote ligament healing with IASTM. Loghmani and Warden [66] investigated the potential utility of manual therapy in the form of IASTM on ligament healing. Results indicate that IASTM-treated ligaments were 43% stronger, 40% stiffer, and able to absorb 57% more energy than contralateral, nontreated, injured ligaments at 4 weeks following injury. These mechanical differences may have resulted from favorable effects of IASTM on the organization of the underlying collagen substructure. IASTM should

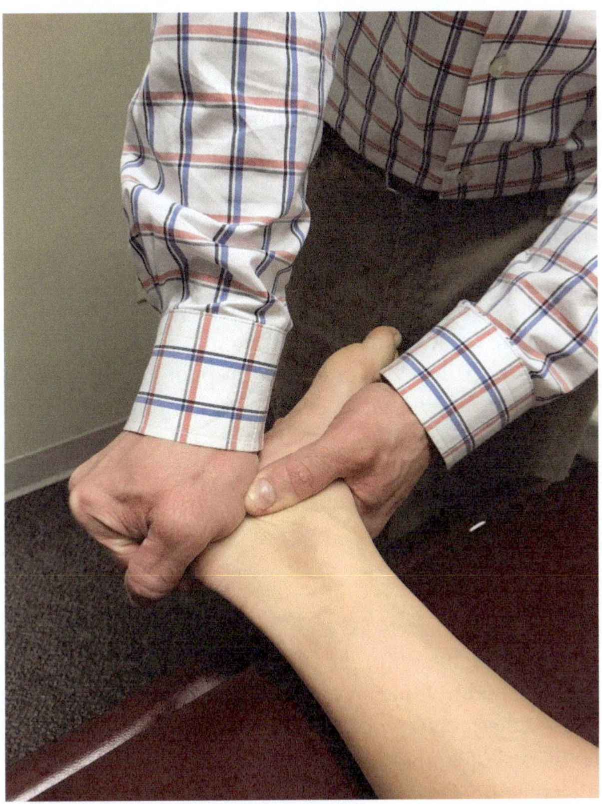

Fig. 7.11 Subtalar lateral mobilization for eversion

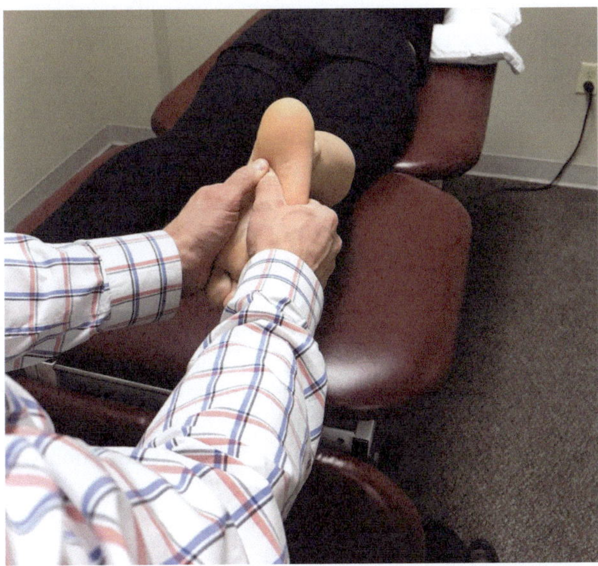

Fig. 7.12 Cuboid whip manipulation technique

NOT be a considered a primary intervention in the treatment of peroneal tendon injuries but may provide some improvement in flexibility in those lacking ankle dorsiflexion. Soft tissue mobilization can be an effective intervention for reducing pain and improving muscle guarding and pain in the region of the peroneal muscles and should be considered in cases of peroneal tendonitis.

Trigger Point Dry Needling

There is some evidence that the inclusion of Trigger Point Dry Needling (TrP-DN) within the lateral peroneus muscle into a proprioceptive/strengthening exercise program results in better outcomes in pain and function 1 month after the end of the therapy in individuals with ankle instability [67]. There is still limited evidence at this time but it should be considered for cases of peroneal tendonitis to help reduce pain and improve function.

Taping/Bracing

With the high incidence and subsequent financial burden of ankle sprains, focus on preventative measures is imperative. Prophylactic taping, bracing, neuromuscular training, and wearing special shoes have all been theorized to positive effects of reducing incidence and severity of ankle sprains. Individuals suffering from a lateral ankle sprain become prone to developing chronic mechanical (such as ligamentous laxity) and functional (neuromuscular deficiency without ligament laxity) ankle instability [68, 69]. Individuals with mechanical and functional ankle instability have been shown to achieve the best sprain recurrence prevention with use of external prophylactic support such as taping and/or bracing, along with neuromuscular training [70, 71].

The impact of taping and brace is unclear. While reports of possible proprioceptive benefits have been made, evidence suggests that neither taping or bracing increases joint position sense or movement sense [72]. Benefits of taping likely revolve around the impact of the external modality on ankle kinematics, particularly during the stance phase of gait.

Nonelastic Athletic Taping

Taping is arguably the most commonly used measure to prevent ankle sprains. The literature have demonstrated significantly lower ankle sprain rates in taped individuals as compared to untaped, most notably in individuals with a previous history of sprain [73, 74]. A variety of forms of taping methods and materials have become prevalent in the market, though the most commonly examined in the literature is nonelastic athletic taping (see Fig. 7.13).

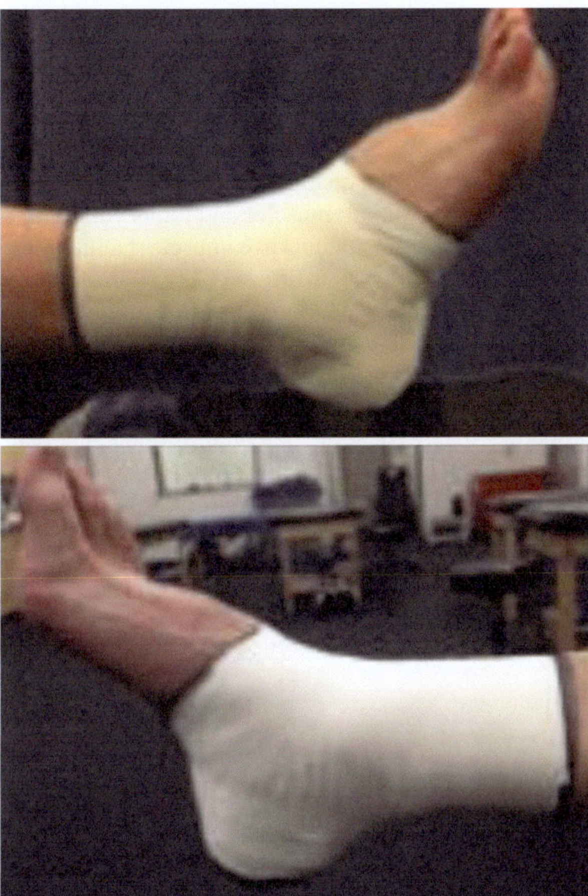

Fig. 7.13 Basket-Weave athletic taping for ankle stability

Practitioners have used a closed basket-weave technique with nonelastic white athletic tape (WAT) as the taping standard for treatment and prevention of ankle injuries [75]. This taping method can effectively limit ankle inversion to avoid strain on the lateral talocrural ligaments [76]. WAT is the current standard for treatment and prevention of ankle injuries, having shown the ability to limit ankle ROM in all directions, which may be advantageous in the prevention of ankle injuries [77–79]. However, previous studies have indicated some faults of this taping method, including discomfort, mechanical loosening after activity, and restriction of ROM in all directions [79, 80]. Other methods including the use of one similar to a lateral wedge orthosis is performed with leukotape. The tape is fixated at the medial calcaneus and pulled across the plantar surface of the foot across the cuboid crossing the talocrural joint. This will help to pull the foot into pronation and reduce the stress on the inflamed peroneal tendons.

Elastic Ankle Taping

There are a variety of forms of elastic tape (kinesiology tape (KT)) that have become prevalent for the treatment of a variety of conditions, particularly in the athletic populations. Unlike typical WAT, KT is made of thin, elastic, adhesive fibers that are intended to mimic the quality of human skin. The theory behind such an elastic tape is to provide stability to muscles and joints without limiting ROM [81, 82]. KT has also been proposed to improve muscle facilitation, enhance joint stability and awareness, and provide a lifting effect to the tissue layers, promoting lymphatic drainage and edema reduction [81, 82]. There is little in the literature supporting the theories of increasing muscle facilitation or inhibiting muscle activation in individuals with ankle pathology. Some evidence suggests that KT may not have proprioceptive benefits in the treatment of ankle injuries [83]. However, the mechanical properties may have some potential in impacting rear foot position during stance, particularly in individuals with chronic ankle instability [84] (see Fig. 7.14).

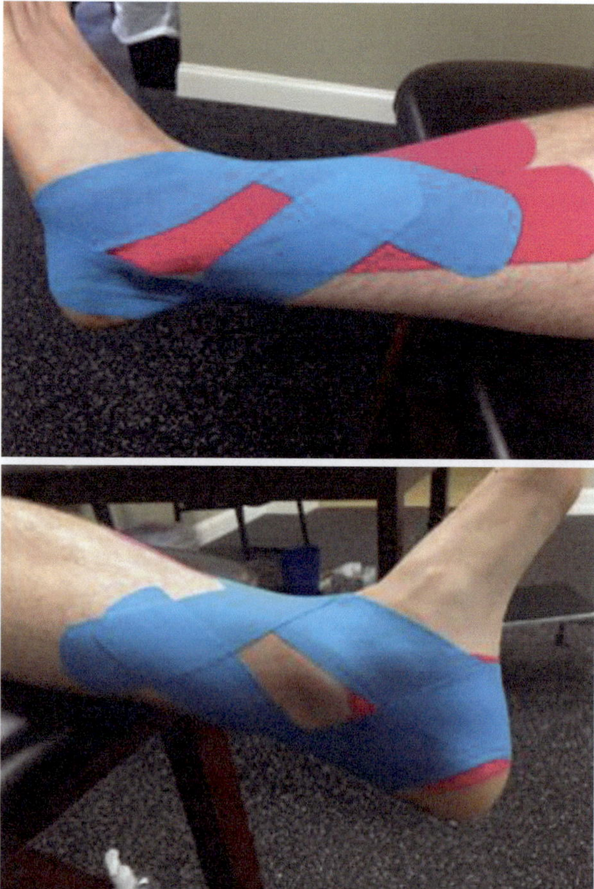

Fig. 7.14 Ankle supportive taping utilizing elastic tape

Ankle Bracing

Bracing has also been demonstrated to be an effective external preventative measure to prevent ankle sprains. Bracing has been shown to be superior to neuromuscular training alone and to have a similar injury rate reduction capacity as ankle taping [85]. Bracing may be the most cost- and time-efficient preventative measure, as the cost and time of application of taping material are limiting factors [73]. Semi-rigid bracing has also been shown to limit ankle ROM, primarily in the frontal plane [86].

Therapeutic Exercise

Prescriptive therapeutic exercise has been demonstrated as perhaps the most important consideration in rehabilitation of tendon pathologies. Considerations must be given to the nature of the pathology and the timing within the rehabilitation process. Biomechanics, muscle performance, ROM, and proprioceptive limitations should all be considered when prescribing therapeutic exercise.

Individuals with injuries impacting the peroneal musculature typically present with weakness in hindfoot eversion. As a result, a propensity toward a more inverted position at initial heel contact in the stance phase may be present, particularly in individuals with chronic ankle instability. Additionally, as the peroneals serve to offset the pull of the muscles that invert the foot, a loss of stability during weight-bearing activities may be demonstrated. Finally, due to the peroneus longus' distal attachments along the medial column of the foot, instability of the first metatarsal and loss of transverse arch height in the fore foot may be present. Exercise progressions to address weakness and the functional manifestations of this weakness are imperative.

Joint proprioception deficits are common with injuries, especially in situations such as chronic ankle instability. Additionally, if immobilization and/or external prophylactic support is utilized to manage a condition, proprioceptive deficits may be present. There are many forms of neuromuscular re-education and proprioceptive exercises to help address some of these deficits. Non-weight-bearing position replication activities are helpful early in the rehabilitation program and, as healing allows, progression to weight-bearing balance including reactive activities will aid in improving proprioception. Finally, progressing to functionally specific activities for the patient is key to return to a prior level of function.

Optimization of biomechanics and function should be involved in the rehabilitation of all foot and ankle injuries. This includes improving strength and function of foot intrinsic musculature to improve stability of the foot arches. This is specifically relevant to the function of the peroneal musculature. An overly pronated foot in weight-bearing is associated with a decrease in the height of the arches in the foot. This can impact the line of pull of the peroneal muscles, creating potential for altered load on the tendon and a decrease in the function of the muscle. There is a subsequent increase in potential for abnormal stress in other areas of the foot. An overly supinated foot has a propensity for increased lateral loading and a higher

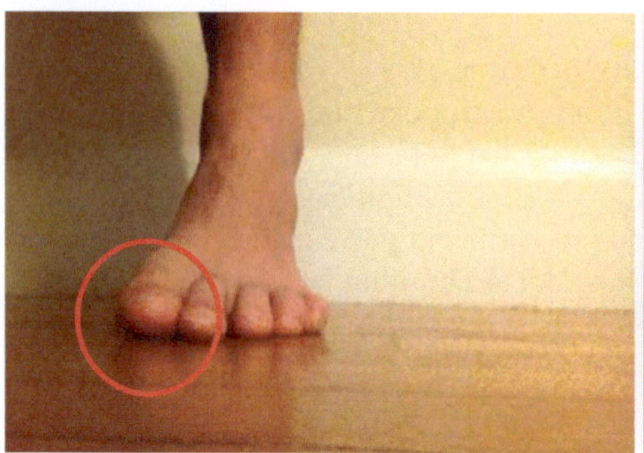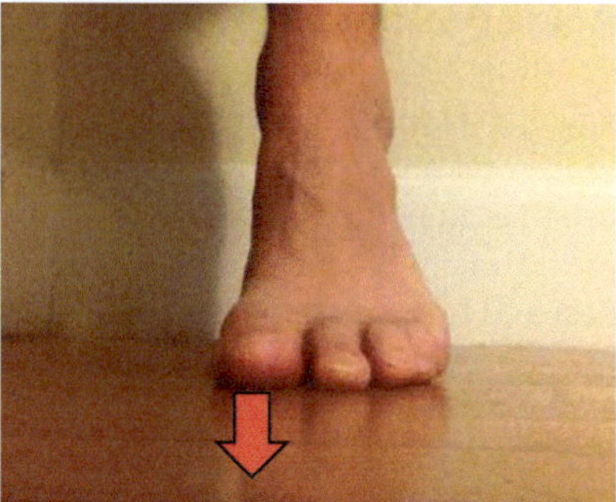

Fig. 7.15 Calf raise exercise with focus on accentuating ground contact of the first metatarsal (peroneus longus focus)

potential for inversion injuries, both of which can subject the peroneal muscles to injury. In addition to intrinsic muscle function, focused exercise addressing the function of the extrinsic muscles is imperative. This includes, but is certainly not limited to, specific exercise to target the functionality of the peroneal muscles in weight-bearing. As the peroneus longus is specifically important to maintaining the stability of the medial column of the foot on the ground during late stance, an exercise such as a heel rise focused on medial column ground contact might be indicated (see Fig. 7.15).

Muscle contraction type, repetition, and load are also very important concepts to consider when prescribing exercise, specifically those pertaining to the injured tissue. Pain may be a limiting factor in exercise prescription. Isolating muscles early with isometric contractions has the potential for improving cortical awareness and may have the potential to improve pain. Eccentric loading exercises have demonstrated success as a strategy in the remodeling phases of rehabilitation, specifically in degenerative tendon pathologies [56].

Prevention

In order to reduce the prevalence of peroneal tendon injuries, we must reduce lateral ankle sprain, lateral ankle sprain recurrence, and development of chronic ankle instability. Activity-specific proprioceptive training, strengthening, and prophylactic bracing as indicated are all potential injury prevention strategies.

Summary

As with any region of the body, the key to successful rehabilitation of peroneal tendon injuries is program specificity. There is no "one size fits all" treatment. Identification of the pathology, associated biomechanics, and functional limitations through a detailed and ongoing evaluation and monitoring of treatment response are all imperative to successful rehabilitation.

References

1. Selmani E, Gjata V, Gjika E. Current concepts review: peroneal tendon disorders. Foot Ankle Int. 2006;27(3):221–8.
2. Perry J, Burnfield J. Gait analysis: normal and pathological function. Thorofare: Slack, Inc; 2010.
3. Kokubo T, Hashimoto T, Nagura T, et al. Effect of the posterior tibial and peroneal longus on the mechanical properties of the foot arch. Foot Ankle Int. 2012;33(4):320–5.
4. Baumhauer JF, Alosa DM, Renstrom AF, Trevino S, Beynnon B. A prospective study of ankle injury risk factors. Am J Sports Med. 1995;23(5):564–70.
5. Arnason A, Sigurdsson SB, Gudmundsson A, Holme I, Engebretsen L, Bahr R. Risk factors for injuries in football. Am J Sports Med. 2004;32(1_suppl):5–16.
6. Bahr R, Bahr IA. Incidence of acute volleyball injuries: a prospective cohort study of injury mechanisms and risk factors. Scand J Med Sci Sports. 1997;7(3):166–71.
7. Noronha M, França LC, Haupenthal A, Nunes GS. Intrinsic predictive factors for ankle sprain in active university students: a prospective study. Scand J Med Sci Sports. 2013;23(5):541–7.
8. Emery CA, Meeuwisse WH. The effectiveness of a neuromuscular prevention strategy to reduce injuries in youth soccer: a cluster-randomised controlled trial. Br J Sports Med. 2010;44(8):555.
9. Engebretsen AH, Myklebust G, Holme I, Engebretsen L, Bahr R. Intrinsic risk factors for acute ankle injuries among male soccer players: a prospective cohort study. Scand J Med Sci Sports. 2010;20(3):403–10.
10. Hiller CE, Refshauge KM, Herbert RD, Kilbreath SL. Intrinsic predictors of lateral ankle sprain in adolescent dancers: a prospective cohort study. Clin J Sport Med. 2008;18(1):44–8.
11. Kofotolis ND, Kellis E, Vlachopoulos SP. Ankle sprain injuries and risk factors in amateur soccer players during a 2-year period. Am J Sports Med. 2007;35(3):458–66.
12. McKay GD, Goldie PA, Payne WR, Oakes BW. Ankle injuries in basketball: injury rate and risk factors. Br J Sports Med. 2001;35(2):103–8.
13. McGuine TA, Keene JS. The effect of a balance training program on the risk of ankle sprains in high school athletes. Am J Sports Med. 2006;34(7):1103–11.
14. Shell IG, Greenberg GH, McKnight R, et al. Decision rules for the use of radiography in acute ankle injuries: refinement and prospective validation. JAMA. 1993;269(9):1127–32.
15. Jonckheer P, Willems T, De Ridder R, et al. Evaluating fracture risk in acute ankle sprains: any news since the Ottawa ankle rules? A systematic review. Eur J Gen Pract. 2016;22(1):31–41.
16. Roth JA, Taylor WC, Whalen J, Roth JA, Taylor WC, Whalen J. Peroneal tendon subluxation: the other lateral ankle injury. Br J Sports Med. 2010;44(14):1047–53.
17. Martin RL, Davenport TE, Paulseth S, Wukich DK, Godges JJ. Ankle stability and movement coordination impairments: ankle ligament sprains. J Orthop Sports Phys Ther. 2013;43(9):A1–40.
18. de Noronha M, Refshauge KM, Herbert RD, Kilbreath SL. Do voluntary strength, proprioception, range of motion, or postural sway predict occurrence of lateral ankle sprain? Br J Sports Med. 2006;40(10):824–8.
19. Pope R, Herbert R, Kirwan J. Effects of ankle dorsiflexion range and pre-exercise calf muscle stretching on injury risk in Army recruits. Aust J Physiother. 1998;44(3):165–72.
20. Andres BM, Murrell GA. Treatment of tendinopathy: what works, what does not, and what is on the horizon. Clin Orthop Relat Res. 2008;466(7):1539–54.
21. Karlsson J, Wiger P. Longitudinal split of the peroneus brevis tendon and lateral ankle instability: treatment of concomitant lesions. J Athl Train. 2002;37(4):463–6.

22. Sobel M, DiCarlo EF, Bohne WH, Collins L. Longitudinal splitting of the peroneus brevis tendon: an anatomic and histologic study of cadaveric material. Foot Ankle. 1991;12(3):165–70.
23. Sobel M, Pavlov H, Geppert MJ, Thompson FM, DiCarlo EF, Davis WH. Painful os peroneum syndrome: a spectrum of conditions responsible for plantar lateral foot pain. Foot Ankle Int. 1994;15(3):112–24.
24. Martin RL, Irrgang JJ. A survey of self-reported outcome instruments for the foot and ankle. J Orthop Sports Phys Ther. 2007;37(2):72–84.
25. Martin RL, Irrgang JJ, Burdett RG, Conti SF, Van Swearingen JM. Evidence of validity for the Foot and Ankle Ability Measure (FAAM). Foot Ankle Int. 2005;26(11):968–83.
26. Binkley JM, Stratford PW, Lott SA, Riddle DL. The Lower Extremity Functional Scale (LEFS): scale development, measurement properties, and clinical application. North American Orthopaedic Rehabilitation Research Network. Phys Ther. 1999;79(4):371–83.
27. Redmond AC, Crane YZ, Menz HB. Normative values for the foot posture index. J Foot Ankle Res. 2008;1(1):6.
28. Redmond AC, Crosbie J, Ouvrier RA. Development and validation of a novel rating system for scoring standing foot posture: the foot posture index. Clin Biomech (Bristol, Avon). 2006;21(1):89–98.
29. Cornwall MW, McPoil TG, Lebec M, Vicenzino B, Wilson J. Reliability of the modified foot posture index. J Am Podiatr Med Assoc. 2008;98(1):7–13.
30. Keenan AM, Redmond AC, Horton M, Conaghan PG, Tennant A. The foot posture index: Rasch analysis of a novel, foot-specific outcome measure. Arch Phys Med Rehabil. 2007;88(1):88–93.
31. McLaughlin P, Vaughan B, Shanahan J, Martin J, Linger G. Inexperienced examiners and the foot posture index: a reliability study. Man Ther. 2016;26:238–40.
32. Delahunt E, Monaghan K, Caulfield B. Altered neuromuscular control and ankle joint kinematics during walking in subjects with functional instability of the ankle joint. Am J Sports Med. 2006;34(12):1970–6.
33. Monaghan K, Delahunt E, Caulfield B. Ankle function during gait in patients with chronic ankle instability compared to controls. Clin Biomech (Bristol, Avon). 2006;21(2):168–74.
34. Martin RL, McPoil TG. Reliability of ankle goniometric measurements: a literature review. J Am Podiatr Med Assoc. 2005;95(6):564–72.
35. Elveru RA, Rothstein JM, Lamb RL. Goniometric reliability in a clinical setting. Subtalar and ankle joint measurements. Phys Ther. 1988;68(5):672–7.
36. Aydog E, Aydog ST, Cakci A, Doral MN. Reliability of isokinetic ankle inversion- and eversion-strength measurement in neutral foot position, using the Biodex dynamometer. Knee Surg Sports Traumatol Arthrosc. 2004;12(5):478–81.
37. Fraser JJ, Koldenhoven RM, Saliba SA, Hertel J. Reliability of ankle-foot morphology, mobility, strength, and motor performance measures. Int J Sports Phys Ther. 2017;12(7):1134–49.
38. Kelln BM, McKeon PO, Gontkof LM, Hertel J. Hand-held dynamometry: reliability of lower extremity muscle testing in healthy, physically active, young adults. J Sport Rehabil. 2008;17(2):160–70.
39. Ancillao A, Palermo E, Rossi S. Validation of ankle strength measurements by means of a hand-held dynamometer in adult healthy subjects. J Sens. 2017;2017:8.
40. Alfuth M, Hahm MM. Reliability, comparability, and validity of foot inversion and eversion strength measurements using a hand-held dynamometer. Int J Sports Phys Ther. 2016;11(1):72–84.
41. Chrintz H, Falster O, Roed J. Single-leg postural equilibrium test. Scand J Med Sci Sports. 1991;1(4):244–6.
42. Forkin DM, Koczur C, Battle R, Newton RA. Evaluation of kinesthetic deficits indicative of balance control in gymnasts with unilateral chronic ankle sprains. J Orthop Sports Phys Ther. 1996;23(4):245–50.
43. Jerosch J, Prymka M. Proprioception and joint stability. Knee Surg Sports Traumatol Arthrosc. 1996;4(3):171–9.

44. Lentell G, Katzman LL, Walters MR. The relationship between muscle function and ankle stability. J Orthop Sports Phys Ther. 1990;11(12):605–11.
45. Bohannon RW, Larkin PA, Cook AC, Gear J, Singer J. Decrease in timed balance test scores with aging. Phys Ther. 1984;64(7):1067–70.
46. Iverson GL, Kaarto ML, Koehle MS. Normative data for the balance error scoring system: implications for brain injury evaluations. Brain Inj. 2008;22(2):147–52.
47. Finnoff JT, Peterson VJ, Hollman JH, Smith J. Intrarater and interrater reliability of the Balance Error Scoring System (BESS). PM R. 2009;1(1):50–4.
48. Plisky PJ, Rauh MJ, Kaminski TW, Underwood FB. Star excursion balance test as a predictor of lower extremity injury in high school basketball players. J Orthop Sports Phys Ther. 2006;36(12):911–9.
49. Gribble PA, Kelly SE, Refshauge KM, Hiller CE. Interrater reliability of the star excursion balance test. J Athl Train. 2013;48(5):621–6.
50. Hertel JMS, Denegar CR. Intratester and intertester reliability during the star excursion balance tests. J Sport Rehabil. 2000;9:104–16.
51. Gribble PA, Hertel J, Denegar CR, Buckley WE. The effects of fatigue and chronic ankle instability on dynamic postural control. J Athl Train. 2004;39:321–9.
52. Hertel J, Braham RA, Hale SA, Olmsted-Kramer LC. Simplifying the star excursion balance test: analyses of subjects with and without chronic ankle instability. J Orthop Sports Phys Ther. 2006;36(3):131–7.
53. Olmsted LC, Carcia CR, Hertel J, Shultz SJ. Efficacy of the star excursion balance tests in detecting reach deficits in subjects with chronic ankle instability. J Athl Train. 2002;37(4):501–6.
54. Hubbard TJ, Kramer LC, Denegar CR, Hertel J. Contributing factors to chronic ankle instability. Foot Ankle Int. 2007;28(3):343–54.
55. Cook JL, Rio E, Purdam CR, Docking SI. Revisiting the continuum model of tendon pathology: what is its merit in clinical practice and research? Br J Sports Med. 2016;50(19):1187–91.
56. Cook JL, Purdam CR. Is tendon pathology a continuum? A pathology model to explain the clinical presentation of load-induced tendinopathy. Br J Sports Med. 2009;43(6):409–16.
57. Galloway MT, Lalley AL, Shearn JT. The role of mechanical loading in tendon development, maintenance, injury, and repair. J Bone Joint Surg Am. 2013;95(17):1620–8.
58. Heckman DS, Gluck GS, Parekh SG. Tendon disorders of the foot and ankle, part 1: peroneal tendon disorders. Am J Sports Med. 2009;37(3):614–25.
59. Krause JO, Brodsky JW. Peroneus brevis tendon tears: pathophysiology, surgical reconstruction, and clinical results. Foot Ankle Int. 1998;19(5):271–9.
60. Redfern D, Myerson M. The management of concomitant tears of the peroneus longus and brevis tendons. Foot Ankle Int. 2004;25(10):695–707.
61. Whitman JM, Cleland JA, Mintken P, et al. Predicting short-term response to thrust and nonthrust manipulation and exercise in patients post inversion ankle sprain. J Orthop Sports Phys Ther. 2009;39(3):188–200.
62. Pellow JE, Brantingham JW. The efficacy of adjusting the ankle in the treatment of subacute and chronic grade I and grade II ankle inversion sprains. J Manipulative Physiol Ther. 2001;24(1):17–24.
63. Vicenzino B, Branjerdporn M, Teys P, Jordan K. Initial changes in posterior talar glide and dorsiflexion of the ankle after mobilization with movement in individuals with recurrent ankle sprain. J Orthop Sports Phys Ther. 2006;36(7):464–71.
64. Cleland JA, Mintken PE, McDevitt A, et al. Manual physical therapy and exercise versus supervised home exercise in the management of patients with inversion ankle sprain: a multicenter randomized clinical trial. J Orthop Sports Phys Ther. 2013;43(7):443–55.
65. Cheatham SW, Lee M, Cain M, Baker R. The efficacy of instrument assisted soft tissue mobilization: a systematic review. J Can Chiropr Assoc. 2016;60(3):200–11.
66. Loghmani MT, Warden SJ. Instrument-assisted cross-fiber massage accelerates knee ligament healing. J Orthop Sports Phys Ther. 2009;39(7):506–14.
67. Salom-Moreno J, Ayuso-Casado B, Tamaral-Costa B, Sánchez-Milá Z, Fernández-de-Las-Peñas C, Alburquerque-Sendín F. Trigger point dry needling and proprioceptive exercises

for the management of chronic ankle instability: a randomized clinical trial. Evid Based Complement Alternat Med. 2015;2015:790209.

68. Hiller CE, Nightingale EJ, Lin CW, Coughlan GF, Caulfield B, Delahunt E. Characteristics of people with recurrent ankle sprains: a systematic review with meta-analysis. Br J Sports Med. 2011;45(8):660–72.

69. Morrison KE, Kaminski TW. Foot characteristics in association with inversion ankle injury. J Athl Train. 2007;42(1):135–42.

70. Verhagen EA, Bay K. Optimising ankle sprain prevention: a critical review and practical appraisal of the literature. Br J Sports Med. 2010;44(15):1082–8.

71. Verhagen EA, van Mechelen W, de Vente W. The effect of preventive measures on the incidence of ankle sprains. Clin J Sport Med. 2000;10(4):291–6.

72. Janssen KW, Kamper SJ. Ankle taping and bracing for proprioception. Br J Sports Med. 2013;47(8):527–8.

73. Olmsted LC, Vela LI, Denegar CR, Hertel J. Prophylactic ankle taping and bracing: a numbers-needed-to-treat and cost-benefit analysis. J Athl Train. 2004;39(1):95–100.

74. Rovere GD, Clarke TJ, Yates CS, Burley K. Retrospective comparison of taping and ankle stabilizers in preventing ankle injuries. Am J Sports Med. 1988;16(3):228–33.

75. Simoneau G. Changes in ankle joint proprioception resulting from strips of athletic tape applied over the skin. J Athl Train. 1997;32:141–7.

76. Beam JW. Orthopedic taping, wrapping, bracing, and padding. 2nd ed. Philadelphia: F. A. Davis Company; 2012.

77. Best R, Mauch F, Bohle C, Huth J, Bruggemann P. Residual mechanical effectiveness of external ankle tape before and after competitive professional soccer performance. Clin J Sport Med. 2014;24(1):51–7.

78. Simoneau GG, Degner RM, Kramper CA, Kittleson KH. Changes in ankle joint proprioception resulting from strips of athletic tape applied over the skin. J Athl Train. 1997;32(2):141–7.

79. Purcell SB, Schuckman BE, Docherty CL, Schrader J, Poppy W. Differences in ankle range of motion before and after exercise in 2 tape conditions. Am J Sports Med. 2009;37(2):383–9.

80. Cordova ML, Takahashi Y, Kress GM, Brucker JB, Finch AE. Influence of external ankle support on lower extremity joint mechanics during drop landings. J Sport Rehabil. 2010;19(2):136–48.

81. Bicici S, Karatas N, Baltaci G. Effect of athletic taping and kinesiotaping(R) on measurements of functional performance in basketball players with chronic inversion ankle sprains. Int J Sports Phys Ther. 2012;7(2):154–66.

82. Briem K, Eythorsdottir H, Magnusdottir RG, Palmarsson R, Runarsdottir T, Sveinsson T. Effects of kinesio tape compared with nonelastic sports tape and the untaped ankle during a sudden inversion perturbation in male athletes. J Orthop Sports Phys Ther. 2011;41(5):328–35.

83. Halseth T, McChesney JW, Debeliso M, Vaughn R, Lien J. The effects of kinesio taping on proprioception at the ankle. J Sports Sci Med. 2004;3(1):1–7.

84. Yen SC, Folmar E, Friend KA, Wang YC, Chui KK. Effects of kinesiotaping and athletic taping on ankle kinematics during walking in individuals with chronic ankle instability: a pilot study. Gait Posture. 2018;66:118–23.

85. Janssen KW, van Mechelen W, Verhagen EA. Bracing superior to neuromuscular training for the prevention of self-reported recurrent ankle sprains: a three-arm randomised controlled trial. Br J Sports Med. 2014;48(16):1235–9.

86. Cordova ML, Ingersoll CD, LeBlanc MJ. Influence of ankle support on joint range of motion before and after exercise: a meta-analysis. J Orthop Sports Phys Ther. 2000;30(4):170–7; discussion 178–182.

87. Chagas-Neto FA, de Souza BN, Nogueira-Barbosa MH. Painful os peroneum syndrome: underdiagnosed condition in the lateral midfoot pain. Case Rep Radiol. 2016;2016:8739362.

88. Oliva F, Frate D, Ferran NA. Peroneal tendons subluxation. Sports Med Arthrosc Rev. 2009;17(2):105–11.

89. Lee JS, Kim KB, Jeong JO, Kwon NY, Jeong SM. Correlation of foot posture index with plantar pressure and radiographic measurements in pediatric flatfoot. Ann Rehabil Med. 2015;39(1):10–7.
90. Kang MH, Lee DK, Park KH, Oh JS. Association of ankle kinematics and performance on the y-balance test with inclinometer measurements on the weight-bearing-lunge test. J Sport Rehabil. 2015;24(1):62–7.
91. Lee DK, Kang MH, Lee TS, Oh JS. Relationships among the Y balance test, berg balance scale, and lower limb strength in middle-aged and older females. Braz J Phys Ther. 2015;19(3):227–34.

Conservative Treatment of Peroneal Tendon Injuries: Peroneal Tendon Sheath Ultrasound-Guided Corticosteroid Injection

8

David I. Pedowitz, Rachel Shakked, Daniel J. Fuchs, and Johannes B. Roedl

Introduction

Orthopedic surgery has a history replete with efforts to enhance nonoperative management in an effort to avoid surgery which brings with it necessary risks and potential morbidity. In this light, corticosteroid injections have been employed to relieve pain related to myriad inflammatory conditions.

Painful peroneal tendon pathologies fall into three primary categories: tendinopathy, tendon instability (subluxation and dislocation), and tendon tears and ruptures. While sometimes self-limited, peroneal tendon pathology may present with acute traumatic or chronic insidious lateral ankle pain that may be accompanied by weakness of ankle eversion. Often subsequent to an inversion ankle injury, the inciting event may be acute or chronic.

There is a high occurrence of peroneal pathology in asymptomatic populations and normal variants can simulate pathology on MRI, such as magic angle phenomenon, pseudosubluxation of the peroneus brevis tendon, bifurcated peroneus brevis tendon, or insertion of the peroneus quartus tendon into the peroneus brevis [1]. Because of this, peroneal tendon sheath (PTS) injection with local anesthetic can be a useful diagnostic modality [2, 3].

For symptomatic peroneal tendinopathy and tears, treatment traditionally begins with nonsteroidal anti-inflammatory drugs, rest/activity modification, physical therapy, and immobilization. Surgery is typically reserved for cases refractory to

D. I. Pedowitz (✉) · R. Shakked · D. J. Fuchs
Sidney Kimmel Medical College, Thomas Jefferson University, The Rothman Institute, Philadelphia, PA, USA

J. B. Roedl
Division of Musculoskeletal Imaging and Intervention, Department of Radiology, Thomas Jefferson University Hospital, Philadelphia, PA, USA

© Springer Nature Switzerland AG 2020
M. Sobel (ed.), *The Peroneal Tendons*,
https://doi.org/10.1007/978-3-030-46646-6_8

"

nonoperative treatment methods [4]. There are no evidence-based guidelines on the treatment of peroneal tendon pathology, though in 2018, a group of European foot and ankle surgeons published a consensus document that included proposed treatment progression based on etiology [4, 5]. They were unable to reach consensus on the use of corticosteroid injections as therapeutic or diagnostic tools because of limited published data [4]. In this light, most orthopedists use corticosteroid injections sparingly because of the fear of spontaneous tendon rupture.

Although there is some evidence of spontaneous tendon rupture when injections are used for lateral epicondylitis or trigger thumb, there are limited case reports supporting an increased risk of spontaneous peroneal tendon rupture following injection [6–8].

At the authors' institution, PTS injections are offered when other nonoperative modalities have failed, and are performed under ultrasound guidance to increase accuracy and avoid intratendinous injection. [2]

A recent investigation at the authors' institution looked at the clinical outcomes and safety of ultrasound-guided corticosteroid injection of the peroneal tendon sheath for chronic tendinopathy or tears. The goal of the intervention was to decrease pain and increase function without seeing a concomitant increased incidence of spontaneous tendon rupture or any other PTS-related complication.

Techniques

Diagnostic Ultrasound

For the diagnostic ultrasound, the patient is in a slightly lateral position leaning over to the contralateral side, as shown in Fig. 8.1. Using a 15 MGHz small foot print ultrasound probe (e.g., hockey stick probe), both peroneal tendons are scanned from their myotendinous junction at the mid fibula to the level of the fibular groove and distally to their insertions on the fifth metatarsal base (peroneus brevis) and on the first metatarsal base (peroneus longus).

Peroneal tendons are assessed for tendinosis (tendon thickening) and tendon tears. Tears are, in general, either partial-thickness or full-thickness split tears and most commonly occur at the level of the fibular groove or just distal to it (in the subfibular region) or at the level of a prominent peroneal tubercle. If it is a partial-thickness tear, further distinction between low-grade partial thickness tears (involving less than 50% of the tendon thickness) and high-grade partial thickness tears (more than 50% of the tendon thickness) is made. For the peroneus brevis tendon, the typical progression of pathology is from thinning of the tendon in a "U" or "boomerang" shape with the peroneus longus "pushing" into the "U" (Fig. 8.2), then development of a partial thickness split tear at the apex of the "U" (Fig. 8.3), and then a full-thickness split tear of the peroneus brevis tendon, resulting in two tendons limbs. The peroneus longus then herniates in between the two peroneus brevis limbs (Fig. 8.4).

Additionally, the presence of tenosynovitis is evaluated (Fig. 8.5) and color flow (Fig. 8.6) is assessed indicating the degree of acute inflammation.

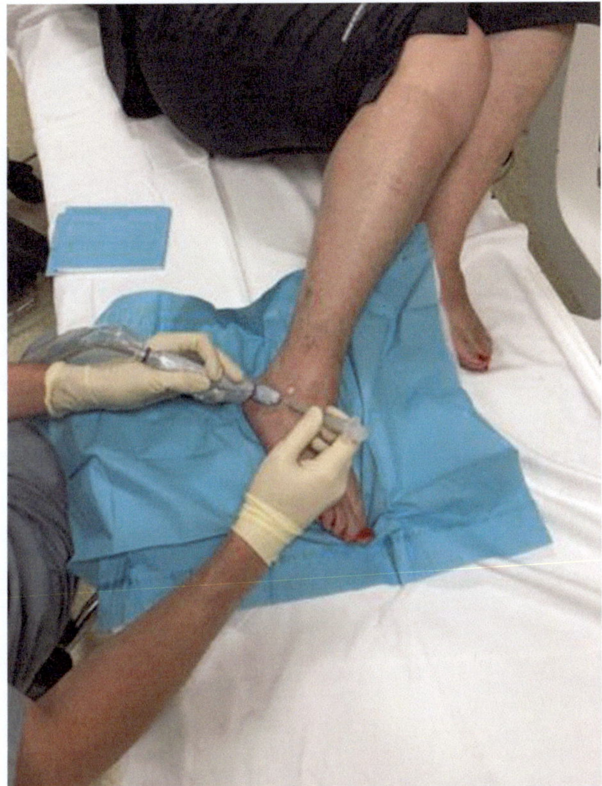

Fig. 8.1 Patient positioning

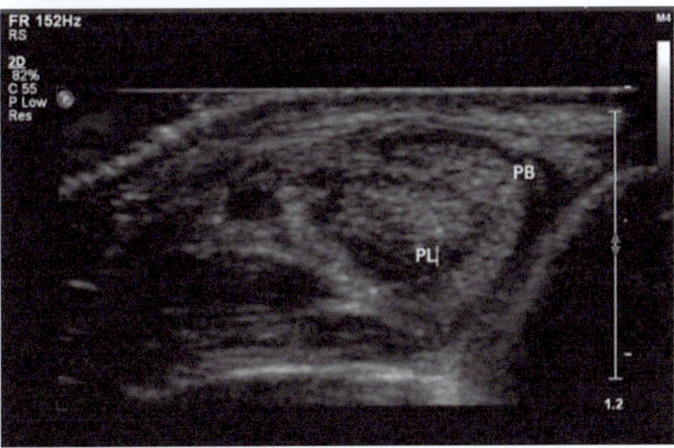

Fig. 8.2 Thinning of the peroneus brevis tendon with a "boomerang" shape

Lastly, intrasheath subluxation of the peroneal tendons is evaluated with dynamic ultrasound by having the patient perform a circumduction movement of the foot by instructing the patient to slowly draw a big circle with the great toe. In patients with subluxation, the peroneus brevis and longus tendons snap around each other and change positions during the circumduction (Figs. 8.7, 8.8, and 8.9).

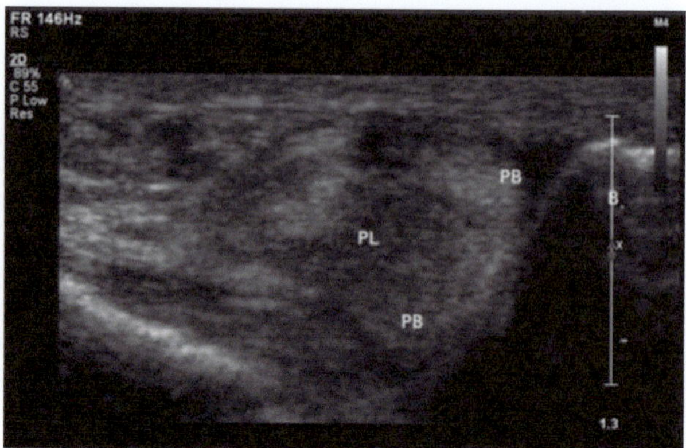

Fig. 8.3 Partial-thickness split tear of the peroneus brevis tendon with the peroneus longus tendon pushing into the peroneus brevis

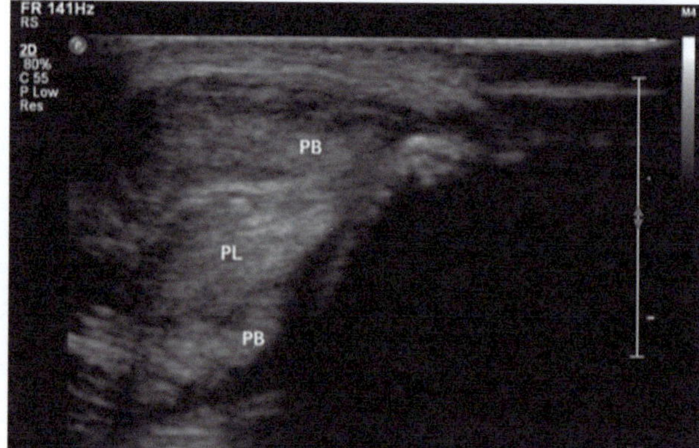

Fig. 8.4 Full-thickness split tear of the peroneus brevis tendon

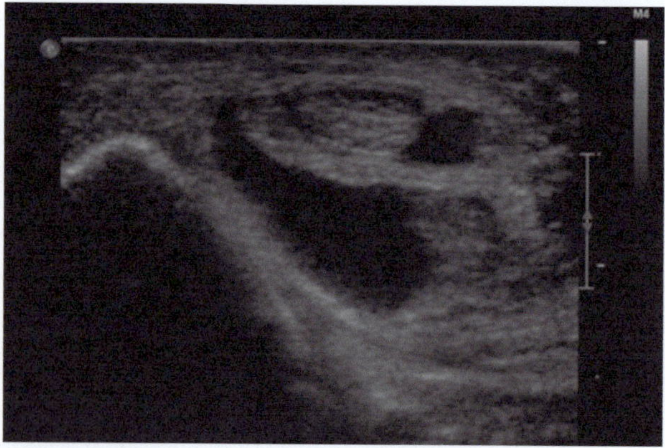

Fig. 8.5 Moderate to severe tenosynovitis of the peroneal tendon sheath

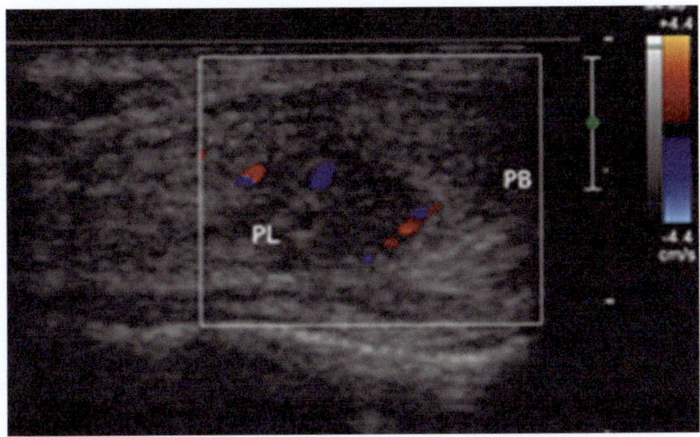

Fig. 8.6 Mild tenosynovitis with increased color flow (indicating acute inflammation)

Ultrasound-Guided Injection

The skin is first prepped in a sterile fashion and all instruments and the working field are draped with sterile coverings (Fig. 8.1). We recommend to inject at the level of the subfibular region between the levels of fibular tip and the peroneal tubercle. At a more proximal level, needle access might be compromised by the nearby fibula, Achilles tendon or sural nerve. A more distal level might not get enough filling of the proximal third of the tendon sheath due to gravity.

Under ultrasound guidance and using a 15 MGHz small foot print ultrasound probe (e.g., hockey stick probe), the tendons are shown in short axis and are easily accessible at that level from a medial approach (Fig. 8.1). A 25-gauge 1.5-inch needle is guided through the subcutaneous fat and is placed in the peroneal tendon sheath, strictly avoiding puncture of the tendons. A 1–2 cm needle track through subcutaneous fat is recommended to avoid back spillage of corticosteroid and subsequent skin depigmentation or atrophy. The track also decreases the risk of infection.

After needle placement in the peroneal tendon sheath, tenosynovial fluid is aspirated (if present) and then a small test injection of local anesthetic is given (0.5 ml) to ensure proper needle placement. A mix of 1% lidocaine and 0.5% bupivacaine is used for the local anesthetic. Then, a mix of 0.5 ml of corticosteroid (3 mg of Betamethasone) and 0.5 ml of local anesthetic is injected into the tendon sheath and appropriate filling is confirmed with ultrasound. Soluble corticosteroid (e.g., Betamethasone or Solumedrol) is recommended for peroneal tendon sheath injections rather than less soluble corticosteroids (e.g., triamcinolone or methylprednisolone) to avoid skin or subcutaneous fat atrophy or skin depigmentation. Pressure is applied (with gauze) on the skin puncture site immediately after the needle is removed and then a bandaid is placed. Patients remove the dressing the next day and have no limitations or restrictions but are seen back at approximately 6 weeks postinjection.

Outcomes

Nonoperative treatment for peroneal tendon tendinopathy or tear typically includes physical therapy, nonsteroidal anti-inflammatory drugs (NSAIDs), activity

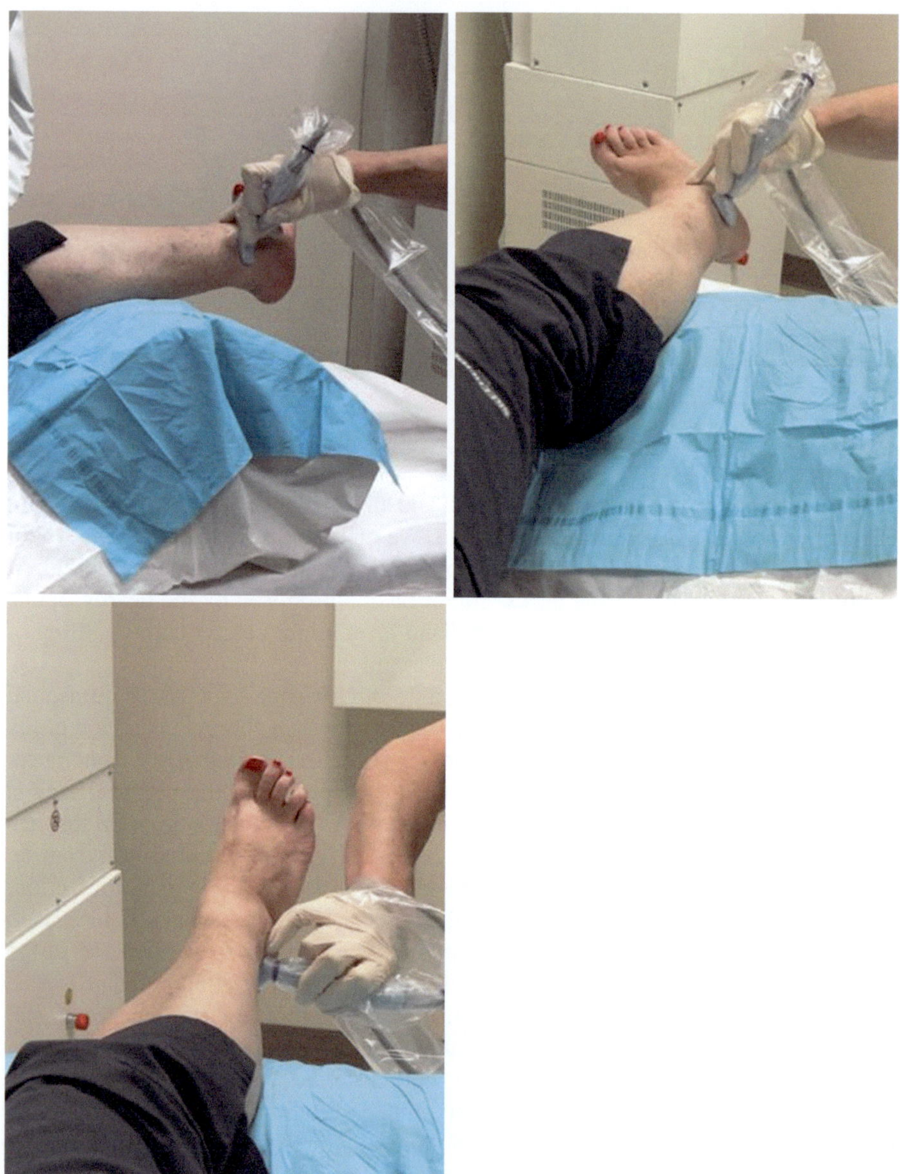

Figs. 8.7, 8.8, and 8.9 Dynamic ultrasound in different phases of foot circumduction to assess for peroneal tendon subluxation

modification, and boot or brace immobilization. Prior to considering surgery, peroneal tendon sheath cortisone injections may be beneficial for diagnostic and therapeutic purposes. There is some concern for spontaneous tendon rupture with cortisone injection adjacent to tendinous structures based on prior case reports [5–7,

9]. However, a recent large retrospective study of 109 injections in 96 patients at the authors' institution found that a single, ultrasound-guided peroneal tendon sheath injection was safe and effective [10]. One injection (0.9%) resulted in peroneus longus tendon tear progression 1 week later; however, the patient had a history of prior amniotic fluid injections at an outside facility as well as prior surgery including peroneus longus tubularization for central tendinopathy. Although most patients only experienced pain relief for a short duration, about one third of patients experienced sustained pain relief for over 3 months. Generally, the injection lasted longest in those patients with shorter duration of symptoms. Multiple injections may increase the risk of tendon rupture [10]. In order to avoid intratendinous injection, which may be associated with higher risk of tendon injury, ultrasound guidance should be utilized. A cadaver study showed 100% accuracy with ultrasound, but only 60% accuracy without ultrasound [2]. A survey study performed in 2011 found that 54% of AOFAS members performed corticosteroid injection for peroneal tendonitis, whereas only 2% performed injections around the midsubstance Achilles tendon [11].

Discussion

Ultrasound-guided peroneal tendon sheath injection is a technique that can be used in the nonoperative treatment of patients with peroneal tendinosis or a peroneal tendon tear. It can be used in conjunction with brace immobilization and physical therapy, and may be helpful in avoiding or delaying surgery. There is a theoretical risk of iatrogenic tendon rupture from corticosteroid injection of tendons about the foot and ankle. However, there is limited evidence available to quantify the risk of iatrogenic rupture of the peroneal tendons or other tendons in the lower and upper extremities. Isolated case reports comprise the bulk of the literature reporting tendon ruptures after corticosteroid injection [5, 12], while a large systematic review of 991 patients reported only one episode of tendon rupture following injection of lateral humeral epicondyle, subacromial bursa, or Achilles tendon [12].

More recent evidence sheds light on the efficacy and risk profile of peroneal tendon sheath corticosteroid injection using ultrasound guidance [10]. Most notably, the risk associated with the injections was very low. There were only two reported complications (1.8%) in 96 patients and 109 injection. These included one sural neuritis and one progression of a peroneus longus tear. Duration of pain relief was mixed with a significant number of patients (44%) only receiving 0–1 weeks of pain relief, while 37% received greater than 12 weeks of relief. Notably, duration of pain relief was related inversely to duration of symptoms prior to the injection. Lastly, 25% of patients went on to have surgery on their peroneal tendons at an average of 151 days after the injection.

Additional investigation is required to better evaluate the efficacy of ultrasound-guided corticosteroid injections of the tendon sheath. Use of a control group of patients who did not receive an injection or received a placebo saline injection would be useful, as well as patient-reported outcome data. Nevertheless, this technique should be considered as part of the nonoperative treatment of peroneal tendon conditions. There is now convincing data that the injection is low risk and can provide sustained relief in a subset of patients. Furthermore, there is diagnostic utility of performing these injections, particularly for the subset of patients who experience temporary pain relief. A temporary positive response to injection has been shown to be predictive of positive long-term results from surgery in other areas of orthopedic surgery [13].

Conclusion

The conservative treatment of peroneal tendon pathology includes a variety of modalities but based on recent data should also include the consideration of ultrasound-guided peroneal tendon sheath corticosteroid injections. Initial data suggest that in recalcitrant cases or in cases in which postoperatively patients develop increased pain and tenderness over the tendons, this technique can be performed safely and with significant symptomatic improvement. While there is a technical skill set involved in performing these injections, they should now be at least considered when traditional nonsurgical modalities have failed to provide adequate relief.

References

1. Wang XT, Rosenberg ZS, Mechlin MB, Schweitzer ME. Normal variants and diseases of the peroneal tendons and superior peroneal retinaculum: MR imaging features. Radiographics. 2005;25(3):587–602.
2. Muir JJ, Curtiss HM, Hollman J, Smith J, Finnoff JT. The accuracy of ultrasound-guided and palpation-guided peroneal tendon sheath injections. Am J Phys Med Rehabil. 2011;90(7):564–71.
3. Resnick D, Goergen TG. Peroneal tenography in previous calcaneal fractures. Radiology. 1975;115(1):211–3.
4. van Dijk PA, Miller D, Calder J, DiGiovanni CW, Kennedy JG, Kerkhoffs GM, et al. The ESSKA-AFAS international consensus statement on peroneal tendon pathologies. Knee Surg Sports Traumatol Arthrosc. 2018;26(10):3096–107.
5. Smith AG, Kosygan K, Williams H, Newman RJ. Common extensor tendon rupture following corticosteroid injection for lateral tendinosis of the elbow. Br J Sports Med. 1999;33(6):423–4. discussion 4-5
6. Borland S, Jung S, Hugh IA. Complete rupture of the peroneus longus tendon secondary to injection. Foot (Edinb). 2009;19(4):229–31.
7. Madsen BL, Noer HH. Simultaneous rupture of both peroneal tendons after corticosteroid injection: operative treatment. Injury. 1999;30(4):299–300.
8. Simpson MR, Howard TM. Tendinopathies of the foot and ankle. Am Fam Physician. 2009;80(10):1107–14.
9. Cigna E, Ozkan O, Mardini S, Chiang PT, Yang CH, Chen HC. Late spontaneous rupture of the extensor pollicis longus tendon after corticosteroid injection for flexor tenosynovitis. Eur Rev Med Pharmacol Sci. 2013;17(6):845–8.
10. Fram BR, Rogero R, Fuchs D, Shakked RJ, Raikin SM, Pedowitz DI. Clinical outcomes and complications of peroneal tendon sheath ultrasound-guided corticosteroid injection. Foot Ankle Int. 2019;40(8):888–94.

11. Johnson JE, Klein SE, Putnam RM. Corticosteroid injections in the treatment of foot & ankle disorders: an AOFAS survey. Foot Ankle Int. 2011;32(4):394–9.
12. Coombes BK, Bisset L, Vicenzino B. Efficacy and safety of corticosteroid injections and other injections for management of tendinopathy: a systematic review of randomised controlled trials. Lancet. 2010;376(9754):1751–67.
13. Green DP. Diagnostic and therapeutic value of carpal tunnel injection. J Hand Surg Am. 1984;9(6):850–4.

Peroneal Tendonitis and Tendonopathy

Kevin A. Schafer, Samuel B. Adams,
and Jeremy J. McCormick

Tendon Structure and Tendinopathy Pathogenesis

Tendinopathies are some of the most common musculoskeletal conditions afflicting both active and more sedentary patients. These pathologies account for as much as 30% of musculoskeletal consultations [1]. "Tendinopathy" is a broad and nonspecific term used to describe a dysfunctional tendon. More specific terms such as tendinosis, tendonitis, and tenosynovitis refer to the distinct process causing the tendon pathology, although these terms are often incorrectly used interchangeably. Tendonitis refers to inflammation of the tendon proper, usually occurring when the tendon is suddenly overloaded either too rapidly or too forcefully such that microtears result (Fig. 9.1) [2]. Tenosynovitis is also an inflammatory process, with the inflammation occurring in both the tendon and its sheath. As such, only sheathed tendons, such as the peroneals, can develop tenosynovitis [3]. Tendinosis, on the other hand, describes degeneration of the collagen bundles without clear evidence of inflammation.

There has been significant research into the various causes of the more common tendinopathies occurring throughout the body. Classically, chronically painful tendons were presumed to be both painful and dysfunctional secondary to inflammatory processes and were thus commonly referred to as "tendonitis." However, early cellular and histochemical research identified absent or low levels of detectable inflammation in chronic injury settings, challenging this theory [4, 5]. These findings suggested that the most common tendinopathies were degenerative conditions

K. A. Schafer · J. J. McCormick (✉)
Department of Orthopedic Surgery, Washington University School of Medicine,
St Louis, MO, USA
e-mail: kaschafer@wustl.edu; McCormickj@wustl.edu

S. B. Adams
Foot and Ankle Division, Department of Orthopedic Surgery,
Duke University Medical Center, Durham, NC, USA
e-mail: Samuel.adams@duke.edu

© Springer Nature Switzerland AG 2020
M. Sobel (ed.), *The Peroneal Tendons*,
https://doi.org/10.1007/978-3-030-46646-6_9

Pathology	Histologic changes	Graphic
Tendinosis	Intratendinous degeneration of collagen fibers	
Tendinitis	Inflammation of tendon proper	

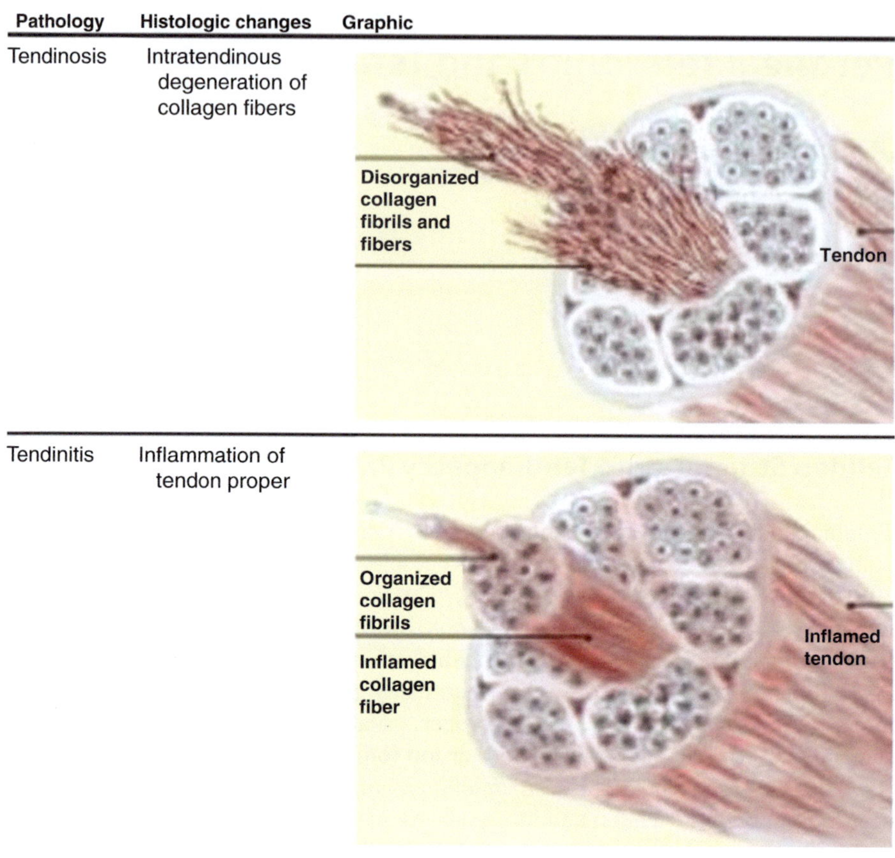

Fig. 9.1 Tendinosis versus tendinitis [3]

secondary to chronic overuse and repetitive strain and were more correctly termed "tendinosis." Nevertheless, more recent investigations in animals and humans suggest a more complex and comprehensive process in which inflammatory mediators alter cellular pathways such that tendon structure changes [6, 7]. As such, the less specific term of "tendinopathy" is currently most appropriately used to discuss this poorly understood process.

Better understanding the pathogenesis of tendinopathy begins with an understanding of the basic structure and function of tendons. Tendons are specialized connective tissues that create motion at joints throughout the body by allowing the transmission of large muscular forces to bone. The peroneal tendons specifically potentiate foot eversion and plantar flexion and stabilize subtalar motion in concert with other dynamic stabilizers. Tendon microstructure is crucial to this function. While tendons are predominantly water (approximately 55% by weight), their dry mass is primarily type I collagen (roughly 70%) [8]. Well-organized type 1 collagen bundles are densely packed and uniformly oriented in tendons, creating a tissue with significant tensile strength [9]. In addition, other molecules such as proteoglycans and elastins help to lubricate and impart elasticity, respectively [10]. Collectively, these biomolecules create a highly specialized tendon matrix and an overall dynamic tissue.

The importance of this overall structure has been highlighted in histopathologic analyses of both healthy and injured tendons. In comparison to healthy tendon, pathologic tendons demonstrate disorganized collagen bundles with loss of parallel alignment, increased proteoglycan and glycosaminoglycan content, and an increase in vascular and nerve ingrowth [9]. Additionally, studies of degenerated tendons have shown significant decreases in total collagen content, an increased proportion of type III to type I collagen, and a number of molecular modifications to the collagen molecules themselves and their interconnections (crosslinks) [11].

While these microscopic changes in tendinopathy have been documented, the ultimate pathogenesis of these changes is poorly understood. Injuries to tendon microstructure and tendon matrix have been shown to induce a remodeling process that is thought to be regulated by destructive and constructive enzymes, growth factors, and signaling molecules [11]. In fact, it is thought that the tendon matrix, similar to bone, is constantly remodeling throughout life. Our current understanding of the pathogenesis of tendinopathy is that a combination of intrinsic and extrinsic factors leads to an imbalance in turnover homeostasis such that the overall tendon structure is altered.

The molecular pathways implicated in this turnover imbalance have not been well defined. One hypothesis, termed the "neurogenic hypothesis," is derived from histologic studies identifying substance P and other neuropeptides in degenerated tendons (Fig. 9.2a) [11–13]. In short, this hypothesis purports that repetitive mechanical strain induces the release of neuromodulators like substance P from afferent nerve fibers, thereby triggering histamine release from mast cells. As a result, several downstream pathways involved in regulating vascular permeability, angiogenesis, cellular differentiation, and extracellular matrix production are altered [11, 14]. Ultimately, tissue homeostasis is disrupted and tendon microstructure is altered such that tendon integrity is impaired. These molecular pathways are thought to be activated in acute injury and function as a normal component of tendon healing and adaptation to exercise (Fig. 9.2b). However, it is hypothesized that chronic activation of these pathways may play a key role in the pathogenesis of degenerative tendinopathies. As such, these pathways may be a potential target for future medical therapies [14]. Overall, these investigations into these pathways highlight that inflammation and chronic tendon degeneration are not exclusive pathologies but rather closely linked processes at the cellular level.

Intrinsic and Extrinsic Factors in Tendinopathy

Although the cellular mechanisms involved in tendinopathy are under active investigation, we must consider why these processes and ultimately tendon failure occur in each individual patient. In each clinical case of tendinopathy, a number of the

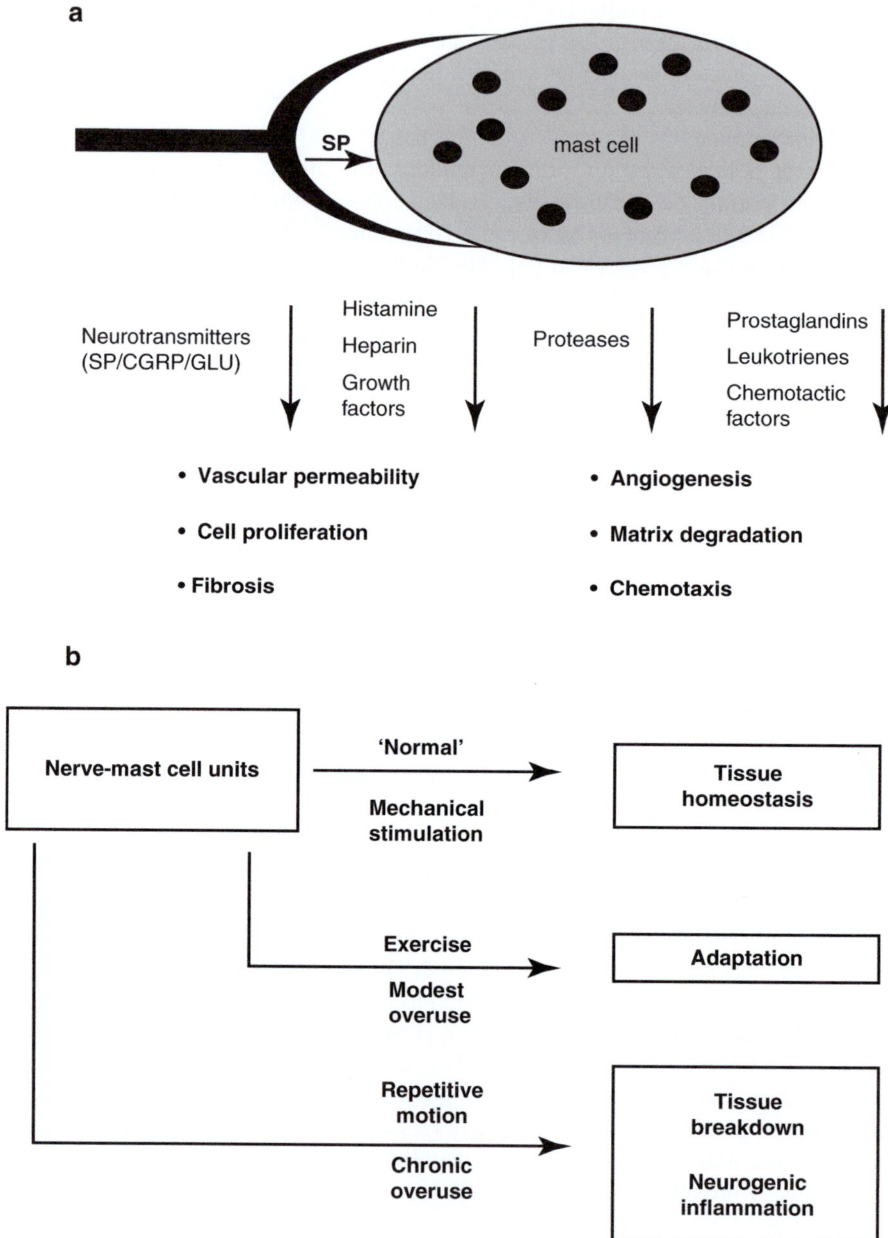

Fig. 9.2 The neurogenic hypothesis of tendinopathy [11]. (**a**) Substance P (SP) is released from sensory neurons, triggering mast cell activation and histamine release. Multiple cellular pathways are affected. (**b**) These pathways are thought to play key roles in normal tissue homeostasis and adaptation to exercise, but they may also damage tendon integrity when chronically activated

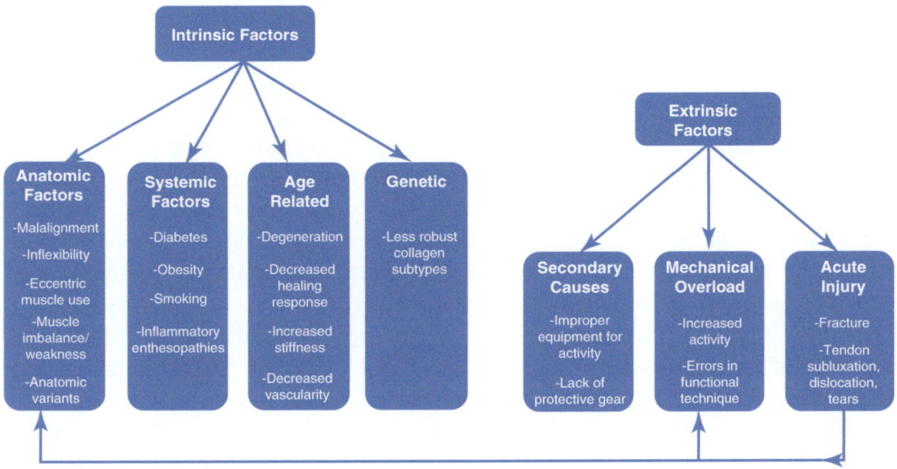

Fig. 9.3 Intrinsic and extrinsic factors in tendinopathy. (Adapted from Federer et al. [3])

following factors likely contribute to a disruption in the remodeling pathways governing tendon homeostasis (Fig. 9.3).

Intrinsic Factors

A number of intrinsic factors can make a patient more susceptible to developing a peroneal tendinopathy. These factors include patient anatomy, vascularity, patient age, genetics, and systemic factors [3, 15].

Each patient's anatomy creates a unique mechanical environment for a tendon. Malalignment, such as in cavovarus foot posture, places increased and repetitive loads on the peroneal tendons in comparison to a more neutral hindfoot alignment in both static and dynamic settings. Similarly, inflexibility, hyperflexibility, muscular weakness, and imbalance can require dynamic stabilizers such as the peroneals to see increased repetitive loads with both basic and more athletic activities.

Additionally, there are several anatomic factors specific to the peroneal tendons that may predispose a patient to injury. A shallow retromalleolar groove has been proposed to alter peroneal tendon stability and potentiate tendon tearing [16]. Also, the superior and inferior peroneal retinaculum can create compression and friction forces on the peroneal tendons, potentially limiting normal tendon gliding and contributing to the development of tenosynovitis. This is particularly common in cases of peroneal tendon or peroneal tendon sheath hypertrophy. Another anatomic variant specific to peroneal tendon pathology is the presence of a prominent peroneal tubercle, a bony projection found on the lateral aspect of the calcaneus that maintains separation between the peroneus longus and brevis tendons [3]. Seen in 40% of individuals, this variant is thought to be associated with tendon tearing and the development of tenosynovitis [17]. Some patients have also been found to have an accessory muscle, termed peroneus quartus, which is thought to contribute to pathology by crowding the peroneus brevis and longus in the peroneal tunnel [18]. Lastly, some patients have been found to have a low-lying muscle belly of the peroneus brevis, with the muscle extending into the fibular groove and crowding the contents of the peroneal tunnel and contributing to the development of tendinopathy [19].

The vascular supply to the tendon is also important to the ability of the tendon to remodel, repair, and maintain its structural integrity. Tendons receive direct vascular supply at both the osseous and musculotendinous junctions. Sheathed tendons such as the peroneals and tibialis posterior receive additional blood supply from the vincula and mesotendon. Both peroneal tendons are primarily vascularized by the peroneal artery, with the peroneus longus also receiving significant vascularization from a branch of the anterior tibial artery at the dorsolateral foot [20]. Despite a robust blood supply, there have been identified zones of each tendon with relatively decreased blood supply, termed watershed or hypovascular zones. These areas are thought to be at increased risk of degeneration secondary to a compromised healing response [3, 21]. However, an anatomic study of the peroneal tendons showed that the entirety of the brevis tendon is well perfused by distal branches of the peroneal artery [20], challenging the theory that the brevis tendon has a hypovascular region at the level of the lateral malleolus [22]. The peroneus longus, however, was found to have a hypovascular zone in 80% of samples (8 of 10 specimens) [20], a finding consistent with prior descriptions of potential watershed regions within the longus tendon at the lateral malleolus or at the cuboid tunnel where the tendon courses past the cuboid toward the plantar aspect of the foot [20, 22].

Increasing age has also been proposed as an intrinsic risk factor for tendon degeneration. Tendon vascularity is known to deteriorate with age, and as such, tendons have decreased resilience and healing potential [23]. Additionally, studies of cellular processes in aging populations have shown that progenitor stem cell counts decrease and that tenocytes have a decreased capacity for protein synthesis [24, 25]. Collectively, these factors make aging tendons less apt to respond to and recover from injury.

A number of recent studies have investigated the role of genetics as an intrinsic factor in tendon and ligament injuries. It has been theorized that genetically driven changes in collagen composition may place certain patients at an increased risk for tendon and ligament injuries. Collagen V, a protein regulating fiber diameter and collagen fiber assembly [26], has been the focus of numerous studies. A recent meta-analysis looked at 11 studies analyzing the role of collagen type V alpha 1 chain (COL5A1) polymorphisms in tendon and ligament injuries, including achilles tendinopathy, lateral epicondylitis, and anterior cruciate ligament rupture [27]. Certain polymorphisms were found to be protective and reduce the risk of tendon and ligament injuries in Caucasian populations. Conversely, other studies have identified particular variants of COL5A1 associated with an increased risk developing tendinopathy [28].

Lastly, systemic factors can result in impaired structural integrity and tendon repair mechanisms. Diabetes mellitus has been studied extensively in both humans and animal models, with diabetics three times more likely to have tendinopathy than nondiabetics [29]. Diabetics have also been shown to have increased tendon size and greater irregularity in fiber bundles in the absence of increased inflammation [30], suggesting a direct disruption of the pathways governing tendon homeostasis and repair. Smoking has similarly been shown to directly affect tendon integrity and to decrease their repair capacity [31]. These findings in both diabetics and smokers are likely due, in part, to the effect of these disease processes on the body's micro- and macrovascular systems [32]. Finally, obesity has been shown to contribute to the development of tendinopathy through weight-driven mechanical overload. Obesity may also have a systemic influence on the development of tendinopathy, as elevated inflammatory mediators such as adipokines and overall dyslipidemia have been investigated in potentially directly altering tendon structure [33, 34].

Extrinsic Factors

The primary extrinsic factor in tendinopathy is mechanical overload. Overload can be secondary to short but high-intensity forces, as well as lower forces experienced with increasing frequency or prolonged durations. As such, overload can occur with both basic lower level and more athletic activities. Factors more commonly seen during athletic activities include technique or training errors (i.e., sudden increases in training intensity or frequency) [35]. Furthermore, improper footwear and certain training surfaces may contribute to overload [35–37]. With regard to mechanical overload, factors creating repetitive loads are of particular concern as these loads are thought to induce repeated microinjuries before the tendon can remodel or repair.

Lastly, acute injuries can disrupt normal tendon health and secondarily create new intrinsic and extrinsic risk factors that were not present prior to injury. Fractures or tendon subluxations or dislocations, for example, can alter static and dynamic anatomy (i.e., inflexibility, muscle imbalance, and altered joint axes), thereby potentiating future injuries and impairing the ability of the tendon to fully recover. These altered anatomic factors may also place a patient at risk for mechanical overload. The acute injury event itself may also disrupt the collagen microstructure in a capacity that is beyond complete remodeling and repair and increase the likelihood of future injury.

Conclusion

In conclusion, peroneal tendinopathies are a complex pathology. The cellular processes governing tendon remodeling and repair are poorly understood, but injury in some way is thought to alter cellular signaling and ultimately tendon microstructure. Practitioners can best approach treatment by considering both the intrinsic and extrinsic patient factors that lead to injury. Identifying these factors, particularly those that are modifiable, can allow for maximal impact on patient recovery and ultimate function. The subsequent chapters in this book will provide a thorough review of the evaluation and treatment of these peroneal tendon problems with the goal of optimizing care for our patients.

References

1. Andarawis-Puri N, Flatow EL, Soslowsky LJ. Tendon basic science: development, repair, regeneration, and healing. J Orthop Res. 2015;33(6):780–4.
2. Bass E. Tendinopathy: why the difference between tendinitis and tendinosis matters. Int J Ther Massage Bodywork. 2012;5(1):14–7.
3. Federer AE, Steele JR, Dekker TJ, Liles JL, Adams SB. Tendonitis and tendinopathy: what are they and how do they evolve? Foot Ankle Clin. 2017;22(4):665–76.
4. Boyer MI, Hastings H 2nd. Lateral tennis elbow: "is there any science out there?". J Shoulder Elb Surg. 1999;8(5):481–91.
5. Khan KM, Cook JL, Kannus P, Maffulli N, Bonar SF. Time to abandon the "tendinitis" myth. BMJ. 2002;324(7338):626–7.
6. Abate M, Silbernagel KG, Siljeholm C, Di Iorio A, De Amicis D, Salini V, et al. Pathogenesis of tendinopathies: inflammation or degeneration? Arthritis Res Ther. 2009;11(3):235.
7. Millar NL, Murrell GA, McInnes IB. Inflammatory mechanisms in tendinopathy – towards translation. Nat Rev Rheumatol. 2017;13(2):110–22.
8. Thorpe CT, Screen HR. Tendon structure and composition. Adv Exp Med Biol. 2016;920:3–10.
9. Xu Y, Murrell GA. The basic science of tendinopathy. Clin Orthop Relat Res. 2008;466(7):1528–38.
10. Chiodo CP. Understanding the anatomy and biomechanics of ankle tendons. Foot Ankle Clin. 2017;22(4):657–64.
11. Riley G. The pathogenesis of tendinopathy. A molecular perspective. Rheumatology (Oxford). 2004;43(2):131–42.
12. Ackermann PW. Neuronal regulation of tendon homoeostasis. Int J Exp Pathol. 2013;94(4):271–86.
13. Ljung BO, Forsgren S, Friden J. Substance P and calcitonin gene-related peptide expression at the extensor carpi radialis brevis muscle origin: implications for the etiology of tennis elbow. J Orthop Res. 1999;17(4):554–9.
14. Han SH, Choi W, Song J, Kim J, Lee S, Choi Y, et al. The implication of substance P in the development of tendinopathy: a case control study. Int J Mol Sci. 2017;18(6).
15. Almekinders LC. Tendinitis and other chronic tendinopathies. J Am Acad Orthop Surg. 1998;6(3):157–64.
16. Heckman DS, Reddy S, Pedowitz D, Wapner KL, Parekh SG. Operative treatment for peroneal tendon disorders. J Bone Joint Surg Am. 2008;90(2):404–18.
17. Bruce WD, Christofersen MR, Phillips DL. Stenosing tenosynovitis and impingement of the peroneal tendons associated with hypertrophy of the peroneal tubercle. Foot Ankle Int. 1999;20(7):464–7.
18. Lui TH. Tendoscopic resection of low-lying muscle belly of peroneus brevis or quartus. Foot Ankle Int. 2012;33(10):912–4.
19. Mirmiran R, Squire C, Wassell D. Prevalence and role of a low-lying peroneus brevis muscle belly in patients with peroneal tendon pathologic features: a potential source of tendon subluxation. J Foot Ankle Surg. 2015;54(5):872–5.
20. van Dijk PA, Madirolas FX, Carrera A, Kerkhoffs GM, Reina F. Peroneal tendons well vascularized: results from a cadaveric study. Knee Surg Sports Traumatol Arthrosc. 2016;24(4):1140–7.
21. McCarthy MM, Hannafin JA. The mature athlete: aging tendon and ligament. Sports Health. 2014;6(1):41–8.
22. Petersen W, Bobka T, Stein V, Tillmann B. Blood supply of the peroneal tendons: injection and immunohistochemical studies of cadaver tendons. Acta Orthop Scand. 2000;71(2):168–74.
23. Funakoshi T, Iwasaki N, Kamishima T, Nishida M, Ito Y, Kondo M, et al. In vivo visualization of vascular patterns of rotator cuff tears using contrast-enhanced ultrasound. Am J Sports Med. 2010;38(12):2464–71.

24. Ippolito E, Natali PG, Postacchini F, Accinni L, De Martino C. Morphological, immunochemical, and biochemical study of rabbit achilles tendon at various ages. J Bone Joint Surg Am. 1980;62(4):583–98.
25. Zhou Z, Akinbiyi T, Xu L, Ramcharan M, Leong DJ, Ros SJ, et al. Tendon-derived stem/progenitor cell aging: defective self-renewal and altered fate. Aging Cell. 2010;9(5):911–5.
26. Birk DE, Fitch JM, Babiarz JP, Doane KJ, Linsenmayer TF. Collagen fibrillogenesis in vitro: interaction of types I and V collagen regulates fibril diameter. J Cell Sci. 1990;95(Pt 4):649–57.
27. Pabalan N, Tharabenjasin P, Phababpha S, Jarjanazi H. Association of COL5A1 gene polymorphisms and risk of tendon-ligament injuries among Caucasians: a meta-analysis. Sports Med Open. 2018;4(1):46.
28. Altinisik J, Meric G, Erduran M, Ates O, Ulusal AE, Akseki D. The BstUI and DpnII variants of the COL5A1 gene are associated with tennis elbow. Am J Sports Med. 2015;43(7):1784–9.
29. Ranger TA, Wong AM, Cook JL, Gaida JE. Is there an association between tendinopathy and diabetes mellitus? A systematic review with meta-analysis. Br J Sports Med. 2016;50(16):982–9.
30. Oliveira RR, Medina de Mattos R, Magalhaes Rebelo L, Guimaraes Meireles Ferreira F, Tovar-Moll F, Eurico Nasciutti L, et al. Experimental diabetes alters the morphology and nanostructure of the achilles tendon. PLoS One. 2017;12(1):e0169513.
31. Lundgreen K, Lian OB, Scott A, Nassab P, Fearon A, Engebretsen L. Rotator cuff tear degeneration and cell apoptosis in smokers versus nonsmokers. Arthroscopy. 2014;30(8):936–41.
32. Chang SA. Smoking and type 2 diabetes mellitus. Diabetes Metab J. 2012;36(6):399–403.
33. Castro AD, Skare TL, Nassif PA, Sakuma AK, Barros WH. Tendinopathy and obesity. Arq Bras Cir Dig. 2016;29 Suppl 1(Suppl 1):107–10.
34. Scott A, Zwerver J, Grewal N, de Sa A, Alktebi T, Granville DJ, et al. Lipids, adiposity and tendinopathy: is there a mechanistic link? Critical review Br J Sports Med. 2015;49(15):984–8.
35. O'Neill S, Watson PJ, Barry S. A Delphi study of risk factors for achilles tendinopathy- opinions of world tendon experts. Int J Sports Phys Ther. 2016;11(5):684–97.
36. Mears AC, Osei-Owusu P, Harland AR, Owen A, Roberts JR. Perceived links between playing surfaces and injury: a worldwide study of elite association football players. Sports Med Open. 2018;4(1):40.
37. Rowson S, McNally C, Duma SM. Can footwear affect achilles tendon loading? Clin J Sport Med. 2010;20(5):344–9.

Acute Subluxation/Dislocation of the Peroneal Tendons

Francesco Oliva, Clelia Rugiero,
Alessio Giai Via, and Nicola Maffulli

Introduction

Peroneal tendon dislocation is an uncommon sport-related injury. The first case was described by Monteggia in 1803 in a ballet dancer [1]. The injury is frequently associated with sports with cutting maneuvers such as judo, gymnastics, soccer, rugby, basketball, ice skating, skiing, water skiing, and mountaineering [2]. Acute subluxation usually occurs while the foot is dorsiflexed with the peroneal muscles strongly contracted [3]. Conservative management of acute subluxation is associated with a high rate of recurrence, and acute peroneal subluxation in high-demand individuals should be primarily managed surgically [4]. Untreated or misdiagnosed acute injury predisposes a patient to pain and recurrent peroneal dislocation [5]. However, recurrent subluxation of the peroneal tendons is uncommon [6].

F. Oliva
Department of Musculoskeletal Disorders, School of Medicine and Surgery,
University of Salerno, Salerno, Italy

C. Rugiero
Orthopaedic and Traumatology Department, University of Roma Tor Vergata,
Tor Vergata Hospital, Rome, Italy

A. Giai Via
Orthopaedic and Traumatology Department, Sant'Anna Hospital, Como, Italy

N. Maffulli (✉)
Department of Musculoskeletal Disorders, School of Medicine and Surgery,
University of Salerno, Salerno, Italy

Queen Mary University of London, Barts and the London School of Medicine and Dentistry,
Centre for Sports and Exercise Medicine, Mile End Hospital, London, UK
e-mail: n.maffulli@qmul.ac.uk

© Springer Nature Switzerland AG 2020
M. Sobel (ed.), *The Peroneal Tendons*,
https://doi.org/10.1007/978-3-030-46646-6_10

Anatomy

The peroneal tendon complex is formed by the tendons of peroneus longus and peroneus brevis. Their insertion is associated with some anatomic variability, which is important to know in order to avoid possible complications [7]. The peroneal tendons share a common tendon sheath proximal to the distal tip of the fibula, with the peroneus brevis medial and anterior to the peroneus longus. More distally, each tendon lies in its own sheath. The common sheath is contained within a sulcus, the fibular groove, on the posterolateral aspect of the fibula, preventing subluxation. The groove is 5–10 mm wide and up to 3 mm deep [8]. The retrofibular groove is formed not by the concavity of the fibula itself but by a relatively pronounced ridge of collagenous soft tissue blended with the periosteum that extends along the posterolateral lip of the distal fibula [4]. The shape of the groove is primarily determined by this thick fibrocartilaginous periosteal cushion, and not by the bone itself [3]. The primary restraint to tendon subluxation is the superior peroneal retinaculum. This fibrous band originates on the posterolateral aspect of the fibula and inserts onto the lateral surface of the calcaneus. It is 10–20 mm wide, is reinforced superficially by transverse fibers, and courses in a posteroinferior direction, although variants in width, thickness, and insertional patterns are not uncommon [8]. The sural nerve is a branch of the tibial nerve [9]. Its proximity to the peroneal groove needs to be considered when planning surgery, as its damage results in loss of sensation to the lateral aspect of the foot.

Pathology

The superior peroneal retinaculum is the primary restraint to subluxation of the peroneal tendons in the fibular groove. Eckert and Davis described three grades of acute tears of the superior retinaculum; a fourth grade was later described by Ogden (Fig. 10.1). In grade 1, the retinaculum is separated from the collagenous lip and lateral malleolus. In grade 2, the collagenous lip is elevated with the retinaculum. In grade 3, a thin sliver of bone, visible on radiographs, is avulsed with the collagenous lip and the retinaculum [4]. In grade 4, the retinaculum is torn away from its posterior attachment on the calcaneus [6]. The superior peroneal retinaculum itself generally remains intact [4]. Clinical determination of injury grade is not possible, except for grade 3 injuries, which can be diagnosed on radiographs.

Clinical Features

Acute dislocation of the peroneal tendons is often misdiagnosed as an ankle sprain and treated by early mobilization, which may increase the risk of chronic dislocation [10]. Patients with recurrent subluxation usually give a history of previous ankle injury often misdiagnosed as a sprain. An unstable ankle that gives way or is associated with a popping or snapping sensation is commonly described. The

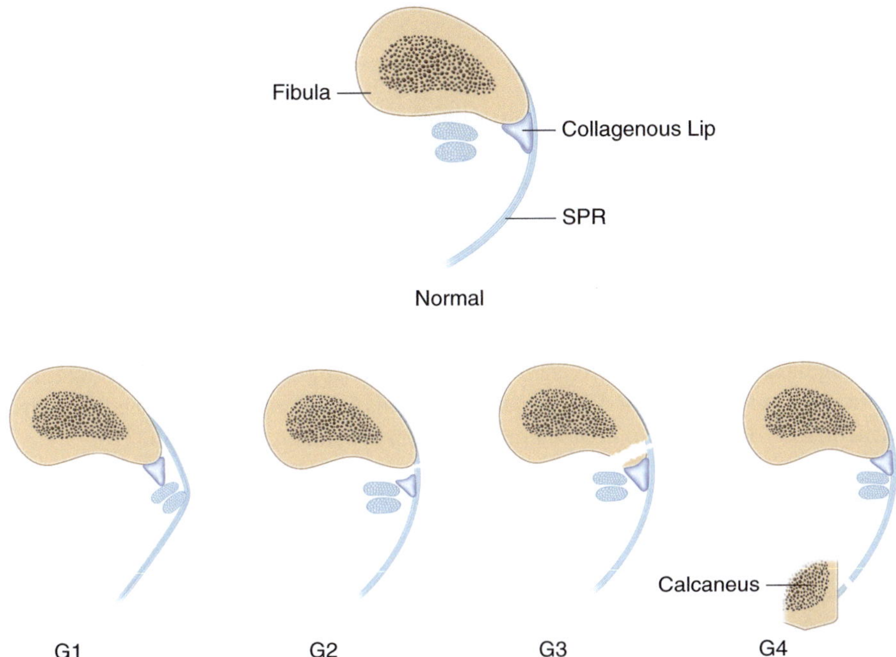

Fig. 10.1 Schematic classification of acute dislocation peroneal tendons according to Ogden. Grade 1: the SPR is ripped from the fibula. Grade 2: the collagenous lip is torn and avulsed together with the retinaculum. Grade 3: a little fragment of bone is avulsed with the retinaculum. Grade 4: the retinaculum is torn from its posterior attachment on the calcaneus. SPR superior peroneal retinaculum, PLT peroneus longus tendon, PBT peroneus brevis tendon

Fig. 10.2 Subluxation of peroneal tendon

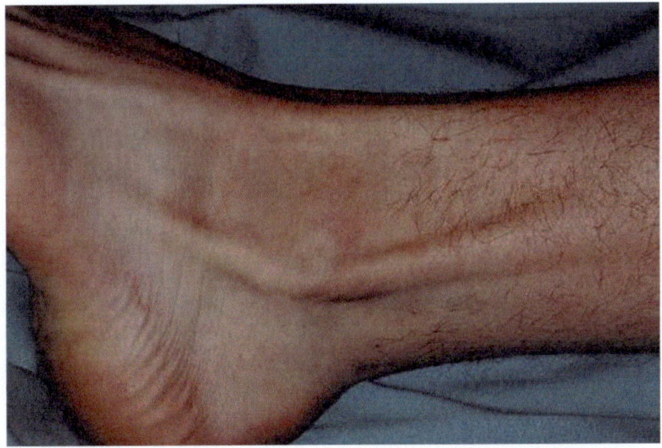

peroneal tendons may actually be seen subluxing anteriorly on the distal fibula during ambulation (Fig. 10.2) [11]. Positioning the patient prone with the knees flexed at 90°, with active dorsiflexion and plantar flexion and eversion against resistance, may demonstrate the dynamic instability of the tendons [12].

Imaging

While radiographs are helpful in diagnosing grade 3 injuries to the superior peroneal retinaculum [13], the roles of ultrasound, CT, and magnetic resonance imaging (MRI) have been debated. These imaging modalities are not widely used. Dynamic high-resolution ultrasound is effective in demonstrating subluxation and associated tendon splits [14–15]. CT may be helpful in assessing the retrofibular groove prior to and postoperatively in groove-deepening procedures [16]. Static MRI is useful in grading superior peroneal retinaculum injuries, identifying splits in the peroneal tendons, diagnosing abnormality in the lateral collateral ankle ligament complex, and demonstrating morphological abnormalities of the fibular groove (flat, convex, or irregular) [17]. When there is clinical suspicion of peroneal tendon subluxation, static MRI with active dorsiflexion of the foot may demonstrate displaced tendons. Kinematic MRI may also demonstrate position-dependent dislocation [18].

Preoperative Planning

Instability is assessed clinically. A comprehensive examination of the ankle and foot is required to exclude other pathology, such as a lesion of the anterior talofibular ligament. Recurrent or chronic dislocation of the peroneal tendons presents with instability and clicking of the lateral aspect of the ankle, with the tendons subluxing anteriorly [19].

Management

There is no consensus on the optimal management of peroneal tendon pathologies [20]. Although conservative management may be attempted in acute dislocations, recurrent dislocations should be managed surgically [21–28]. Conservative management of acute subluxation is associated with a high rate of recurrence, and acute peroneal subluxation in high-demand individuals should be primarily managed surgically [4]. Various surgical techniques have been described. However, no randomized studies have been conducted to determine which method of treatment is superior, and the available literature is limited to case reports and small case series. There are five categories of surgical repair: [1] anatomic reattachment of the retinaculum, (2) reinforcement of the superior peroneal retinaculum with local tissue transfers, [3] rerouting the tendons behind the calcaneofibular ligament, [4] bone block procedures, and [5] groove-deepening procedures [2].

The aim of anatomic reattachment of the retinaculum is restoration of the primary restraint to the peroneal tendons. Reattachment with sutures brought through drill holes in the distal fibula has been described [4, 29–33]. As an alternative, Beck [23] brought the retinaculum through a slit created in the distal fibula and fixed this with a screw, and treated nine patients without complication. Eighteen of twenty one patients treated with the "Singapore operation" at 9 years had excellent results.

However, three patients experienced postoperative pain and neuromas; no recurrence was noted [34]. Karlsson et al. reported 13 patients with good to excellent results who were able to return to full activity and two patients whose activity was limited by pain; no recurrence was noted at follow-up. They did, however, employ groove deepening in conjunction with reattachment if the posterior surface of the fibula was flat or convex [33].

Different procedures were described to augment or reinforce an attenuated retinaculum with tissue transfers consisting of either tendon or periosteal flaps. Ellis Jones [35] first described restraining the peroneal tendons with a strip of Achilles tendon anchored through a drill hole in the fibula. No recurrences were noted in a long-term follow-up of 15 patients who underwent the Ellis-Jones repair [36]. Thomas et al. [5] described a modification to this procedure that allowed the use of a smaller strip of Achilles tendon, reducing the risk of weakening the tendon. The use of the tendon of peroneus brevis [37–39], plantaris [40–41], and peroneus quartus [42] has been described for the same purpose. Zoellner and Clancy [43] and Gould [44] used periosteal flaps to restrain the peroneal tendons in a deepened peroneal grove with satisfactory results. In patients treated with a periosteal flap from the retrofibular grove on its own or incorporated with groove deepening, no postoperative complications were noted [45]. The use of the calcaneofibular ligament (CFL) as an alternative restraint has been considered. Platzgummer [46] described dividing the CFL and transposing the tendons behind it; 13 patients operated with this technique showed good or excellent results, with no evidence of recurrence or instability. Sarmiento and Wolf [47] later divided the peroneal tendons and reattached them after rerouting them behind the CFL [48]; 11 patients showed no evidence of recurrence or instability at follow-up, although two patients suffered sural nerve injury [49]. Both methods may potentially weaken these structures. To preserve CFL integrity, a bone block of the ligamentous insertion on the fibula [50] or the calcaneus [26] is mobilized, the tendons are transposed, and the bone block is reattached with a screw. Pozo and Jackson [50] reported no complications and return to full level of activity in a case report. Poll and Duijfjes [26] reported 10 patients with no recurrence or instability.

Bone block procedures were developed to deepen the retrofibular groove using a bone graft as a physical restraint to the peroneal tendons. In 1920, Kelly [51] described a bone block procedure using screw fixation for the sliding veneer graft but later designed a wedge-shaped graft that avoided the use of screws near the ankle joint. DuVries [52] and Watson-Jones [53] modified Kelly's technique. Watson-Jones [53] used an osteoperiosteal flap anchored by a soft-tissue pedicle and secured it posteriorly with sutures. DuVries [52] anchored a posteriorly displaced wedge with a screw. Other authors reported on patients with chronic subluxation operated with a modified Kelly technique with no recurrence [22, 24, 54]. Larsen et al. [25] and Lowy et al. [55] reported on the DuVries technique. Larsen et al. [25] reported many complications including intraarticular screw, fracture of the malleolus, fracture of the graft, nonunion, redislocation, and pain associated with the screw, but Lowy et al. [55] noted no complications in a case report. In 1989, Micheli et al. [56] treated 12 patients with an inferiorly displaced fibula bone graft fixed with screws; one suffered a traumatic fracture of the graft, and two required exploration for pain; no recurrences were noted. Tendon adhesion to the fresh bone wound, fractures of bone grafts, and the need for metalwork are major disadvantages of bone block procedures [23].

The depth of the retrofibular sulcus was previously thought to play an important role in the restraint of the peroneal tendons, thus leading to the development of procedures to deepen the sulcus when it was found to be flat or convex. Zoellner and Clancy [43] elevated an osteoperiosteal flap posteriorly on the distal fibula and removed cancellous bone with a gauge. The flap was then reduced into the deepened sulcus, and the tendons replaced into this. Their nine patients had excellent results with no recurrence or instability. Hutchinson and Gustafson described a similar method in combination with superior peroneal retinaculum (SPR) reattachment. Of twenty patients, three patients had poor results with resubluxation, and one of these patients developed reflex sympathetic dystrophy [57]. Gould [44] reported a single patient in whom groove deepening was incorporated with restraint of the peroneal tendons by reflection of elevated osteoperiosteal flaps. Mendicino et al. [58] employed intramedullary drilling and cortical impaction to achieve groove deepening. Cho et al. [59] compared the operative outcome between retinaculum repair with and without fibular groove deepening for the treatment of recurrent traumatic peroneal tendon dislocation in young and active patients. Both techniques showed good outcomes for the treatment of recurrent traumatic peroneal tendon dislocation; however, isolated retinaculum repair compared to retinaculum repair with fibular groove deepening was a faster and simpler technique. Also, Maffulli et al. [60] emphasized that the low incidence of peroneal tendon dislocation suggests that the bony sulcus is not a predisposing factor for dislocation.

The need for groove deepening has been questioned. Anatomic studies demonstrate the incidence of a flat or convex sulcus as high as 18% [7], 28% [24], and 30% [61]. The low incidence of peroneal tendon subluxation would suggest that the bony sulcus is not a predisposing factor to subluxation [7]. Histologic studies demonstrating that the peroneal groove is defined by the fibrocartilaginous periosteal cushion and not by the bony sulcus add weight to this argument [3].

Endoscopic anatomical retinacular repair is a more recent technique, which offers an attractive alternative to open repair and may reduce complications and allow early return to sports [58]. Tendoscopy is a useful tool to detect and treat peroneal tendon pathology [62–63]. It shows several advantages over conventional open surgery, including less pain, shorter hospital stays, better cosmesis, and faster recovery [63–67]. Endoscopic superior peroneal retinaculum reconstruction is not technically difficult and can be attempted by foot and ankle arthroscopists. However, if a suture anchor other than a Mitek anchor is used, the length of the anchor should not be longer than the diagonal of the cross-section of the lateral malleolus to avoid extrusion of the anchor tip into the lateral ankle gutter or the distal tibiofibular syndesmosis [68]. The advantages of this minimally invasive approach include better cosmesis, less soft-tissue dissection, no wound retraction needed, better assessment of retinaculum integrity, grading of injury, detection of coexisting pathology, less postoperative pain, less peritendinous fibrosis, and less subjective tightness at peroneal tendons [63–67]. The potential risk of this procedure includes sural nerve injury, iatrogenic fracture of the lateral malleolus, iatrogenic tear of the superior peroneal retinaculum, peroneal tendon injury, recurrence of peroneal tendon dislocation, and implant protrusion into the distal tibiofibular syndesmosis or the ankle joint [69].

In conclusion, treatment of peroneal tendon dislocation should be based on whether it is an acute or chronic injury and if the patient is or not an athlete. The nonathlete with an acute dislocation may be offered conservative management but should be warned that there a 50% possibility of recurrent dislocation. In case of failure of conservative management or chronic instability, surgical intervention is advised. Surgery is recommended for elite athletes having sustained either acute or chronic dislocation. Surgery in nonathletes with acute peroneal instability consists of reduction of the tendons into the retrofibular groove and repair of the superior peroneal retinaculum. In addition, there was agreement that both endoscopic and open treatments are appropriate surgical modalities. However, endoscopic treatment may allow earlier functional rehabilitation and earlier return to play. In all types of peroneal instability managed by open stabilization, the superior peroneal retinaculum should always be repaired, but extra care should be taken not to over-tighten the superior peroneal retinaculum, which could result in stenosis of the retromalleolar space [70].

Authors' Preferred Surgical Technique

Under general or spinal anesthesia, the patient is placed supine on the operating table with a sandbag under the buttock of the operative side to internally rotate the affected leg. A tourniquet is applied to the thigh, the leg exsanguinated, and the cuff inflated to 250 mmHg. A 3–5 cm longitudinal incision is made along the course of the peroneal tendons. The incision starts posterior to the tip of the lateral malleolus and progresses proximally, staying well anterior to the sural nerve. The incision is deepened to the peroneal tendon sheath, which is incised longitudinally 3 mm posterior to the posterior border of the fibula. The superior peroneal retinaculum is normally thin and deficient, especially anteriorly. The peroneal tendons are identified by blunt dissection and protected. The lateral aspect of the lateral malleolus is exposed, and the "pouch" formed between the bony surface of the lateral malleolus and the superior peroneal retinaculum, where the tendons sublux, becomes visible. The bony surface of the lateral malleolus is roughened up with a periosteal elevator to produce a bleeding surface, and three or four anchors are inserted along the posterior border of the lower fibula. After manual testing that the anchors cannot be dislodged, the superior peroneal retinaculum is reconstructed in a "vest over pants" fashion, making sure that the pouch between the bony surface of the lateral malleolus and the superior peroneal retinaculum is totally obliterated. The ankle is kept in eversion and slight dorsiflexion so that the peroneal tendons are in the "worst possible position." The strength of the repair is tested moving the ankle through the whole range of motion.

If a tear of the peroneal tendons is found, this is repaired with fine absorbable sutures. The wound is closed in layers with 2/0 Vicryl for the subcutaneous fat, subcuticular undyed 3/0 Vicryl and Steristrips. Dressing swabs, dressing, and crepe bandage are applied. A below-knee walking synthetic cast is applied with the ankle in neutral and slight eversion. Weight bearing is allowed from the day after the operation, and the plaster is removed 4 weeks after the procedure, when rehabilitation is started. Gradual return to activities and to sport is allowed over the course of 3–4 months from the procedure [71].

Postoperative Care

Patients are discharged the day after surgery, after having been taught to use crutches by an orthopedic physical therapist. No thromboprophylaxis is normally used. Patients are allowed to bear weight on the operated leg as tolerated but are told to keep the leg elevated as much as possible for the first 2 postoperative weeks. Patients are reviewed at the second postoperative week, and the cast is removed 4 weeks from the operation. At that stage, patients mobilize the ankle with physical therapy guidance. Immediately after removal of the cast, regardless of their weight-bearing status in the cast, patients are allowed to only partially weight bear and commence gradual stretching and strengthening exercises during 8–10 weeks after surgery. Cycling and swimming are started 2 weeks after removal of the cast, when patients are allowed to fully bear weight on the operated leg. Patients are allowed to return to their sport at 5 months postoperatively [60].

Conclusions

Acute dislocation of the peroneal tendons is often misdiagnosed as an ankle sprain and treated by early mobilization, which may increase the risk of chronic dislocation. Surgical reconstruction for recurrent subluxation of the peroneal tendons poses a challenge. Many procedures have been described, but some are nonphysiological and have marked postoperative morbidity. For example, bone block procedures may lead to fracture of the graft or of the lateral malleolus, intraarticular placement of the screws, and recurrence of the subluxation [9].

Intraoperative problems may include damage to the sural nerve, which is usually between 7 and 14 mm posterior to the tip of the fibula. This risk can be minimized by formal identification and protection of the nerve, which can be retracted posteriorly with the short saphenous vein at the beginning of the procedure [72]. However, the approach that we described is safely anterior to the nerve, and it is not necessary to formally identify and protect it.

Early postoperative problems may include hematoma and wound infection. Inflammatory foreign-body reaction related to the use of biodegradable anchors has been described, but in most instances, this runs subclinically and passes unnoticed [73–74]. We have not experienced any clinical complications related to the anchors, whether metallic or bioabsorbable, using this technique [19].

Though seldom indicated given the rarity of patients presenting with such pathology, the procedure recommended is technically easy, with minimal disturbance of the local anatomy, is safe, and restores the normal relationship of the peroneal tendons in their groove [19].

Recurrent peroneal tendon subluxation is a relatively rare sports-related injury that occurs when the acute injury is misdiagnosed or not adequately managed. The primary pathology is failure of the superior peroneal retinaculum, the principal restraint to the peroneal tendons. While diagnosis remains dependent on clinical suspicion and clinical examination, there is an emerging role for imaging to determine the classification of the retinaculum injuries and associated tendon injuries to plan surgery. There is no standardized method to report the severity of the condition, and therefore, it is difficult to compare the various studies. Many surgical techniques have been described, but it is impossible to determine from the relatively small series which procedure is superior. If an anatomical approach to treating the pathology is utilized, reattachment of the superior retinaculum, as we have described, seems a most appropriate technique. Rarely, the retinaculum in recurrent cases may not be robust enough to withstand repair and a different approach to the problem may be required. Randomized controlled trials may be the way forward in determining the best surgical management method. However, the relative rarity of the condition and the large number of surgical techniques described make such study difficult [71].

References

1. Monteggia GB. Istituzioni chirurgiche, parte III. Milan; 1803. p. 336–41.
2. Mizel MS. Orthopedic knowledge update. Foot and ankle 2. Rosemont: American Academy of Orthopedic Surgeons; 1998.
3. Kumai T, Benjamin M. The histological structure of the malleolar groove of the fibula in man: its direct bearing on the displacement of the peroneal tendons and their surgical repair. J Anat. 2003;203:257–62.
4. Eckert WR, Davis EA. Acute rupture of the peroneal retinaculum. J Bone Joint Surg Am. 1976;58(5):670–2.
5. Thomas JL, Sheridan L, Graviet S. A modification of the Ellis Jones procedure for chronic peroneal subluxation. J Foot Surg. 1992;31(5):454–8.
6. Oden RR. Tendon injuries about the ankle resulting from skiing. Clin Orthop Relat Res. 1987;216:63–9.
7. da Rocha GM, Pereira Pinto A, Fabián AA, et al. Insertional anatomy of peroneal brevis and longus tendon – a cadaveric study. Foot Ankle Surg. 2018. Article in press; https://doi.org/10.1016/j.fas.2018.07.005.
8. Edwards MM. The relation of the peroneal tendons to the fibula, calcaneus and cuboideum. Am J Anat. 1928;42:213–53.
9. Williams PL. Gray's anatomy. 38th ed. Churchill. Livingstone: Edinburgh; 1995.
10. Du Vries H. Surgery of the foot. 2nd ed. St Louis: C.V. Mosby Company; 1965. p. 256–7.
11. Niemi WJ, Savidakis J Jr, DeJesus JM. Peroneal subluxation: a comprehensive review of the literature with case presentations. J Foot Ankle Surg. 1997;36(2):141–5.
12. Safran MR, O'Malley D Jr, Fu FH. Peroneal tendon subluxation in athletes: new exam technique, case reports, and review. Med Sci Sports Exerc. 1999;31(7 Suppl):S487–92.
13. Church CC. Radiographic diagnosis of acute peroneal tendon dislocation. AJR Am J Roentgenol. 1977;129(6):1065–8.

14. Neustadter J, Raikin SM, Nazarian LN. Dynamic sonographic evaluation of peroneal tendon subluxation. AJR Am J Roentgenol. 2004;183(4):985–8.
15. Magnano GM, Occhi M, Di Stadio M, et al. High-resolution US of non-traumatic recurrent dislocation of the peroneal tendons: a case report. Pediatr Radiol. 1998;28(6):476–7.
16. Szczukowski M Jr, St Pierre RK, Fleming LL, et al. Computerized tomography in the evaluation of peroneal tendon dislocation: a report of two cases. Am J Sports Med. 1983;11(6):444–7.
17. Rosenberg ZS, Bencardino J, Astion D, et al. MRI features of chronic injuries of the superior peroneal retinaculum. AJR Am J Roentgenol. 2003;181(6):1551–7.
18. Shellock FG, Feske W, Frey C, et al. Peroneal tendons: use of kinematic MR imaging of the ankle to determine subluxation. J Magn Reson Imaging. 1997;7(2):451–4.
19. Oliva F, Ferran N, Maffulli N. Peroneal retinaculoplasty with anchors for peroneal tendon subluxation. Bull Hosp Joint Dis;2006. 63(3 & 4).
20. van Dijk PA, Miller D, Calder J, DiGiovanni CW, Kennedy JG, et al. The ESSKA-AFAS international consensus statement on peroneal tendon pathologies. Knee Surg Sports Traumatol, Arthroscopy. 2018;26:3096. https://doi.org/10.1007/s00167-018-4971-x.
21. Brage ME, Hansen ST Jr. Traumatic subluxation/dislocation of the peroneal tendons. Foot Ankle. 1992;13(7):423–31.
22. McLennan JG. Treatment of acute and chronic luxations of the peroneal tendons. Am J Sports Med. 1980;8(6):432–6.
23. Beck E. Operative treatment of recurrent dislocation of the peroneal tendons. Arch Orthop Trauma Surg. 1981;98(4):247–50.
24. Wobbes T. Dislocation of the peroneal tendons. Arch Chir Neerl. 1975;27(3):209–15.
25. Larsen E, Flink-Olsen M, Seerup K. Surgery for recurrent dislocation of the peroneal tendons. Acta Orthop Scand 1984;55(5):554–5.
26. Poll RG, Duijfjes F. The treatment of recurrent dislocation of the peroneal tendons. J Bone Joint Surg Br. 1984;66(1):98–100.
27. Tan V, Lin SS, Okereke E. Superior peroneal retinaculoplasty: a surgical technique for peroneal subluxation. Clin Orthop. 2003;410:320–5.
28. Kollias SL, Ferkel RD. Fibular grooving for recurrent peroneal tendon subluxation. Am J Sports Med. 1997;25(3):329–35.
29. Alm A, Lamke LO, Liljedahl SO. Surgical treatment of dislocation of the peroneal tendons. Injury. 1975;7(1):14–9.
30. Das De S, Balasubramaniam P. A repair operation for recurrent dislocation of peroneal tendons. J Bone Joint Surg Br. 1985;67(4):585–7.
31. Smith TF, Vitto GR. Subluxing peroneal tendons. An anatomic approach. Clin Podiatr Med Surg. 1991;8(3):555–77.
32. Mason RB, Henderson JP. Traumatic peroneal tendon instability. Am J Sports Med. 1996;24(5):652–8.
33. Karlsson J, Eriksson BI, Sward L. Recurrent dislocation of the peroneal tendons. Scand J Med Sci Sports. 1996;6(4):242–6.
34. Hui JH, Das De S, Balasubramaniam P. The Singapore operation for recurrent dislocation of peroneal tendons: long-term results. J Bone Joint Surg Br. 1998;80(2):325–7.
35. Jones E. Operative treatment of chronic dislocation of the peroneal tendons. Bone Joint Surg. 1932;14:574–6.
36. Escalas F, Figueras JM, Merino JA. Dislocation of the peroneal tendons. Long-term results of surgical treatment. J Bone Joint Surg Am. 1980;62(3):451–3.
37. Arrowsmith SR, Fleming LL, Allman FL. Traumatic dislocations of the peroneal tendons. Am J Sports Med. 1983;11(3):142–6.
38. Gurevitz SL. Surgical correction of subluxing peroneal tendons with a case report. J Am Podiatry Assoc. 1979;69(6):357–63.
39. Stein RE. Reconstruction of the superior peroneal retinaculum using a portion of the peroneus brevis tendon. A case report. J Bone Joint Surg Am. 1987;69(2):298–9.
40. Miller JW. Dislocation of peroneal tendons: a new operative procedure. A case report. Am J Orthop. 1967;9(7):136–7.

41. Hansen BH. Reconstruction of the peroneal retinaculum using the plantaris tendon: a case report. Scand J Med Sci Sports. 1996;6(6):355–8.
42. Mick CA, Lynch F. Reconstruction of the peroneal retinaculum using the peroneus quartus. A case report. J Bone Joint Surg Am. 1987;69(2):296–7.
43. Zoellner G, Clancy W Jr. Recurrent dislocation of the peroneal tendon. J Bone Joint Surg Am. 1979;61(2):292–4.
44. Gould N. Technique tips: footings. Repair of dislocating peroneal tendons. Foot Ankle. 1986;6(4):208–13.
45. Lin S, Tan V, Okereke E. Subluxating peroneal tendon: repair of superior peroneal retinaculum using a retrofibular periosteal flap. Tech Foot Ankle Surg. 2003;2(4):262–7.
46. Platzgummer H. Uber ein einfaches Verfahren zur operativen Behandlung der habituellen Peronaeussehnenluxation. Arch Orthop Unfallchir. 1967;61:144–50.
47. Sarmiento A, Wolf M. Subluxation of peroneal tendons. Case treated by rerouting tendons under calcaneofibular ligament. J Bone Joint Surg Am. 1975;57(1):115–6.
48. Steinbock G, Pinsger M. Treatment of peroneal tendon dislocation by transposition under the calcaneofibular ligament. Foot Ankle Int. 1994;15(3):107–11.
49. Martens MA, Noyez JF, Mulier JC. Recurrent dislocation of the peroneal tendons. Results of rerouting the tendons under the calcaneofibular ligament. Am J Sports Med. 1986;14(2):148–50.
50. Pozo JL, Jackson AM. A rerouting operation for dislocation of peroneal tendons: operative technique and case report. Foot Ankle. 1984;5(1):42–4.
51. Kelly RE. An operation for the chronic dislocation of the peroneal tendons. Br J Surg. 1920;7:502.
52. DuVries HL. Surgery of the foot. 4th ed. St. Louis: C.V. Mosby Co.; 1978.
53. Watson-Jones R. Fractures and joint injuries. 4th ed. Williams &Wilkins: Baltimore; 1956.
54. Marti R. Dislocation of the peroneal tendons. Am J Sports Med. 1977;5(1):19–22.
55. Lowy A, Kruman N, Kanat IO. Subluxing peroneal tendons. Treatment with the use of an autogenous sliding bone graft. J Am Podiatr Med Assoc. 1985;75(5):249–53.
56. Micheli LJ, Waters PM, Sanders DP. Sliding fibular graft repair for chronic dislocation of the peroneal tendons. Am J Sports Med. 1989;17(1):68–71.
57. Hutchinson BL, Gustafson LS. Chronic peroneal tendon subluxation. New surgical technique and retrospective analysis. J Am Podiatr Med Assoc. 1994;84(10):511–7.
58. Mendicino RW, Orsini RC, Whitman SE, et al. Fibular groove deepening for recurrent peroneal subluxation. J Foot Ankle Surg. 2001;40(4):252–63.
59. Cho J, Kim JY, Song DG, Lee WC. Comparison of outcome after retinaculum repair with and without fibular groove deepening for recurrent dislocation of the peroneal tendons. Foot Ankle Int. 2014;35(7):683–9. https://doi.org/10.1177/1071100714531233.
60. Maffulli N, Ferran NA, Oliva F, Testa V. Recurrent subluxation of the peroneal tendons. Am J Sports Med. 2006;34:986. originally published online Feb 1, 2006. https://doi.org/10.1177/0363546505283275.
61. Mabit C, Salanne PH, Blanchard F, et al. The retromalleolar groove of the fibula: a radioanatomical study. Foot Ankle Surg. 1999;5:179–86.
62. Guillo S, Calder JD. Treatment of recurring peroneal tendon subluxation in athletes: endoscopic repair of the retinaculum. Foot Ankle Clin. 2013;18(2):293–300. https://doi.org/10.1016/j.fcl.2013.02.007. Epub 2013 Mar 22
63. van Dijk CN, Kort N. Tendoscopy of the peroneal tendons. Arthroscopy. 1998;14:471–8.
64. Jerosch J, Aldawoudy A. Tendoscopic management of peroneal tendon disorders. Knee Surg Sports Traumatol Arthrosc. 2007;15:806–10.
65. de Leeuw PA, van Dijk CN, Golanó P. A 3-portal endoscopic groove deepening technique for recurrent peroneal tendon dislocation. Tech Foot Ankle Surg. 2008;7:250–6.
66. Lui TH. Endoscopic peroneal retinaculum reconstruction. Knee Surg Sports Traumatol Arthrosc. 2006;14:478–81.
67. Lui TH. Endoscopic management of recalcitrant retrofibular pain without peroneal tendon subluxation or dislocation. Arch Orthop Trauma Surg. 2012;132:357–61.

68. Lui TH. Eckert and Davis grade 3 superior peroneal retinaculum injury: treated by endoscopic peroneal retinaculum reconstruction and complicated by malposition of the suture anchors. J Orthop Case Rep. 2015;5:73.
69. Hau WWS, Lui TH, Ngai WK. Endoscopic superior peroneal retinaculum reconstruction. Arthrosc Tech. 2018;7(1):e45–51. Published online 2017 Dec 18. PMCID: PMC5852255. PMID: 29552468. https://doi.org/10.1016/j.eats.2017.08.050.
70. van Dijk PA, Miller D, Calder J, DiGiovanni CW, Kennedy JG, et al. The ESSKA-AFAS international consensus statement on peroneal tendon pathologies, vol. 26. Sports Traumatology, Arthroscopy: Knee Surgery; 2018. p. 3096. https://doi.org/10.1007/s00167-018-4971-x.
71. Ferran NA, Oliva F, Maffulli N. Recurrent subluxation of the peroneal tendons. Sports Med. 2006;36(10):839–46. 0112-1642/06/0010-0839/$39.95/0
72. Lawrence SJ, Botte MJ. The sural nerve in the foot and ankle: an anatomic study with clinical and surgical implications. Foot Ankle Int. 1994;15(9):490–4.
73. Bostman O, Pihlajamaki H. Clinical biocompatibility of biodegradable orthopaedic implants for internal fixation: a review. Biomaterials. 2000;21:2615–21.
74. Weiler A, Hoffmann RF, Stahelin AC, Helling HJ, Sudkamp NP. Biodegradable implants in sports medicine: the biological base. Arthroscopy. 2000;16:305–21.

Peroneus Brevis Tears

11

P. Kvarda, P. A. D. Van Dijk,
G. R. Waryasz, and C. W. DiGiovanni

Introduction

The peroneal tendons play an important role in dynamic stabilization of the lateral ankle and hindfoot and, therefore, subsist under substantial tension even during routine activity. Repetitive ankle sprains may increase this tension and can eventually lead to tearing or rupture. Peroneal tendon tears are often associated with sporting activities that require rapid foot and ankle movement or eccentric loading, such as skiing, soccer, American football, running, basketball, and ice-skating [1]. Superimposed peroneal tendon injury after an acute ankle or foot sprain can be overlooked due to surrounding soft-tissue swelling and exam difficulty and must, therefore, always be considered as part of the differential diagnosis—particularly when "isolated" sprains fail to improve as expected [2].

Historically, the first case of peroneal tendinopathy was reported by Monteggia in 1803, and the first peroneal tendon split tear localized to the area of the distal fibula was noted by Meyers in 1924 in three anatomic specimens [3, 4].

P. Kvarda (✉)
Massachusetts General Hospital, Harvard Medical School, Boston, MA, USA

University Hospital of Basel, Department of Orthopedics and Traumatology,
Basel, Switzerland
e-mail: pkvarda@mgh.harvard.edu

P. A. D. Van Dijk
Orthopedic Research Department, Academisch Medisch Centrum,
Universiteit van Amsterdam, Amsterdam, The Netherlands
e-mail: p.a.vandijk@amc.uva.nl

G. R. Waryasz · C. W. DiGiovanni
Massachusetts General Hospital, Harvard Medical School, Boston, MA, USA

Newton-Wellesley Hospital, Newton, MA, USA
e-mail: gwaryasz@partners.org; cwdigiovanni@partners.org

© Springer Nature Switzerland AG 2020
M. Sobel (ed.), *The Peroneal Tendons*,
https://doi.org/10.1007/978-3-030-46646-6_11

"""

Anatomy

The PB muscle originates from the inferior two-thirds of the fibula and intermuscular septum and runs immediately posterior to the lateral malleolus, superficial to the calcaneofibular ligament, anterior to the PL tendon, and superior to the peroneal tubercle of the calcaneus within its own sheath. The shape is a flattened ovoid as it inserts into the styloid process of the fifth metatarsal base [5]. The PL emerges from the proximal two-thirds of the fibula, lateral tibia condyle, and intermuscular septum and inserts on the plantar side of the first metatarsal base and medial cuneiform. Both tendons run in the retrofibular groove at the level of lateral malleolus. This fibro-osseous tunnel is created by the dorsal aspect of the distal fibula, superior peroneal retinaculum (SPR), the posterior talofibular ligament, the posterior tibiotalar ligament, and the calcaneofibular ligament [6]. The PB has a long musculotendinous junction that may extend inferior to the ankle joint and occupy increased volume within the tendon sheath that can lead to tenosynovitis, superior peroneal retinaculum damage, or chronic tearing. This is referred to commonly as a "low-lying muscle belly," although the presence of this distinct anatomic finding has not been proven consistently pathologic. Fifteen percent of patients have a peroneal tendon sheath that communicates to the ankle or subtalar joint.

The retinacula consist fascia and synovial sheath. The SPR originates from the posterolateral distal fibula directly above the tip of it and inserts on the lateral wall of the calcaneus or Achilles and has the most important role in stabilizing the peroneal tendons. The IPS has a relatively smaller role in stabilization, and it holds the tendons around the peroneal tubercle in their separate subsheaths. It originates from the inferior extensor retinaculum and insertion the lateral surface of the calcaneus. The calcaneofibular ligament lies inferior to the peroneal tendons and stabilizes the tendons in the retrofibular groove [7]. Furthermore, a fibrocartilaginous ridge is located at the posterolateral border of the distal fibula, which acts to deepen the retrofibular groove by 2–4 mm and also functions as a bumper to prevent subluxation [5] (Fig. 11.1).

The PL and PB share a synovial tendon sheath 2.5–3.5 cm proximal to the tip of the fibula and then separate into their own at the level of the peroneal tubercle [5]. Both tendons are innervated by the superficial peroneal nerve and receive blood supply through the posterior peroneal artery and the medial tarsal artery [8]. Three avascular zones have been reported in the literature: one in the PB at level of the lateral malleolus and two in the PL as it passes around the lateral malleolus and under the cuboid where mostly tendinopathy occurs [8, 9]. More recently, however, a study by van Dijk et al. found well-vascularized peroneal tendons via a common vincula by the peroneal artery and lack of any hypovascular zones [10].

The PB plantar flexes and everts the foot and is also a primary abductor of the forefoot. Twenty-eight percent of eversion power comes from the PB and 35% of power comes from the PL [5]. Both tendons are active stabilizers of the ankle during inversion–supination [11]. Moreover, the SPR and tendons together are also static stabilizers of anterior talar displacement in a neutral ankle position [12].

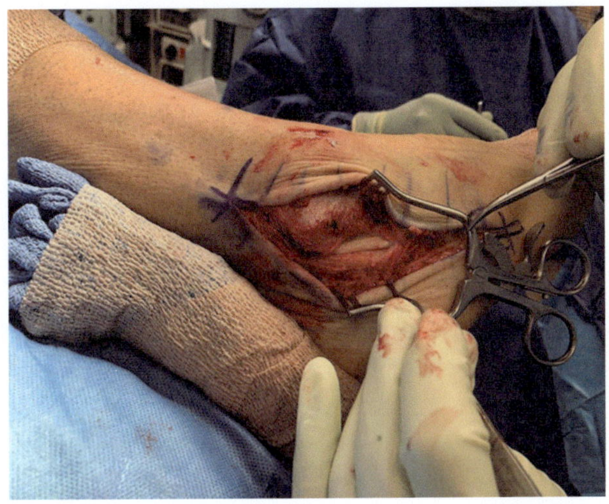

Fig. 11.1 Extended lateral approach to explore the peroneal tendons. Longitudinal opening the peroneal tendon sheath with the peroneus brevis tendon in view and excessive synovitis

Anatomic variants can include a low-lying PB muscle belly, presence of an accessory peroneus muscle/tendon, a flat or shallow retrofibular groove, laxity of the retinaculum, and hypertrophy of the peroneal tubercle. The most common anatomical muscle variant is the peroneus quartus (PQ) muscle, with an incidence of 10–22% [13–15]. The PQ has different attachment sites, but commonly, it originates from the PB and inserts on the retrotrochlear eminence of the heel bone. PQ may cause different pathological conditions, such as pain, tendon tear, tenosynovitis, and snapping [16]. Low-lying PB muscle occurs when the muscle belly reaches below the superior margin of the SPR and can be present up to 33% in individuals; it has been reported to lead to tendon tear [17, 18]. Hyer et al. investigated the morphology of the peroneal tubercle as a risk factor for peroneal tendon tears [19].

Epidemiology, Etiology, Mechanism, and Histology

Due to its vulnerable position within the retromalleolar groove, the PB is more prone than the PL to tear. Dombek et al. found PB tear in 88% and PL tear in 13% of 40 patients in a retrospective case series. They also noted concomitant tendon lesions in 15 of 40 patients [20]. In cadaveric studies, the prevalence of peroneus brevis tears has been reported to exist between 11% and 37% [18].

Acute peroneal injuries usually occur in plantar flexion of 15–25 degrees with inversion of the foot. In this position, the tendons are exposed to high mechanical loads at the level of the fibula. Recurrent ankle sprains exacerbate these loads, predisposing the tendons to hypertrophic tendinopathy, recurrent stenosis, and eventually tearing [21, 22]. Two possible injury mechanisms are compression of the PB in between the fibula and the PL, or subluxation of the tendon because of either SPR tear or laxity. Primary luxation of the PB tendon is the main reason for chronic tears with underlying pathological conditions, such as shallow or convex fibular groove.

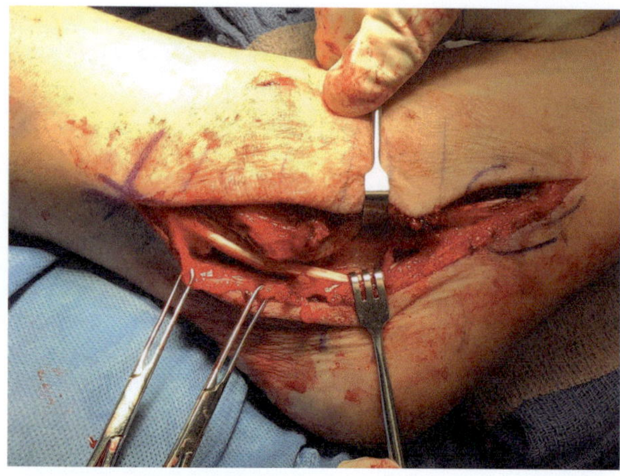

Fig. 11.2 Lateral approach to the peroneal tendons with an enlarged peroneal tubercle in view

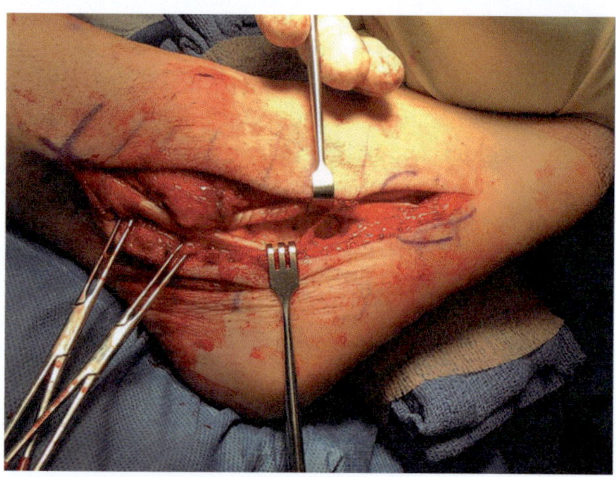

Fig. 11.3 Lateral approach to the peroneal tendons. After excision of a hypertrophied peroneal tubercle and tubularization of a peroneus brevis tear

PB pathology has also been reported as one of the most common associated findings that exist in patients who present with chronic lateral ankle instability [22–24]. One of the more common anatomic variations that predisposes the PB to pathology is hindfoot malalignment such as subtle or overt cavus foot deformity [25, 26] (Figs. 11.2 and 11.3).

Unfortunately, varying terms are still being used today to describe peroneal tendon pathology. In a recent international consensus statement, it was clarified that the term "tear" should denote a longitudinal tear in the presence of partial tendon integrity, whereas "rupture" should denote complete tendon discontinuity (separation of the ends) [2].

The most common type of PB pathology is the isolated "tear," usually being 2.5–5 cm in length. Bucket handle tears can occur when the PL acts like a wedge between the two split ends of the PB. A PB tear can also occur at its insertion along the base of the fifth metatarsal sometimes as a result of fracture or as a result of an

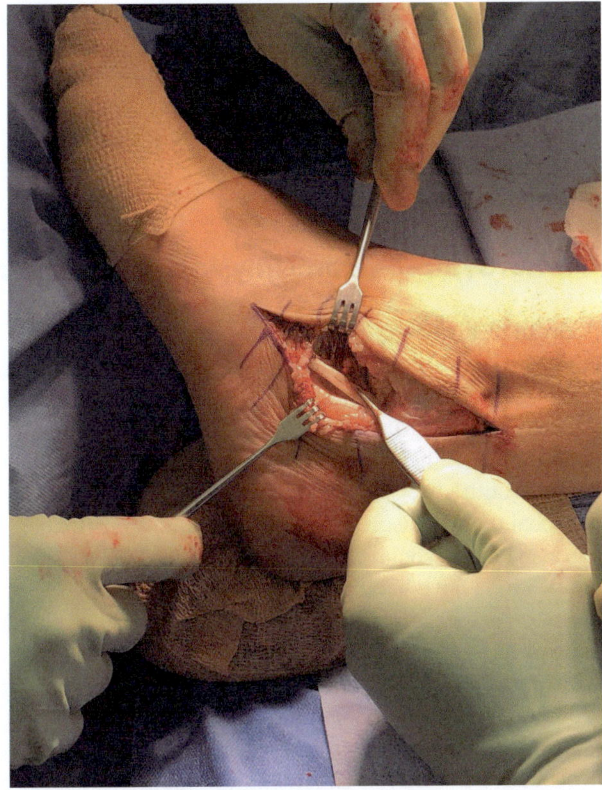

Fig. 11.4 Longitudinal partial tear of the peroneus brevis tendon, shown with the tip of the forceps

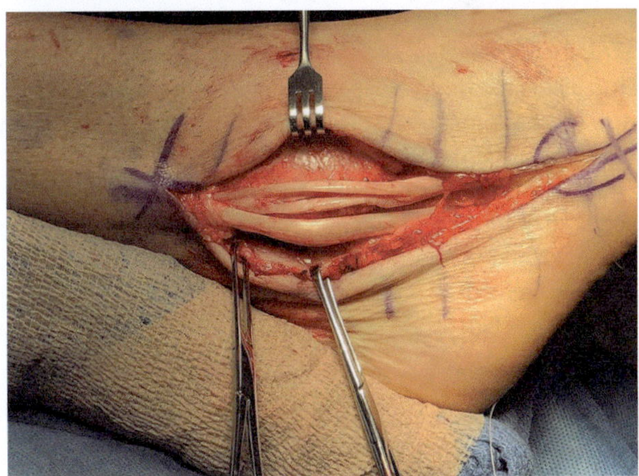

Fig. 11.5 Intraoperative findings of a large, complex longitudinal tear of the peroneus brevis tendon. The peroneal tendons are luxated out of the retrofibular groove after opening the peroneal sheath

os vesalianum [1, 27]. While peroneal tendon tears are well documented in the current literature, there are few case reports describing peroneal tendon ruptures [28] (Figs. 11.4 and 11.5).

Few articles to date have studied the histology of the peroneal tendon tears. Sobel et al. observed in a cadaveric study vascular proliferation, collagen bundle splaying, and developing of fibrovascular connective tissue without inflammatory activity [29]. In the Japanese population, Miura et al. found similar histologic change, including collagen bundle separation with blood vessel proliferation in a cadaveric study of 112 dissected ankles [30].

Clinical Symptoms and Physical Examination

A detailed history is the most important aspect of the initial assessment of every patient with an extensive history of the injury mechanism being essential for an adequate differential diagnosis. Documenting comorbidity is also an important step during evaluation, including at-risk disease states such as rheumatoid arthritis, psoriasis, diabetic neuropathy, calcaneal fractures, local steroid injections, Charcot–Marie–Tooth disease, and other neuromuscular disorders that can contribute to peroneal tendon disorder [27]. The use of ciprofloxacin and other fluoroquinolones has also been associated with tendinopathy and may lead to rupture [31]. Congenital dislocations have been reported [32].

In the acute setting, patients usually complain of sudden onset of pain, swelling, and warmth in the posterolateral ankle. In case of a PB tear, patients usually present with pain around the distal fibula, whereas PL tears typically present with pain around the cuboid tunnel and the peroneal tubercle [33].

A dislocated tendon or in situ snapping can also be identified via palpation with provocative maneuver. Ligamentous stability and neurovascular status should also be assessed, accompanied by a complete assessment of the excursion and strength of the PB. Peroneal subluxation is tested by flexing the knee and having the patient actively plantar flex and dorsiflex against resisted eversion. The peroneal compression test is useful to evaluate for peroneal brevis tendonitis by observing pain, crepitus, or snapping by everting the foot and dorsiflexion while manual pressure is placed against the fibular groove [34].

Assessment of ankle alignment, especially hindfoot varus or other congenital/acquired deformity, is required since hindfoot varus is a common predisposing factor for peroneal tendon injury [35]. Flexibility of the foot and ankle is important factor to plan the management. Patients with hindfoot varus should be assessed for possible underlying factors, such as Charcot–Marie–Tooth disease and related motor neuropathies.

Imaging

It can sometimes be challenging to differentiate peroneal tendon tear from other associated lateral ankle pathologies, such as lateral ligament rupture or syndesmotic injury. In a recent international consensus statement, therefore, it was agreed that initial assessment should follow the Ottawa ankle guidelines [36]. These include AP and lateral weight-bearing radiographs of the affected ankle and, if foot pathology is suspected, an oblique view. These views enable the clinician to evaluate possible fifth metatarsal base fracture, distal fibular fleck avulsion indicating traumatic subluxation/luxation of the peroneal tendons, fracture of the os peroneum, bipartite or multipartite os peroneum, and hypertrophy of peroneal tubercle [37]. Review by an (orthopedic) specialist is reserved only for cases where imaging reveals a "fleck sign" or fracture of the distal fibula, or in case of a clear history of a popping sensation or frank dislocation of the tendons. Moreover, if the patient is unable to weight bear by 1–2 weeks post injury, referral to the specialist is warranted [2]. The panel agreed that specialist evaluation should also consider and evaluate for other causes for lateral ankle pain. The literature supports several diagnostic modalities for thereafter diagnosing peroneal tendon tear.

X-Ray

Besides differentiation in the acute phase, plain weight-bearing radiographs are critical for the evaluation of the bony alignment and morphology of the ankle and foot. Radiographs of the contralateral side may be helpful to compare. A Harris heel view is also a useful radiographic tool to assess hindfoot alignment and peroneal tubercle hypertrophy as well as the retromalleolar groove [38].

Ultrasound

Dynamic sonography has enjoyed a growing role in the diagnosis of foot and ankle maladies, and its use in identifying peroneal pathology has been among those leading these applications. Tendon thickening, fluid collection, tears, and eventually adhesions can be observed (Fig. 11.6). Ultrasound is suitable to evaluate dynamic peroneal function especially for intrasheath peroneal tendon subluxation. Sonography-guided

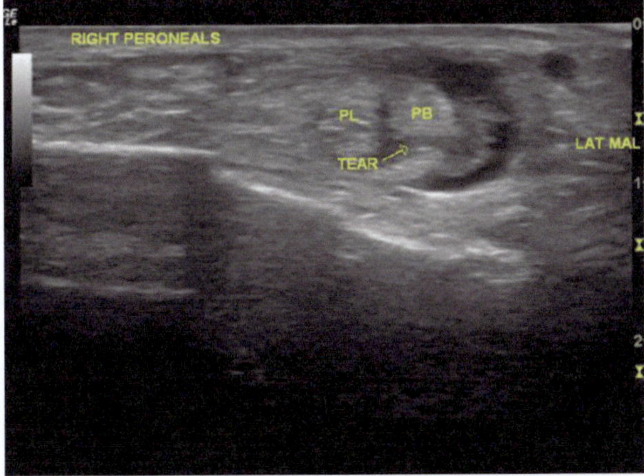

Fig. 11.6 Ultrasound illustration of the right peroneal tendons. The examination showed a transmural tear of the peroneus brevis tendon

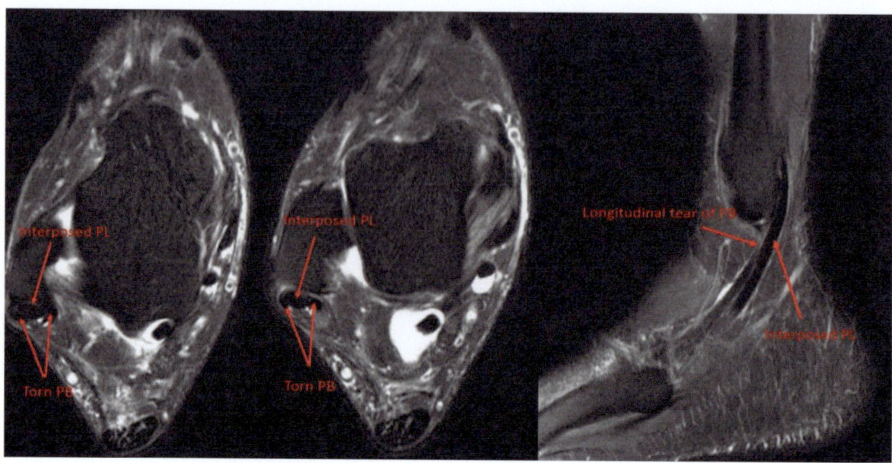

Fig. 11.7 A 57-year-old man with right posterior ankle pain. The MRI shows a longitudinal tear of the peroneus brevis (PB) tendon with an interposed peroneus longus tendon (PL) with associated tenosynovitis

tendon sheath injection with local anesthetics can also be helpful in differentiating pathology at this level. Ultrasound remains a safe, noninvasive, quick, and cheap imaging modality, but its effectiveness and usefulness still depend on the experience of the examiner. Grant et al. reported that sensitivity, specificity, and accuracy of ultrasonography for peroneal tendon injuries were 100%, 85%, and 90%, respectively [39].

Magnetic Resonance Imaging

Magnetic resonance imaging (MRI) is probably still today's diagnostic modality of choice. This method allows the most detailed assessment of the peroneal tendons and further structures around the tendons. Healthy tendons have homogenous low-signal intensity in T1- and T2-weighted and STIR (short tau inversion recovery) images [40]. Pathological changes, such as tenosynovitis or tear, may be associated with increased signal intensity on T2 or STIR images or loss of signal homogeneity [41] (Figs. 11.7 and 11.8). In a study by Kijowski et al., it has been reported that the presence of predominantly or uniform intermediate-signal intensity within the peroneal tendons on three consecutive axial proton density-weighted images is a highly sensitive and moderately specific indicator of symptomatic peroneal tendinopathy. The presence of intermediate T2 signal within the peroneal tendons and the presence of circumferential fluid within the peroneal tendon sheath greater than 3 mm in maximal width are highly specific indicators of peroneal tendinopathy and peroneal tenosynovitis, respectively [42]. Attention must be paid to the so-called magic angle effect of MRI, which is a false-positive interpretation. The "magic angle effect" occurs as the tendons follow the curved path around the lateral malleolus and the fibers are 55° to the magnetic axis resulting in artifactual signal. The effect may

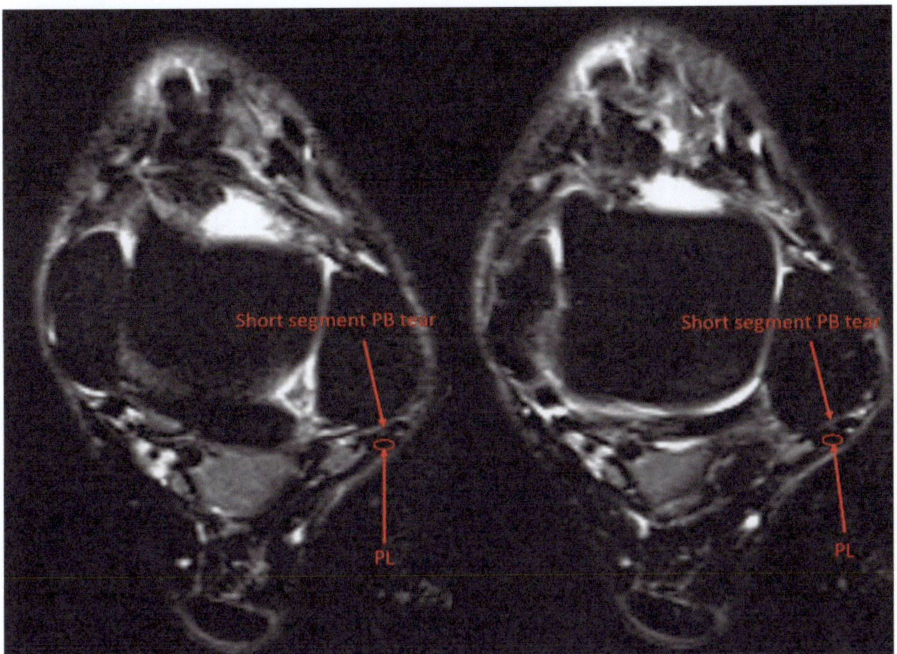

Fig. 11.8 A 37-year-old woman with left ankle pain after she slipped on wet steps. The MRI shows a short segmental longitudinal tear of the peroneus brevis (PB) tendon

mask subtle tendinosis and has been shown to decrease sensitivity and specificity to about 80% and 75%, respectively [18]. Normal anatomic variants, such as low-lying PB muscle belly, peroneus quartus muscle, and hypertrophy peroneal tubercle, can also be well visualized with MRI [40].

Res et al. investigated the peroneal muscle quality and found significantly higher fatty degeneration in patients with a PB tendon tear than in patients without tendon pathology. Res et al. highlighted the potential diagnostic and treatment defining value of the preoperative MRI. Imaging the peroneal musculotendinous complex in whole may become in future as a practical tool in diagnostic and treatment algorithm for peroneal tendon tears [43].

Computer Tomography

Computer tomography (CT) is not currently part of the standard protocol for imaging peroneal tendon disorders due its limited soft-tissue resolution. It enables, however, the best reconstruction and assessment of bony structures, such as retrofibular groove, distal fibula morphology, calcaneal fracture, and peroneal tubercle. With calcaneal fractures, the peroneal tendons should be visualized to ensure that they are not dislocated or entrapped [44].

Tendoscopy

Arthroscopic and endoscopic techniques have become well-established diagnostic and treatment modalities for foot and ankle surgery. Development of particular arthroscopic equipment has permitted better tendon visualization and minimally invasive treatment of certain tendon disorders. Pioneers of the tendoscopy technique were Wertheimer et al. and van Dijk et al. in the late 1990s [45, 46]. Currently, the most common uses of foot/ankle tendoscopy have been for the visualization of the posterior tibial tendon, Achilles tendon, and peroneal tendons. A recent systematic review by Cychosz et al. showed a comprehensive description of tendoscopy in the foot and ankle surgery with evidence-based recommendation for or against intervention [47]. There is weak evidence in the current literature (Level IV and V studies), and the technique is used on a regular basis due to its relative safety and efficiency and usually in combination with other surgical methods [47–54]. The main advantage of tendoscopy is purported to be minimal soft-tissue damage, lower risk, and shorter recovery and rehabilitation time—although prospective comparative data with open approaches are still lacking. Using this technique, the PB tendon can be visualized and evaluated from the myotendinous junction to the peroneal tubercle. Dynamic evaluation of the tendons during tendoscopy is not influenced by excessive incision of the tendon sheath and allows an in situ evaluation.

With the development of the available equipment and the surgical techniques, the spectrum of indications for peroneal tendoscopy has been widened. It includes diagnostic purposes by posterolateral ankle pain, retrofibular pain, impingement at the peroneal tubercle, and snapping. As treatment, tendoscopy is indicated for tenosynovitis, peroneal tendon subluxation/dislocation, intrasheath subluxation, adhesions and scarring and tendon tear, the removal of a low-lying muscle belly, excision of an enlarged peroneal tubercle, and excision of a peroneus quartus tendon [47, 48]. According to several published reports, the complication rate remains relatively low after peroneal tendoscopy, although general complications can occur, such as hematoma, deep venous thrombosis, infection, hyposensitivity around the portals, adhesions, and seroma. Procedure-specific complications, such as iatrogenic tear of tendon sheath, sural nerve damage, peroneal superficial nerve damage, peroneal tendon instability, or fracture of distal fibula through excessive burring, are also possible. This form of intervention, however, remains a good option for patients who present with normal imaging but have recalcitrant pain directly over the peroneal tendons without alternative explanation, and this can always easily be converted to an open procedure if necessary. Tendoscopy can also be effective in avoiding open dislocation of the tendon if a tear is known to be distal to the tip of the fibula.

Surgical Technique: Peroneal Tendoscopy

Peroneal tendoscopy can be performed in the outpatient clinic under local, regional, epidural, or general anesthesia. Patients are usually placed in the lateral decubitus position allowing optimal access to the anterior and posterior aspect of the tendon in case an open procedure is required eventually. Patients can also be placed, however, in supine or prone position, depending on the planned procedure and the surgeon's preference. A thigh tourniquet is useful to improve the visual quality during the procedure and avoid impedance of instrument excursion from proximal to distal. Bony landmarks are the distal fibula, peroneal tubercle, and fifth metatarsal, while soft-tissue landmarks are the peroneal tendons. Before administration of the anesthetics, the patient is asked to actively evert the foot. In this way, the peroneal tendon can be identified and its course can be marked on the skin along with ideal portal location superiorly and inferiorly.

Superior, middle, and inferior portals can be utilized. The superior portal is located 2–3 cm proximal to the tip of the lateral malleolus. The distal portal is located 2 cm distally from the tip of the lateral malleolus. Depending on the location of the disorder and working space, an additionally middle portal can be used, dorsolateral to the tip of the lateral malleolus.

First, the distal portal is created by making an incision through the skin, followed by penetration of the tendon sheath. A 30° 4.0-, 2.7-, or 1.9-mm trocar is then inserted depending on surgeon preference, and the tendon sheath is injected with saline to increase the working space. Passing the larger diameter scope through a relatively small retinaculum, however, can be challenging [55]. The superior portal is made under direct vision of the scope by introducing a spinal needle, approximately 2–3 cm proximal to the posterior edge of the lateral malleolus.

Visual inspection of the structures is then initiated. A working instrument is introduced through the superior working portal. Releasing scar, debridement of synovitis, identifying a tear and confirming its length, and ruling out subluxation/dislocation are standard steps during tendoscopy. The portals may be changed depending on the location of the disorder and planned procedure. Making the incisions in line with the open approach will allow the surgeon to convert to an extensive incision by connecting the portal sites when necessary for more complex tears or bone/tendon pathology (Fig. 11.9).

Regardless of approach, attention must always be paid for the sural nerve and the superficial peroneal nerve, which can be injured introducing instrument in distal and superior portals.

Treatment

Conservative Management

Surgical treatment should be reserved for symptomatic patients when conservative measures fail [2]. In general, nonoperative treatment contains NSAIDs, resting, ice, wearing of below-knee boot/cast or splint, bracing, lateral wedge orthosis to offload peroneal tendons, physical therapy, steroid, or NSAID intrasheath injection. Recently, ultrasound-guided PRP intrasheath injection has been described as a successful treatment in tendinopathy (Fig. 11.10). Dallaudière et al. reported significant improvement of pain (VAS score, $P < 0.01$), functional outcome score (WOMAC

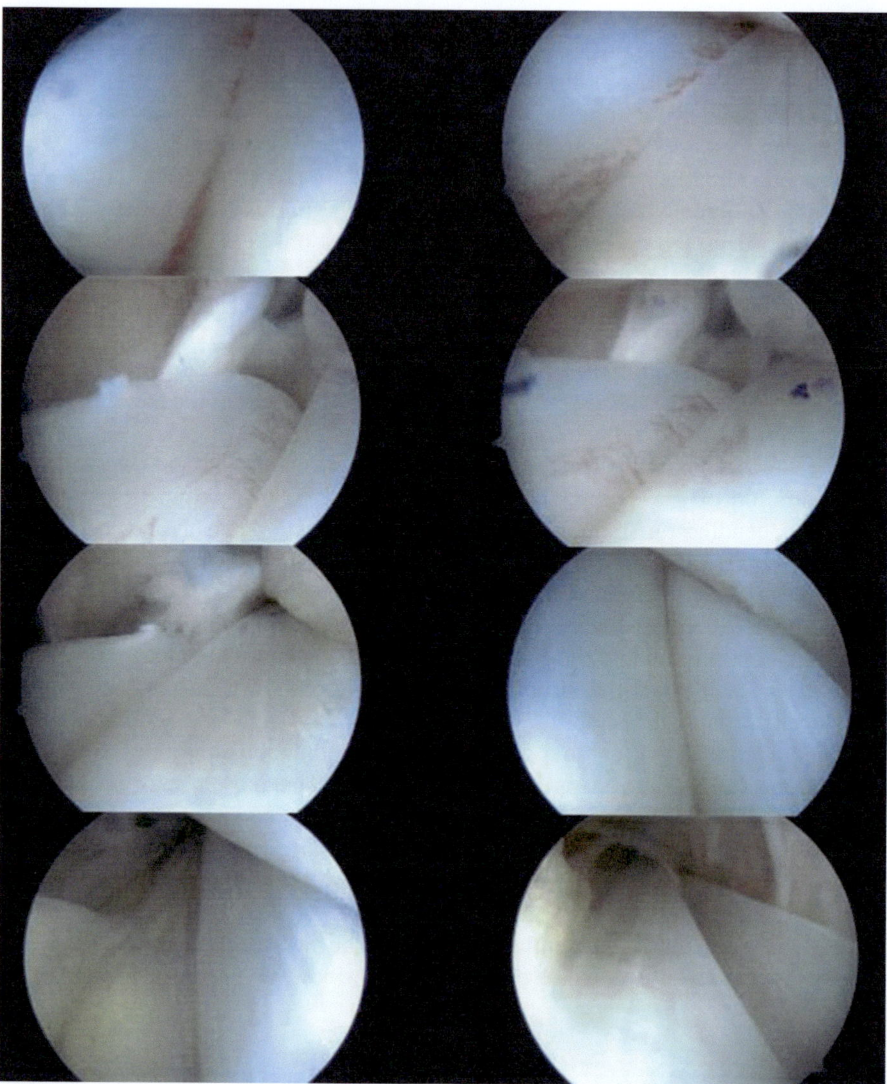

Fig. 11.9 Intraoperative images of peroneal tendoscopy. Looking from proximal to distal inflammation and red inflamed synovium on the peroneus brevis tendon is shown. No clear sign of a tendon tear was visualized

score, $P < 0.001$), and ultrasound measurement of tendinopathy ($P < 0.001$) [56]. There is, however, no evidence regarding the effectiveness in peroneal tendon tears and to date, therefore, not recommended as a standard treatment [2]. While conservative management is often successful in treating peroneal tendinopathy, it often fails to resolve symptoms of overt peroneal tendon tearing or rupture. Krause and Brodsky reported that conservative treatment failed in 83% of the patients with PB

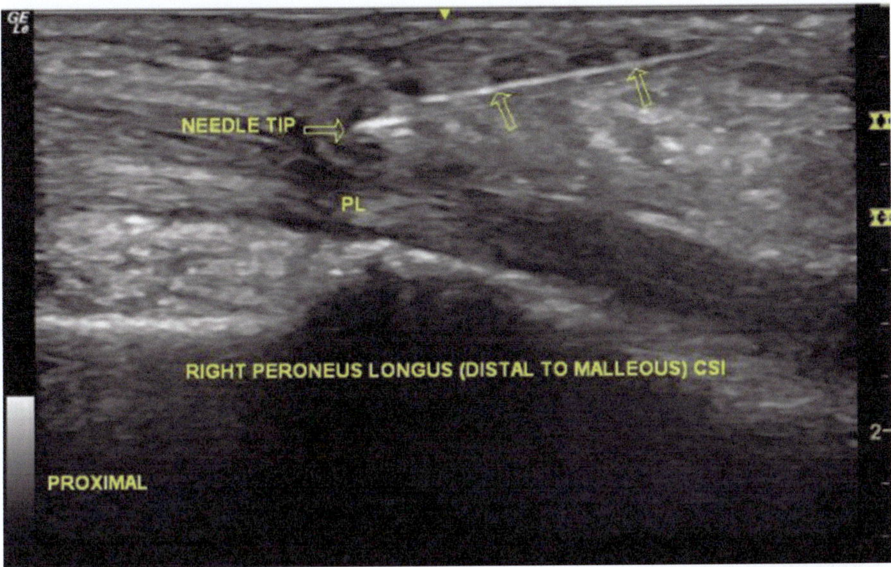

Fig. 11.10 Ultrasound-guided intrasheath injection of local anesthetics, an additional diagnostic tool

tears [57]. In case of tenderness over the peroneal tendons and negative imaging results, an ultrasound-guided intrasheath injection of local anesthetics can be useful in differentiating intrasheath and other posterolateral ankle pathologies (Fig. 11.10).

Surgical Management/Basic Principles/Repair/Tubularization/End to End/Tenodesis

When addressing peroneal tendon tears surgically, it is necessary to treat both the tendon pathology itself and its underlying cause when identifiable (shallow fibular groove, avulsed peroneal sheath, lateral ligamentous laxity, varus hindfoot, prominent peroneal tubercle, presence of low-lying peroneal brevis muscle belly, accessory peroneal, etc.). Care must be taken to not disrupt the fibrocartilaginous ridge of the fibula and leave a good cuff of tissue to repair the sheath or use bone tunnels/anchors.

Surgical treatment of acute simple or complex longitudinal split tearing is debridement with or without tubularized repair, while transverse rupture can be treated with classic end-to-end repair when identified in the acute setting. Both absorbable and nonabsorbable suture material can be used (Fig. 11.11). Advocates of nonabsorbable sutures promote its ongoing mechanical assist, but proponents of absorbable material express concern about these sutures causing surrounding tissue irritation and friction that can potentially lead to synovitis.

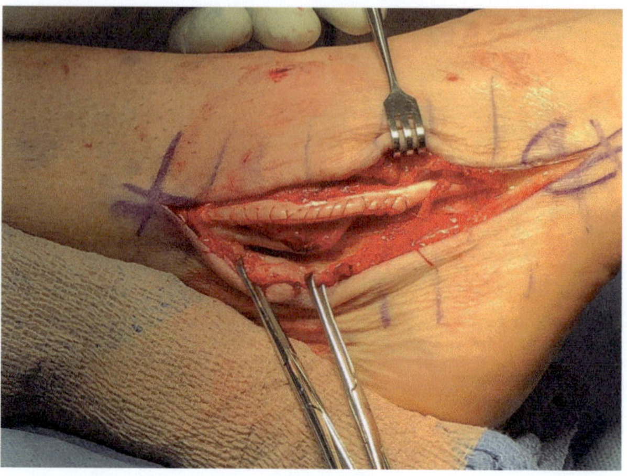

Fig. 11.11 Debridement and tubularization of a complex tear of the peroneus brevis tendon with absorbable suture material

Several treatment algorithms have been proposed in the literature, generally suggesting that if <50% of the cross-sectional area of the tendon is damaged, then all affected tissue can be debrided and tubularized [20, 57, 58]. This 50% threshold, however, is not based on substantiated data and remains clinically unproven and somewhat arbitrary in nature. Currently, it is now generally preferred to preserve and repair remaining tendon tissue with primary debridement and tubularization whenever there is at least some degree of reasonable native tendon left following debridement, even if this is significantly less than 50% [2].

Tenodesis is an option for larger, more complex PB tears or for tears with potential muscle atrophy, and can be performed both proximal and distal to the PL tendon after resection of the damaged area, either by direct side-to-side anastomosis or via Pulvertaft-type weave. Tendon interposition/replacement with graft (allograft or autograft) is an alternative option for extensive, irreparable tears if the proximal muscle is still reasonably healthy. Semitendinosus autograft or allograft can be used for this procedure, with good proximal muscle quality being required to this procedure. In cases when both tendon and muscle are unsalvageable, complete tendon transfer via insertion of the FHL or FDL has also been described.

Recent findings by Res et al. indicated the potential value of MRI investigating the muscle quality to help determine surgical treatment method and predict outcome after peroneal tendon surgery. In addition to the tendon tear morphology, defining the fatty degeneration and atrophy of the peroneal muscles based on the Goutallier classification should be part of the preoperative assessment and planning [43].

Surgical Technique: Autograft Interposition or Transfer

Autograft harvest is made by an oblique 3-cm longitudinal incision 2–3 cm distal to the joint line over the pes anserine tendons. The pes tendons should be palpable deep to sartorial fascia. The fascia is then incised. The tendons are located on the deep aspect of the sartorial fascia. After identification of the tendons, the semitendinosus is stitched with a nonabsorbable suture. A tendon stripper is then used to harvest the tendon. The graft is prepared by removing muscle fibers and then tubularized and sutured to the base of the fifth metatarsal with suture anchor placed under fluoroscopic guidance. If distal tendon is present, the graft can instead be secured to the stump with a Pulvertaft weave. The tension for proximal stabilization is determined with the foot and ankle neutral position. The graft should be secured to the proximal muscle tendon unit with the foot and ankle in this neutral position. The peroneal sheath is then closed, followed by wound closure [59]. Pellegrini et al. reported significant restored distal tension ($P \leq 0.022$) after PB allograft reconstruction versus tenodesis in five different foot positions under axial loading [60]. In a retrospective case series of 14 patients with allograft reconstruction of peroneal tendons, Mook et al. noted significant improvement of pain, eversion strength, and functional outcome scores [61].

In cases of irreparable and/or concomitant tendon lesions, reconstruction is also possible with tendon transfer. Flexor digitorum longus (FDL) and flexor hallucis longus (FHL) tendons have been used for this technique, which is suitable for both acute and chronic injuries as well. In cases of muscular atrophy or fatty infiltration, this technique has the advantage of the attached additional muscular power source. Neurological muscular conditions including Charcot–Marie–Tooth disease affecting the peroneal muscle quality should be considered for this type of reconstruction [62]. Harvesting of the FHL or FDL will be performed at or below the knot of Henry, usually through an incision on the sole of the foot plantar to the cuneiform and first metatarsal. When less tendon length is needed, the section can be performed proximally to the insertion point. Through a second incision medially and proximally to the medial malleolus, the harvested tendon will be retracted proximally and then transferred to the lateral side. The tendon will be passed through the peroneal tendon sheath and attached to the previously implanted anchor at the base of the fifth metatarsal [63]. Jockel et al. described increased AOFAS hindfoot scores, improved pain scores, and good or excellent patient satisfaction after a single-stage FDL or FHL transfer for severe concomitant peroneal tendon tears [64]. Seybold et al. examined nine patients with FDL or FHL transfer for concomitant PB and PL tears in a retrospective case series and reported successful outcomes postoperatively and good patient satisfaction, however remaining significant deficit in strength and balance [65]. In an anatomic comparison study, Seybold et al. preferred FHL tendon transfer over FDL for concomitant PB and PL tears, due to its longer length. They also reported visible compression of the neurovascular bundle after FDL transfer in contrast to FHL transfer [65, 66]. Redfern and Myerson suggested in 2004 a treatment algorithm for concomitant tears based on intraoperative assessment of both tendon quality [58].

Postoperative Treatment

After primary repair of the peroneal tendon, immobilization for 2 weeks is required to allow incisional healing in a non-weight-bearing below-knee splint with the foot and ankle in neutral. Thereafter, a walking boot and crutch ambulation is typically allowed with progressive weight-bearing and formal physiotherapy. Range of motion exercises is allowed except for resisted eversion up to 6 weeks postoperatively when the tendon sheath is taken down proximal to the tip of the fibula. This helps to protect the tendon sheath repair and reduce dislocation risk. Usually, strengthening exercises start at 8 weeks postoperatively. A stirrup brace can be used for 3 months during stressful activities.

A 6-week non-weight-bearing period is considered for tendon-transfer procedures with physiotherapy similar to other methods. However, there is no clear consensus in the available literature of an ideal postoperative rehabilitation program. van Dijk et al. reported, in a systematic review of 49 studies, a median of 6- to 8-week immobilization and physiotherapeutic exercises that began within 4 weeks after surgery [67].

After tendoscopy, the postoperative treatment may differ and implement shorter immobilization period and earlier weight-bearing, still based on the intraoperative diagnosis and completed surgery. Tendoscopy does not violate the integrity of the tendon sheath, and therefore, a more aggressive rehab is likely safe. A tenoscopic-assisted open surgery where the sheath is not opened proximal to the tip of the fibula can have a more aggressive physical therapy program since there is no theoretical concern of tendon dislocation since the proximal sheath is intact.

Conclusion

Peroneal brevis tendon tears are common and often overlooked. A precise history and physical examination are essential first steps in the diagnostic algorithm, alongside with a combination of imaging modalities including radiographs, MRI, and ultrasonography. Treatment should be reserved for symptomatic patients only, with conservative management being the first step. By choosing and conducting the surgical treatment, addressing both the tendon pathology and the underlying disorder is the basic principle to achieve the best outcome. Various surgical methods can be used, based on the etiology and specific pathology. The postoperative treatment includes usually a short-period immobilization and early physiotherapeutically exercises; however, it can differ according to the undertaken surgical method.

References

1. Rebecca A, Cerrato MSM. Peroneal tendon tears, sSurgical manageament and its complications. Foot Ankle Clin N Am. 2009;14:299–312.
2. van Dijk PA, Miller D, Calder J, DiGiovanni CW, Kennedy JG, Kerkhoffs GM, et al. The ESSKA-AFAS international consensus statement on peroneal tendon pathologies. Knee Surg Sports Traumatol Arthrosc. 2018; epub ahead of print.
3. Meyers A. Further evidences of attrition in the human body. Am J Anat. 1924;34:241–67.
4. Monteggia G. Instiuzini chirurgiche parte secondu; 1803. p. 336–41.
5. Piper S. Foot and ankle sports medicine. J Can Chiropractic Assoc. 2014;58(4):481.
6. Southerland JT, Boberg JS, Downey MS, Nakra A, Rabjohn LV. McGlamry's comprehensive textbook of foot and ankle surgery, vol. 1. 4th ed; 2013. p. 1165–6.

7. Roster B, Michelier P, Giza E. Peroneal tendon disorders. Clin Sports Med. 2015;34(4):625–41.
8. Sobel M, Geppert MJ, Hannafin JA, Bohne WH, Arnoczky SP. Microvascular anatomy of the peroneal tendons. Foot Ankle. 1992;13(8):469–72.
9. Petersen W, Bobka T, Stein V, Tillmann B. Blood supply of the peroneal tendons: injection and immunohistochemical studies of cadaver tendons. Acta Orthop Scand. 2000;71(2):168–74.
10. van Dijk PAD, Madirolas FX, Carrera A, Kerkhoffs GMMJ, Reina F. Peroneal tendons well vascularized: results from a cadaveric study. Knee Surg Sports Traumatol Arthrosc. 2016;24:1140–7.
11. Ziai P, Benca E, von Skrbensky G, Graf A, Wenzel F, Basad E, et al. The role of the peroneal tendons in passive stabilisation of the ankle joint: an in vitro study. Knee Surg Sports Traumatol Arthrosc. 2013;21(6):1404–8.
12. Hatch GF, Labib SA, Rolf RH, Hutton WC. Role of the peroneal tendons and superior peroneal retinaculum as static stabilizers of the ankle. J Surg Orthop Adv. 2007;16(4):187–91.
13. Hecker P. Study on the peroneus on the tarsus. Anat Rec. 1923;26:79–82.
14. Sobel M, Levy ME, Bohne WH. Congenital variations of the peroneus quartus muscle: an anatomic study. Foot Ankle. 1990;11(2):81–9.
15. Cheung YY, Rosenberg ZS, Ramsinghani R, Beltran J, Jahss MH. Peroneus quartus muscle: MR imaging features. Radiology. 1997;202(3):745–50.
16. Bilgili MG, Kaynak G, Botanlioglu H, Basaran SH, Ercin E, Baca E, et al. Peroneus quartus: prevalence and clinical importance. Arch Orthop Trauma Surg. 2014;134(4):481–7.
17. Geller J, Lin S, Cordas D, Vieira P. Relationship of a low-lying muscle belly to tears of the peroneus brevis tendon. Am J Orthop (Belle Mead NJ). 2003;32(11):541–4.
18. Davda K, Malhotra K, O'Donnell P, Singh D, Cullen N. Peroneal tendon disorders. EFORT Open Rev. 2017;2(6):281–92.
19. Hyer CF, Dawson JM, Philbin TM, Berlet GC, Lee TH. The peroneal tubercle: description, classification, and relevance to peroneus longus tendon pathology. Foot Ankle Int. 2005;26(11):947–50.
20. Dombek MF, Lamm BM, Saltrick K, Mendicino RW, Catanzariti AR. Peroneal tendon tears: a retrospective review. J Foot Ankle Surg: Off Publ Am Coll Foot Ankle Surg. 2003;42(5):250–8.
21. Larsen E. Longitudinal rupture of the peroneus brevis tendon. J Bone Joint Surg. 1987;69(2):340–1.
22. BF DG, Fraga CJ, Cohen BE, Shereff MJ. Associated injuries found in chronic lateral ankle instability. Foot Ankle Int. 2000;21(10):809–15.
23. Sammarco GJ, DiRaimondo CV. Chronic peroneus brevis tendon lesions. Foot Ankle. 1989;9(4):163–70.
24. Sobel M, Warren RF, Brourman S. Lateral ankle instability associated with dislocation of the peroneal tendons treated by the Chrisman-Snook procedure. A case report and literature review. Am J Sports Med. 1990;18(5):539–43.
25. Saupe N, Mengiardi B, Pfirrmann CW, Vienne P, Seifert B, Zanetti M. Anatomic variants associated with peroneal tendon disorders: MR imaging findings in volunteers with asymptomatic ankles. Radiology. 2007;242(2):509–17.
26. Chilvers M, Manoli A 2nd. The subtle cavus foot and association with ankle instability and lateral foot overload. Foot Ankle Clin. 2008;13(2):315–24, vii.
27. Selmani E, Gjata V, Gjika E. Current concepts review: peroneal tendon disorders. Foot Ankle Int. 2006;27(3):221–8.
28. Borton DC, Lucas P, Jomha NM, Cross MJ, Slater K. Operative reconstruction after transverse rupture of the tendons of both peroneus longus and brevis. Surgical reconstruction by transfer of the flexor digitorum longus tendon. J Bone Joint Surg. 1998;80(5):781–4.
29. Sobel M, DiCarlo EF, Bohne WH, Collins L. Longitudinal splitting of the peroneus brevis tendon: an anatomic and histologic study of cadaveric material. Foot Ankle. 1991;12(3):165–70.
30. Miura K, Ishibashi Y, Tsuda E, Kusumi T, Toh S. Split lesions of the peroneus brevis tendon in the Japanese population: an anatomic and histologic study of 112 cadaveric ankles. J Orthop Sci. 2004;9(3):291–5.

31. Sharma P, Maffulli N. Tendon injury and tendinopathy: healing and repair. J Bone Joint Surg Am. 2005;87(1):187–202.
32. Kojima Y, Kataoka Y, Suzuki S, Akagi M. Dislocation of the peroneal tendons in neonates and infants. Clin Orthop Relat Res. 1991;266:180–4.
33. Cerrato RA, Myerson MS. Peroneal tendon tears, surgical management and its complications. Foot Ankle Clin. 2009;14(2):299–312.
34. Sobel M, Geppert MJ, Olson EJ, Bohne WH, Arnoczky SP. The dynamics of peroneus brevis tendon splits: a proposed mechanism, technique of diagnosis, and classification of injury. Foot Ankle. 1992;13(7):413–22.
35. Manoli A 2nd, Graham B. The subtle cavus foot, "the underpronator". Foot Ankle Int. 2005;26(3):256–63.
36. Stiell IG, McKnight RD, Greenberg GH, McDowell I, Nair RC, Wells GA, et al. Implementation of the Ottawa ankle rules. JAMA. 1994;271(11):827–32.
37. Philbin TM, Landis GS, Smith B. Peroneal tendon injuries. J Am Acad Orthop Surg. 2009;17(5):306–17.
38. Heckman DS, Gluck GS, Parekh SG. Tendon disorders of the foot and ankle, part 1: peroneal tendon disorders. Am J Sports Med. 2009;37(3):614–25.
39. Grant TH, Kelikian AS, Jereb SE, McCarthy RJ. Ultrasound diagnosis of peroneal tendon tears. A surgical correlation. J Bone Joint Surg Am. 2005;87(8):1788–94.
40. Wang XTRZ, Mechlin MB, Schweitzer ME. Normal variants and diseases of the peroneal tendons and superior peroneal retinaculum: MR imaging features. Radiographics. 2005;25:587–602.
41. Lee SJ, Jacobson JA, Kim SM, Fessell D, Jiang Y, Dong Q, et al. Ultrasound and MRI of the peroneal tendons and associated pathology. Skelet Radiol. 2013;42(9):1191–200.
42. Kijowski R, De Smet A, Mukharjee R. Magnetic resonance imaging findings in patients with peroneal tendinopathy and peroneal tenosynovitis. Skelet Radiol. 2007;36(2):105–14.
43. Res LCS, Dixon T, Lubberts B, Vicentini JRT, van Dijk PA, Hosseini A, et al. Peroneal tendon tears: we should consider looking at the muscle instead. J Am Acad Orthop Surg. 2018;26(22):809–15.
44. Wong-Chung J, Marley WD, Tucker A, O'Longain DS. Incidence and recognition of peroneal tendon dislocation associated with calcaneal fractures. Foot Ankle Surg: Off J Eur Soc Foot Ankle Surg. 2015;21(4):254–9.
45. Wertheimer SJWC, Loder BG, Calderone DR, Frascone ST. The role of endoscopy in treatment of stenosing posterior tibial tenosynovitis. J Foot Ankle Surg. 1995;34:15–22.
46. van Dijk CNSP, Kort N. Tendoscopy (tendon sheath endoscopy) for overuse tendon injuries. Oper Tech Sports Med. 1997;5:170–8.
47. Cychosz CC, Phisitkul P, Barg A, Nickisch F, van Dijk CN, Glazebrook MA. Foot and ankle tendoscopy: evidence-based recommendations. Arthroscopy. 2014;30(6):755–65.
48. Marmotti A, Cravino M, Germano M, Del Din R, Rossi R, Tron A, et al. Peroneal tendoscopy. Curr Rev Musculoskelet Med. 2012;5(2):135–44.
49. Scholten PE, van Dijk CN. Tendoscopy of the peroneal tendons. Foot Ankle Clin. 2006;11(2):415–20. vii
50. Scholten PE, Breugem SJ, van Dijk CN. Tendoscopic treatment of recurrent peroneal tendon dislocation. Knee Surg Sports Traumatol Arthrosc. 2013;21(6):1304–6.
51. Michels F, Jambou S, Guillo S, Van Der Bauwhede J. Endoscopic treatment of intrasheath peroneal tendon subluxation. Case Rep Med. 2013;2013:274685.
52. Lui TH. Endoscopic resection of the peroneal tubercle. J Foot Ankle Surg. 2012;51(6):813–5.
53. Lui TH. Tendoscopic resection of low-lying muscle belly of peroneus brevis or quartus. Foot Ankle Int. 2012;33(10):912–4.
54. Panchbhavi VKM, Trevino SG. The technique of peroneal tendoscopy and its role in management of peroneal tendon anomalies. Tech Foot Ankle Surg. 2003;2(3):192–8.
55. Sammarco VJ. Peroneal tendoscopy: indications and techniques. Sports Med Arthrosc Rev. 2009;17(2):94–9.

56. Dallaudiere B, Pesquer L, Meyer P, Silvestre A, Perozziello A, Peuchant A, et al. Intratendinous injection of platelet-rich plasma under US guidance to treat tendinopathy: a long-term pilot study. J Vasc Intervent Radiol: JVIR. 2014;25(5):717–23.
57. Krause JO, Brodsky JW. Peroneus brevis tendon tears: pathophysiology, surgical reconstruction, and clinical results. Foot Ankle Int. 1998;19(5):271–9.
58. Redfern D, Myerson M. The management of concomitant tears of the peroneus longus and brevis tendons. Foot Ankle Int. 2004;25(10):695–707.
59. Ellis SJ, Rosenbaum AJ. Hamstring autograft reconstruction of the peroneus brevis. Techn Foot Ankle Surg. 2018;17(1):3–7.
60. Pellegrini MJ, Glisson RR, Matsumoto T, Schiff A, Laver L, Easley ME, et al. Effectiveness of allograft reconstruction vs tenodesis for irreparable peroneus brevis tears: a cadaveric model. Foot Ankle Int. 2016;37(8):803–8.
61. Mook WR, Parekh SG, Nunley JA. Allograft reconstruction of peroneal tendons: operative technique and clinical outcomes. Foot Ankle Int. 2013;34(9):1212–20.
62. Coughlin MJ, Saltzman CL, Anderson RB. Mann's surgery of the foot and ankle, vol. 1. 9th ed; 2014. p. 1250.
63. Coughlin MJ, Saltzman CL, Anderson RB. Mann's surgery of the foot and ankle, vol. 1. 9th ed; 2014. p. 1257–9.
64. Jockel JR, Brodsky JW. Single-stage flexor tendon transfer for the treatment of severe concomitant peroneus longus and brevis tendon tears. Foot Ankle Int. 2013;34(5):666–72.
65. Seybold JD, Campbell JT, Jeng CL, Short KW, Myerson MS. Outcome of lateral transfer of the FHL or FDL for concomitant peroneal tendon tears. Foot Ankle Int. 2016;37(6):576–81.
66. Seybold JD, Campbell JT, Jeng CL, Myerson MS. Anatomic comparison of lateral transfer of the long flexors for concomitant peroneal tears. Foot Ankle Int. 2013;34(12):1718–23.
67. van Dijk PA, Lubberts B, Verheul C, DiGiovanni CW, Kerkhoffs GM. Rehabilitation after surgical treatment of peroneal tendon tears and ruptures. Knee Surg Sports Traumatol Arthrosc: Off J ESSKA. 2016;24(4):1165–74.

Peroneus Brevis Tears Associated with Chronic Lateral Ankle Instability

12

Jon Karlsson, Louise Karlsson, Eleonor Svantesson, and Eric Hamrin Senorski

Introduction

An ankle sprain is defined as a tear of the ankle ligaments, most of ten the anterior talofibular ligament (ATFL) and, secondarily, the calcaneofibular ligament (CFL). It has been repeatedly shown that ankle sprains are the most common sports-related injury. The injury can vary in severity, between partial and complete ligament ruptures. It is also well known that approximately 85–90% of all ankle ligament injuries involve the lateral ligament complex.

Treatment of an ankle sprain is often standardized, with nonsurgical approach, consisting of short rest, compression and range-of-motion training until the swelling subsides. Weightbearing is recommended as early as tolerated by the patient. This is followed by strength, stability, and agility training, preferably with the patient fully loading the injured joint. Return to sports is possible after 7–10 days, depending on the extent of injury and residual swelling and pain. Return to sports can be aided by an external support (sports tape or similar, like ankle brace) during at least the first 3 months after injury. External support has been associated with reducing the risk of secondary ankle sprain but is not superior to strength and stability training. Such an early return to sports is possible due to the fact that ankle injury seldom leads to serious sequelae in the long term, like osteoarthritis of the joint. Returning to sports should be gradual after resolution of initial impairment in the range of motion and swelling, as well as after having recovered symmetrical strength and coordination.

However, chronic ankle instability – leading to repeated giving way and sense of insecurity – may ensue in approximately 10–20% of all cases after an acute ankle sprain. It should also be born in mind that recurrent ankle sprains may in the

J. Karlsson (✉) · L. Karlsson · E. Svantesson · E. H. Senorski
Department of Orthopaedics, Sahlgrenska University Hospital, Sahlgrenska Academy, Gothenburg University, Gothenburg, Sweden
e-mail: jon.karlsson@vgregion.se; eric.hamrin.senorski@gu.se

medium-to-long term alter the biomechanics of the ankle joint and this may ultimately lead to cartilage degeneration and osteoarthritis [1, 2]. It has also been shown that more than 90% of patients with ankle instability have associated intraarticular pathology, such as osteochondral injuries, free bodies, and subchondral cysts.

Extraarticular pathology is also encountered in several cases [3–10]. Longitudinal tear or attrition of the peroneus brevis tendon has been mentioned as a cause of lateral ankle pain [11]. This is especially relevant in patients who have recurrent and/or chronic pain after acute ankle ligament injury. Peroneus brevis injury should always be considered as a relevant differential diagnosis in patients with longstanding problems (especially pain) after an otherwise noncomplicated ankle ligament injury. It is noteworthy that the peroneus longus tendon is very seldom involved [12]. An inversion ankle injury may thus produce not only ligament damage to the ATFL and CFL as well, but also injury to the Superior Peroneal Retinaculum (SPR) and/or the peroneal tendons.

Most probably, pathological conditions of the peroneal tendon(s) are underreported reasons of lateral ankle pain and dysfunction. They may be difficult to distinguish from lateral ankle ligament injuries [4, 5, 7, 9, 13].

Anatomy

The peroneal muscles form the lateral compartment of the lower leg. They are innervated by the superficial peroneal nerve. The peroneus brevis muscle originates from the distal two-thirds of the fibula, and the tendons start (with anatomic variations) approximately 2–3 cm proximal to the tip of the fibula. The peroneus longus arises not only from the proximal two-thirds of the fibula but also from the lateral condyle of the tibia. Finally, the peroneus tertius is distinct to the peroneus brevis and longus tendons and is located within the anterior compartment of the leg [5]. The peroneus brevis is relatively flat and runs directly posterior to the distal fibula, while the peroneus longus is more rounded and runs behind the peroneus brevis tendon. Both tendons are located in the retromalleolar groove, which is a fibro-osseous tunnel. The superior peroneal retinaculum (SPR) is the boundary of the groove, and both tendons are located under the SPR [6]. The SPR is a very important structure that creates the stability of the tendons in the retromalleolar groove. The retinaculum is composed of both fascia and synovial sheaths, which form both inferior and superior bands, spanning the Achilles tendon and the calcaneus, respectively. The superior band is the main restraint to tendon subluxation/dislocation [7]. The shape of the retromalleolar groove is important as well. It is concave in approximately 80% of all people, and flat in 11%. The depth is 2–4 mm with an average width of 9 mm [11].

Below the retromalleolar groove, the tendons run in two distinct synovial sheaths. They cross the lateral calcaneal wall and are separated by the peroneal tubercle [12].

Peroneus Brevis Tendon Tear and Ligament Injury

Longitudinal tear of the peroneus brevis tendon was first reported almost 100 years ago [13–22]. In later days, it has been shown that the lesion is more common than previously believed.

There are researchers who have reported peroneus tendon lesions, both in clinical and cadaveric studies, in up to 37% of specimens. The clinical relevance of the autopsy studies is, however, not known. Several studies have shown the anatomical correlation between the longitudinal tear of the peroneus brevis tendon and chronic lateral ankle instability. Accordingly, the inversion injury leads not only to ligament tear/rupture, but also – either primarily but more probably secondarily – injury/attrition of the SPR and the peroneal tendons. In most cases, the central portion of the tendon is damaged and in most cases (probably around 90–95%), the SPR is damaged. The vascularity of the tendon in the retromalleolar groove is compromised and tissue damage ensues [6].

The biomechanical explanation is that the peroneus longus tendon pulls on the peroneus brevis tendon during walking and running (i.e., during the eversion of the swing phase of the step) over the sharp posterior edge of the fibula. This leads to minor, but repeated, posterior dislocation (subluxation) of the most anterior part of the peroneus brevis tendon; the tendon tear starts and increases as further tendon damage ensues. This almost always leads to pain at the posterior margin of the fibula.

The cause of the tendon injury is inversion ankle injury, with secondary insufficiency of the lateral ankle ligament(s) and rupture/attrition/elongation of the SPR. As time goes, the damaged retinaculum does not restrain the peroneus brevis tendon behind the sharp posterior fibular edge.

Clinical Presentation

The patient almost always reports an inversion lateral ankle injury. The tendon damage, which is present from the start, is most often overlooked and the diagnosis missed or at least delayed. Due to the recurrent instability of the peroneus brevis tendon and the damage to the SPR, the tendon degeneration is aggravated over time, and the patient never recovers. Nonsurgical treatment is usually nonsuccessful at this stage.

The patient describes acute ligament injury, with nonsuccessful recovery and thereafter, recurrent lateral instability of the ankle [23, 24]. In addition, a typical presentation is retromalleolar pain and chronic retromalleolar swelling [23]. At this stage, it should be borne in mind that a longitudinal tear in the peroneus brevis tendon has been described more distally along the lateral calcaneus wall and the narrow passage around the peroneal tubercle. Moreover, a fracture of the os peroneum has been reported – more seldom, though – with associated pain, as the reason for recurrent lateral ankle pain [16].

The pain is typically located posterior to the lateral malleolus, while recurrent lateral instability is the primary problem [25]. This combination of recurrent instability and pain is typical and is in clear contrast to the clinical presentation of chronic ankle instability alone, where giving way is the main problem, and pain is usually a secondary problem only and might have a different location, caused by anterior tibial and/or talar osteophytes and/or loose intraarticular bodies (cartilage).

Physical examination includes assessment of ligament integrity, for instance anterior drawer test and increased inversion of the talus. Most important is, however, the palpable swelling behind the lateral malleolus and pain at the same location [25, 26].

Both Magnetic Resonance Imaging (MRI) and/or Ultrasonography (US) can be helpful to increase the diagnostic accuracy of the tendon injury and also to determine the extent of tendon damage. Such modalities are recommended when surgery is planned.

Treatment

Nonsurgical treatment alone is usually not successful. The surgical approach is anterolateral, with the incision behind the lateral malleolus. The typical finding is that the anterior half of the peroneus brevis tendon is subluxed over the sharp posterior edge of the fibula. This is not to be mistaken for a primary recurrent peroneus brevis tendon dislocation. In case of concomitant ligament injury, stabilization of the ligaments should be performed as well [22, 23, 25–31].

Several different approaches have been reported, e.g., a modified Broström-Gould procedure or a modified Chrisman-Snook procedure. One problem, both theoretical and clinical, when using the Chrisman-Snook procedure is the tendon damage, making this procedure less reliable [32, 33].

Anatomical ankle ligament reconstruction is recommended as a safe procedure and has been shown to constantly produce stable ankles and restore laxity, with secure restoration of ligament laxity. The risk of surgical complications is low [34–36]. Anatomical reconstruction of the injured ligaments and reconstruction of the SPR and tendon rupture can be technically accomplished using the same skin incision. The incision is approximately 8 cm long along the posterior edge of the fibula, with an exposure of the peroneal tendons and the ATFL and CFL at the same time. The ligaments are tested for integrity/laxity and are thereafter shortened as needed in order to tighten them as necessary during the anatomic reconstruction. The peroneal tendon sheath is divided approximately 5–6 mm posterior to the fibular attachment. Thereafter, the peroneus brevis tendon is examined for tendon damage. In most cases, the damage is obvious; however, on some occasions the damage may be intratendinous and more difficult to locate [22, 33–38].

Thereafter, the degenerative tendon tissue is carefully excised. It is noteworthy that on some (or even many) occasions the tendon tear is double or triple [36–38]. On very few occasions, the tendon is so damaged that it is difficult or almost impossible to repair/reconstruct. Moreover, complete rupture of the peroneus brevis tendon is very uncommon (Fig. 12.1).

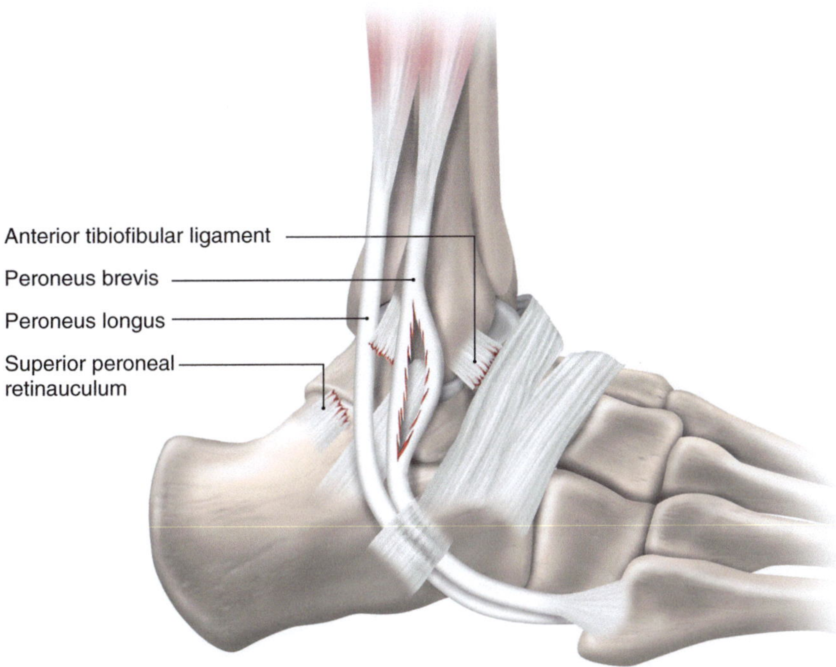

Fig. 12.1 Longitudinal tear of the peroneus brevis tendon. The tendon is torn over the sharp posterior edge of the fibula. The superior peroneal retinaculum (SPR) and the anterior talofibular ligament are injured. The peroneus longus tendon is normal

After excision of the damaged tendon tissue, the tendon is repaired with absorbable side-to-side sutures. The first suture line is deep, closing the posterior gap of the tendon, if any. A second and more superficial suture line is then used to close and tubularize the tendon. It is very important to excise all damaged tendon tissue, and, in some cases, the most anterior part of the peroneus brevis tendon needs to be excised (Figs. 12.2 and 12.3), [22, 35].

Thereafter, reconstruction of the SPR is performed, using small drill holes at the posterior aspect of the fibular edge. Thereby, the peroneal system is stabilized, which is very important. Finally, anatomical reconstruction of both the ATFL and CFL is performed. It is strongly recommended to always reconstruct both ligaments at the same time (Fig. 12.4), [22, 35, 38–40].

Postoperatively, a plaster cast is applied for 2–3 weeks and full weightbearing is recommended. After approximately 3 weeks, when sutures have been removed, range-of-motion training is started. As quickly as tolerated by the patient, light balance/coordination training with full weightbearing is advised [40, 41]. More progressive rehabilitation is then commenced at 6–8 weeks, including isolated

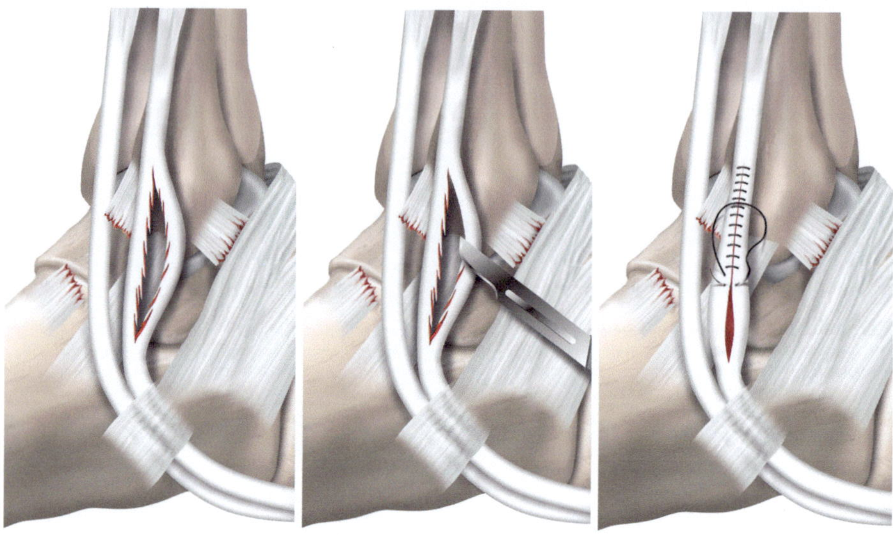

Fig. 12.2 Reconstruction of the peroneus tendon, with side-to-side sutures. The anterior talofibular ligament is reconstructed after the tendon injury is repaired

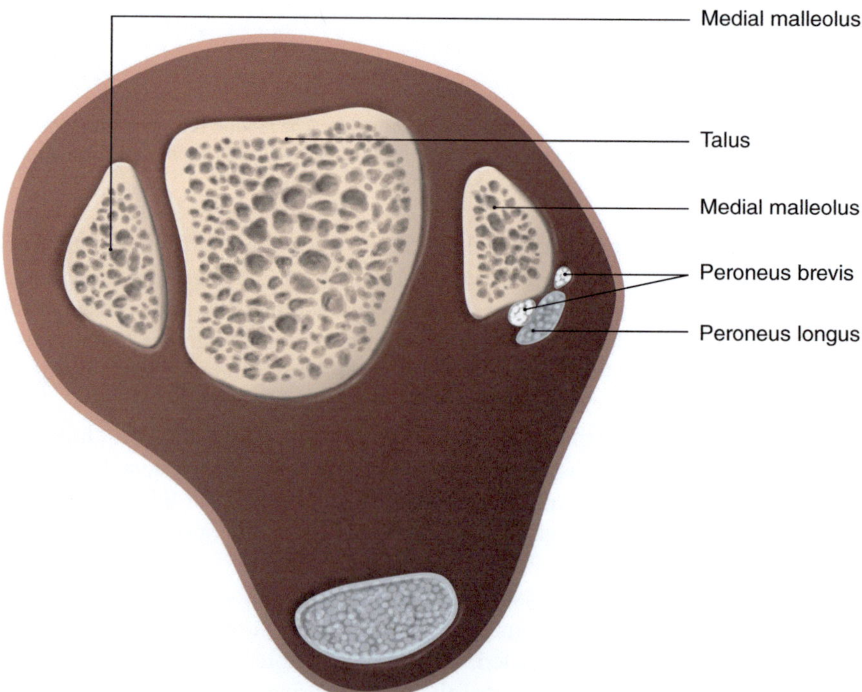

Fig. 12.3 Injury to the peroneus brevis tendon. The peroneus longus tendon is normal

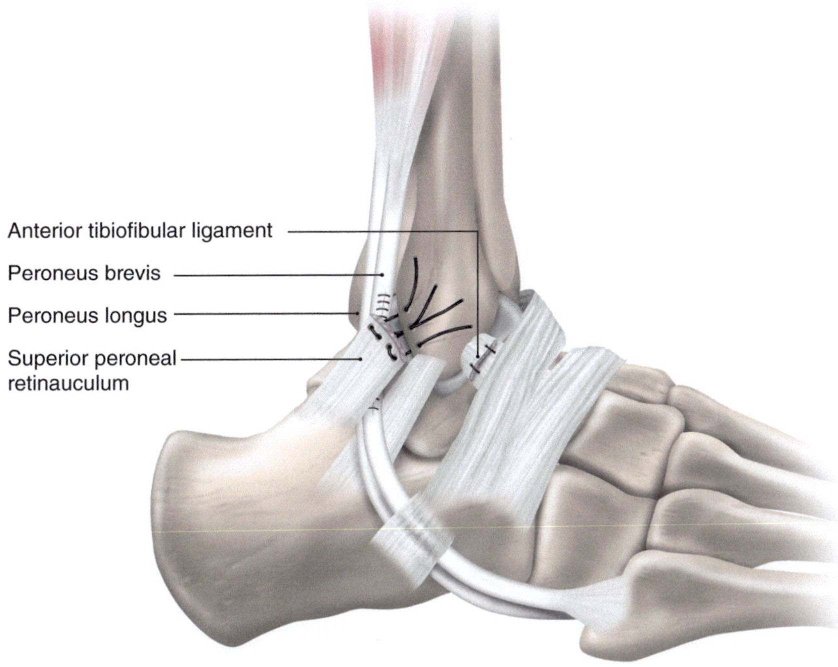

Fig. 12.4 Reconstruction of the superior peroneal retinaculum is performed after repair/reconstruction of the peroneus brevis tendon behind the lateral malleolus. The superior peroneal retinaculum is reconstructed, using sutures through drill channels in the posterior edge of the lateral fibula, in order to avoid recurrent subluxation of the peroneal tendon(s). Finally, anatomical reconstruction of the ankle ligaments (in this case, the anterior talofibular ligament) is performed

strength training of ankle joint eversion, where the load on the reconstructed peroneus brevis tendon is gradually increased, and closed-chain exercises using bilateral and unilateral loading of the lower extremity. Balance and coordination training can be progressed using variation balance boards; jumping and pivoting exercises, however, should be limited to every 2–3 days to help ensure sufficient recovery. Monitoring increases in swelling and pain is advised to ensure that load capacity is not exceeded.

Return to sports activities is individual, and more criteria-based than time-based. Resolving limitations in range of motion and swelling is recommended before initiating jumping, running, or sport-specific training. Ankle joint strength, jumping ability, and balance should be symmetrical between limbs before full return to sports. Return to sports may take time. It usually takes around 4–6 months until full recovery and should be introduced gradually [22, 35, 36, 42–45].

Prognosis

The results have been reported as satisfactory in the majority of cases. Repeated surgery is not frequent, and once the rehabilitation period is over, the risk of recurrence is low.

References

1. Larsen E. Longitudinal rupture of the peroneus brevis tendon. J Bone Joint Surg. 1987;69-B:340–1.
2. Sobel M, DiCarlo E, Bohne WHO, Collins L. Longitudinal splitting of the peroneus brevis tendon; an anatomic and histologic study of cadaveric material. Foot Ankle. 1991;12:165–70.
3. Sobel M, Levy ME, Bohne WHO. Congenital variations of the peroneus quartus muscle: an anatomic study. Foot Ankle. 1991;11:81–9.
4. Sobel M, Bohne WHO, Markisz JA. Cadaver correlation of peroneal tendon changes with magnetic resonance imaging. Foot Ankle. 1991;11:384–8.
5. Sobel M, Geppert MJ, Warren RF. Chronic ankle instability as a cause of peroneal tendon injury. Clin Orthop Relat Res. 1993;296:187–91.
6. Meyers AW. Further evidence of attrition of the human body. Am J Anat. 1924;34:241–8.
7. Brodsky JW, Zide JR, Kane JM. Acute peroneal injury. Foot Ankle Clin. 2017;22(4):833–41.
8. Cerrato RA, Myerson MS. Peroneal tendon tears, surgical management and its complications. Foot Ankle Clin. 2009;14(2):299–312.
9. Dombek MF, Orsini R, Mendicion RW, Saltrick K. Peroneus brevis tendon tears. Clin Podiatr Med Surg. 2001;18(3):409–27.
10. Gomes MDR, Pinto AP, Fabian AA, Gomes TJM, Navarro A, Olivia XM. Insertional anatomy of peroneal brevis and longus tendons – a cadaveric study. Foot Ankle Surg. 2018; https://doi.org/10.1016/fas.2018.07.005.
11. Roster B, Michelier P, Giza E. Peroneal tendon disorders. Clin Sports Med. 2015;34(4):625–41.
12. Patterson MJ, Cox WK. Peroneus longus tendon rupture as a cause of chronic lateral ankle pain. Clin Orthop Relat Res. 1999;365:163–6.
13. Bassett FH III, Speer KP. Longitudinal rupture of the peroneus tendons. Am J Sports Med. 1993;21:354–7.
14. Sobel M, Bohne WHO, Levy ME. Longitudinal attrition of the peroneus brevis tendon in the fibular groove: an anatomic study. Foot Ankle. 1990;11:124–8.
15. Bonnin M, Tavernier T, Bouysset M. Split lesions of the peroneus brevis tendon in chronic ankle laxity. Am J Sports Med. 1997;25:699–703.
16. Wander DS, Ludden JW, Galli K, Mayer DP. Surgical management of a ruptured peroneus longus tendon with a fractured multipartite os peroneum. J Foot Ankle Surg. 1994;33:124–8.
17. Sobel M, Geppert MJ, Hannafin JA, Bohne WHO, Arnoczky SP. Microvascular anatomy of the peroneal tendons. Foot Ankle. 1992;13:469–72.
18. Sobel M, Geppert MJ, Olsen EJ, Bohne WHO, Arnoczky SP. The dynamics of peroneus brevis tendon splits: a proposed mechanism, technique of diagnosis and classification of injury. Foot Ankle. 1992;13:413–22.
19. Slater HK. Acute peroneal tendon tears. Foot Ankle Clin. 2007;12(4):659–74.
20. Squires N, Myerson MS, Gamba C. Surgical treatment of peroneal tendon tears. Foot Ankle Clin. 2007;12(4):675–95.
21. Ziai P, Benca E, von Skrbensky G, Graf A, Wenzel F, Basad E, Windhager R, Buchhorn T. The role of the peroneal tendons in passive stabilisation of the ankle joint: an in vitro study. Knee Surg Sports Traumatol Arthrosc. 2013;21:1404–8.
22. Karlsson J, Wiger P. Longitudinal split of the peroneus brevis tendon and lateral ankle instability: treatment of concomitant lesions. J Athl Train. 2002;37(4):463–6.

23. Sobel M, Warren RF, Brourman S. Lateral ankle instability associated with dislocation of the peroneal tendons treated by the Chrisman-Snook procedure: a case reports and literature review. Am J Sports Med. 1990;18:539–43.
24. Sobel M, Bohne WHO, O'Brien SJ. Peroneal tendon subluxation in a case of anomalous peroneus brevis muscle. Acta Orthop Scand. 1992;63:682–4.
25. Evans JD. Subcutaneous rupture of the tendon of peroneus longus; report of a case. J Bone Joint Surg. 1966;48-B:507–9.
26. Minoyama O, Uahiyama E, Iwaso H, Hiranuma K, Takeda Y. Two cases of peroneus brevis tendon tear. Br J Sports Med. 2002;36:65–6.
27. Sammarco GJ, DiRaimondo CV. Chronic peroneus brevis tendon lesions. Foot Ankle. 1989;9:163–70.
28. CV DR. Overuse conditions of the foot and ankle. In: Sammarco GJ, editor. Foot and ankle manual. Philadelphia: Lea & Febiger; 1991. p. 266–8.
29. Munk RL, David PH. Longitudinal rupture of the peroneus brevis tendon. J Trauma. 1976;10:803–6.
30. Sobel M, Geppert MJ. Repair of concomitant lateral ankle ligament instability and peroneus brevis splits through a posteriorly modified Broström-Gould. Foot Ankle. 1992;13:224–5.
31. Chauban B, Panchal P, Szabo E, Wilkins T. Split peroneus brevis tendon: an unusual case of ankle pain and instability. J Am Board Fam Med. 2014;27:297–302.
32. Chrisman OD, Snook GA. Reconstruction of lateral ligament tears of the ankle. J Bone Joint Surg. 1969;51-A:904–11.
33. Snook GA, Chrisman OD, Wilson TC. Long-term results of Chrisman-Snook operation for reconstruction of lateral ligaments of the ankle. J Bone Joint Surg. 1985;67-A:1–8.
34. Araoye I, Pinter Z, Netto CDC, Hudson P, Shah A. Revisiting the prevalence of associated copathologies in chronic ankle instability. Are there any predictors of outcome? Foot Ankle Specialist. 2018; https://doi.org/10.1177/1938640018793513.
35. Karlsson J, Brandsson S, Kälebo P, Eriksson BI. Surgical treatment of concomitant chronic ankle instability and longitudinal rupture of the peroneus brevis tendon. Scand J Med Sci Sports. 1998;8:42–9.
36. Arrowsmith SR, Fleming LL, Allman FL. Traumatic dislocations of the peroneal tendons. Am J Sports Med. 1983;11:142–6.
37. Gould N, Seligson D, Gassman J. Early and later repair of lateral ligament of the ankle. Foot Ankle. 1980;1:84–9.
38. Karlsson J, Bergsten T, Lansinger O, Peterson L. Reconstruction of the lateral ligaments of the ankle for chronic lateral ligament instability of the ankle joint. J Bone Joint Surg. 1988;70-A:581–8.
39. Steginsky B, Riley A, Lucas DE, Philbin TM, Berlet GC. Patient-reported outcome and return to activity after peroneus brevis rupture. Foot Ankle Int. 2016;37(2):178–85.
40. Sammarco GJ, Mangone PG. Diagnosis and treatment of peroneal tendon injuries. Foot Ankle Surg. 2000;6:197–205.
41. Kane JM, Zide JR, Brodsky JW. Acute peroneal tendon injuries in sports. Oper Tech Sports Med. 2017;25:113–9.
42. Housley SN, Lewis JE, Thompson DL, Warren G. A proximal Fibularis brevis muscle is associated with longitudinal split tendons: a cadaveric study. J Foot Ankle Surg. 2017;56:34–6.
43. Shakked RJ, Karnovsky S, Drakos MC. Operative treatment of lateral ligament instability. Curr Rev Musculoskelet Med. 2017;10:113–21.
44. Drakos M, Behrens SB, Mulcahey MK, Paller D, Hoffman E, DiGiovanni CW. Proximity of arthroscopic ankle stabilization procedures to surrounding structures. An anatomic study. Arthroscopy. 2013;26:1089–94.
45. Andersson KJ, LeCocq JF. Operative treatment of injury to the fibular collateral ligament of the ankle. J Bone Joint Surg. 1954;36-A:825–30.

Groove Deepening Procedures and Approaches to Treatment of Peroneal Tendon Dislocations

David A. Porter and Joseph E. Jacobson

Introduction

Peroneal tendon dislocation is often associated with athletic activity. It was first popularized as a diagnosis in the sport of downhill skiing [20]. It was surmised that the tip of the ski itself would get caught in the snow and the athlete dorsiflexes and evert the ankle while the momentum carries them down the hill. The tip of the ski would remain lodged in the snow and cause the peroneal tendon to seek a more direct path from the lateral foot to the retrofibular area and dislocate anteriorly and laterally around the fibular tip. This dislocation has now been noted in almost all sports and can be associated with similar activity that commonly causes an ankle sprain. From personal observation, lateral ankle instability and peroneal tendon dislocation together is uncommon, occurring in only 10% of cases. It is speculated that a smooth or convex posterior fibula contributes to instability of the peroneal tendons. Nonoperative treatment for peroneal tendon dislocation historically has been proven to be unsuccessful. However, surgical procedures for stabilization have historically shown excellent outcomes. With appropriate rehabilitation and avoidance of some common pitfalls, such as extensive immobilization which leads to scarring, a successful return to recreational or competitive athletics is typically attainable.

D. A. Porter (✉)
Methodist Sports Medicine, Indianapolis, IN, USA
e-mail: davidaporter@sbcglobal.net

J. E. Jacobson
Department of Orthopedics, Indiana University, Indianapolis, IN, USA
e-mail: jacobsje@iu.edu

© Springer Nature Switzerland AG 2020
M. Sobel (ed.), *The Peroneal Tendons*,
https://doi.org/10.1007/978-3-030-46646-6_13

Historical Perspective

Peroneal tendon injury is a common problem in both the athletic and nonathletic populations. Most peroneal tendon injuries occur in the middle-aged patient. Peroneal tendon tear and tendinopathy is the most common injury to the peroneal tendon complex. The degenerative tearing of the peroneal tendon occurs in the older population, while the younger athletic population has a much lower incidence of peroneal tendon injury. However, in the younger population, and especially the athletic population, peroneal tendon dislocation is much more common [4, 10]. In fact, peroneal tendon dislocation may be the most common presentation for peroneal tendon complex injury in the teenage and young adult athlete [7]. A great deal of attention has been given to instability of the peroneal tendons, but true dislocation remains uncommon. Pseudosubluxation or intrasheath peroneal tendon instability is also another cause of peroneal tendon pain [26, 27, 37]. This involves the peroneal tendons subluxing within the sheath. Intrasheath subluxation involves the peroneus longus tendon displacing lateral to the brevis within a stretched-out sheath and "loose" superior peroneal retinaculum.

The Anatomy of the Tissue (Peroneals, Retinaculum, and Posterior Fibula) [6]

The peroneus brevis originates off the proximal intermuscular septum and middle third fibula, descends distally in the lateral compartment of the lower leg, and then positions itself in the peroneal sulcus on the posterior distal fibula. The peroneus longus tendon, in a similar manner, originates off the proximal tibia lateral condyle and proximal fibula, is also in the lateral compartment of the lower leg, and positions itself just posterior to the brevis tendon. The longus is slightly more lateral and is more prone to dislocation than the brevis. The posterior sulcus of the fibula has a variable contour; thus, a flat or convex contour is considered a predisposition to dislocation [1, 14]. The two tendons exist in a fibro-osseous tunnel bordered anteriorly by the posterior fibular fibrocartilaginous sulcus (distal 4 cm), posteriorly and laterally by the superior peroneal retinaculum (primary constraint to dislocation) and medially primarily by the calcaneal fibular ligament (CFL), though the posterior talofibular ligament and posterior–inferior tibiofibular ligament form part of the medial border also. There is a posterolateral fibrocartilaginous meniscal-like structure that adds depth and lateral constraint to the retromalleolar groove [1, 14]. This structure is often avulsed with acute tendon dislocations and degenerated in chronic dislocations. The posterior fibular anatomy has a varied surface contour: 82% are concave, 11% are "flat," and 7% are convex [6, 15]. The flat and convex anatomy, in association with peroneal dislocation, requires a formal fibular osteotomy for groove deepening in addition to reconstruction of the superior peroneal retinaculum, regardless of the acuteness of the dislocation. It should be noted, however, Adachi and coworkers [1] did not find a difference between the inherent anatomy between subjects treated for peroneal dislocation and a similar population of subjects that have not had a peroneal tendon instability history. Schon's lab has demonstrated that a peroneal groove deepening procedure can reduce the pressure within the peroneal sheath [38], and presumably decrease the risk of recurrent instability.

The Nature of the Problem

A shallow, flat, or convex posterior fibula is thought to lead to poor bony stability of the peroneal tendons. After a dislocation of the peroneal tendon, lack of inherent bony stability puts a significant strain on the repaired or reconstructed superior peroneal retinaculum. It has been concluded that groove deepening of the posterior fibula is not only helpful, but also necessary, in situations where there is no deep bony stability. Even a mild concavity to the posterior fibula is typically enough to prevent redislocation after appropriate superior peroneal repair in the acute settings. However, in the chronic recurring dislocation setting, more concavity is needed to the posterior groove requiring fibular osteotomy for deepening to support the retinacular reconstruction.

Routine ankle imaging does not assess the posterior fibular sulcus. Advanced imaging with MRI, often used in the chronic setting to assess for peroneal tendon tears, can also evaluate the posterior groove, and, in the acute setting, assess the integrity of the superior peroneal retinaculum [35] Thomas has utilized ultrasound (U/S) to evaluate the dislocating peroneal tendons and the integrity of the superior peroneal retinaculum [37]. We have not commonly used this imaging modality but think it will have a more common role as U/S becomes more prevalent in the office practice.

A common question facing the surgeon is Do I need to deepen the groove? And if I do, how deep does it need to be? Also, if I am going to do bony work, does that lead to potential scarring of the tendon? If I choose a groove deepening procedure, should I perform an indirect method? Or is a direct groove deepening procedure more reliable and effective? Further, how does undergoing a groove deepening procedure impact my rehabilitation and return to sports and activity? To further answer these questions, let us examine historically the different groove deepening approaches. Each approach requires some form of an osteotomy of the fibula. See also Ferran's [8], Heckman's [10], and Marti's [17] review on this topic for other approaches and opinions. The earliest approach was described by Kelly [12] and involved a true rotational fibular osteotomy. We have organized our discussion by classifying the approaches as direct and indirect osteotomies/groove deepening's. We should note here that another approach taken by several authors (covered in another chapter in this book) involves rerouting the peroneal tendons under the CFL by osteotomizing the CFL attachment to the distal fibula [16, 25, 31, 32].

Direct Groove Deepening Approaches

RE Kelly, in 1920 reporting from Liverpool England in the British Journal of Surgery [12], first proposed groove deepening for a recurrent peroneal tendon dislocation. He reported making a posterolateral approach to the fibula, remaining anterior to the peroneal groove, and staying out of the peroneal sheath. He

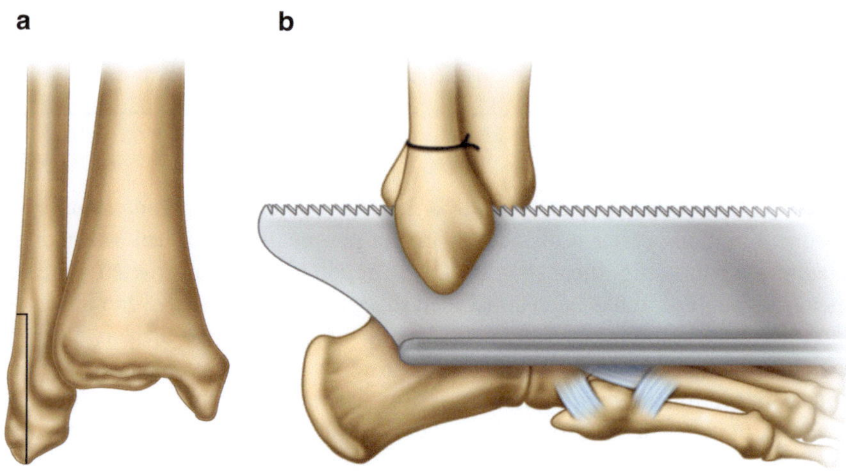

Fig. 13.1 (a, b) Kelly [12] Veneer graft in lateral malleolus, lateral aspect of fibula is rotated posterior to deepen posterior malleolar sulcus. (Cited with permission)

performed a sagittal "veneer"-type osteotomy of the distal 2 inches above the distal fibular tip and then rotated the lateral bony "veneer" posteriorly to create a deepened groove (Fig. 13.1). The procedure was performed on a sergeant in the Salatonika army and reported a 1-year follow-up with no recurrence to the dislocation.

Zoellner and Clancy [43] proposed and reported on approaching groove deepening via a direct groove approach also. However, rather than a true rotational osteotomy of the fibula, they approached the groove deepening via a hinged posterior flap of the retromalleolar groove which results in a more direct posterior deepening. Their technique involved "*the groove for the (peroneal) tendons is deepened by removal of some inner fibular substance, while the smooth tenosynovial channel is maintained as an intact periosteal flap on the fibula*" [43] (Fig. 13.2). The authors desired "*a simple procedure that corrects the basic deformity of a shallow peroneal groove, without the use of metallic fixation or transfer of a tendon or ligament.*"

Slatis and coworkers [30] modified the Zoellner and Clancy [43] report of direct deepening by removing the cartilaginous gliding layer of bone from the retromalleolar fibular groove, removing further cancellous bone using a curved chisel, and replacing the cartilaginous gliding bone by impacting it into the deepened groove [30] (Fig. 13.2a–c). The tendons are then replaced. No fixation is utilized to secure the replaced posterior bone. Plaster cast immobilization was required to allow healing of the replanted bone. Four case reports were reported and return to sports was 4–5 months postoperative without any redislocations (Fig. 13.3).

Porter, McCarroll, and coworkers [24] also modified the Zoellner and Clancy approach by removing the posterior corticocancellous retromalleolar groove with the intact serosa surface, deepened the distal posterior groove by removing cancellous bone with a motorized 4.0 egg burr, and then replaced the gliding surface by reattaching it with sutures in the depth of the deepened groove [24] (Fig. 13.4a–d).

Recurrent dislocation of the peroneal tendon

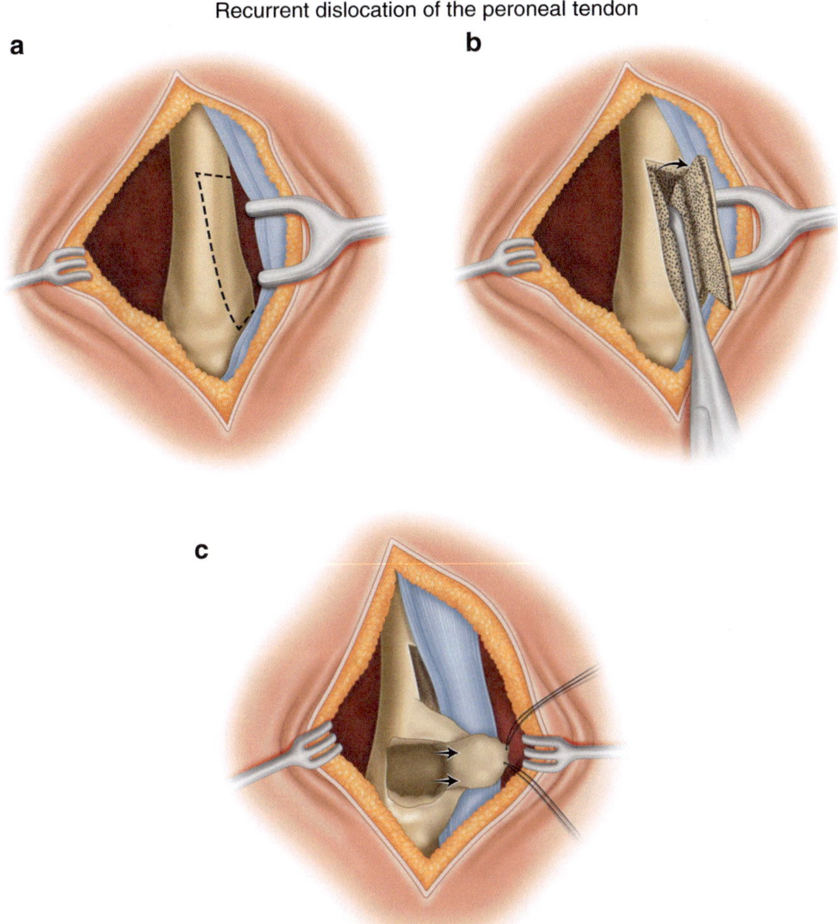

Fig. 13.2 Direct Groove deepening procedure as reported by Zoellner and Clancy [43]. (**a**) Demarcation of osteotomy off posterior fibular with peroneal tendons posteriorly retracted. (**b**) Hinged posterior flap raised initially to allow removal of cancellous bone and then swinging back of the posterior hinged bony flap into area of removed bone to allow "deepen the groove". (**c**) Periosteal flap off lateral fibula with posterolateral hinge to re-inforce and reconstruct the superior peroneal retinaculum after peroneal tendons replaced in deepened groove (cited with permission [43])

The authors note the degree of deepening within the posterior fibula must be enough such that the posterior border of the peroneal tendons lies flush with, or anterior to, the posterior border of the deepened groove. This degree of depth and concavity to the posterior fibula gives a strong bony resistance to recurrent dislocation. This detailed groove deepening and a standard superior peroneal retinacular reconstruction allowed the authors to be more accelerated in their rehabilitation. The authors reported on 13 athletes (14 ankles) allowed early weight bearing (1–2 weeks PO), only used intermittent immobilization with a walking boot (4 weeks total and then

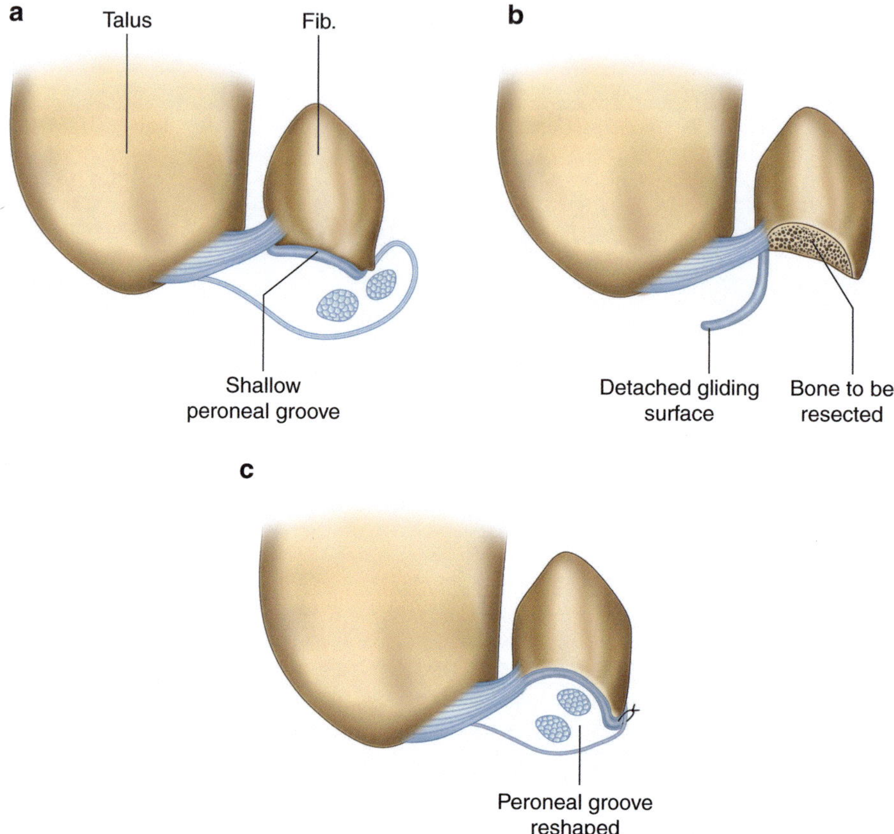

Fig. 13.3 (**a–c**) Slatis and coworker's method of surgical repair of chronic dislocation of the peroneal tendons. The retromalleolar groove is reshaped and the cartilaginous gliding layer is at the same time maintained. First, the retromalleolar groove is exposed (**a**), then the bone is resected under the displaced serosal surface (**b**), then the groove deepened, the serosal surface replaced, and the tendons replaced in the deepened groove. The SPR then is reattached (**c**). (Cited with permission [30])

2 weeks wean into a stirrup brace), and reported earlier return to sports (3 months). No dislocations were observed and near-normal ROM was achieved.

Zhenbo and colleagues [42] report in 2014 an approach reminiscent of the Kelly procedure. Their approach also involved a sagittal osteotomy in the fibula with a posterior slide of the osteotomy fixed with absorbable screws [42] (Fig. 13.5). After the posterolateral approach to the fibula and incision of the peroneal tendon sheath, the peroneals are inspected and repaired as indicated, with excision of any low-lying muscle belly. *"The periosteum (is) then detached anteriorly, keeping the anterior talofibular ligament and calcaneofibular ligament attached to the distal fibula. An oblique 20-degree (toward the sagittal plane) osteotomy was made anteromedially with a small oscillating saw extending from about 3 cm above the lateral malleolus*

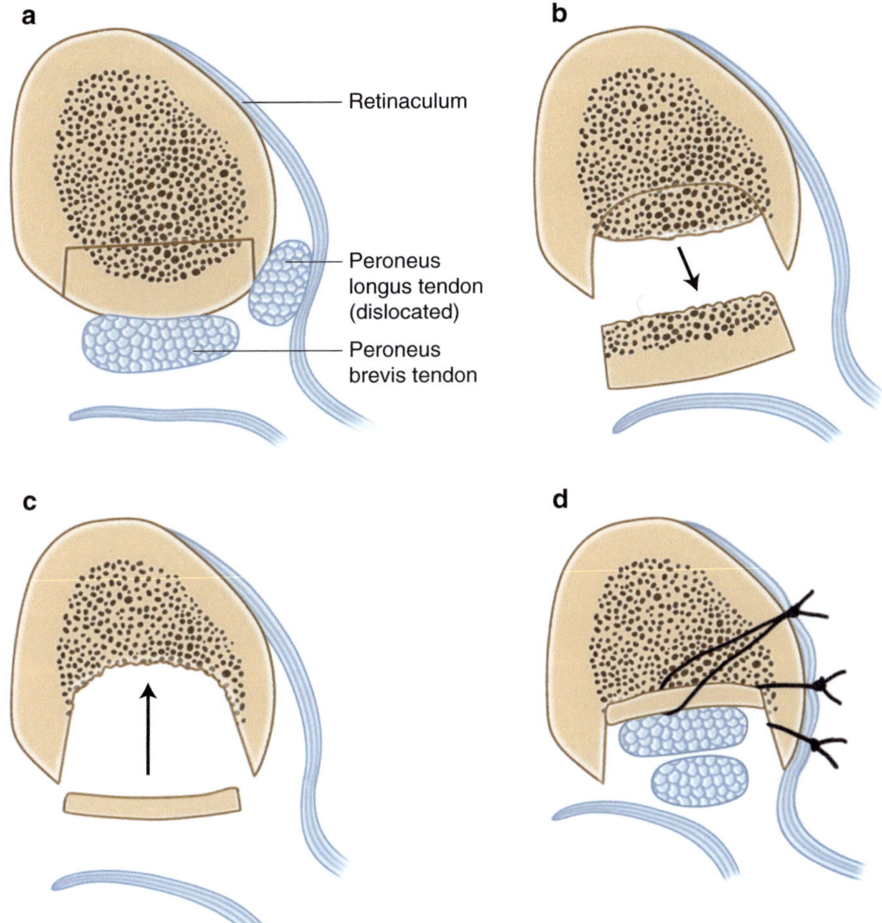

Fig. 13.4 (**a–d**) Porter and associates approach to direct fibular osteotomy for groove deepening. A modified approach to the Zoellner and Clancy [43] approach involves removing the posterior cortical cancellous sulcus (**a, b**: rather than hinging), deepening the cancellous groove, and replacing the posterior sulcus in the deepened cancellous bed with reattachment of the superior peroneal retinaculum (**c, d**). [Cited with permission FAI [24]]

to the fibular apex. When the saw nearly reached the posterior edge, the osteotomy exit(s) posterolaterally without damaging the cartilaginous ridge. The graft (3 × 2 × 0.5 cm) (is) slid 20 to 30 degrees (3–5 mm) posteriorly to ensure an adequate block to dislocation (Fig. 13.5). After application of bone wax to the raw surface, the tendons were manipulated into their correct position while the graft was secured to the distal fibula with 2 or 3 absorbable self-reinforced polylactide (SR-PLLA) screws (Conmed Biofix SmartScrew, ConmedLinvatec, Espoo, Finland), taking care to avoid intraarticular screw insertion. To protect the tendons from being frayed by the coarse interface, the SPR and tendon sheath were fastened to

Fig. 13.5 Sagittal Oblique osteotomy of the fibula/lateral malleolus is undertaken, positioned posteriorly, and fixed with absorbable screws. The tendon sheath and superior peroneal retinaculum is attached to the periosteal sleeve on the posterior surface of the distal fibula while the needle was rerouted back to affix the SPR and sheath through 5 drill holes in the graft, using the modified Das De technique [39]

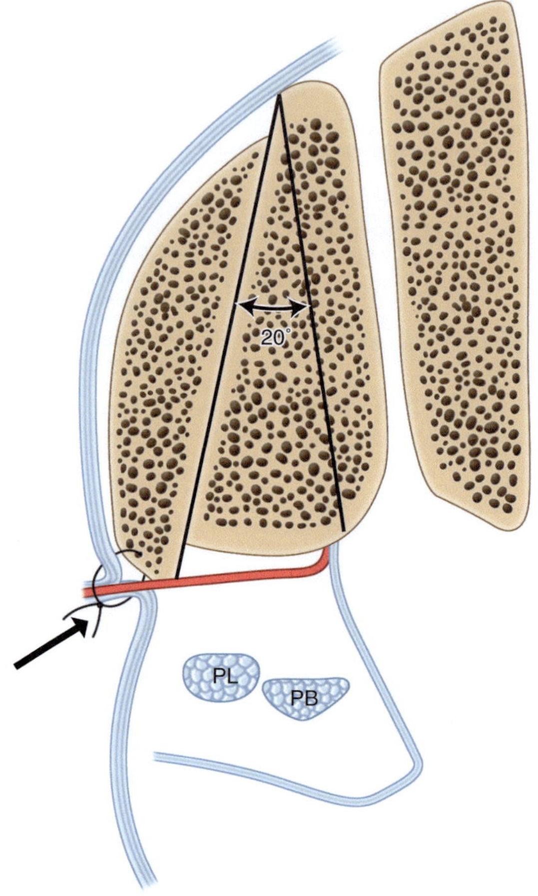

the periosteal sleeve on the posterior surface of the distal fibula with nonabsorbable suture (2–0 Ethibond, Ethicon Endosurgery, Somerville, NJ), while the needle was rerouted back to affix the SPR and sheath through 5 drill holes in the graft, using the modified Das De technique [39]. Finally, the periosteum (is) affixed to the SPR/sheath insertion with the graft enveloped in a soft tissue capsule."

Routine closure is utilized with 4 weeks in a below knee cast in neutral followed by NWB in a boot for an additional 2 weeks. The greater caution in rehabilitation is secondary to the true fibular osteotomy.

Indirect Groove Deepening Approachesv

Shawen and Anderson first described the indirect approach [29]. These authors prefer a "sloppy lateral position" with a 10-pound sand bag under the ipsilateral hip. A standard posterolateral approach is undertaken to access the groove and peroneal

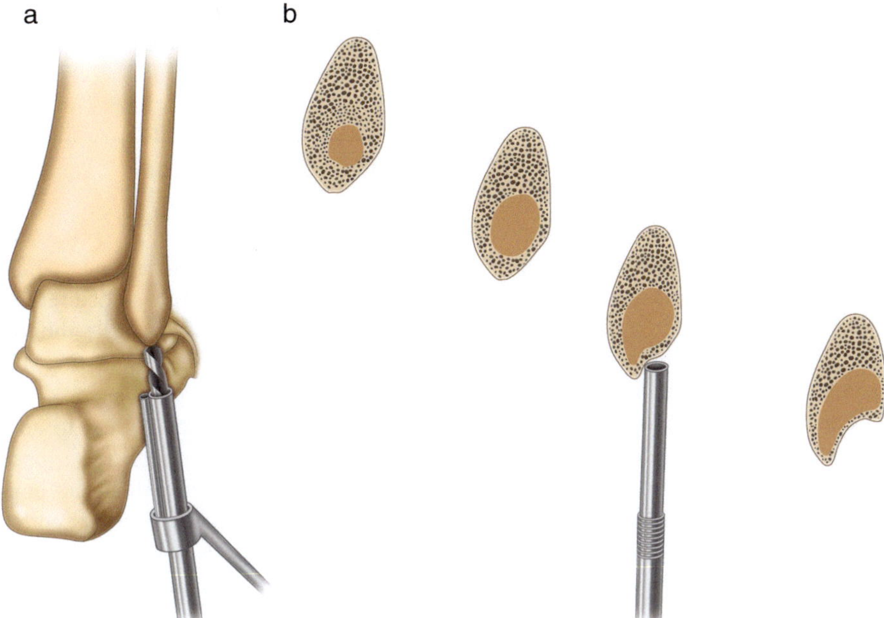

Fig. 13.6 (**a**) Indirect method of retrofibular groove deepening for treatment of dislocating peroneal tendons with inadequate bony stability [29]. An "appropriately sized reamer" is utilized to thin the retromalleolar, subcortical bone through the exposed fibular tip. (**b**) The thinned retromalleolar bone then allows a blunt 3–4-mm impactor to deepen the groove to provide enhanced bony stability

tendons. The peroneal tendons are repaired if indicated. The tip of the fibula is exposed, and the "reamer from the Arthrex bio-tenodesis screw set" and a "suitably sized" reamer are used to "thin" the posterior cortex of the groove. A moderate, wide bone impactor is used to deepen the posterior surface in an indirect manner, recreating the concavity needed to insure stability. The superior retinaculum was sewn back and imbricated to give soft tissue restraint to redislocation (Fig. 13.6).

Walters and coworkers, from Germany, reported in The American Journal of Sports Medicine (AJSM) on their technique for groove deepening via an indirect approach [41]. The authors describe the patient in a lateral position with the operative side up. A standard approach is made to the fibular groove. The peroneal tendon sheath is taken directly off the posterior border of the fibula to enter the peroneal sheath and expose the posterior fibular groove. After determining that groove deepening is required, the authors describe their indirect approach (Figs. 13.7) [41].

The fibular tip is identified and exposed. A 3.5-mm drill is used to make multiple passes under the posterior cortex as shown in Fig. 13.7a. Then, a "small" osteotome is utilized to perforate the medial and lateral border of the retromalleolar groove. The posterior cortical serosal surface can then be impacted/"compacted" to "deepen" the groove to a depth of at least 5 mm utilizing a wide blunt bone tamp/impactor.

The posterior cartilage rim is retained, if it is present. The superior peroneal retinaculum is then sewn into the medial border of the cancellous surface (Fig. 13.7b) to further inhibit redislocation of the peroneal tendons [41].

Intrasheath Peroneal Dislocation Without SPR Avulsion

Intrasheath dislocations typically present as a "snapping tendon" [26, 27, 37]. There may or may not be a definable history of a lateral ankle injury. It is proposed that the SPR has been either torn or stretched but not avulsed, and thus there is added redundancy to the superior peroneal retinaculum. Thus, the peroneus longus subluxes laterally around the brevis but still within the retinaculum and sheath, creating this "snapping" sensation that can, at times, be audible.

Our approach is the same as the chronic dislocation. We surmise that, to adequately return the tendons permanently to their rightful position (longus posterior to the brevis), a deep groove is required to provide both bony and soft tissue constraints to subluxation. We have not attempted to treat these athletes/patients with a soft tissue correction only. Vega, Guelfi, and coworkers [9, 40] from Barcelona have reported experience with tendonoscopy for treatment with 6 of the 8 patients not requiring a fibular osteotomy but resection of a peroneus quartus and/or resection of low-lying peroneus brevis muscle with good results. Our rehabilitation of these surgically treated intrasheath subluxations is the same as the chronic dislocation and is discussed below.

Rehabilitation Principles and Approaches

There is a significant difference in the rehabilitation protocols used. Some have utilized non-weightbearing for 2–6 weeks [3, 21], but Porter et al. [24] advocated early weight bearing and early ROM. We utilize an ankle block anesthetic with a Monitored Anesthesia Care (MAC) approach. We believe this gives excellent immediate postoperative pain control. To augment efficacy and duration of the ankle block, we utilize cold-compression therapy (AircastCryocuff DJO, Carlsbad, CA) in conjunction with removable boot intermittent immobilization [24]. The cold compression therapy, in conjunction with the block, gives 12–16 hours of effective anesthesia. We use NSAIDs and acetaminophen on a scheduled basis to give a baseline of continuous pain control. We believe this cold therapy with these scheduled over-the-counter medications reduces the need for oral opioids and certainly negates the need for overnight stay.

Fig. 13.7 Indirect method of groove deepening as described by Walter and coworkers [43]. A 3.5-mm drill is used to make multiple passes under the posterior cortex with the peroneal tendons displaced laterally, and a "small" osteotome is then utilized to perforate the medial and lateral border of the retromalleolar groove. This alteration is made at the level shown by the middle diagram of the posterior fibula (**a**). The posterior sulcus can then be impacted to deepen the groove and the peroneal tendons placed fully within the bony groove and the SPR sewn into the medial lip of the lateral border of the deepened groove as shown (**b**). PB Peronaeus brevis tendon, PL Peronaeus longus tendon

The intermittent immobilization allows us to initiate ROM (DF, PF, and inversion, but we hold DF with eversion until after 6 weeks) after the sutures are removed at 2 weeks. We also begin a stationary bike program with the boot immobilization starting at 1–2 weeks depending on how the ankle looks. Balance in the boot can be

a

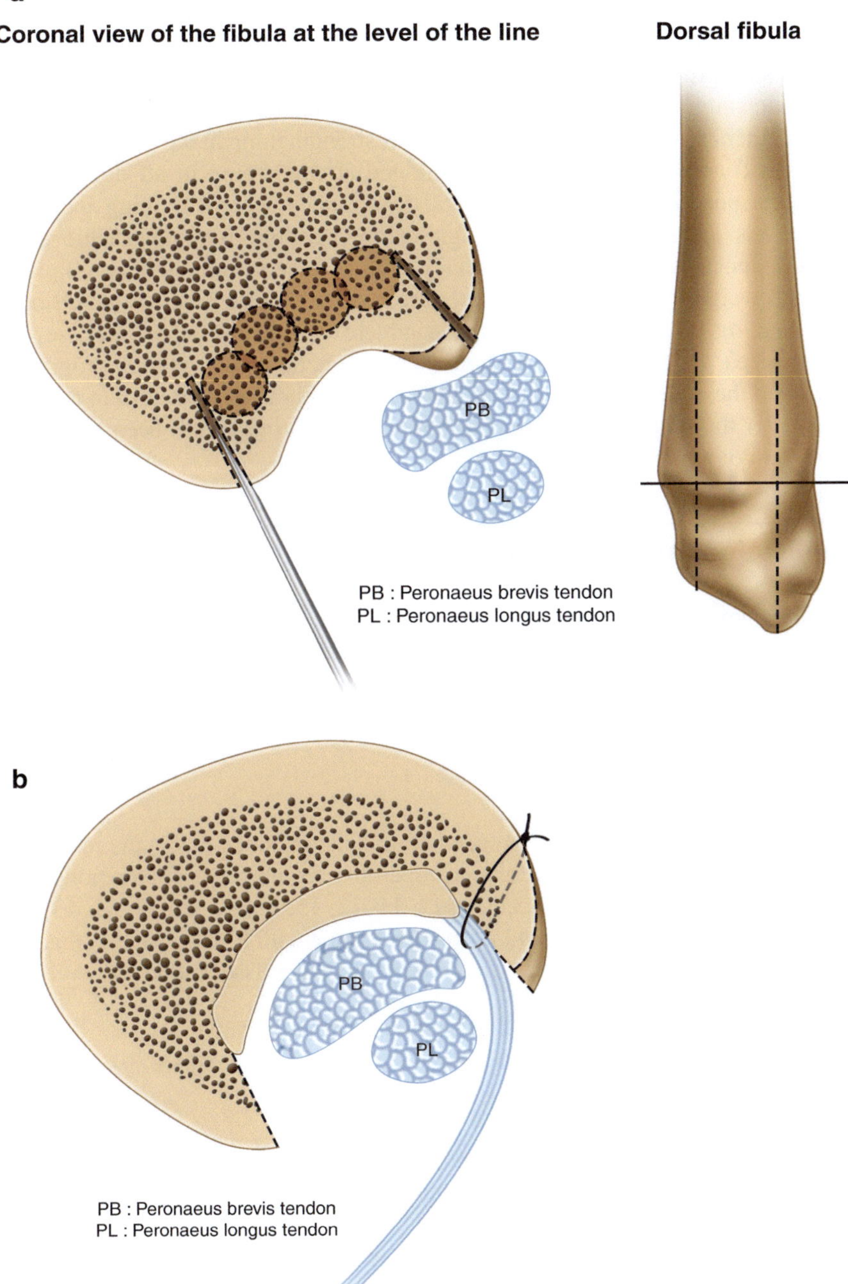

initiated at 2 weeks. We instruct the athlete on how to wean off crutches over the first 10–14 days. We start desensitization massage immediately to reduce causalgia/neuralgia risk. We believe early weight bearing serves as initial proprioception retraining, but also aids as a form of desensitization.

We use boot immobilization for 6 weeks, then wean the athlete out of the boot into a stirrup brace between weeks 6 and 8. We do allow stationary biking with a stirrup brace and double standing toe-raise at 4 weeks. At the 6-week appointment, we instruct the athlete how to wean out of the boot into the stirrup brace for daily activities, start proprioception retraining in the brace, and go from double standing toe-raises to single standing toe-raises as well. We then allow dorsiflexion and eversion strengthening with elastic bands as well as strengthening in the other directions as mentioned above. We progress to weighted strengthening in all directions at 2–3 months postoperative. We allow full lower body weight training including squats, cleans, and lunges after full weightbearing treadmill running is achieved.

At 6–8 weeks, we progress from biking with a brace to stair stepper, elliptical, and partial weight bearing treadmill exercises (Alter-G). We progress to full body weight running on a treadmill when the athlete can do the other exercises for 30–40 minutes, 4–5 days a week without pain. A functional progression program is begun when the athlete can run full weightbearing without pain. Return to sports is allowed after the sports-specific function progression program has been completed without pain or apprehension.

Complications and Potential Pitfalls

Generally, complications are uncommon after groove deepening and superior peroneal retinacular reconstruction regardless of the technique used. No deep venous thrombotic events have been reported in the literature [2, 13, 24].

Recurrent Dislocation

Recurrent dislocation is the most dreaded complication, since this is the reason for the surgery to begin with. Fortunately, postoperative instability is uncommon, especially with groove deepening procedures [2, 11–13, 15, 17, 19, 21, 39, 41–43]. We have only had one redislocation and it was in a female with Ehlers-Danlos (that was not in our study report-24) that we tried using her native tissues. She did well with revision and use of allograft tissue.

Infection and Wound Healing

Infection is also rare after these procedures [2, 3, 14, 39, 41, 42] and should be less than 0.5%. Kollias did report 2 of 11 patients had a suture abscess that resolved with local treatment.

Complications surrounding wound healing is also rare in the athlete, but can be common if the patient is a smoker or diabetic. Even with early ROM, we did not see a high propensity for wound healing issues [24]. Walther and coworkers did report that one-third of their patients noted "suture knot irritability, but it resolved uneventfully over time." Other studies either did not mention wound healing or did not mention wound-healing problems [3, 39, 41].

Peroneal Tendon Tear

A peroneal tendon tear can be common at the time of surgery in chronic cases, and in our experience direct repair and/or tubularization has a high success rate in our experience. None of the prior reports have indicated a peroneal tendon tear postoperative as a common problem after groove deepening procedures [2, 3, 11–13, 15, 19, 21, 29, 39, 41–43]. Only Marti noted, "continued peroneal pain" in 2/12 patients [17]; however, the authors did not mention further workup or surgery. Raikin, in his report on intrasheath subluxation, reported there were 4 patients that had a peroneus brevis tear at the time of surgery, [26] which would be considered a complication of the injury, but not of the surgery.

Nonunion

Nonunion should be uncommon, and none were reported in the nonrotational osteotomies [24, 39, 41]. The osteotomy is performed in well-vascularized cancellous bone. If secured, we have found no nonunions even with early weight bearing and early ROM. Higher risks for nonunion exist, in theory, with the earlier rotational osteotomies, but there were none reported [12, 17, 39].

Stiffness

We see this as a real potential for disability of the ankle due to stiffness if the ankle is immobilized for a prolonged period of time. To counteract this potential complication/risk, we choose to secure the bone flap in the deepened groove, fully place the posterior bone flap in the groove, maintain the serosa surface on the posterior flap, and encourage and allow early ROM. Boot immobilization, rather than casting, has now shown to be both reliable and near complication free [24]. Three additional authors [2, 3, 17] noted "good or full range-of-motion," and the other noted a 10% rate of "stiffness" [13]. Most authors did not report on range-of-motion (ROM).

Fibula Fracture

Large fragment fractures requiring ORIF are rare. Small fracturing of the posterior lateral lip of the lateral deepened groove can [39] and has occurred in our series [24], but responds well to boot immobilization for 3–4 weeks and then back into a stirrup brace with rare long-term difficulty and no requirements for further surgery.

Significant fracture after these fibular osteotomies for groove deepening is not reported [3, 21]. Zhenbo did report 3/21 patients suffered a "stress fracture" after their rotational osteotomy.

Sural Nerve Injury/Neuritis

Sural nerve irritability is rarely reported [2, 13, 24, 41]. The sural nerve is potentially in the operative field for all peroneal tendon surgery approaches. If the surgeon stays close to the posterior border of the fibula, this takes the surgical field anterior to the sural nerve. Drifting the incision or dissection more posterior certainly puts the nerve at risk. Desensitization massage (DSSM) is routinely instituted postoperatively in our practice. Mafulli did note 3/14 patients with "nerve irritability" that resolved after 6 months [15]. Interestingly, Ogawa [21] noted 4/5 worker compensation patients reported "nerve irritability," but none of the 10 nonworker compensation patients reported nerve irritability. We believe that with careful incision placement and early DSSM, nerve irritability should be avoided and resolve quickly in the postoperative period.

Principles of Groove Deepening

In summary, once it has been determined that a groove deepening is necessary, we think the following principles are crucial to an optimal outcome:

1. A fibular osteotomy is necessary to give adequate groove deepening if not inherently present.
2. The fibular osteotomy must be deepened to point that the posterior border of the peroneal tendons, when replaced within the deepened groove, must be flush with, or anterior to, the posterior border of the resultant groove.
3. Tightening and imbrication of the superior peroneal retinaculum must be undertaken also to give appropriate soft tissue constraint to dislocation. Reattachment of the SPR must be undertaken in instances of true dislocation (intrasheath dislocations do not require reattachment of SPR, just imbrication and tightening since SPR not detached).
4. Rehabilitation must include early ROM to prevent scarring and subsequent pain from tendon restriction. We believe that early weight bearing is also advantageous for accelerated recovery.

The Author's Preferred Approach

We first determine if there is an acute dislocation. That is, are we seeing the athlete/patient within the first 1–2 weeks of injury, or is this a chronic dislocation that has been reoccurring greater than 4 weeks from the time of initial injury?

For the acute dislocation, we still believe that operative treatment is the treatment of choice. In some situations, the posterior lateral cartilaginous rim is still intact and the posterior fibular anatomy has a reasonable concave contour. In this situation with a good underlying groove, we will initially try acute repair of the superior peroneal retinaculum. We have had good success when there is a naturally good deep groove in the acute setting. We do not take this acute repair approach without groove deepening in the chronic setting however.

For the chronic recurring dislocation, there are numerous techniques described [2, 3, 5, 9, 11–13, 15, 16, 18, 19, 21–26, 28–31, 33, 34, 36, 39, 41–43]. We always perform a groove deepening procedure. In this chronic setting, the posterior lateral cartilaginous rim is almost always absent and we have not found the posterior fibula to have enough concavity to support the peroneal tendons and their position. Thus, we do the fibular osteotomy described above by Porter et al. [24] and imbricate and reattach the superior peroneal retinaculum to the posterolateral fibula. We utilize the same rehabilitation protocol described above for all our procedures. Regarding intrasheath subluxations, our approach is the same as that of the chronic dislocation, but they do not require reattachment of the SPR; however, we tighten the SPR by overlapping the cut SPR fibers to those attached to the posterolateral fibula. For those patients/athletes with inherent ligament laxity (Ehlers-Danlos and its variants), we utilize gracilis allograft to reconstruct and augment the SPR and do a thorough groove deepening procedure. We attach the gracilis graft to the posterior tibia with a suture anchor and bone groove, then wrap it around the peroneal tendons and attach it to the typical SPR site on the posterolateral fibula.

Conclusion

In conclusion, groove deepening is a very satisfactory procedure with a high success rate in conjunction with superior peroneal retinacular reconstruction for the patient/athlete with acute or chronic peroneal dislocation. The surgeon has multiple approaches that have been documented to be successful. As noted, a fibular osteotomy is required to further deepen a shallow, flat, or convex fibula. We have described both direct and indirect approaches, as well as rotational approaches. Direct and indirect seem more popular today than the rotational osteotomies. Peroneal tendon dislocation/subluxation is not common; therefore, we recommend familiarizing with one or two of these groove deepening approaches and rely on that approach. Familiarity will serve the surgeon well in this approach and the success rate should be high with little risk of complications.

Bibliography

1. Adachi N, Fukuhara K, Kobayashi T, Nakasa T, Ochi M. Morphologic variations of the fibular malleolar groove with recurrent dislocation of the peroneal tendons. Foot Ankle Int. 2009;30(6):540–4.

2. Adachi N, Fukuhara K, Tanaka H, Nakasa T, Ochi M. Superior retinaculoplasty for recurrent dislocation of peroneal tendons. Foot Ankle Int. 2006;27(12):1074–8.
3. Cho J, Kim J, Song D, Lee W. Comparison of outcome after retinaculum repair with and without fibular groove deepening for recurrent dislocation of the peroneal tendons. Foot Ankle Int. 2014;35(7):683–9. https://doi.org/10.1177/1071100714531233.
4. Dijk PA, Gianakos AL, Kerkhoffs GM, Kennedy JG. Return to sports and clinical outcomes in patients treated for peroneal tendon dislocation: a systematic review. Knee Surg Sports Traumatol Arthrosc. 2016;24(4):1155–64. https://doi.org/10.1007/s00167-015-3833-z.
5. Dijk PA, Vopat BG, Guss D, Younger A, Digiovanni CW. Retromalleolar groove deepening in recurrent peroneal tendon dislocation: technique tip. Orthop J Sports Med. 2017;5(5):232596711770667. https://doi.org/10.1177/2325967117706673.
6. Edwards M. The relations of the peroneal tendons to the fibula, calcaneus, and cuboideum. Am J Anat. 1928;42:213–53.
7. Ferran NA, Oliva F, Maffulli N. Recurrent subluxation of the peroneal tendons. Sports Med. 2006;36(10):839–46. https://doi.org/10.2165/00007256-200636100-00003.
8. Ferran NA, Maffulli N, Oliva F. Management of recurrent subluxation of the peroneal tendons. Foot Ankle Clin. 2006;11(3):465–74. https://doi.org/10.1016/j.fcl.2006.06.002.
9. Guelfi M, Vega J, Malagelada F, Baduell A, Dalmau-Pastor M. Tendoscopic treatment of peroneal intrasheath subluxation: a new subgroup with superior peroneal retinaculum injury. Foot Ankle Int. 2018;39(5):542–50. https://doi.org/10.1177/1071100718764674.
10. Heckman DS, Reddy S, Pedowitz D, Wapner KL, Parekh SG. Operative treatment for peroneal tendon disorders. J Bone Joint Surg. 2008;90(2):404–18. https://doi.org/10.2106/jbjs.g.00965.
11. Hu M, Xu X. Treatment of chronic subluxation of the peroneal tendons using a modified posteromedial peroneal tendon groove deepening technique. J Foot Ankle Surg. 2018;57(5):884–9. https://doi.org/10.1053/j.jfas.2018.03.009.
12. Kelly RE. An operation for the chronic dislocation of the peroneal tendons. Br J Surg. 1920;7:502–4.
13. Kollias SL, Ferkel RD. Fibular grooving for recurrent peroneal tendon subluxation. Am J Sports Med. 1997;25(3):329–35.
14. Kumai T, Benjamin M. The histological structure of the malleolar groove of the fibula in man: its direct bearing on the displacement of peroneal tendons and their surgical repair. J Anat. 2003;203(2):257–62. https://doi.org/10.1046/j.1469-7580.2003.00209.
15. Maffulli N, Ferran NA, Oliva F, Testa V. Recurrent subluxation of the peroneal tendons. Am J Sports Med. 2006;34:986–92.
16. Martens MA, Noyez JF, Mulier JC. Recurrent dislocation of the peroneal tendons. Results of rerouting the tendons under the calcaneofibular ligament. Am J Sports Med. 1986;14(2):148–50.
17. Marti R. Dislocation of the peroneal tendons. Am J Sports Med. 1977;5:19–22.
18. Maqdes A, Steltzlen C, Pujol N. Endoscopic fibular groove deepening for stabilisation of recurrent peroneal tendons instability in a patient with open physes. Knee Surg Sports Traumatol Arthrosc. 2017;25(6):1925–8. https://doi.org/10.1007/s00167-016-4210-2.
19. McLennan JG. Treatment of acute and chronic luxations of the peroneal tendons. Am J Sports Med. 1980;8:432–6.
20. Oden RR. Tendon injuries about the ankle resulting from skiing. Clin Orthop Relat Res. 1987;216:63–9.
21. Ogawa BK, Thordarson DB, Zalavras C. Peroneal tendon subluxation repair with an indirect fibular groove deepening technique. Foot Ankle Int. 2007;28(11):1194–7. https://doi.org/10.3113/fai.2007.1194.
22. Oliva F, Ferran N, Maffulli N. Peroneal retinaculoplasty with anchors for peroneal tendon subluxation. Bull Hosp Joint Dis. 2006;63(3–4):113–6.
23. Poll R, Duijfres F. The treatment of recurrent dislocation of the peroneal tendons. J Bone Joint Surg. 1984;66-B:98–100.
24. Porter D, McCarroll J, Knapp E, Torma J. Peroneal tendon subluxation in athletes: fibular groove deepening and retinacular reconstruction. Foot Ankle Int. 2005;26:436–41.

25. Pozo JL, Jackson AM. A rerouting operation for dislocation of peroneal tendons: operative technique and case report. Foot Ankle. 1984;5(1):42–4.
26. Raikin SM. Intrasheath subluxation of the peroneal tendons. Surgical technique. J Bone Joint Surg. 2009;91:146–55. https://doi.org/10.2106/JBJS.H.01356.
27. Raikin SM, Elias I, Nazarian LN. Intrasheath subluxation of the peroneal tendons. J Bone Joint Surg Am. 2008;90(5):992–9.
28. Saxena A, Ewen B. Peroneal subluxation: surgical results in 31 athletic patients. J Foot Ankle Surg. 2010;49(3):238–41.
29. Shawen SB, Anderson RB. Indirect groove deepening in the management of chronic peroneal tendon dislocation. Tech Foot Ankle Surg. 2004;3:118–25.
30. Slätis P, Santavirta S, Sandelin J. Surgical treatment of chronic dislocation of the peroneal tendons. Br J Sports Med. 1988;22:16–8.
31. Stenquist DS, Gonzalez TA, Tepolt FA, Kramer DE, Kocher MS. Calcaneofibular ligament transfer for recurrent peroneal tendon subluxation in pediatric and young adult patients. J Pediatr Orthop. 2018;38(1):44–8. https://doi.org/10.1097/bpo.0000000000000731.
32. Steinbock G, Pinsger M. Treatment of peroneal tendon dislocation by transposition under the calcaneofibular ligament. Foot Ankle Int. 1994;15:107–11.
33. Stover C, Bryan D. Traumatic dislocation of the peroneal tendons. J Bone Joint Surg. 1962;61-A:292–4.
34. Suh JW, Lee JW, Park JY, Choi WJ, Han SH. Posterior fibular groove deepening procedure with low-profile screw fixation of fibrocartilaginous flap for chronic peroneal tendon dislocation. J Foot Ankle Surg. 2018;57(3):478–83. https://doi.org/10.1053/j.jfas.2017.10.033.
35. Taljanovic MS, Alcala JN, Gimber LH, Rieke JD, Chilvers MM, Latt LD. High-resolution US and MR imaging of peroneal tendon injuries. Radiographics. 2015;35(1):179–99. https://doi.org/10.1148/rg.351130062.
36. Tan V, Lin SS, Okereke E. Superior peroneal retinaculoplasty: a surgical technique for peroneal subluxation. Clin Orthop Relat Res. 2003;410:320–5. https://doi.org/10.1097/01.blo.0000063594.67412.32.
37. Thomas JL, Lopez-Ben R, Maddox J. A preliminary report on intra-sheath peroneal tendon subluxation: a prospective review of seven patients with ultrasound verification. J Bone Joint Surg Am. 1989;71:293–5.
38. Title CI, Jung H, Parks BG, Schon LC. The peroneal groove deepening procedure: a biomechanical study of pressure reduction. Foot Ankle Int. 2005;26(6):442–8. https://doi.org/10.1177/107110070502600603.
39. Tomihara T, Shimada N, Yoshida G, Kaneda K. Comparison of modified Das De procedure with Du Vries procedure for traumatic peroneal tendon dislocation. Arch Orthop Trauma Surg. 2010;130(8):1059–63.
40. Vega J, Batista JP, Golanó P, Dalmau A, Viladot R. Tendoscopic groove deepening for chronic subluxation of the peroneal tendons. Foot Ankle Int. 2013;34(6):832–40. https://doi.org/10.1177/1071100713483098.
41. Walther M, Morrison R, Mayer B. Retromalleolar groove impaction for the treatment of unstable peroneal tendons. Am J Sports Med. 2009;37(1):191–4. https://doi.org/10.1177/0363546508324310.
42. Zhenbo Z, Jin W, Haifeng G, Huanting L, Feng C, Ming L. Sliding fibular graft repair for the treatment of recurrent peroneal subluxation. Foot Ankle Int. 2014;35(5):496–503. https://doi.org/10.1177/1071100714523271.
43. Zoellner G, Clancy W Jr. Recurrent dislocation of the peroneal tendon. J Bone Joint Surg Am. 1979;61(2):292–4.

Intrasheath Subluxation of the Peroneal Tendons

14

Steven M. Raikin and Rabun Fox

Background

In 1803, Monteggia published a brief discourse on instability of the peroneal tendons. In his writing, he discussed a patient presenting with frank dislocations of the peroneus brevis and longus tendons [1]. In the modern era, peroneal instability involving dislocation of the tendons from the confines of the retrofibular groove through the superior peroneal retinaculum (SPR) has been well studied. Eckert and Davis' work classified the pathology according to the lesion of the retinaculum, or its attachment, which produces instability [2]. This was later added by Ogden into four grades depending on the degree of SPR injury or bony avulsion [3].

In contrast to dislocation of the peroneal tendons from their anatomic location posterior to the fibula, intrasheath peroneal subluxation involves alteration of the normal relationship of the peroneal brevis and longus tendons relative to each other, but with the tendons remaining within the confines of the superior peroneal retinaculum. Published work by Raikin et al. was the first to clearly define intrasheath subluxation [4]. Isolated case reports discussing mechanical symptoms about the peroneal tendons without gross instability had demonstrated this clinical entity [5, 6]. These publications did not, however, provide adequate cohorts size and were presented without systematic approach. In his initial work, Raikin et al. identified a cohort of patients presenting with peroneal mechanical symptoms who did not have dislocation of the tendons on clinical examination [4]. Dynamic sonographic imaging investigation demonstrated that there was a reversal of the normal relationship of the peroneus longus and brevis within their groove or displacement of the peroneus longus into a longitudinal tear of the brevis during range of motion as opposed to traditional displacement of the tendons from within the groove [4, 7]. These patients did not demonstrate any lesions of the SPR which characterized traditional

S. M. Raikin (✉) · R. Fox
Anchorage Fracture and Orthopedic clinic, Anchorage, AL, USA
e-mail: steven.raikin@rothmaninstitute.com; Rabin.Fox@Rothmaninstitute.com

© Springer Nature Switzerland AG 2020
M. Sobel (ed.), *The Peroneal Tendons*,
https://doi.org/10.1007/978-3-030-46646-6_14

253

peroneal instability. A standard imaging and surgical protocol were presented in conjunction with outcome measures with mostly good to excellent results [4] Thomas et al. published their own series of seven patients who presented in similar fashion and with similar imaging findings [8].

Clinical Presentation and Physical Examination

The most common mechanism of injury resulting in peroneal instability is an inversion-type ankle sprain injury. The peroneus brevis muscle, functioning as the primary dynamic stabilizer of the ankle, fires aggressively in an attempt to protect the ankle. This is thought to alter the normal mechanics of the peroneus brevis and longus tendons relative to each other resulting in subsequent dysmotility and instability. In the largest published cohort on intrasheath subluxation, all patients sustained an injury to the ankle within 6 months [4]. The cohort presented was an average of 25 years of age and the majority female. Patients are frequently initially diagnosed as and treated for an ankle sprain with immobilization and/or physical therapy, which may result in delayed diagnosis and management.

The chief complaint on presentation is usually pain posterior to the distal fibula along the path of the peroneal tendons, more so than over the anterior talofibular ligament. Patients will frequently be aware of a clicking or popping feeling (which they will frequently state they can hear) behind the fibula, which is painful. Ankle instability is not an associated complaint, but may be a concomitant injury. Patients are usually able to ambulate without difficulty, but develop pain and clicking with athletic activity.

Clinical examination of intrasheath subluxation may demonstrate swelling in the posterior lateral ankle. Patients will usually have tenderness to palpation over the course of the peroneal tendons at the level of the SPR behind the distal fibula It is important to palpate the region of the anterior talofibular ligament, anterior syndesmosis, inframalleolar region, and the Achilles insertion to identify or rule-out concomitant pathology. Patient's clinical alignment should be evaluated for cavovarus which could potentiate the tendon pathology. During active circumduction of the ankle with the examiner's fingers applying pressure over the SPR attachment to the posterior distal fibula, a clicking sensation can usually be palpated during eversion and dorsiflexion of the ankle joint. This will usually be accompanied by a report of pain from the patient. Testing of peroneal strength should also be performed and compared to the contralateral side. Strength loss may be due to injury to the peroneal tendon or secondary to painful inhibition. This may additionally limit the ability to feel the dysmotility making the clinical diagnosis more difficult. It is important to note that with active testing reproduces the mechanical symptom, the peroneal tendons are not felt to dislocate from their anatomic location posterior to fibula, as is found with classical classic peroneal dislocation / instability.

Diagnostic Imaging

Initial imaging evaluation for suspected peroneal pathology should include standard weight-bearing ankle radiographs. While no specific radiographic findings have been correlated with intrasheath subluxation, radiographs may demonstrate associate pathologies such as cavovarus alignment, tarsal coalitions, avulsion fractures, and osteochondral lesions.

Definitive diagnosis requires utilization of advanced imaging modalities. Dynamic ultrasound has been demonstrated to be the modality of choice to confirm the diagnosis of peroneal intrasheath subluxation. This should be performed utilizing a high-resolution ultrasonography (US) with high-frequency linear transducers by a musculoskeletal ultrasonographer experienced in performing dynamic studies, as the results can be very operator dependent. Static images are reported as part of the complete imaging assessment to evaluate for tendon tears and tendinosis. Characterization of tendonitis and tears may be useful for surgical planning when other advanced imaging is not performed. Dynamic ultrasound has been demonstrated to definitively identify peroneal instability and confirm intrasheath subluxation [7, 9]. The technique includes axial and longitudinal images of the peroneal tendons as they course posterior to the fibula particularly during active eversion and dorsiflexion of the ankle joint. It is essential that testing include hindfoot inversion and eversion during dorsiflexion and plantar flexion to mimic the motion which most commonly elicits symptoms and clinical findings and patient should be instructed to attempt to replicate their symptoms. Testing should be performed both passively and actively. During the imaging, the peroneus longus may be visualized to reverse its natural position posterior and medial to the peroneus brevis at the level of the superior peroneal retinaculum (Fig. 14.1). The peroneus longus may also be

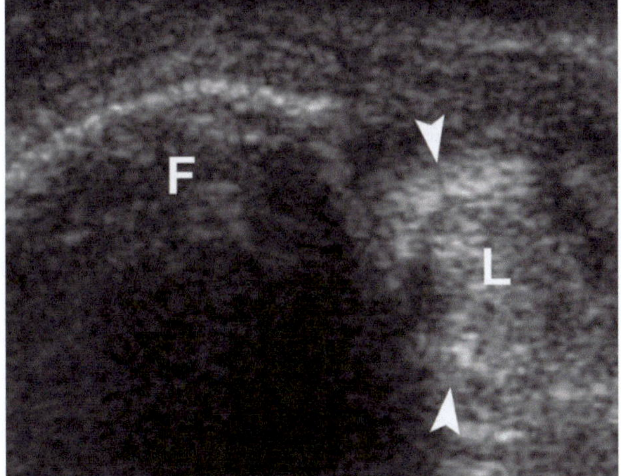

Fig. 14.1 Dynamic ultrasonography showing type-B intrasheath subluxation. The peroneus longus tendon has subluxated through the split peroneus brevis tendon. The white arrowheads point to the two split portions of the peroneus brevis tendon. F = fibula, and L = peroneus longus tendon. (With permission from Wolters Kluwer Publisher)

observed displacing into a longitudinal tear of the peroneus brevis. Morphologic variants are discussed in the following section. The integrity of the lateral ankle ligaments, particularly the anterior talofibular ligament, can be assessed during the same study with the ultrasonographer performing an anterior drawer and varus stress test on the ankle while visualizing the ligament and talar shift with the ultrasound probe.

Computerized tomography is generally unnecessary unless concomitant pathology such as fracture, malunion, nonunion, or other deformities are suspected. Magnetic resonance imaging (MRI) evaluation can be an important adjunct to the workup of suspected peroneal tendon pathology. For the specific evaluation of intrasheath subluxation, MRI is limited, as it is a static study that cannot visualize the change in relationship of the tendons that occurs with this pathologic process. Sensitivity and specificity of MRI in assessing structural derangement of the peroneal tendons has been demonstrated [10], but 35% of patients with no peroneal symptomatology will have incidental peroneal pathology seen on their MRI study [11]. Further limitations of this modality exist due to the magic angle effect, though this can be improved with extremity position [12]. Concomitant soft tissue pathology, including those of superior peroneal retinaculum, lateral ligament complex, syndesmosis, or synovitis of the ankle joint can also be well visualized. It is important to correlate clinical examination and findings with the imaging to limit distractors of incidental findings. Despite general limitations of magnetic resonance imaging, this can be useful in assessing the osseous morphology of the posterior fibular groove. In a patient cohort presenting with intrasheath subluxation, Raikin et al. demonstrated a convex groove in 70% of patient and a flattened groove in 21% of patient [4]. This information can further aid in surgical planning. Unless there is need to evaluate for unrelated concerns such as osteochondral lesions of the talus, we do not recommend MRI as part of the routine evaluation for suspected intrasheath peroneal subluxation.

Classification

The original classification for peroneal instability was defined by Eckert and Davis [2], with subsequent modification by Ogden [3]. This classification scheme was for a diagnosis of peroneal dislocation out of the retrofibular groove and characterized the essential lesion to the superior peroneal retinaculum or its attachment. The four grades each allowed for dislocation of the peroneal tendon from anatomic location behind the fibula either under or through the SPR completely out of the retrofibular groove. In contrast, intrasheath subluxation is defined by an intact superior peroneal retinaculum, with the peroneus brevis and longus tendons both remaining within the SPR and the groove but reverse their natural anatomic positions. That is, the round peroneus longus tendon comes to temporarily lie anterior and deep to the flat peroneus brevis tendon. Two subtypes have been described [4]. Type A pathology (Fig. 14.2) is defined by the peroneus longus tendon subluxing around an intact peroneus brevis tendon. Type B (Fig. 14.3)

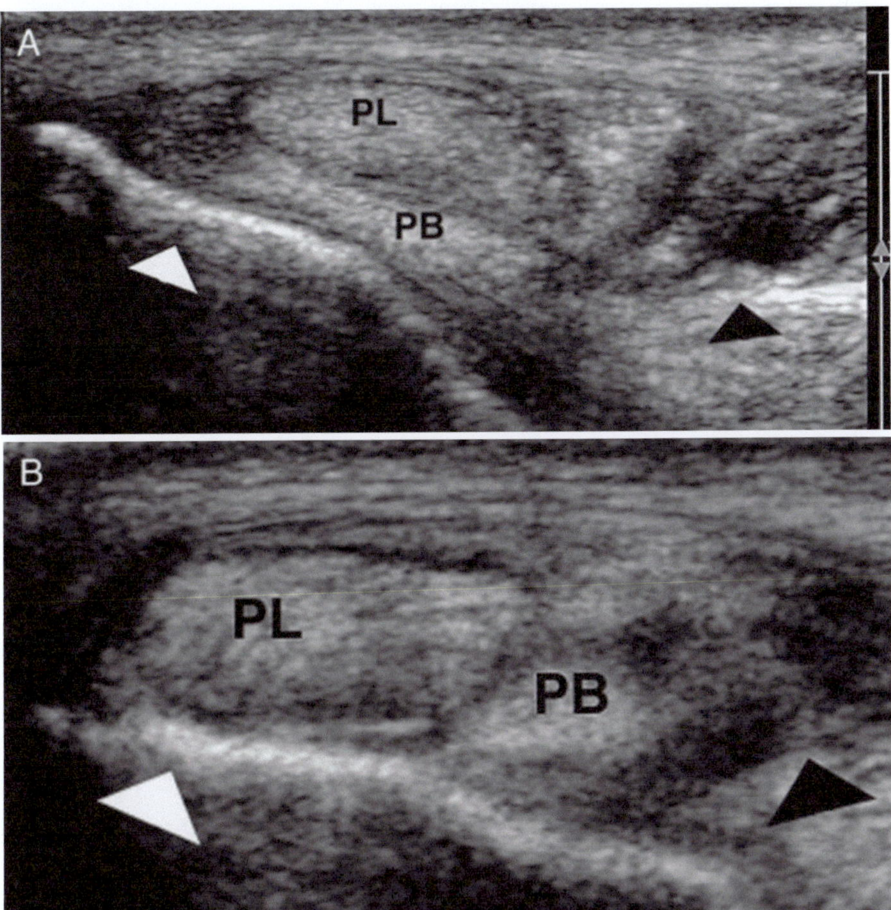

Fig. 14.2 (**a**) Transverse ultrasound image at the fibular groove showing normal relationship of echogenic tendons of peroneus brevis (PB) adjacent to fibula cortex (white arrowhead) and peroneus longus (PL) posterior and lateral to it. Note hypoechoic adjacent peroneus brevis muscle belly (black arrowhead). (**b**) Transverse ultrasound image immediately after intrasheath subluxation shows the peroneus brevis tendon (PB) now medial from prior location in Fig. 14.2a, and peroneus longus tendon (PL) now immediately adjacent to the fibula cortex (white arrowhead). Again, note hypoechoic adjacent peroneus brevis muscle belly (black arrowhead). (With permission from Elsevier Publisher)

pathology involves a peroneus longus tendon which subluxing through a longitudinal split tear within the peroneus brevis tendon to reverse its position (Fig. 14.4). Raikin et al. demonstrated that Type A injuries occur at a rate of 2.5:1 compared to Type B injuries [4] (Table 14.1). The classification of these injuries was described initially on dynamic ultrasound and confirmed via intraoperative assessment. Further study is warranted to determine sensitivity and specificity of this study in larger cohorts.

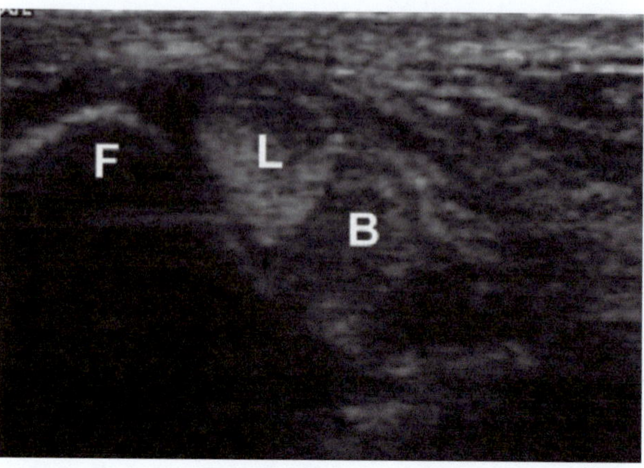

Fig. 14.3 Dynamic ultrasonography showing type-A intrasheath subluxation: the reversal of the normal peroneal tendon position with the peroneus longus tendon lying deep to the brevis tendon. (F = fibula, B = peroneus brevis tendon, and L = peroneus longus tendon). (With permission from Wolters Kluwer Publisher)

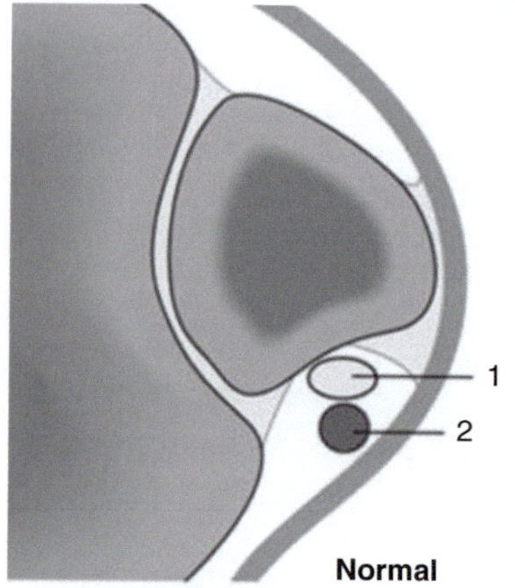

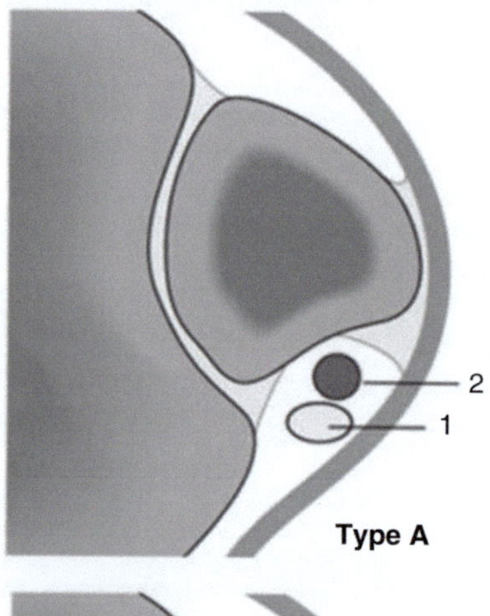

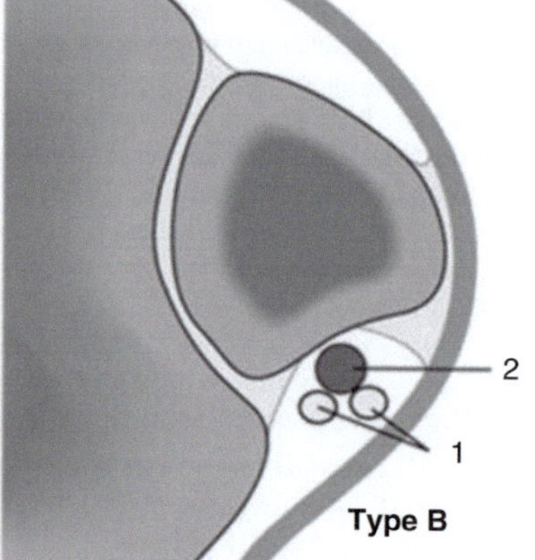

Fig. 14.4 Graphic replication of the Oden modification7 of the Eckert and Davis classification of true peroneal subluxation 2 (grades 1 through 4) (see text). 1 = peroneus brevis tendon, and 2 = peroneus longus tendon. (With permission from Wolters Kluwer Publisher)

Table 14.1 Demographic data and distribution of patients according to the Classification System of Peroneal Subluxation by Eckert and Davis and the Intrasheath Subluxation Classification

	No. of patients	Gender (F:M)
Total	57	42:15
Grade according to system of Eckert and Davis		
1	24 (42%)	17:7
2	8 (14%)	6:2
3	11 (19%)	5:6
4	0 (0)	
Intrasheath subluxation type	14 (25%)	14:0
A	10 (18%)	
B	4 (7%)	

With permission from Wolters Kluwer Publisher

Management

Currently, there are no published data on nonoperative management protocols in a cohort of patients with intrasheath subluxation, or the natural history of acute traumatic subluxation. Authors on this topic have discussed the various modalities that have been attempted in their respective populations [4–6]. Generally, nonsurgical management for suspected peroneal pathology is initiated with a course of immobilization, followed by attempted physical therapy. However, this has a limited role in instability as immobilization alone will not address the retinacular pathology which allows for peroneal displacement or prevent further intrasheath subluxation. Other modalities such as bracing and physical therapy may provide some benefit in peroneal tears and tendonitis, though again they will not impart stability to the tendons as a definitive solution for the pathology. Most cases, at the time of diagnosis after being treated initially as an ankle sprain, are already chronic in nature and will be recalcitrant to additional nonoperative modalities.

Surgical management of intrasheath subluxation has been described by multiple authors. The early publications on this pathology utilized various techniques without systematic approach and presented isolated cases. Harper illustrated two cases wherein he performed open approaches combined with debridement, tenodesis, and a rerouting procedure which involved the peroneal tendons placed deep in the calcaneofibular ligament [5]. Another published case series with similar open surgical debridement of peroneus brevis have demonstrated this approach [6]. Although follow up and outcome reporting in these cases were limited, no early complications or recurrence were noted.

In the largest published cohort on intrasheath subluxation, Raikin et al. described their surgical approach to intrasheath subluxation [4]. Through a standard open posterior-lateral approach, the superior peroneal retinaculum was incised and the tendons inspected. Concurrent pathology of the tendons was addressed and a fibular groove deepening procedure was performed. The groove deepening was performed on all patients, irrespective of fibular groove morphology. The peroneal tendons were then placed into the groove and the superior peroneal retinaculum closed. The technique is described in detail below. With this approach, patient self reported outcomes as good to excellent in 13 of 14 patient and fair in 1 patient. Significant improvements were recorded for AOFAS scores, with an average of 61 preoperatively to 93 postoperatively, and visual analog which decreased from 5.6 to 1.2. Outcomes of surgical management have also been presented by Thomas et al. though there were only three surgically managed patients [8]. These patients underwent open management of concurrent peroneal tendon tears, low-lying muscle belly, or peroneus quartus. It was noted that all patients had concave fibular groove morphology and thus, no deepening procedure was performed. Outcomes published were clearly limited by size of cohort, but statistically significant improvements from preoperative to postoperative American College of Foot and Ankle Surgeons scores were noted and each of the operative patients returned to their respective preoperative activities following rehabilitation.

Tendoscopic management of peroneal subluxation has also been published. In their study, Vega et al. demonstrated the technical approach to using this modality for intrasheath subluxation [13]. In a cohort of six patients, tendoscopy was performed via standard proximal and distal portals. Concurrent pathology of tenosynovitis, peroneus brevis tears, low-lying muscle belly, and peroneus quartus was addressed. In two patients, a fibular groove deepening was also performed without need for open approach. Although cohort size is limited, marked improvements in the AOFAS scores from 79 to 99 were noted, along with coinciding improvements in visual analog scores from an average of 7.6 to 0 postoperatively. Another case series of three patients has been published using this approach with good results and early return to activity, but outcome reporting was very limited [12]. Tendoscopic management is a highly technical approach and this may limit its utility in all clinical settings depending on the concomitant pathology.

Surgical Technique [14]

The author performs the surgical management on an outpatient basis with a combination of general anesthesia and popliteal nerve block. A longitudinal incision along the course of the peroneal tendons posterior to the fibula is made centered over the level of the superior peroneal retinaculum (Fig. 14.5). Care should be taken to curve the incision distally to avoid the sural nerve which will lie in the superficial layer of the posterior soft tissue. The superior peroneal retinaculum should then be identified and examined for any injuries either intrasubstance or at its attachment to the fibula. The retinaculum is then incised to expose the peroneal tendons. A cuff of tissue approximately 1–2 millimeters should be left at the fibular attachment to aid in repair, although the SPR may be repaired via bone tunnels if poor quality tissue or inadequate cuff remains. The peroneal tendons should be explored and inflamed tenosynovium excised. The peroneus brevis with frequently have a low-lying muscle belly extending into under the SPR, or a peroneus quartus may be present, both

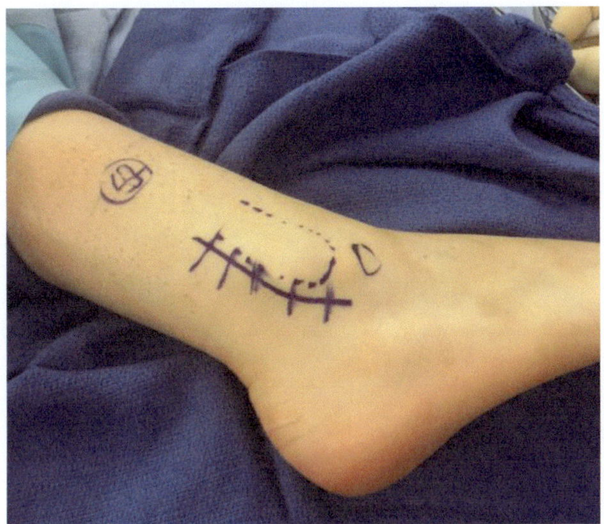

Fig. 14.5 Standard posterior-lateral incision placement

taking up room within the groove. When present, these should be debrided or resected to a level at least 2 cm above the fibular groove to allow for normal tendon excursion. Longitudinal tears of the peroneus brevis tendon (or longus if present) should be debrided and repaired with tubularization.

At this point, the fibular groove is inspected. The senior author elects to deepen the fibular groove on all patients to aid in peroneal stability, though other authors have demonstrated that perhaps this is not essential unless there is palpable convexity to the retrofibular region. The fibular groove deepening procedure performed was originally described by Zoellner and Clancy [15], and subsequently modified by Raikin for this application. A thin osteotome is utilized to osteotomize the posterior retrofibular groove (Fig. 14.6). The osteotomy preserves the smooth fibroosseous sheath against which the peroneal tendons run behind the fibula, which is repaired at the end of the procedure to protect tendon gliding. The osteotomy includes only the fibro-osseous sheath and a very this sliver of bone to allow reincorporation. The cortical window is then hinged along its medial side to expose the underlying cancellous bone. The underlying cancellous bone is then removed with a burr and curettes to a depth of 6–9 mm, creating an evenly deepened groove (Fig. 14.7). The cortical flap including the fibro-osseous sheath is then replaced and impacted into the depth of the new groove (Fig. 14.8). The peroneal tendons are placed within this groove and the ankle is placed through a gentle range of motion to assess stability. A k-wire or small drill is then utilized to create 3–4 holes in the lateral overhanging lip of the fibula. These are utilized to repair the superior peroneal retinaculum to the underside of the exposed fibula utilizing nonabsorbable braided suture (Fig. 14.9). Range of motion is again tested to ensure smooth motion within the retinacular repair. A layered closure is performed and the patient is placed into a splint.

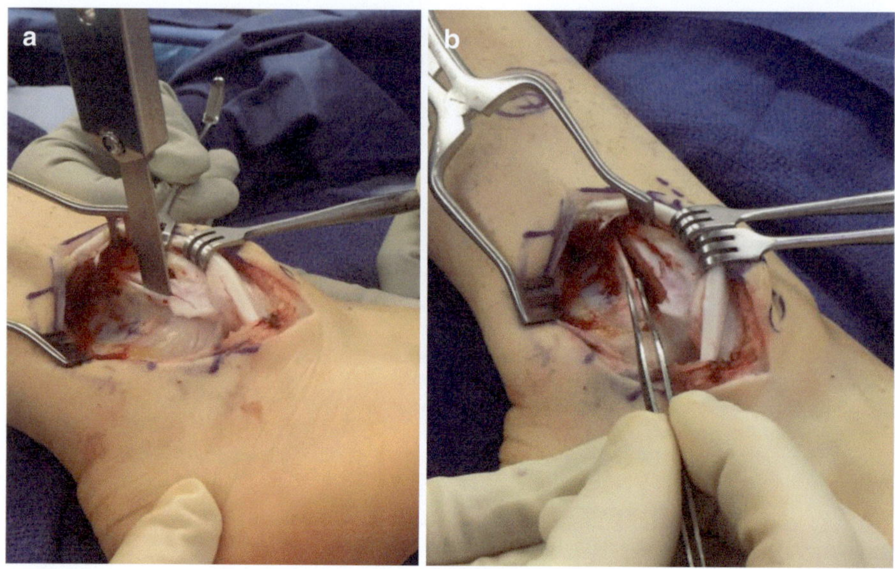

Fig. 14.6 (**a**) Use of thin osteotome to create the posterior fibular window prior to deepening. (**b**) Demonstration of the size and thickness of the ideal fibular osteotomy

Fig. 14.7 Use of Burr to create a trough into which the osteotomized fibula will be depressed

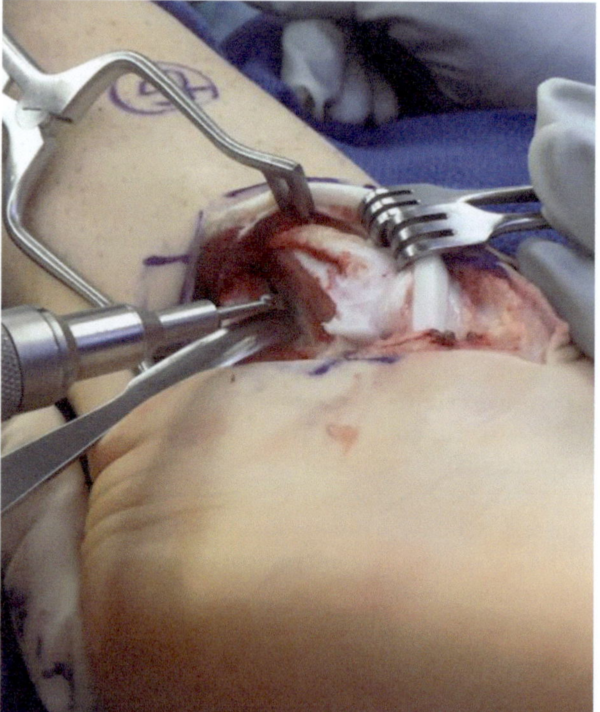

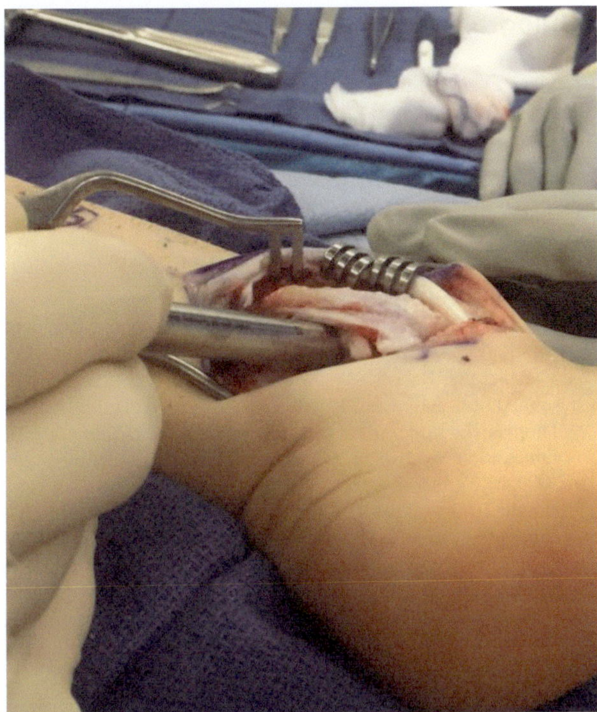

Fig. 14.8 Replacement of the cortical window of the fibula into a deepened position

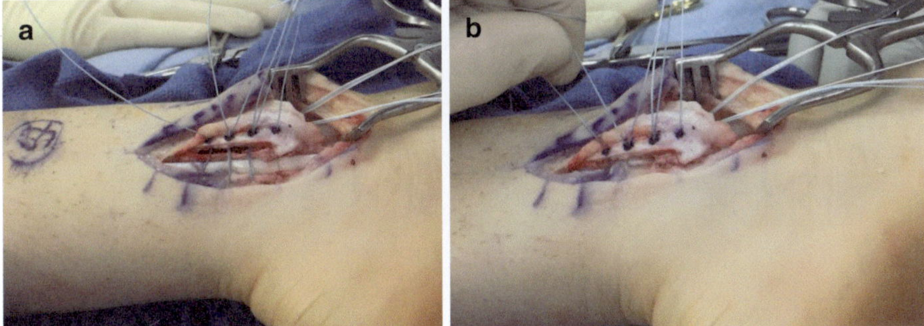

Fig. 14.9 (**a**) Demonstration of the location of drill holes and superior peroneal retinaculum. (**b**) Once tightened, the superior peroneal retinacular repair provides a strong construct to prevent further instability

Postoperative protocol includes nonweight bearing for 6 weeks. The patient is allowed to transition to a CAM walker boot at the 2-week period to allow for plantar and dorsiflexion. At 6 weeks postoperatively, the patients are transitioned to weight bearing as tolerated in the boot and physical therapy is initiated with an early focus on range of motion and graduated return to strengthening.

Bibliography

1. Monteggia GB. Instituzini chirurgiche. Parte Secondu. Milan; 1803, p 336–41.
2. Eckert WR, Davis EA Jr. Acute rupture of the peroneal retinaculum. J Bone Joint Surg Am. 1976;58:670–2.
3. Oden RR. Tendon injuries about the ankle resulting from skiing. Clin Orthop Relat Res. 1987;216:63–9.
4. Raikin SM, Elias I, Nazarian LM. Intrasheath subluxation of the peroneal tendons. J Bone Joint Surg Am. 2008;90:992–9.
5. Harper MC. Subluxation of the peroneal tendons within the peroneal groove: a report of two cases. Foot Ankle Int. 1997;18:369–70.
6. McConkey JP, Favero KJ. Subluxation of the peroneal tendons within the peroneal tendon sheath. A case report. Am J Sports Med. 1987;15:511–3.
7. Neustadter J, Raikin SM, Nazarian LN. Dynamic sonographic evaluation of peroneal tendon subluxation. AJR Am J Roentgenol. 2004;183(4):985–8.
8. Thomas JL, Lopez-Ben R, Maddox J. A preliminary report on intra-sheath peroneal tendon subluxation: a prospective review of 7 patients with ultrasound verification. J Foot Ankle Surg. 2009;48(3):323–9.
9. Draghi F, Bortolotto C, Draghi A, Gitto S. Intrasheath instability of the peroneal tendons: dynamic ultrasound imaging. J Ultrasound Med. 2018;37(12):2753–8.
10. Park H, Lee S, Park N, Rho M, Chung E, Kwag H. Accuracy of MR findings in characterizing peroneal tendons disorders in comparison with surgery. Acta Radiol. 2012;53(7):795–801.
11. O'Neil JT, Pedowitz DI, Kerbel YE, Codding JL, Zoga AC, Raikin SM. Peroneal tendon abnormalities on routine magnetic resonance imaging of the foot and ankle. Foot Ankle Int. 2016;37(7):743–7.
12. Michels F, Jambou S, Guillo S, Van Der Bauwhede J. Endoscopic treatment of intrasheath peroneal tendon subluxation. Case Rep Med. 2013;2013:1–4.
13. Vega J, Golanó P, Dalmau A, Viladot R. Tendoscopic treatment of intrasheath subluxation of the peroneal tendons. Foot Ankle Int. 2011;32(12):1147–51.
14. Raikin SM. Intrasheath subluxation of the peroneal tendons surgical technique. J Bone Joint Surg Am. 2009;91(Suppl 2 (Part 1)):146–55.
15. Zoellner G, Clancy W Jr. Recurrent dislocation of the peroneal tendon. J Bone Joint Surg Am. 1979;61:292–4.

Arthroscopy and Tendoscopy in the Treatment of Peroneal Tendon Pathology

15

Cristian Ortiz, Jorge Batista, Manuel Pellegrini, and Ana Butteri

Introduction

Advances in arthroscopic techniques and equipment have allowed surgeons to be able to perform different kinds of arthroscopies and tendoscopies around the foot and ankle.

Arthroscopy is a well-established procedure to treat foot and ankle disorders, but the relatively novel tendoscopic technique was first published by Wertheimer in 1995 [1].

In 1997, Van Dijk published a paper on endoscopy of Achilles, anterior tibialis, and peroneal tendons and named it "tendoscopy." This minimally invasive approach that can be used for diagnostic or treatment purposes and may have the advantages of producing less postoperative pain, fewer soft tissue complications, earlier return to daily activities and sports, and better patient satisfaction [2].

Electronic Supplementary Material The online version of this chapter (https://doi.org/10.1007/978-3-030-46646-6_15) contains supplementary material, which is available to authorized users.

C. Ortiz (✉)
Clínica Universidad de los Andes, Universidad de los Andes, Santiago, Chile
e-mail: caortiz@clinicauandes.cl

J. Batista
Centro Artroscópico Jorge Batista SA, Club Atlético Boca Juniors, Buenos Aires, Argentina

M. Pellegrini
Clínica Universidad de los Andes, Universidad de los Andes, Santiago, Chile

Hospital JoséJoaquín Aguirre, Universidad de Chile, Santiago, Chile
e-mail: mpellegrini@clinicauandes.cl

A. Butteri
Fellowship Foot and Ankle, Universidad de los Andes, Santiago, Chile
e-mail: abutteri@clinicauandes.cl

© Springer Nature Switzerland AG 2020
M. Sobel (ed.), *The Peroneal Tendons*,
https://doi.org/10.1007/978-3-030-46646-6_15

Although there is poor evidence for the majority of the common indications of foot and ankle tendoscopies, it is a relatively safe and effective procedure that can be used as an isolated technique or combined with open procedures. The most commonly performed tendoscopies in the foot and ankle are for Achilles, flexor hallucis longus, and peroneal tendons.

Accurate clinical diagnosis of these disorders is often difficult, and they are frequently underdiagnosed. Because arthroscopy of the ankle is now a well-established procedure used for diagnosis and treatment of foot and ankle disorders, peroneal tendoscopy could also be an effective tool for accurately diagnosing peroneal tendon abnormalities and treating some of these disorders [3].

We are going to focus on described indications of tendoscopy for the peroneal tendons.

Indications

Most common problems of the peroneal tendons can be summarized into three main categories:

1. Inflammation
2. Subluxation or dislocation
3. Tears and ruptures

Indications for peroneal tendoscopy including retrofibular pain, tenosynovitis, subluxation or dislocation, intrasheath subluxation, partial tears, impingement of peroneus longus at the peroneal tubercle, postoperative adhesions and scarring, and resection of a peroneus quartus tendon or a bifid peroneus brevis or a low-lying peroneal muscle, superior retinaculum reconstruction, and endoscopic groove deepening [4–9].

Tendon repair has also been described in longitudinal tears and complete tendon ruptures. Although we must say that this last indication is not performed by most authors in a reliable way [10, 11] (Table 15.1).

In order to have proper indications and adequate surgical technique, some specific aspects of basic science must be kept in mind. These include anatomy, physiopathology, history and physical examination, and appropriate use of imagenological studies.

Anatomy

The peroneal muscles lie in the lateral compartment of the leg and are innervated by the superficial peroneal nerve. The peroneus longus tendon originates proximally from the lateral condyle of the tibia and at the head of the fibula, and the peroneus brevis tendon originates from superior 2/3 of the fibula and the interosseous membrane.

Table 15.1 Indications for peroneal tendoscopy

Indication	Author	Outcome
Snapping, diagnostic	Van Dijk and Klort [12]	3 of 4 no recurrence after adhesiolysis, 1 peroneal tubercle successfully removed, 1 longitudinal tear successfully treated
Tenosynovitis	Scholten and Ven Dijk [13]	10 successfully treated
Tenosynovitis	Jerosch and Aldawoudy [14]	7 successfully treated
Postoperative adhesion and scarring	Marmotti et al. [15]	5 of 5 successful results
Subluxation or dislocation	Guillo and Calder [16]	7 out of 7 returned to previous activity level
Subluxation or dislocation	Vega et al. [17]	6 out of 6 successful intrasheath dislocation
Partial tear	Vega et al. [17]	24 patients; 15 symptoms free, 6 partially, 3 no change
Endoscopic resection of peroneal tubercle	Lui et al. [18]	One case in zone 2 with good results
Superior peroneal retinaculum repair	Wataru [19]	5 patient with 6 months f/u good results
Peroneus quartus resection	Opdam [20]	Case report with good result

Typically, the musculotendinous unit of the peroneus brevis tendon is located proximal to the superior peroneal retinaculum; however, it may occasionally present with a lower insertion and generating a continent-contained conflict at the retromalleolar groove, increasing pressure in this space and producing pathology [21]. Under the same perspective, a peroneus quartus muscle can be located inside this space and produce a similar situation. The prevalence of this muscle oscillates between 10% and 22% and typically originates from the muscle belly of the peroneal brevis and inserts into the peroneal trochlea of the calcaneus [22–25].

The peroneal tendons are synovialized tendons that allow performing an endoscopy to introduce liquid and expand the space between both synovial sheath layers. Both tendons enter in a common synovial sheath approximately 4 cm proximal to the tip of the lateral malleolus. They run posterior to the lateral malleolus through a fibrous bone tunnel called the retromalleolar groove, with the peroneus longus tendon located posterolateral with respect to the peroneus brevis tendon. Distal to the articulation of the ankle, the synovial sheath separates upon reaching the peroneal trochlea on the lateral face of the calcaneus. The peroneus longus tendon passes underneath the peroneal trochlea, and the peroneus brevis tendon passes over the top. The peroneal tendons traverse under the inferior retinaculum, which lays approximately 2–3 cm distal from the tip of the fibula. The peroneus brevis tendon continues directly until its insertion in the tuberosity at the base of the fifth metatarsal. The peroneus longus tendon rotates medially between the groove of the cuboid and the long plantar ligament and inserts in the superficial plantar of the first metatarsal and the lateral aspect of the medial cuneiform.

There are two critical zones for the pathology of the peroneal tendons: the retromalleolar groove for both tendons and the cuboid notch for the peroneus longus tendon.

The retromalleolar groove is limited by the superior peroneal retinaculum posterolaterally, anteriorly by the fibula, and medially by both talofibular (anterior and posterior) and calcaneofibular ligaments [26, 27]. This groove is lined by fibrocartilage and varies in depth and shape [28], potentially affecting the stability of the peroneal tendons when they pass behind the fibula. In a cadaveric study of 178 fibulas, 82% presented a concave retromalleolar groove, 11% flat, and 7% convex [29]. The groove measures between 6 and 7 mm in width and between 2 and 4 mm of depth and is reinforced by a fibrocartilage ridge. The shape of the groove is determined more by its fibrocartilage ridge than by the concavity of the fibula [30, 31]. Although the morphology of the retromalleolar groove can contribute to the subluxation and consequent injury of the peroneal tendons [23, 29, 32], apparently there are no clinical differences considering groove type in patients with and without instability of the peroneal tendons [33]. The superior peroneal retinaculum is the primary restraint to the subluxation of the peroneal tendons in the ankle. This structure corresponds to a band of fibrous tissue approximately 1–2 cm of width, which originates from the posterolateral aspect and distal fibula, with great variety in its insertion [34].

The passage of the peroneus longus tendon at the level of the cuboid notch represents a zone of direction change, and therefore of maximum stress for the tendon. The os peroneum, a fibrocartilaginous enlargement, is a structure that increases the resistance of the peroneus longus tendon in this zone of maximum stress [35], and it is estimated that it ossifies in approximately a 20% of the general population [36, 37]. The hypertrophy of the os peroneum is considered a cause of tenosynovitis in the peroneal tendons [24, 37–39], given the mechanical stress trauma and thinning of the sheath, which can secondarily alter normal excursion [40].

The peroneal arteries and the perforating branches of the anterior tibial artery irrigate the lateral compartment of the leg. Additionally, they receive irrigation through links that originate from the posterior peroneal artery and from branches of the medial tarsal. These links penetrate the posterolateral aspect of each tendon of its route to the retromalleolar groove. It has been proposed that the peroneal tendons present critical avascular zones that can contribute to tendinopathy [41]. However, the presence of avascular zones has been refuted by many authors [42, 43].

In order to plan endoscopic portal, it is useful to separate peroneal anatomy into three zones.

A recent article by Hull shows that the vast majority of the length of the peroneal tendons can be seen during routine peroneal tendoscopy. A more distal skin portal site may improve visualization of zone 3 of the peroneus longus [44].

Physiopathology

Tendinosis and tenosynovitis of the peroneal tendons correspond to an alteration of the normal tendon structure and inflammation of the synovial sheath, respectively [27]. Considering that both conditions can coexist in greater or lesser extent, the term tendinopathy is used to refer to all spectrums of the illness. Among its causes are repetitive and prolonged activities, severe sprains, chronic instability of the ankle, direct traumas, and fractures of the ankle or calcaneal [23, 40, 45, 46]. The tendinopathy of the peroneals usually originates in patients who take part in prolonged or repetitive activities over time and is particularly frequent in its presentation after a period of relative inactivity [27].

Multiple injury mechanisms have been described: sprain of the ankle by forced inversion, chronic tendon hyperlaxity of the ankle, and peroneal tendon subluxation. Although the etiology of peroneal tendon tears is not completely understood [47], many authors have documented the presence of predisposing anatomical factors that can contribute to tears in the peroneal tendons: a convex or flat fibula groove, low or abnormal muscle belly, incompetence of the superior peroneal retinaculum, presence of a posterolateral fibular osteophyte, and a cavus foot have been associated directly with injury of the peroneal tendons [48, 49].

The primary function of these muscles is the eversion and plantar flexion of the ankle, as they are in a retromalleolar position. Secondarily, the long peroneal produces the plantar flexion of the first metatarsal. Besides, they participate in the dynamic stability of the ankle, especially during the partial support and elevation of the heel on the gait [28, 50].

The presence of anatomical variants related to the retromalleolar trochlea, as in the tendons themselves, can predispose the presence of pathology of the peroneal tendons. The hypertrophy of the peroneal trochlea also has been implicated in the etiopathogenesis of this problem increasing the mechanical stress in the peroneal tendons, potentially leading to tendinopathy and restriction of the normal displacement between the synovial sheaths [23, 51, 52].

The presence of cavus and/or varus of the foot predisposes to biomechanical alterations of both peroneal tendons, reducing the lever arm and increasing forces of displacement in the lateral malleolus, peroneal trochlea, and in the cuboid notch [53, 54], so the addition of other stress agents can raise the probability of producing disorders at the level of peroneal tendons.

Tendinopathy and/or tear of the peroneal tendons can cause lateral instability of the ankle. It has been described that the patients submitted to surgery for chronic lateral instability of the ankle, 77% presented tenosynovitis of the peroneal tendons, 54% presented an attenuated superior peroneal retinaculum, and 25% presented tears of the peroneus brevis tendon [54].

Tears of the peroneal tendons can occur in a chronic or acute form. During acute inversion of the ankle, an impingement of the peroneus brevis tendon is produced between the peroneus longus tendon and the posterior aspect of the fibula, which can lead to a longitudinal tear (split tear) or a complete tear of the peroneus brevis tendon [55, 56]. However, frequently, this results after damage caused by repetitive subluxation. The posterolateral border of the fibula can create a defect in the tendon while it is repeatedly subluxated over the crest. This defect often evolves into a longitudinal break of approximately 2.5–5 cm in length [57]. Occasionally, a bucket handle tear may appear where the peroneus longus tendon is luxated through the split tear in the peroneus brevis tendon [58].

Tears of the peroneus longus tendon can occur in an isolated form or in conjunction with tears of the peroneus brevis tendon. Acute tears of the peroneus longus tendon result from sports injuries, lateral instability of the ankle, instability of the peroneal tendons, or traumatic injuries such as tendon avulsion at the level of the os peroneum and/or traumatic lacerations of the tendon [32, 39, 46, 59–61]. Classically, these tears occur at the level of the cuboid, in the os peroneum, in the peroneal trochlea, or at the level of the tip of the lateral malleolus [62, 63]. However, the presence of os peroneum does not predispose to tears of the peroneus longus tendon [64, 65].

The mechanical stress that affects the synovial sheath when elapsed over the peroneal trochlea and the cuboid notch can be considered a relevant factor in the physiopathology of longitudinal tears in the peroneus longus tendon. Brandes y and Smith in its study defined three anatomical zones where tears of the peroneus longus tendon are most frequent [53]. Zone A extends from the tip of the lateral malleolus until the peroneal trochlea, zone B from the peroneal trochlea up to the inferior peroneal retinaculum, and zone C from the inferior peroneal retinaculum to the cuboid notch [53, 58]. In the same study, it was reported that 77% of tears of the peroneus longus tendon are located at the level of zone C.

Although longitudinal tears are the most frequent, there have also been documented transverse tears of both tendons. These tears occur most frequently in acute injuries and are located distal to the os peroneum and also can occur at the level of the muscle-tendon unit [66].

The instability of the peroneal tendons occurs under physiological load, the tendons alter their position and/or habitual anatomical location producing symptoms. This condition can be subdivided depending on the competence of the superior peroneal retinaculum and the grade of dislocation (complete or incomplete) of the tendons with respect to the retromalleolar groove.

The most frequent form of presentation occurs with a rupture of the retinaculum and where the tendons dislocate outside of the retromalleolar groove. The most common mechanism is an abrupt contracture of the peroneal tendons during a forced inversion of the ankle or during a forced dorsiflexión of the foot while is in eversion [31, 67]. This produces disruption of the superior peroneal retinaculum and allows that the peroneal tendons subluxate anteriorly over the lateral malleolus [26, 68]. This condition is frequently associated with lateral instability of the ankle, considering that the rupture of the complex lateral ligamentary increases the tension over the superior peroneal retinaculum [69, 70]. A dysplastic retromalleolar groove, a hyperlaxity of the superior peroneal retinaculum for a retropie as a result of cavovarus cavovarus or a congenital absence of the superior peroneal retinaculum, can contribute to the subluxation mechanism of the peroneal tendons [46, 71, 72].

The subluxation of the peroneal tendons is classified into four grades. In grade 1, the superior peroneal retinaculum is elevated from the fibula at the subperiosteal level. In grade 2, the fibrocartilage crest comes off from the anterior aspect of the fibula; In grade 3, the superior peroneal retinaculum is avulsed from the fibula with a small cortical fragment; and in grade 4, the superior peroneal retinaculum is disinserted at the level of its posterior insertion in the calcaneal and/or the Achilles tendon [30, 73].

Another form of instability occurs when position of the tendons are altered inside the synovial sheath, without producing a dislocation with respect to the retromalleolar groove, with an unscathed retinaculum. This condition is known as intrasheath dislocation of the peroneal tendons. Described for the first time by Raikin et al., it is characterized by the presence of pain and swelling in the posterior zone of the distal fibula but is not possible to clinically reproduce a subluxation outside of the retromalleolar groove. Patients often describe a click of the peroneal tendons during maximum eversion and dorsiflexion of the foot. Ultrasound allows a dynamic evaluation, demonstrating subluxation of the peroneus brevis and longus tendon within the retromalleolar groove with an intact superior peroneal retinaculum [74]. Additionally, tears of the inferior peroneal retinaculum could produce distal dislocation of the peroneus longus tendon over the peroneal trochlea [75].

History and Physical Exam

A detailed medical history and a thorough physical exam are essential, in particular in patients presenting with chronic pain and instability of the ankle. Frequently, patients experience repetitive sprains of the ankle or fractures of the ankle and/or calcaneus, among other injuries. Associated conditions such as rheumatoid arthritis, psoriasis, hyperparathyroidism, diabetic neuropathy, use of fluoroquinolones, and history of infiltration with corticosteroids should be investigated [66, 76, 77].

Differential diagnoses include lateral instability of the ankle, tarsal sinus syndrome, fractures at the base of the fifth metatarsal or cuboid and fibula, stress fractures of the calcaneus, cuboid tunnel syndrome, osteochondral injuries of the talus, loose bodies (tibiotalar or subtalar), degenerative joint disease, tarsal coalition, sural neuritis, radiculopathy, malignant tumor, and accessory muscle or bone [72].

Peroneal tendinopathy is defined as acute if the symptoms are present for less than 2 weeks, subacute if the symptoms are present for between 2 and 6 weeks, and chronic if the symptoms persist for more than 6 weeks [27].

Tendinopathy can present itself as a gradual and insidious pain associated with edema of variable amounts referred to the posterolateral zone of the ankle [72].

Patients with a history of subluxation of the peroneal tendons often describe it as a painful clicking sensation. Tears of the peroneus brevis tendon are often referred to a persistent increase of volume along the trajectory of the tendon, while with tears of the peroneus longus tendon pain can flow around the cuboid notch and extend to the plantar aspect of the foot in relation to its distal insertion zone. However, many patients can complain more of instability in the posterolateral region of the ankle than of pain, and therefore their presence should be suspected [72, 78].

The inspection and palpation with active load of the peroneal tendons is a relevant aspect of the physical exam. The evaluation of the alignment of the hindfoot and forefoot is fundamental due to the coexistence of cavovarus can predispose it to injuries in the peroneal tendons [50]. Coleman's block test can be useful for determining if the cavovarus hindfoot is the primary problem or if it is secondary to a valgus forefoot or to a plantar flexed first metatarsal.

During palpation of the course of the peroneal tendons, sensitivity can be elicited. The strength of the peroneal tendons should be evaluated for weakness, pain, or both while performing counter-resistance eversion of the foot, maintaining the ankle in plantar flexion, with and without plantar flexion of the first metatarsal.

The presence of instability can be evaluated with flexion of 90° and requesting the patient to actively perform movements of plantar flexion and dorsiflexion of the ankle while counter resistance is performed. The test is considered positive when you can see or feel the anterior subluxation of the tendons over the lateral malleolus. Sobel et al. [37] described the compression test of the peroneal tendons in the peroneal grove to evaluate the presence of tendinopathy.

Radiology

Clinical diagnosis of peroneal tendon problems is based upon history and physical examination since radiological studies could be misleading. In most cases, radiological study is useful in a patient presenting with lateral pain of the ankle, and in which there is a suspected tear in the peroneal tendons. It should always start with simple X-rays. In that sense, a weightbearing anteroposterior, lateral, and Saltzman projections of both ankles should be obtained. Abnormal findings indicating pathology of the peroneal tendons include an avulsion at the base of the fifth metatarsal, an avulsion of the distal fibula denominated "fleck sign" (that indicates a grade 3 injury of the superior peroneal retinaculum, which is in turn pathognomonic of traumatic subluxation of the peroneal tendons) [79], hypertrophy of the peroneal trochlea, or presence of an os peroneum [50]. The simple X-rays can also reveal fractures of the os peroneum or an os peroneum or a bi or multipartite os peroneum.

Ultrasonography (US) is a noninvasive method allowing dynamic evaluations of the tendons [79], which is useful to evaluate competence of the superior peroneal. In that sense, the positive predictive value to detect subluxation of peroneal tendons has been reported to reach 100% [80, 81]. The US can identify tears of the peroneal tendons with an 85–100% of specificity and with 100% of sensitivity [62, 81, 82]. However, this modality also allows performing invasive procedures such as infiltration under direct vision of the synovial sheath of the peroneal tendons with 100% of precision [83]. Despite this, it should be taken into consideration that US is operator-dependent and has a substantial learning curve. A study comparing US and MRI in the diagnosis of peroneal tendon tears reported a sensitivity/specificity of 100%/90% and 23%/100% for US and MRI, respectively [82].

Computed tomography is a useful method to define with greater accuracy those bone abnormalities associated with tendinopathy of the peroneal tendons such as hypertrophy of the peroneal trochlea, calcaneum fractures, os peroneum, or lateral malleolus. However, the poor resolution for defining soft tissues limits its usefulness for identifying intrinsic injuries of the peroneal tendons [84].

MRI is the standard method for evaluating disorders in tendons, since it provides a tridimensional evaluation of the peroneal tendons [85]. Axial views with the foot in slight plantar flexion provides the best definition of the contour of the peroneal tendons, the content of the synovial sheath, and the adjacent structures such as the superior peroneal retinaculum or the retromalleolar groove [86, 87].

The tendons normally present with a homogenous intensity in signal T1, T2, and in STIR (short tau inversion recovery). In tenosynovitis, tendinosis, or in tears in tendons, high intensity signal in T2 or in STIR decrease in the homogeneity of the signal, and thinning of the tendons can be observed [58, 88].

The presence of a thin area with signal increase surrounding the peroneal tendons inside the synovial sheath in T2 and STIR is considered normal. However, a great quantity of fluid can be indicative of tenosynovitis [88].

It has been reported that an immediate signal in T2 inside the peroneal tendons possesses a sensitivity of 92% and a specificity of 79% for detecting peroneal tendinopathy, and that the presence of circumferential fluid larger than 3 mm of diameter inside the synovial sheath presents a sensitivity of 17% and a specificity of 100% for identifying tenosynovitis [89]. However, correct diagnosis can often be difficult; due to the presence of fluid inside the synovial sheath of the tendon can also be present in asymptomatic patients [90]. This can also be partially explained by the presence of a phenomenon called the magic angle, which signalizes an increase of intratendinous signal or artifact that occurs when the fibers are located in 55° of the axis of the magnetic field [90, 91].

A tear of the peroneus brevis tendon can be appreciated in the shape of a V ("chevron-shaped"), bisected or with a signal increase in T2 [86]. In a tear of the peroneus longus tendon, there can appear an increase of signal inside the tendon in a linear or circular shape, a synovial sheath with excessive fluid, bone edema in the lateral wall of the calcaneus, or a hypertrophy of the peroneal trochlea [64, 92]. Additionally, loss of homogeneity can be seen in the MRI, with discontinuity of the tendon or with fracture and/or an increase of intensity of the signal in the os peroneum [72].

A study reported a specificity of 80% for MRI in detection of tears of the peroneal brevis tendon, 100% in tears of the peroneal longus tendon, and 60% in tears of both tendons. However, this study demonstrated less usefulness for diagnosing anatomical abnormalities such as a low muscle belly of the peroneal brevis tendon or a peroneal quartus [93]. MRI can reveal injury of the superior peroneal retinaculum with or without dislocation of the peroneal tendons [88].

In a recent article by Kennedy, he looked for results with a correlation between tendoscopy and MRI. They found good clinical outcomes in 23 patients with peroneal tendon disorders, treated with peroneal tendoscopy. Although a relatively small number of patients were included, the study suggests good correlation between tendoscopic findings and preoperative MRI findings of peroneal tendon pathology, supporting the usefulness of MRI as a diagnostic modality for suspected peroneal tendon disorders [94].

Conservative Treatment

Despite the fact that conservative treatment in patients with chronic peroneal tendon injuries has shown a failure rate of up to 50%, particularly in peroneal tendon instability [30, 95], a short period of this treatment modality continue to be performed in anticipation to surgical treatment.

Several conditions should be taken into consideration: chronicity of the injury, the moment of the injury, associated clinical findings, and the level of activity/expectations of the patient [96]. Alternatives of conservative treatment include non-steroidal anti-inflammatories (AINES), ice, compression, physiotherapy with stretching, strengthening and proprioception exercises, modification of the activity, and variable methods of immobilization. In refractory cases, you can temporarily use MAFO (metatarsal foot orthosis) and/or orthotics with control of ankle mobility (CAM-boot).

Infiltration with NSAIDs or corticosteroids inside the synovial sheath of the tendon can be diagnostic and therapeutic. However, infiltration with corticosteroids should be limited to avoid iatrogenic tears of tendon [50, 97].

Finally, platelet-rich plasma (PRP) has been used in peroneal tendon pathology. A recent study of 408 patients in whom infiltration with PRP under US vision was used for the treatment of tendinopathies, 23 of them suffered tendinosis of peroneal tendons; it also reported a statistically significant clinical improvement in functional scores [98].

Surgical Treatment

If pain persists after a prolonged conservative treatment of a minimum of 3 months and the imaging study shows evidence of tendinopathy of the peroneal tendons, subluxation or dislocation, tendon tears, accessory peroneus quartus, or other accessory, low-lying muscle of the peroneus brevis, accessory os peroneus, or prominent peroneal tubercle, then tendoscopy of the peroneal tendons may be used for diagnostic purposes or actually completely treat most of these pathologies.

Surgical Technique

Preoperative Planning

If there are any doubts about peroneal tendon problems, a diagnostic tendoscopy may be performed to rule out its pathology or to proceed with further treatment. This approach allows to better plan final incisions to treat the remaining problems of the ankle (impingement, osteochondral defect, etc.), the foot (cavus, flat foot, etc.), or even remaining problems of the peroneal tendons, which are not suitable to be solved by an isolated tendoscopy (massive rupture of both peroneal tendons).

Patient Positioning

Patient may be positioned lateral, prone, or supine depending on the concomitant procedures that are planned to be performed. The preferred position for most surgeons is lateral [3] (Fig. 15.1).

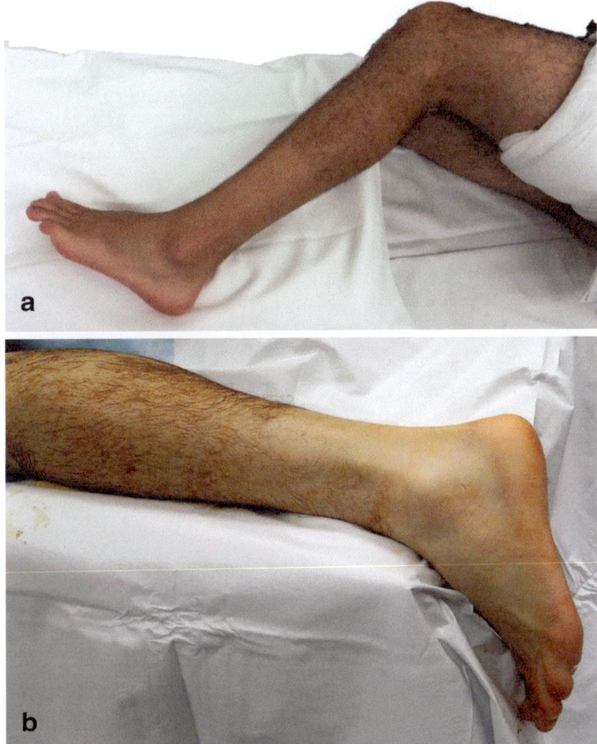

Fig. 15.1 Patient positioning. (**a**) Lateral. (**b**) Prone

Portals

Peroneal tendoscopy is performed with the proximal and distal portals along the course of the peroneal tendons. Most commonly, they are placed 3 cm proximal and 1 cm distal to the lateral malleolar tip. They are better located coaxial to inter-changed portals; depending on the location of the problem, the portal may be changed.

The standard portals described are useful for zone A, and it must be considered that since they cross the ankle joint but the tendons cross the ankle in a curved fashion, so ankle dorsiflexion and plantar flexion may be used for better visualization (Fig. 15.2).

For tendoscopy in zone B, two tendons must be addressed separately. In this zone, the space is tight, so a 2.7 arthroscope is typically recommended. If the patient has a big calf, a more distal proximal portal is recommended for better mobility of the instrumentation.

For zone C, the peroneus longus must be approached through the plantar-lateral and plantar-medial portals. The distal portal is located distal to the turn of the ten-don around the cuboid; this is 1–1.5 cm proximal and 1 cm plantar to the tip of the base of the fifth metatarsal. The medial portal is located at the lateral plantar side of

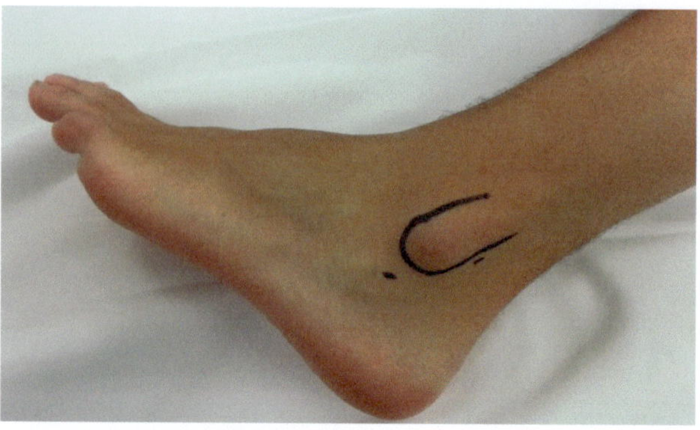

Fig. 15.2 Portals. The standard portals are placed 3 cm proximal and 1 cm distal to the lateral malleolar tip

the base of the first metatarsal. Fluoroscopy is useful to identify the precise location as has been described by Lui. He also recommends not interchanging portals.

Finally the distal portion of the peroneus brevis can be approached through the lateral Lisfranc portal, which is at the lateral corner of the fifth metatarsocuboid joint [99, 100].

Surgical Procedure

A 3 cm skin wound is made, with a blunt dissection of the subcutaneous tissue with a dissector like a hemostat. Then the tendon sheath is open until the white fibers of the tendon are seen.

A 4.0 or a 2.7 arthroscope is introduced at the distal portal. Introduction of the scope must be made smoothly in order to avoid penetrating inside the tendon substance.

Tendons are inspected for inflammation, dislocation, tears, muscle abnormality, or any of the other pathologies already described.

Surgical Options

- Synovectomy: Endoscopic synovectomy may be performed with a 4.0 shaver and radiofrequency. It is one of the easiest and a most commonly performed procedures. It can be isolated or part of the whole endoscopic surgery. Sometimes, a distal insertion of the peroneus brevis is found or an accessory muscle like the peroneus quartus. They can be excised as well (Figs. 15.3, 15.4, and 15.5).
- Groove deepening: In order to perform this procedure, the tendons are dislocated anteriorly and kept in place by a K wire. In this way, the fibular groove is fully exposed. This procedure can be performed with the three portal approaches as was described by Van Dijk [5].
- We prefer to use the classical two portal approach described by Vega, Batista et al. [101], because it is easier to achieve a smooth groove when using the acromionizer in an axial position.

Fig. 15.3 Tenosynovitis

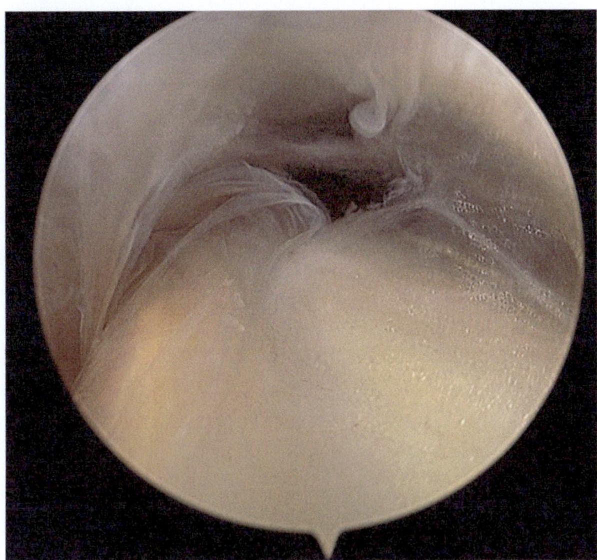

Fig. 15.4 Vyncula

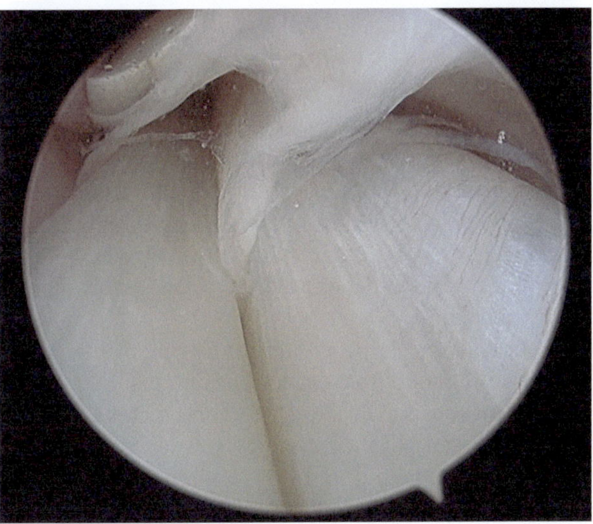

- The lateral cortical rim is left intact, and the groove deepening extends from the most proximal end of distal fibular expansion down to the tip of the lateral malleolus. The distal talofibular ligament and the posterior distal tibiofibular ligaments are left intact (Figs. 15.6, 15.7, 15.8, and 15.9/Video 15.1).
- Repair of a longitudinal tear: Repair of a longitudinal tear is more demanding and has been nicely described by Lui [3]. Percutaneous suturing of the tendon tear can be performed with a curved eyed needle. The limbs of the suture are then retrieved to the portal wound under arthroscopic guidance. Knotting can then be

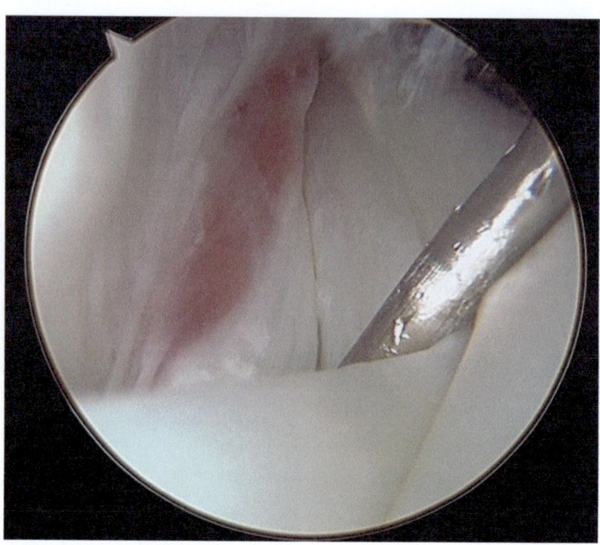

Fig. 15.5 Peroneus quartus

performed. Lui recommends that in the case of an incomplete longitudinal tendon split, the limbs of suture should be retrieved at the same side of the tear to ensure that the knot is over the tear.

After the paper was published by our group in 2018, proving in a cadaveric model that even one-third of the tendon can withstand cyclic loading similar to a normal tendon [102], we strongly believe that the old and baseless rule that 50% of a peroneal tendon rupture should force one to remove the whole tendon is obsolete. Our current management considers removing even more than 50% of a peroneal tendon degenerative damage arthroscopically (up to two thirds of the tendon width).

In another article published by one of the authors, it was demonstrated in a cadaveric model that tendon tension can be restored by an allograft [103]. This supports the clinical experience of the Duke's group in terms of replacing the old tenodesis approach in case of severe degenerative changes in tendons (now it means more than two thirds of the tendon) for tendon graft in order to achieve better clinical results without removing a tendon [104].

- Superior peroneal retinaculum reconstruction: For some authors, peroneal groove deepening is not necessary in most cases. We think that patients who have a flat posterior aspect of the fibular wall without a groove may benefit from a groove deepening procedure. The same would be true for a recurrent case. In a primary case in which the fibular groove is near normal, just a superior peroneal retinaculum reconstruction should be enough and possibly will have less complications and less recovery time.

The technique is clearly explained by Lui [3]. The distal portal is made just distal to lateral malleolar tip. The proximal portal is made at the proximal end of retinaculum, which is about 2 cm from the lateral malleolar tip. The tendons

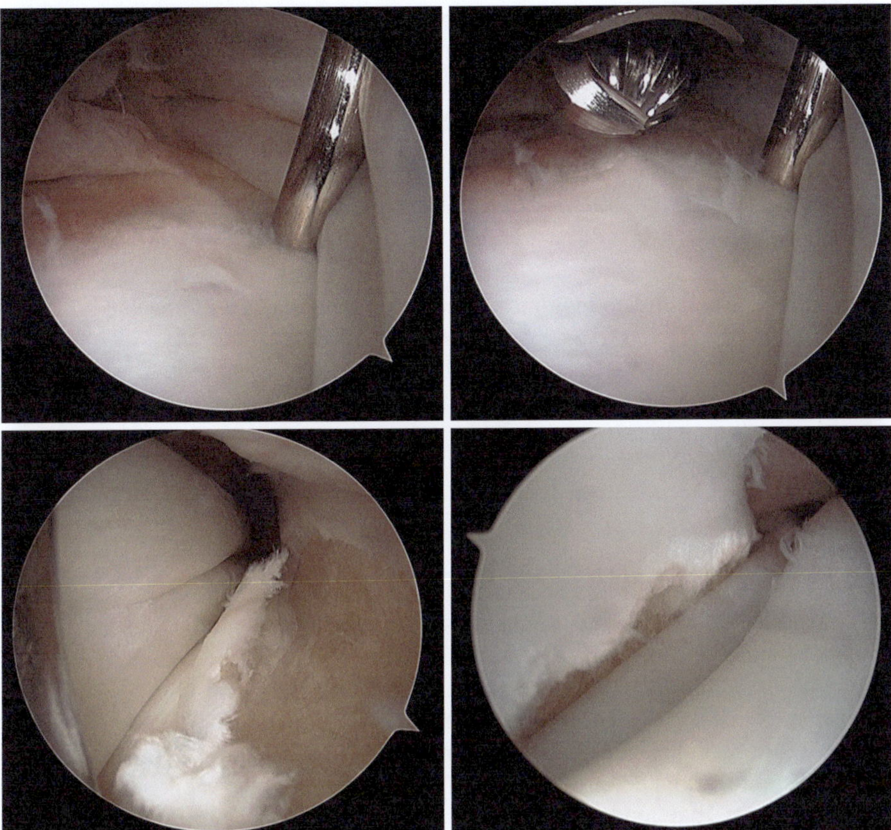

Figs. 15.6, 15.7, 15.8, and 15.9 Groove deepening. The tendons are dislocated anteriorly and kept in place by a K wire. In this way, the fibular groove is fully exposed

are pushed medially and splinted with K wires. The lateral surface of lateral malleolus where retinaculum was stripped off is roughened with arthroscopic burr. Two to three suture anchors are inserted to the fibular ridge through the portals and are evenly spaced out along the span of elevated retinaculum. The suture limbs are passed through the retinaculum by means of an eyed needle through the portals. Sutures are retrieved at the surface of retinaculum to the portal wounds. The retinaculum is pushed back to the bone manually and the sutures are tightened.

Complications

Most patients experience mild pain and quick recovery time. Wound complications are easily controlled with postoperative wound care. We have seen tendon tear secondary to a poorly performed groove deepening in the first series of cases.

There is also a chance to miss a tendon rupture if peroneal tendon exploration is not accurate enough. There is also a potential damage to tendons during the procedure.

General surgical complications such as hematoma, superficial infection, delayed wound healing, hypertrophic scar, deep venous thrombosis, and some others may also happen.

Postoperative Care

Most patients can be treated with tolerated weightbearing in a removable boot or a brace to control eversion (ASO) depending on patient tolerance. Lui recommends non-weightbearing for 4 weeks in case of tendon repair. We think that weightbearing as tolerated should be safe enough to encourage a faster recovery time and return to sports activities.

Results and Outcome

There are not many published articles in literature and none of them have level one evidence. In 2014, Glazebrook made a first approach to find out the present level of evidence for foot and ankle tendoscopy [105]. They reported poor evidence (grade C) in support of Achilles, flexor hallucis longus, and peroneal tendoscopy. This recommendation is mainly based in reports of series with small number of cases.

In a more recent paper by Bernasconi in 2017, better level of evidence was found to support this technique [106]. They concluded that recent scientific evidence suggests that tendoscopy and endoscopic-assisted percutaneous procedures are a safe and effective treatment in chronic and acute disorders of tendons around the ankle (Level of Evidence – Level IV – Systematic review of level II to IV studies).

One of the first reports comes from a paper published in 2006 by Scholten and Van Dijk showing 23 cases of peroneal tendon synovectomy with good results and no complications after 2 years of follow-up [13].

Vega et al. [17] published a larger series with 52 patients with different indications including tenosynovitis – 13, tendon tears – 24, recurrent dislocation – 7, and intrasheath subluxation – 6. After 1 year of follow-up, they reported complete symptom relief in 15 out of 24 tendon ruptures, 6 with partial relief, and 3 with no change; 5 of the 7 tendon subluxation were able to return to their normal activities. Patients with intrasheath subluxation had excellent results.

Mattos et al. describe one case of tenodesis with good results [107].

Summary

Foot and ankle tendoscopy has been growing in terms of indications in the last few years. Peroneal tendoscopy is useful for final diagnosis in order to achieve better incision and timing/planning considering the common associated pathology that

Table 15.2 Diagnostic and treatment algorithm

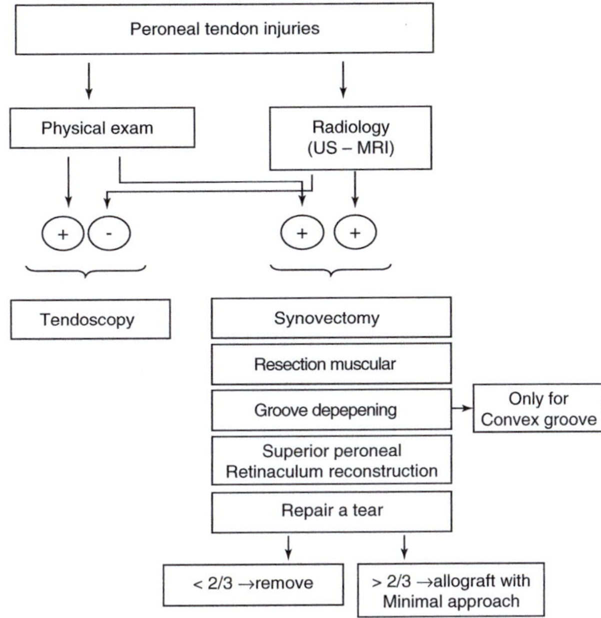

typically needs to be treated at the same time. Patients also benefit from all the advantages of minimally invasive procedures including less recovery time, earlier sports return, shorted hospital stay, better cosmetics, and finally, higher patient satisfaction.

Peroneal tendoscopy seems to be useful for synovectomy and biopsy, resection of symptomatic peroneus quartus or distal insertion of peroneus brevis, for the management of intrasheath peroneal subluxation, excision of enlarged peroneal tubercle tendon partial resection of less than two thirds, and for fibular groove deepening.

However, for most common indication for peroneal surgery (longitudinal tears), we still recommend an open approach to repair or reconstruction with allografts (Table 15.2).

References

1. Wertheimer SJ, Weber CA, Loder BG, Calderone DR, Frascone ST. The role of endoscopy in treatment of stenosing posterior tibial tenosynovitis. J Foot Ankle Surg. 1995;34:15–22.
2. Van Dijk CN, Sholten PE, Kort N. Tendoscopy (tendon sheath endoscopy) for overuse tendon injuries. Oper Tech Sports Med. 1997;5:170–17.
3. Tun Hing Lui, Lung Fung Tse. Peroneal tendoscopy. Foot Ankle Clin N Am. 2015;20:15–25.
4. Bauer T, Deranlot J, Hardy P. Endoscopic treatment of calcaneo-fibular impingement. Knee Surg Sports Traumatol Arthrosc. 2011;19:131–6.
5. De Leeuw PA, Van Dijk CN, Golano P. A 3-portal endoscopic groove deepening technique for recurrent peroneal tendon dislocation. Tech Foot Ankle Surg. 2008;7:250–6.
6. Porter D, McCarroll J, Knapp E, et al. Peroneal tendon subluxation in athletes: fibular groove deepening and retinacular reconstruction. Foot Ankle Int. 2005;26:436–41.
7. Lui TH. Endoscopic lateral calcaneal ostectomy for calcaneofibular impingement. Arch Orthop Trauma Surg. 2007;127:265–7.

8. Lui TH, Lui TH. Endoscopic peroneal retinaculum reconstruction. Knee Surg Sports Traumatol Arthrosc. 2006;14:478–81.

9. Title CI, Jung HG, Parks BG, et al. The peroneal groove deepening procedure: a biomechanical study of pressure reduction. Foot Ankle Int. 2005;26:442–8.

10. Ho KK, Chan KB, Lui TH, et al. Tendoscopic-assisted repair of complete rupture of the peroneus longus associated with displaced fracture of the os peroneum: case report. Foot Ankle Int. 2013;34:1600–4.

11. Lui TH. Endoscopic management of recalcitrant retrofibular pain without peroneal tendon subluxation or dislocation. Arch Orthop Trauma Surg. 2012;132:357–61.

12. van CN D, Kort N. Tendoscopy of the peroneal tendons. Arthroscopy. 1998;14:471–8.

13. Scholten PE, Van Dijk CN. Tendoscopy of the peroneal tendons. Foot Ankle Clin. 2006;11:415–20.

14. Jerosch J, Aldawoudy A. Tendoscopic management of peroneal tendon disorders. Knee Surg Sports Traumatol Arthrosc. 2007;15:806–10.

15. Marmotti A, Cravino M, Germano M, et al. Peroneal tendoscopy. Curr Rev Musculoskelet Med. 2012;5:135–44.

16. Guillo S, Calder JDF. Treatment of recurring peroneal tendon subluxation in athletes. Endoscopic repair of the retinaculum. Foot Ankle Clin. 2013;18:293–300.

17. Vega J, Golano P, Batista JP, et al. Tendoscopic procedure associated with peroneal tendons. Tech Foot Ankle Surg. 2013;12:39–48.

18. Tun Hing Lui. Endoscopic resection of peroneal tubercle. Arthrosc Tech. 2017;6(5):e1489–93.

19. Wataru M, Yotros. Tendoscopic repair of the superior peroneal retinaculum via 2 portals for: peroneal tendon instability. Foot Ankle Int. 2015;36:1243–50.

20. Opdam KTM, van Dijk PAD, SAS S. The peroneus quartus muscle in a locking phenomenon of the ankle: a case report. J Foot Ankle Surg. 2017;56(1):108–11.

21. Freccero DM, Berkowitz MJ. The relationship between tears of the peroneus brevis tendon and the distal extent of its muscle belly: an MRI study. Foot Ankle Int. 2006;27:236–9.

22. Cheung YY, Rosenberg ZS, Ramsinghani R, Beltran J, Jahss MH. Peroneus quartus muscle: MR imaging features. Radiology. 1997;202:745–50.

23. Lamm BM, Myers DT, Dombek M, Mendicino RW, Catanzariti AR, Saltrick K. Magnetic resonance imaging and surgical correlation of peroneus brevis tears. J Foot Ankle Surg. 2004;43:30–6.

24. Sobel M, Levy ME, Bohne WH. Congenital variations of the peroneus quartus muscle: an anatomic study. Foot Ankle. 1990;11:81–9. Erratum in: Foot Ankle. 1991;11:342.

25. Zammit J, Singh D. The peroneus quartus muscle. Anatomy and clinical relevance. J Bone Joint Surg Br. 2003;85:1134–7.

26. Brage ME, Hansen ST Jr. Traumatic subluxation/dislocation of the peroneal tendons. Foot Ankle. 1992;13:423–31.

27. Molloy R, Tisdel C. Failed treatment of peroneal tendon injuries. Foot Ankle Clin. 2003;8:115–29, ix.

28. Roster B, Michelier P, Giza E. Peroneal tendon disorders. Clin Sports Med. 2015;

29. Edwards. The relations of the peroneal tendons to the fibula, calcaneus, and cuboideum. Am J Anat. 1928;42:213–53.

30. Eckert WR, Davis EA Jr. Acute rupture of the peroneal retinaculum. J Bone Joint Surg Am. 1976;58:670–2.

31. Kumai T, Benjamin M. The histological structure of the malleolar groove of the fibula in man: its direct bearing on the displacement of peroneal tendons and their surgical repair. J Anat. 2003;203:257–62.

32. Sobel M, et al. The dynamics of peroneus brevis tendon splits: a proposed mechanism, technique of diagnosis, and classification of injury. Foot Ankle. 1992;13(7):413–22.

33. Adachi N, Fukuhara K, Kobayashi T, et al. Morphologic variations of the fibular malleolar groove with recurrent dislocation of the peroneal tendons. Foot Ankle Int. 2009;30(6):540–4.

34. Davis WH, Sobel M, Deland J, Bohne WH, Patel MB. The superior peroneal retinaculum: an anatomic study. Foot Ankle Int. 1994;15:271–5.

35. LeMinor. Comparative anatomy and significance of the sesamoid bone of the peroneus longus muscle (os peroneum). J Anat. 1987;151:85–99.
36. Anatomical Society. Collective investigations, sesamoids in the gastrocnemius and peroneus longus. J Anat Physiol. 1897;32:182–6.
37. Sobel M, Pavlov H, Geppert MJ, Thompson FM, DiCarlo EF, Davis WH. Painful os peroneum syndrome: a spectrum of conditions responsible for plantar lateral foot pain. Foot Ankle Int. 1994;15:112–24.
38. Burman. Stenosing tendovaginitis of the foot and ankle. Arch Surg. 1953;67:686–98.
39. Sobel M, Geppert MJ, Warren RF. Chronic ankle instability as a cause of peroneal tendon injury. Clin Orthop Relat Res. 1993;296:187–91.
40. Wind WM, Rohrbacher BJ. Peroneus longus and brevis rupture in a collegiate athlete. Foot Ankle Int. 2001;22:140–3.
41. Petersen W, Bobka T, Stein V, Tillmann B. Blood supply of the peroneal tendons: injection and immunohistochemical studies of cadaver tendons. Acta Orthop Scand. 2000;71:168–74.
42. Sobel M, Geppert MJ, Hannafin JA, Bohne WH, Arnoczky SP. Microvascular anatomy of the peroneal tendons. Foot Ankle. 1992;13:469–72.
43. van Dijk PA, Madirolas FX, Carrera A, Kerkhoffs GM, Reina F. Peroneal tendons well vascularized: results from a cadaveric study. Knee Surg Sports Traumatol Arthrosc. 2016;24(4):1140–7.
44. Hull M, Campbell JT, Jeng CL, Henn RF, Cerrato RA. Measuring visualized tendon length in peroneal tendoscopy. Foot Ankle Int. 2018:39:990–93.
45. Abraham E, Stirnaman JE. Neglected rupture of the peroneal tendons causing recurrent sprains of the ankle. Case report. J Bone Joint Surg Am. 1979;61:1247–8.
46. Bonnin M, Tavernier T, Bouysset M. Split lesions of the peroneus brevis tendon in chronic ankle laxity. Am J Sports Med. 1997;25:699–703.
47. Redfern D, Myerson M. The management of concomitant tears of the peroneus longus and brevis tendons. Foot Ankle Int. 2004;25:695–707.
48. Alanen J. Peroneal tendon injuries. Report of thirty-eight operated cases. Ann Chir Gynaecol. 2001;90(1):43–6.
49. Dombek MF, Lamm BM, Saltrick K, Mendicino RW, Catanzariti AR. Peroneal tendon tears: a retrospective review. J Foot Ankle Surg. 2003;42:250–8.
50. Philbin T, Landis G, Smith B. Peroneal tendon injuries. J Am Acad Orthop Surg. 2009;17:306–17.
51. Bruce WD, Christofersen MR, Phillips DL. Stenosing tenosynovitis and impingement of the peroneal tendons associated with hypertrophy of the peroneal tubercle. Foot Ankle Int. 1999;20:464–7.
52. Pierson JL, Inglis AE. Stenosing tenosynovitis of the peroneus longus tendon associated with hypertrophy of the peroneal tubercle and an os peroneum. A case report. J Bone Joint Surg Am. 1992;74:440–2.
53. Brandes CB, Smith RW. Characterization of patients with primary peroneus longus tendinopathy: a review of twenty-two cases. Foot Ankle Int. 2000;21:462–8.
54. DiGiovanni BF, Fraga CJ, Cohen BE, et al. Associated injuries found in chronic lateral ankle instability. Foot Ankle Int. 2000;21(10):809–15.
55. Bassett FH 3rd, Speer KP. Longitudinal rupture of the peroneal tendons. Am J Sports Med. 1993;21:354–7.
56. Munk RL, Davis PH. Longitudinal rupture of the peroneus brevis tendon. J Trauma. 1976;16:803–6.
57. Cerrato RA, Myerson MS. Peroneal tendon tears, surgical management and its complications. Foot Ankle Clin. 2009;14(2):299–312.
58. Squires N, Myerson MS, Gamba C. Surgical treatment of peroneal tendon tears. Foot Ankle Clin. 2007;12(4):675–95, vii.
59. Krause JO, Brodsky JW. Peroneus brevis tendon tears: pathophysiology, surgical reconstruction, and clinical results. Foot Ankle Int. 1998;19(5):271–9.

60. Pelet S, Saglini M, Garofalo R, Wettstein M, Mouhsine E. Traumatic rupture of both peroneal longus and brevis tendons. Foot Ankle Int. 2003;24:721–3.
61. Sammarco. Peroneal tendon injuries. Orthop Clin North Am. 1994;25:135–45.
62. Grant TH, Kelikian AS, Jereb SE, McCarthy RJ. Ultrasound diagnosis of peroneal tendon tears. A surgical correlation. J Bone Joint Surg Am. 2005;87:1788–94.
63. Hyer CF, Dawson JM, Philbin TM, Berlet GC, Lee TH. The peroneal tubercle: description, classification, and relevance to peroneus longus tendon pathology. Foot Ankle Int. 2005;26:947–50.
64. Rademaker J, Rosenberg ZS, Delfaut EM, Cheung YY, Schweitzer ME. Tear of the peroneus longus tendon: MR imaging features in nine patients. Radiology. 2000;214:700–4.
65. Sammarco. Peroneus longus tendon tears: acute and chronic. Foot Ankle Int. 1995;16:245–53.
66. Borton DC, Lucas P, Jomha NM, et al. Operative reconstruction after transverse rupture of the tendons of both peroneus longus and brevis. Surgical reconstruction by transfer of the flexor digitorum longus tendon. J Bone Joint Surg Br. 1998;80(5):781.
67. Safran MR, O'Malley D Jr, Fu FH. Peroneal tendon subluxation in athletes: new exam technique, case reports, and review. Med Sci Sports Exerc. 1999;31(7 Suppl):S487–92.
68. Zoellner G, Clancy W Jr. Recurrent dislocation of the peroneal tendon. J Bone Joint Surg Am. 1979;61:292–4.
69. Geppert MJ, Sobel M, Bohne WH. Lateral ankle instability as a cause of superior peroneal retinacular laxity: an anatomic and biomechanical study of cadaveric feet. Foot Ankle. 1993;14:330–4.
70. Maffulli N, Ferran NA, Oliva F, Testa V. Recurrent subluxation of the peroneal tendons. Am J Sports Med. 2006;34:986–92.
71. Purnell ML, Drummond DS, Engber WD, Breed AL. Congenital dislocation of the peroneal tendons in the calcaneovalgus foot. J Bone Joint Surg Br. 1983;65:316–9.
72. Selmani E, Gjata V, Gjika E. Current concepts review: peroneal tendon disorders. Foot Ankle Int. 2006;27:221–8.
73. Altchek DW, CW DG, Dines JS, et al. Foot and ankle sports medicine. Philadelphia: Lippincott Williams & Wilkins; 2013.
74. Raikin SM, Elias I. Intrasheath subluxation of the peroneal tendons. J Bone Joint Surg Am. 2008;90:992–9.
75. Staresinic M, Bakota B, Japjec M, et al. Isolated inferior peroneal retinaculum tear in professional soccer players. Injury. 2013;44(Suppl 3):S67–70.
76. Rosenberg ZS, Feldman F, Singson RD, Price GJ. Peroneal tendon injury associated with calcaneal fractures: CT findings. AJR Am J Roentgenol. 1987;149:125–9.
77. Sharma P, Maffulli N. Tendon injury and tendinopathy: healing and repair. J Bone Joint Surg Am. 2005;87:187–202.
78. Heckman DS, Gluck GS, Parekh SG. Tendon disorders of the foot and ankle, part 1: peroneal tendon disorders. Am J Sports Med. 2009;37(3):614–25.
79. Church. Radiographic diagnosis of acute peroneal tendon dislocation. AJR Am J Roentgenol. 1977;129:1065–8.
80. Magnano GM, Occhi M, Di Stadio M, Toma' P, Derchi LE. High-resolution US of non-traumatic recurrent dislocation of the peroneal tendons: a case report. Pediatr Radiol. 1998;28:476–7.
81. Neustadter J, Raikin SM, Nazarian LN. Dynamic sonographic evaluation of peroneal tendon subluxation. AJR Am J Roentgenol. 2004;183:985–8.
82. Rockett MS, Waitches G, Sudakoff G, Brage M. Use of ultrasonography versus magnetic resonance imaging for tendon abnormalities around the ankle. Foot Ankle Int. 1998;19:604–12.
83. Muir JJ, Curtiss HM, Hollman J, et al. The accuracy of ultrasound-guided and palpation-guided peroneal tendon sheath injections. Am J Phys Med Rehabil. 2011;90(7):564–71.
84. Rosenberg ZS, Feldman F, Singson RD. Peroneal tendon injuries: CT analysis. Radiology. 1986;161:743–8.
85. Mitchell M, Sartoris DJ. Magnetic resonance imaging of the foot and ankle: an updated pictorial review. J Foot Ankle Surg. 1993;32:311–42.

86. Major NM, Helms CA, Fritz RC, Speer KP. The MR imaging appearance of longitudinal split tears of the peroneus brevis tendon. Foot Ankle Int. 2000;21:514–9.
87. Wang XT, Rosenberg ZS, Mechlin MB, Schweitzer ME. Normal variants and diseases of the peroneal tendons and superior peroneal retinaculum: MR imaging features. Radiographics. 2005;25:587–602. Erratum in: Radiographics. 2005;25:1436. Radiographics. 2006.
88. Lee SJ, Jacobson JA, Kim SM, et al. Ultrasound and MRI of the peroneal tendons and associated pathology. Skelet Radiol. 2013;42(9):1191–200.
89. Kijowski R, De Smet A, Mukharjee R. Magnetic resonance imaging findings in patients with peroneal tendinopathy and peroneal tenosynovitis. Skelet Radiol. 2007;36:105–14.
90. Rosenberg ZS, Bencardino J, Mellado JM. Normal variants and pitfalls in magnetic resonance imaging of the ankle and foot. Top Magn Reson Imaging. 1998;9:262–72.
91. Erickson SJ, Cox IH, Hyde JS, Carrera GF, Strandt JA, Estkowski LD. Effect of tendon orientation on MR imaging signal intensity: a manifestation of the "magic angle" phenomenon. Radiology. 1991;181:389–92.
92. Khoury NJ, el-Khoury GY, Saltzman CL, Kathol MH. Peroneus longus and brevis tendon tears: MR imaging evaluation. Radiology. 1996;200:833–41.
93. Steel MW, DeOrio JK. Peroneal tendon tears: return to sports after operative treatment. Foot Ankle Int. 2007;28:49–54.
94. Kennedy Y. Functional outcomes after peroneal tendoscopy in the treatment of peroneal tendon disorders. Knee Surg Sports Traumatol Arthrosc. 2016;24(4):1148–54.
95. Stover CN, Bryan DR. Traumatic dislocation of the peroneal tendons. Am J Surg. 1962;103:180–6.
96. Chiodo. Acute and chronic tendon injury. In: Richardson EG, editor. Orthopaedic knowledge update: foot and ankle 3. Rosemont: American Academy of Orthopaedic Surgeons; 2003. p. 81–9.
97. Taki K, Yamazaki S, Majima T, Ohura H, Minami A. Bilateral stenosing tenosynovitis of the peroneus longus tendon associated with hypertrophied peroneal tubercle in a junior soccer player: a case report. Foot Ankle Int. 2007;28:129–32.
98. Dallaudiere B, Pesquer L, Meyer P, et al. Intratendinous injection of platelet-rich plasma under US guidance to treat tendinopathy: a long-term pilot study. J Vasc Interv Radiol. 2014;25(5):717–23.
99. Lui TH. Lateral foot pain following open reduction and internal fixation of the fracture of the fifth metatarsal tubercle: treated by arthroscopic arthrolysis and endoscopic tenolysis. BMJ Case Rep. 2014; https://doi.org/10.1136/bcr-2014-204116.
100. Lui TH. Tendoscopy of peroneus longus in the sole. Foot Ankle Int. 2013;34:299–302.
101. Vega, et al. Tendoscopic groove deepening for chronic subluxation of the peroneal tendons. Foot Ankle Int. 2015;34(6):832–40.
102. Wagner E, Wagner P, Ortiz C, Radkievich R, Palma F, Guzmán-Venegas R. Biomechanical cadaveric evaluation of partial acute peroneal tendon tears. Foot Ankle Int. 2018 Jun;39(6):741–5.
103. Pellegrini MJ, Glisson RR, Matsumoto T, Schiff A, Laver L, Easley ME, Nunley JA. Effectiveness of allograft reconstruction vs tenodesis for irreparable peroneus brevis tears. A cadaveric model. Foot Ankle Int. 2016;37(8):803–8.
104. Mook WR, Parekh SG, Nunley JA. Allograft reconstruction of peroneal tendons: operative technique and clinical outcomes. Foot Ankle Int. 2013 Sep;34(9):1212–20.
105. Cychosz Y. Foot and ankle tendoscopy: evidence-based recommendations. Arthroscopy. 2014;(Nov):1–11.
106. Bernasconi A, Sadile F, Smeraglia F, Mehdi N, Laborde J, Lintz F. Tendoscopy of achilles, peroneal and tibialis posterior tendons: an evidence-based update. Foot Ankle Surg. 2018;24(5):374–82.
107. e Dinato M, Freitas F, Filho P. Peroneal tenodesis with the use of tendoscopy: surgical technique and report of 1 case. Arthrosc Tech. 2014;3(1):107–10.

Stenosing Tenosynovitis of the Peroneal Tendons Along the Lateral Wall of the Calcaneus

16

Ezequiel Palmanovich, Meir Nyska, Nissim Ohana, Matias Vidra, and Ran Atzmon

Introduction

The primary action of the peroneus longus and peroneus brevis tendons is to serve as plantar flexors and evertors of the foot. Both muscles are active stabilizers in inversion–supination movement and protect the ankle from sprain injury. The close proximity of the tendons to the lateral calcaneal wall may lead to a stenosing tenosynovitis and cause an injury to the tendons [1, 20, 21, 25, 34, 37, 40, 41, 43]. Due to the long route and adjacency of the tendons to soft tissue and bony structures, such as the inferior peroneal retinaculum or the calcaneus, the tendons may be injured at any area along their course.

At the level of the lateral wall of the calcaneus, the two tendons share a synovial sheath, which separates into two different sheaths more distally, at the level of the peroneal tubercle on the calcaneus. In some cases, the shared peroneal tendon sheath can communicate with the ankle or subtalar joint, through which the synovial fluid can pass [1, 5]. Pathology at this level may produce overflow of the sheath that may lead to eventual stenosis and injury to the tendons. The peroneus brevis has a long musculotendinous muscle belly, which in some cases may extend distal to the lateral malleolus and narrow the space of the tendon sheath. This may lead to pathology such as tenosynovitis or even to a tendon tear. The peroneus quartus muscle can

E. Palmanovich (✉) · M. Nyska · N. Ohana
Meir Medical Center, Department of Orthopaedic Surgery,
Affiliated with the Sackler Faculty of Medicine and Tel Aviv University, Kefar Sava, Israel
e-mail: ohanan@clalit.org.il

M. Vidra
Tel Aviv Medical Center, Department of Orthopaedic Surgery,
Affiliated with the Sackler Faculty of Medicine and Tel Aviv University, Tel Aviv-Yafo, Israel

R. Atzmon
Assuta Medical Center, Department of Orthopaedic Surgery,
Affiliated with the Faculty of Health and Science and Ben Gurion University, Ashdod, Israel

© Springer Nature Switzerland AG 2020
M. Sobel (ed.), *The Peroneal Tendons*,
https://doi.org/10.1007/978-3-030-46646-6_16

also act as an occupying mass producing stenosing tenosynovitis, which usually affects the peroneus brevis tendon [5]. An enlarged peroneal tubercle was also described as a possible cause for peroneal stenosis and subsequent injury to the peroneal tendon. Furthermore, acute or chronic injury of the os peroneum, with concomitant callus formation, can produce peroneal stenosis and tenosynovitis of the peroneus longus tendon [5, 33, 34, 36, 37, 39].

In conclusion, the associated structures and restraints of the lateral calcaneal wall are essential for understanding the patterns of injury and pathology to the peroneal tendons. The objective of this chapter is to review the anatomy, structures, and other contributing factors involved in the stenosis of the peroneal tendons, along with the clinical presentation and treatment options for each condition.

Anatomy of the Lateral Wall of the Calcaneus Bone

The lateral surface of the calcaneus can be divided into thirds. The posterior third is flat and is found subcutaneously. The anterior third articulates with the cuboid bone and, superiorly, with the anterior surface of the talus bone. The middle third is composed of a bony protrusion in its lower segment, named the "eminentia retrotrochearis," which is a large oval eminence with variable dimensions (Fig. 16.1).

In 1860, Hyrtl was the first to identify the peroneal tubercle. After studying 987 calcanei, he named the tubercle "The Processus Trochlearis Calcanei" [3]. In 1928, Edwards et al. described in dry cadaver specimens two osteologic landmarks with distinct anatomical presentations, namely the "Peroneal Tubercle" and the "Retrotrochlear Eminence," the latter of which was found in 98% of the subjects [2]. The retrotrochlear eminence can be located below the angle formed between the lateral border of the sinus tarsi and the lateral border of the posterior articular facet on the talus. It was identified by Gruber et al. and Edwards et al. in 39% and 44% of their participants, respectively. In an MRI study by Saupe et al. from 2007, which

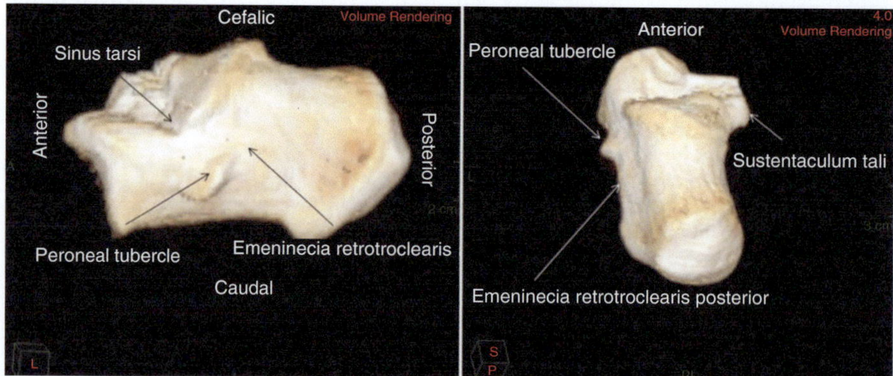

Fig. 16.1 CT showing the peroneal tubercle (also known as processus trochlearis) anterior to the retrotrochlear eminence

tested only asymptomatic patients, the peroneal tubercle was identified in 55% of the 65 patients, whereas the retrotrochlear eminence was identified in all of them [5].

The peroneal tubercle, which is the second osseous prominence on the lateral aspect of the calcaneus, is obliquely inclined, with its longitudinal axis running in a posterosuperior to anteroinferior direction. Whereas some reports indicate that it forms a 45-degree angle with a horizontal reference line [4], Edwards et al. reported the range of the angle to be between 35 and 50 degrees [2].The measured dimensions of the peroneal tubercle are its length, base width, and height. The mean length was measured by Sarrafian at 9–10 mm, mean base width was 6 mm, and the mean height was 3 mm [7]; additional measurements are shown in Table 16.1. A cutoff of 5 mm can be used to define an enlarged peroneal tubercle [8].

In 1904, Laidlaw published the first morphological classification of the peroneal tubercle [4]. The author divided the tubercles into three groups: Group α was described as having a novel and well-isolated portion, group β was described as having a ridge-like portion, and group γ contained tubercles with an imperfectly developed portion. Agarwal et al., who studied 1040 calcanei, also reported morphological variations of the peroneal tubercle, which were classified into four different types [6]. Type I presents with a single peroneal tubercle, anteroinferior to the insertion site of the calcaneofibular ligament. Type II is characterized by a single peroneal tubercle, which is incompletely divided by a smooth groove into anterior and posterior parts. Type III is composed of two peroneal tubercles, which are completely separated by a centrally located rough area. Finally, Type IV lacks a peroneal tubercle altogether (Table 16.2). Hyer et al. also studied peroneal tubercle morphology in 114 calcanei. It was present in 90.4% of patients, and no significant differences were found between males and females [9].

Close examination of the peroneal tubercle reveals that the peroneus brevis tendon slides along its superior surface, which is relatively smooth, whereas the peroneus longus tendon glides along the tubercle's inferior surface. The peroneus longus tendon has a groove to facilitate its gliding. This groove leaves a distinct footprint on the lateral aspect of the calcaneus in 85% of the population. This footprint is also present in the absence of the peroneal tubercle. Moreover, in order to further reduce the friction and aid the gliding of the peroneus longus tendon, a cartilage-covered facet may be present along the course of the tendon. This facet can be found on the

Table 16.1 The dimensions of the peroneal tubercle as described by Edwards et al. [2]

Dimension	Size range	Average
Length	2–17 mm	13.04 mm
Width	2–10 mm	3.13 mm
Height	1–7 mm	3 mm (rarely exceed 5 mm)

Table 16.2 The classification of peroneal tubercles by Agarwal et al. [6]

Type	Description	Comments
I	Single intact tubercle	Antero-inferior to the tubercle of insertion
II	Single, partially divided tubercle	Divided (anterior–posterior) by a smooth groove
III	Two separate tubercles	Separated by a rough-ended area
IV	Absent tubercle	

posterior slope of the peroneal tubercles, and is partly found on the lateral surface of the calcaneus. A groove for the peroneus brevis tendon is rarely seen. The inferior peroneal retinaculum, which is attached superiorly to the calcaneus and inferiorly to the peroneal tubercle, serves to guide both peroneal tendons by attaching them to the calcaneus and by creating a septum to separate the tendons [7].

Anatomy of the Peroneal Tendons Over the Lateral Calcaneal Wall

The peroneus longus muscle originates from the head of the fibula and the lateral femoral condyle of the tibia. It runs along the lateral side of the shin and makes a sharp turn at the cuboid groove toward the medial side of the foot, until its insertion into the plantar-lateral aspect of the first metatarsal and medial cuneiform of the foot. The fifth metatarsal bone is the insertion site of the peroneus brevis muscle, which originates from the middle third of the fibula. The musculotendinous junctions of both tendons are commonly located proximal to the superior peroneal retinaculum [10]. The os peroneum, which is an ossified sesamoid bone, is presented roughly in 20% of the population and is located at the calcaneocuboid joint [11]. The presence of the os peroneum may predispose to the development of stenosing tenosynovitis of the peroneus longus tendon at the region of the cuboid tunnel [12].

The peroneus longus and brevis muscles are innervated by the superficial peroneal nerve and receive their blood supply from the posterior peroneal artery and branches of the medial tarsal artery. The peroneus longus has two avascular zones, one around the cuboid and another around the lateral malleolus, extending to the peroneal tubercle. This creates uneven distribution of blood vessels supplying the peroneal tendons. Therefore, the most frequent sites of peroneal tendinopathy are found in these two avascular zones [10].

In their presentation of the endoscopic approach to the peroneal tendons, Van Dijk [13] depicted the relationship between the peroneal tendons and their bordering structures. They identified a membranous mesotendineal "vincula-like" structure between the peroneal tendons. This structure is attached to the dorsolateral aspect of the fibula and continues along the length of the tendons until their distal insertion site.

Sobel et al. examined 124 legs from 65 fresh human cadavers that were dissected under loupe magnification [14]. In 27 legs (21.7% of specimens), the accessory peroneus quartus muscle was present. The muscle originated from the muscular portion of the peroneus brevis and inserted into the peroneal tubercle of the calcaneus in 17 legs (63%). As a result, in most cases the peroneal tubercle was large and hypertrophied at the insertion site.

Etiology, Biomechanics, and Mechanism of Injury

Peroneal tendon disorders are primarily divided into three types: peroneal tendinopathy without subluxation of the tendons, which may be associated with attritional rupture; peroneal tendinopathy associated with instability of the peroneal tendons at the level of the superior peroneal retinaculum, accompanied by stenosing tenosynovitis of the peroneus longus tendon; and peroneal tendinopathy associated with instability of the peroneal tendons, which may appear with an acute rupture of the superior peroneal retinaculum. The latter occurs when the pathology is at the level of the superior peroneal retinaculum. Stenosing tenosynovitis of the peroneal longus tendon may clinically present with a painful os peroneum, pathological changes at the calcaneal cuboid joint, and an enlarged peroneal tubercle. In some cases, the peroneus longus tendon may be trapped inside a bony tunnel at the level of the cuboid [13].

The etiology and pertinence of the hypertrophied peroneal tubercle are not completely clear, but have been associated with various causes, such as rupture or tenosynovitis of the peroneus brevis or longus tendons that usually occur at the narrowest area of the sheath, the presence of peroneus quartus muscle, flatfoot, osteochondroma lesion, pes cavus, and intra-articular calcaneal fracture [15]. Other studies showed that a supinated foot is associated with peroneal tendon injury in 82% of patients [17, 20, 21]. Dombek et al. suggest that a cavovarus foot and ankle structure may predispose to peroneal tendon injury [21]. structure ankle may predispose to peroneal tendon injury [21].

One case report described an uncommon cause of stenosing tenosynovitis, namely a thick, inflamed, and fibrotic peroneal tendon sheath caused by extrapulmonary tuberculosis. Another case report depicted *Coccidioides immitis* treated with fluconazole to be the cause for stenosing tenosynovitis [42].

Martin et al. [16] described two cases of an osteochondroma lesion of the peroneal tubercle, which were presented with pain on the lateral side of the ankle and foot due to stenosing tenosynovitis of the peroneal tendons. They reported that surgical treatment yielded good results in both cases. A cavovarus foot was also described in the literature as a predisposing factor for stenosing tenosynovitis [17]. A cavovarus position of the foot may reduce the moment arm created by the peroneus longus and increase frictional forces on the tendon at the levels of the peroneal tubercle, lateral malleolus, and cuboid notch, thereby placing the tendon at a mechanical disadvantage. An enlarged peroneal tubercle can produce chronic friction at the anterior aspect of the peroneus longus tendon over the bony prominence, leading to direct tendon injury [10].

With regard to biomechanics, the peroneal tubercle appears to have three different functions: (a) To serve as the insertion of the inferior peroneal retinaculum; (b) to physically separate the common peroneal sheath into two distinct sheaths for the peroneal longus and peroneal brevis tendons; and (c) to function as a fulcrum or pulley for the peroneal tendons [15].

Lateral ankle stability, especially during the midstance and heel rise, is gained primarily due to the combining forces of the peroneus longus and peroneus brevis muscles. Furthermore, the primary action of the peroneus longus tendon is eversion and plantar flexion of the foot [16].

In 1933, McMaster et al. concluded that even in the face of severe strain at the area of normal musculotendinous junction, the tendon does not rupture. Nonetheless, the authors assumed that rupture might occur at other areas such as the insertion of the tendon to the bone, the muscle belly, or its proximal origin in the bone. Moreover, many systemic or local diseases may predispose the tendon to a spontaneous rupture, which often follows a relatively slight strain [18].

Tendon injury can be classified as either direct or indirect. Direct traumatic injury usually involves a sharp object. The mechanism of indirect trauma varies and is often multifactorial and depends on the vascularity, skeletal maturity, and the anatomic location of the injury, in conjunction with the extent of the applied forces. Failure occurs at the weakest link of the bone-tendon-muscle complex when the force exceeds the tolerance of this structure. The tendons can generally endure larger tensile forces than those sustained by the bone or utilized by the muscles. Subsequently, rupture of the tendon or avulsion fractures at the musculotendinous junction occur much more frequently than midsubstance tendon ruptures [19]. There are three typical and distinct anatomic zones where peroneal longus tears typically occur: the peroneal tubercle of the calcaneus, the lateral malleolus, and the cuboid notch [17, 20, 21]. While the true incidence of peroneal tendon tear is still unknown, the estimated range is 11–37% as seen in cadaver dissections and up to 30% in patients undergoing surgery for ankle instability [22].

Clinical Presentation

Prior to the clinical examination, it is important to receive the patient's full medical history and to inquire for any associated conditions and systemic diseases. Among these are diabetes, psoriasis, rheumatoid arthritis, previous calcaneal fractures or local steroid injections, and hyperparathyroidism. It is also important to ask about the use of antibiotics such as quinolone, which has been associated with an increased rate of tendon injury and tear [10, 12, 23, 24]. The common clinical presentation of patients with peroneal tendinitis is gradual onset of pain accompanied by swelling and warmth along the course of the peroneals in the posterolateral area of the ankle. The pain is usually worsened by ankle plantar flexion, passive hindfoot inversion, and by active hindfoot eversion and ankle dorsiflexion [10]. Athletes or people involved in recreational sports may present with lateral ankle swelling and discomfort leading to decreased performance.

Physical examination should start with inspection and may reveal limping or swelling posterior to the lateral malleolus. The entire extremity and specifically the foot should also be inspected for malalignment deformities such as hindfoot varus. Muscle strength may be decreased due to pain and tendon rupture. Nonetheless, even in case of notable eversion or lack of peroneal weakness, peroneal tendon tear or rupture cannot be ruled out. Peroneus longus tendon dysfunction may present with loss or limitation of plantar flexion of the first ray. It is also recommended to palpate the tendon along its course looking for thickening, tenderness, and pain [10]. Additional symptoms and findings include ankle "weakness" and frequent episodes of ankle "giving way," with chronic symptoms of tendinitis, which may indicate longitudinal tear of the peroneus longus [12]. Furthermore, tenosynovitis that does not respond to conservative treatment should raise the suspicion of partial tear.

Imaging and Diagnosis

The use of simple X-ray or advanced imagine such as computed tomography could demonstrate bony structures that might cause stenosing tenosynovitis, such as hypertrophied peroneal tubercle. Sobel et al. suggested the Harris heel view for demonstration of an enlarged peroneal tubercle [11]. A simple plane radiograph, such as Harris-Beath view, may disclose semilunar bony protrusions arising from the expected location of the peroneal tubercle [25]. Ultrasonography has the advantages of being a noninvasive, nonradiating, and inexpensive test. In two different studies, the diagnostic use of ultrasound produced 90–94% accuracy and 85–90% specificity [26, 28, 29]. Yet, the most important advantage of ultrasound is a dynamical demonstration of the tendon's gliding and friction over the peroneal tubercle (Fig. 16.2).

Computed tomography (CT) is considered the best imaging method for visualization of bony structures and bony abnormality, such as an os peroneum, an enlarged peroneal tubercle and, in acute injury, calcaneal, or lateral malleolus fractures (Fig. 16.3). Three-dimensional (3D) reconstruction can provide a more accurate and detailed view of bony anatomy, especially of the calcaneal lateral wall.

Magnetic resonance imaging (MRI) is better for demonstrating soft tissue structure, especially when an increased signal appears on T2-weighted and STIR images. Moreover, loss of homogeneous signal may indicate tenosynovitis, tendinosis, or a tendon tear [26] (Fig. 16.4). Signs that indicates tendon anomaly are gadolinium enhancement and complete obliteration of the fluid, and bone marrow edema along the calcaneal lateral wall or within bony protuberances, such as the peroneal tubercle [27]. Additional findings suggestive of peroneal tendon tear

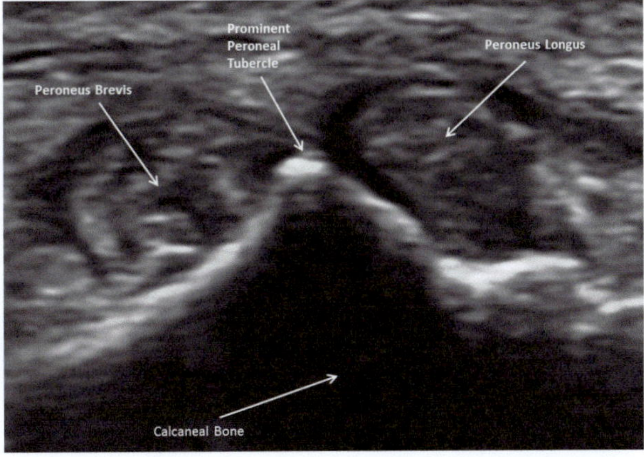

Fig. 16.2 An ultrasonograph demonstrating enlarged peroneal tubercle and the peroneal tendons

Fig. 16.3 CT scan showing sagittal view of bony abnormality, namely an enlarged peroneal tubercle

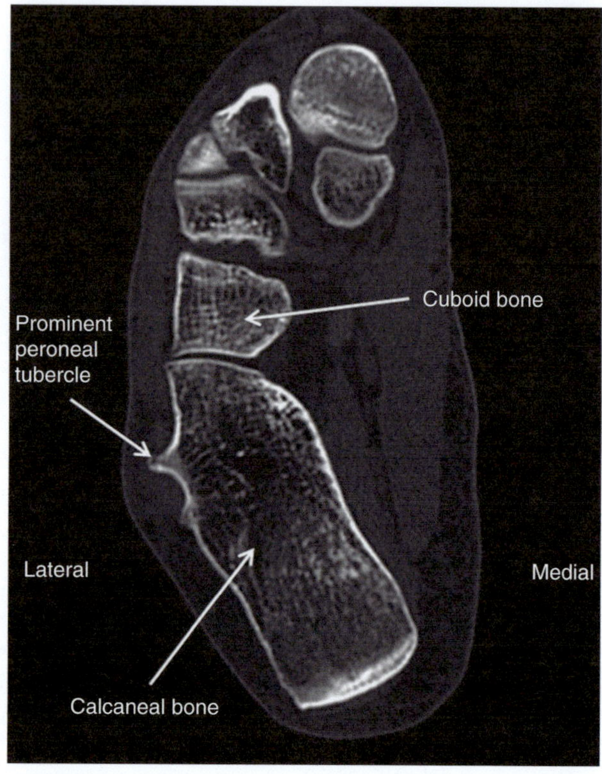

Fig. 16.4 A magnetic resonance imaging (MRI) image showing a pathological peroneal anatomy

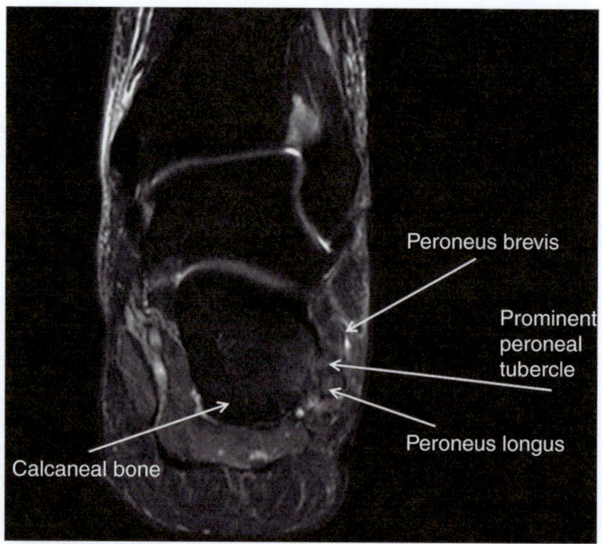

include discontinuity of the tendon or heterogeneity, and a tendon sheath full of fluid. Furthermore, MRI is useful in detecting longitudinal split tears of the peroneal tendons and differentiating this finding from other causes of chronic lateral ankle pain [30]. Rademaker et al. [31] showed an MRI series of nine patients between the ages of 37 and 62 years, with an imaging finding of a partial or a complete tear of the middle portion of the peroneal longus tendon. Of note, five patients denied precedent trauma. Partial tear was diagnosed in four patients, and a complete tear in five patients. The MRI studies demonstrated an empty peroneus longus tendon sheath at the level of the cuboid tunnel, with the tendon retracted proximally. Furthermore, while performing this exam, the "magic angle effect" should be taken into consideration. This phenomenon refers to signal variations of the MRI due to the acute angle created by the peroneus longus while it passes in the foot from the lateral side to the medial-plantar side. The angle, which has a "chevron-like" appearance, is mostly seen in T1 images of tendons that have acute angulations, approximately 55 degrees to the magnetic field [26]. The main disadvantage of MRI examination is that its high sensitivity may lead to a false positive diagnosis [30].

Lidocaine test injection guided by ultrasound was recently described by Watson [44] in cases of stenosing tenosynovitis suspicious. In this series of 11 patients, the lidocaine injection relieves the pain confirming the diagnosis. Surgical release of the peroneal tendon sheath improves the Foot and Ankle Outcome Score (FAOS) in all 11 cases.

Treatment

The treatment is based on the severity of symptoms, imaging demonstrating a positive rupture, and the patient's age, daily function and demands. Treatment options range from conservative treatment to surgical excision and debridement of the tendon and the nearby structure causing the symptoms. Usually, conservative treatment is used as the first line and includes protected weightbearing, cast immobilization, activity modifications, physical therapy, orthotics with a lateral heel wedge, and pharmacological treatment such as NSAID and corticosteroids injection. Surgical treatment is generally reserved for patients who failed a conservative therapy and have severe and chronic symptoms, with clear evidence of peroneal tendon rupture [17]. The surgical procedures vary and are tailored to each patient individually. Pierson, Ingis et al. published a case report describing a congenital calcified hypertrophic peroneal longus associated with a hypertrophic peroneal tubercle and an os peroneum [33]. They described a stenotic fibro-osseous tunnel due to hypertrophied peroneal tubercle. The patient did not respond to conservative treatment, including protected weightbearing, immobilization in a cast, and corticosteroid injections, and symptoms even worsened. Only surgical intervention with excision of the hypertrophied tubercle, which caused the pain, clicking, and symptoms of instability to be completely resolved.

When the cause of stenosing tenosynovitis is an enlarged bony prominence, the most commonly accepted treatment was a complete surgical excision. In 1989, however, Berenter, Goldman et al. published a case report describing a surgical technique that preserves both the gliding capacity of the peroneal tendon and the cartilaginous gliding facet of the peroneal tubercle. According to the authors, this technique has proved to be superior to the acceptable technique [32].

Another short series involving six patients with stenosing tenosynovitis due to hypertrophic peroneal tubercle was published by Chen et al. In that study, the authors reported good outcome after treating the stenosing tenosynovitis with synovectomy and peroneal tubercle resection [35]. Similar results were also reported by Sugimoto et al. in 2009, after treating three patients with surgical resection of an enlarged peroneal tubercle [36].

A case of recurrent hypertrophic peroneal tubercle was published in 2007 by Ochoa, Banerjee et al. This phenomenon was seen in a young patient 4 months following surgical resection [37]. The second surgical resection was performed 10 months after the first operation. The postoperative protocol included non-weight-bearing for 4 weeks and indomethacin treatment due to its ability to interfere with bone healing in heterotrophic ossification [37, 38].

Redfern, Myerson et al. developed a treatment algorithm for a peroneal tendon tear based on the ability to repair the tendon and the amount of tendons involved. The tear is classified as type I when both tendons are grossly intact and repairable, type II when only one tendon is unstable but reparable, while the other tendon is torn and requires tenodesis, and type III when both tendons are torn and unstable. Type III can be further divided into subtypes IIIa and IIIb. Type IIIa describes a condition where both tendons are irreparable with no proximal muscle excursion, treated with tendon transfer. In type IIIb, both tendons are irreparable with proximal muscle excursion, which is treated with an allograft reconstruction [30].

Another classification system to guide surgical decision-making in patients with peroneal tendon tears was proposed by Krause and Brodsky et al. [29]. The classification is intraoperative and is based on the transverse (cross-sectional) area of the viable tendon that remains after debridement of the damaged portion of the tendon, presuming that the retained portion of the tendon has no longitudinal tears. Grade I lesions mean that less than 50% of the cross-sectional area of the tendon is involved, and as such, tendon repair is recommended. In grade II lesions, more than 50% of the cross-sectional area is involved, and tenodesis is recommended.

Saxena et al. described 49 patients with peroneal tendon tear, of whom 11 patients suffered from an isolated peroneus longus tear, and 7 patients suffered from a double tendon tear. Longitudinal tears comprised the majority of the cases. Six patients underwent tendon repair and bony exostectomy of the peroneal tubercle, base of the fifth metatarsal, or distal fibula. The authors reported clinical improvement of 38.7 points in the American Orthopaedic Foot and Ankle score (AOFAS) after surgery. Postoperative protocol included below-knee cast or splint for 2–3 weeks and non-weightbearing. Transition into below-knee removable cast boot was allowed for another 3–5 weeks. Range of motion exercises were initiated at

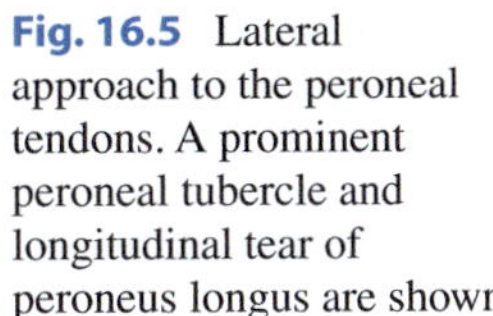

Fig. 16.5 Lateral approach to the peroneal tendons. A prominent peroneal tubercle and longitudinal tear of peroneus longus are shown

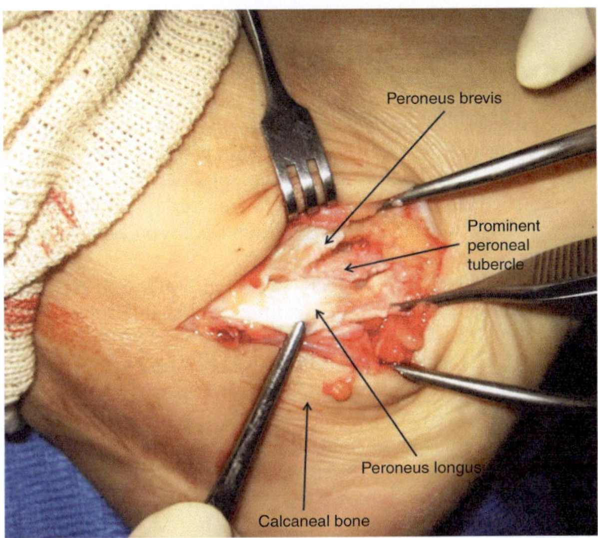

3 weeks postoperatively, and physical therapy was started at approximately 6 weeks [39].

Our experience shows that using the lateral approach to the peroneal longus, excision of the peroneal tubercle and primary tendon repair using absorbable or nonabsorbable suture, in order to recover the tubular fashion of the tendon sutures when possible, yields the best results in long distance runners (Fig. 16.5) [40]. In case of failure or inability for primary tendon repair, we recommend tendon reconstruction using an autogenous graft or allograft. When reconstruction is also impossible, or in case of reconstruction failure, our recommendation is to do triple arthrodesis in order to stabilize the hindfoot and midfoot.

Conflict of Interest All Authors (Palmanovich Ezequiel, Nyska Meir, Ohana Nissim, Vidra Matias, Atzmon Ran) declare that they have no conflict of interest.

References

1. Altchek DW, DiGiovanni CW, Dines JS, et al. Foot and ankle sports medicine. Philadelphia: LippinCott Williams & Wilkins; 2013.
2. Edwards M. The relations of the peroneal tendon to the fibula, calcaneous, and cuboideum. Am J Anat. 1928;42:213–53.
3. Hyrtl J. cited by Burman M. Stenosing tendovaginitis of the foot and ankle: studies with special references to the stenosing tendovaginitis of the peroneal tendos at the peroneal tubercle. AMA Arch Surg. 1953;67:686.
4. Laidlaw PP. The varieties of the oscalcis. J Anat Physiol. 1904;38:133.
5. Saupe N, Mengiardi B, Pfirrmann CW, Vienne P, Seifert B, Zanetti M. Anatomic variants associated with peroneal tendon disorders: MR imaging findings in volunteers with asymptomatic ankles. Radiology. 2007;242:509–17.

6. Agarwal AK, Jeyasingh P, Gupta SC, Gupta CD, Sahai A. Peroneal tubercle and its variations in the Indian calcanei. AnatAnz. 1984;156:241–4.
7. Kelikian RS. Osteology/Myology. In Sarrafian's Anatomy of the foot and ankle. Third edition. Philadelphia, PA: William & Wilkins; 2011.
8. Zanetti M. Founder's lecture of the ISS 2006: borderlands of normal and early pathological findings in MRI of the foot and ankle. Skelet Radiol. 2008;37:875–84.
9. Hyer C, Dawson J, Philbin T, Berlet G, Lee T. The peroneal tubercle: description, classification, and relevance to peroneus longus tendon pathology. Foot Ankle Int. 2005;26:947–50.
10. Selmani E, Gjata V, Gjika E. Currents concepts review: peroneal tendon disorders. Foot Ankle Int. 2006;27:221–8.
11. Sobel M, Pavlov H, Geppert MJ, Thompson FM, DiCarlo EF, Davis WH. Painful osperoneum syndrome: a spectrum of condition responsible for plantar lateral foot pain. Foot Ankle Int. 1994;15:112–24.
12. Clarke HD, Kitaoka HB, Ehman RL. Peroneal tendon injury. Foot Ankle Int. 1998;19:280–8.
13. van Dijk N. NanneKort: tendoscopy of the peroneal tendons. Arthroscopy. 1998;14:471–8.
14. Sobel M, Levy ME, Bohne WH. Congenital variations of the peroneus quartus muscle: an anatomic study. Foot Ankle. 1990;11:81–9. Erratum in: Foot Ankle 1991;11:342.
15. Ruiz JR, Christman RA, Hilstrom HJ. 1993 William J. Stickel Silver Award. Anatomical considerations of the peroneal tubercle. J Am Podiatr Med Assoc. 1993;83:563–75.
16. Martin MA, Garcia L, Hijazi H, Sanchez MM. Osteochondroma of the peroneal tubercle. A report of two cases. Int Orthop. 1995;19(6):405–7.
17. Brandes CB, Smith RW. Characterization of patients with primary longus tendinopathy: a review of twenty-two cases. Foot Ankle Int. 2000;21:462–8.
18. McMaster PE. Tendon and muscle ruptures: clinical and experimental studies on the causes and location of subcutaneous ruptures. J Bone Joint Surg. 1933;15:705–22.
19. Buckwalter J, Einhorn T, Simon S, American Academy of Orthopaedic Surgeons. Orthopaedic basic science. 2nd ed. Rosemont, IL: American Academy of Orthopaedic Surgeons, 2000;24(2):591.
20. Sammarco GJ. Peroneus longus tendon tears: acute and chronic. Foot Ankle Int. 1995;16:245–53.
21. Dombek MF, Lamm BM, Saltrick K, Mendicino RW, Catanzariti AR. Peroneal tendon tears: a retrospective review. J Foot Ankle Surg. 2003;42:250–8.
22. Squires N, Meyerson M, Gamba C. Surgical treatment of peroneal tendon tears. Foot Ankle Clin. 2007;12:675–95.
23. Troung DT, Dussault RG, Kaplan PA. Fracture of the os perineum and rupture of the peroneus longus tendon as a complications of diabetic neuropathy. Skeletal Radiol. 1995;24:626–8.
24. Sharma P, Maffulli N. Tendon injury and tendinopathy: healing and repair. J Bone Joint Surg. 2005;87:187–202.
25. Boles MA, Lomasney LM, Demos TC, Sage RA. Enlarged peroneal process with peroneus longus tendon entrapment. Skelet Radiol. 1997;26:313–5.
26. Major NM, Helms CA, Fritz RC, Speeer KP. The MR appearance of longitudinal split tears of the peroneal brevis tendon. Foot Ankle Int. 2000;21:514–9.
27. Wang XT, Rosenberg ZS, Mechlin MB, Schweitzer ME. Normal variants and diseases of the peroneal tendons and superior peroneal retinaculum: MR imaging features. Radiographics. 2005;25:587–602. Erratum in: Radiographics. 2006;26:640. Radiographics. 2005;25:1436.
28. Grant TH, Kelikian AS, Jereb SE, McCarthy RJ. Ultrasound diagnosis of peroneal tendon tears: a surgical correlation. J Bone Joint Surg. 2005;87:1788–94.
29. Krause JO, Brodsky JW. Peroneus brevis tendon tears: pathophysiology, surgical reconstruction and clinical results. Foot Ankle Int. 1998;19:271–9.
30. Redfern D, Myerson M. The management of concomitant tears of the peroneus longus and brevis tendons. Foot Ankle Int. 2004;25:695–707.
31. Rademaker J, Rosemberg Z, Cheung Y, Schweitzer M. Tear of the peroneus longus tendon: MR imaging features in nine patients. Radiology. 2000;214:700–4.

32. Berenter JS, Goldman FD. Surgical approach for enlarged peroneal tubercles. J Am Podiatr Med Assoc. 1989;79:451–4.
33. Pierson JL, Inglis AE. Stenosing tenosynovitis of the peroneus longus tendon associated with hypertrophy of peroneal tubercle and os perineum. A case report. J Bone Joint Surg Am. 1992;74:440–2.
34. Bruce WD, Christofersen MR, Phillips DL. Stenosing tenosynovitis and impingement of the peroneal tendons associated with hypertrophy of the peroneal tubercle. Foot Ankle Int. 1999;20:464–7.
35. Chen YJ, Hsu RW, Huang TJ. Hypertrophic peroneal tubercle with stenosing tenosynovitis: the results of surgical treatment. Changgeng Yi Xue Za Zhi. 1998;21:442–6.
36. Sugimoto K, Takakura Y, Okahashi K, Tanaka Y, Ohshima M, Kasanami R. Enlarged peroneal tubercle with peroneus longus tenosynovitis. J Orthop Sci. 2009;14:330–5.
37. Ochoa LM, Banerjee R. Recurrent hypertrophic peroneal tubercle associated with peroneus brevis tendon tear. Foot Ankle Surg. 2007;46:403–8.
38. Burd TA, Hughes MS, Anglen JO. Heterotopic ossification prophylaxis with indometacion increases the risk of long bone nonunion. J Bone Joint Surg Br. 2003;85:700–5.
39. Saxena A, Cassidy A. Peroneal tendon injuries: an evolution of 49 tears in 41 patients. J Food Ankle Surg. 2003;42(4):215–20.
40. Palmanovich E, Laver L, Brin YS, Hetsroni I, Nyska M. Tear of peroneus longus in long distance runners due to enlarged peroneal tubercle. BMC Sports Sci Med Rehabil. 2014;6(1):1.
41. Ajoy SM, Samorekar B, Soman S, Jadhav M. Isolated tuberculous peroneal tenosynovitis: a case report. J Clin Diagn Res. 2015;9(7):RD01–2.
42. Majeed A, Ullah W, Hamadani AA, Georgescu A. First reported case of peroneal tenosynovitis caused by Coccidioides immitis successfully treated with fluconazole. BMJ Case Rep. 2016;2016. pii: bcr2016216804.
43. Ziai P, Benca E, von Skrbensky G, et al. The role of the peroneal tendons in passive stabilisation of the ankle joint: an in vitro study. Knee Surg Sports Traumatol Arthrosc. 2013;21(6):1404–8.
44. Watson G, Karnovsky S, Levine D, Drakos M. Surgical treatment for syenosing peroneal tenovinovitis. Foot Ankle Int. 2019;40(3):282–6.

Peroneus Longus Tears Associated with Pathology of The Os Peroneum

17

Kristopher Stockton

Anatomy

The origin of the peroneus longus muscle is on the lateral head and upper fibula, the intermuscular septum, and variably on the lateral tibial condyle and inserts onto the plantar first cuneiform and base of the first metatarsal. The muscle belly lies posterior and lateral to the peroneus brevis muscle belly in the leg. The tendinous portion of the longus begins proximal to the ankle joint and runs posterior to the brevis in the fibular groove. It then runs inferior to the peroneal tubercle of the calcaneus and curves plantar medially through the cuboid tunnel and across the plantar foot. The innervation is by the superficial peroneal nerve. The action of the peroneus longus is to plantarflex the first metatarsal and evert the foot. Both peroneals share a common sheath starting about 4 cm proximal to the tip of the fibula down to level of the peroneal tubercle on the calcaneus at which point the tendons diverge and the brevis continues superior to the tubercle and on to its insertion on the fifth metatarsal base. The longus travels inferior to the tubercle and continues toward the cuboid tunnel and the plantar foot [5]. The peroneal tubercle of the calcaneus separates the tendons and can be variable in size [6]. There is a cartilaginous septum between the tendons at that level, which is attached to the tubercle and this tissue, and the sheath has been referred to as the inferior peroneal retinaculum.

The os peroneum has been reported to be present in 4–30% of the population and can vary in size and density of ossification. It also may be multipartite or present unilaterally. If it is absent, there is a thickening of the tendon into a fibrocartilaginous section at the level of the cuboid tunnel [1, 7–9].

K. Stockton (✉)
Texas Orthopedics, Sports & Rehabilitation Associates, Austin, TX, USA

Department of Orthopaedics, Dell Medical School – The University of Texas at Austin, Austin, TX, USA
e-mail: kstockton@txortho.com

© Springer Nature Switzerland AG 2020
M. Sobel (ed.), *The Peroneal Tendons*,
https://doi.org/10.1007/978-3-030-46646-6_17

Brandes and Smith described three anatomic areas at which the peroneus longus tendon changes direction and thus vulnerable to tears. Zone A is at the tip of the fibula and is least associated with tears. Zone B is at the peroneal tubercle of the calcaneus and had the highest incidence of partial ruptures. Zone C is at the cuboid tunnel and had the highest incidence of complete ruptures [7].

History and Physical Exam

In regard to the specific pathology at the level of the cuboid tunnel involving an os peroneum, patients may present with either an acute onset of pain and dysfunction after a recognizable injury of varying severity or can present with chronic pain with or without any known trauma. The injury is commonly an inversion sprain of the ankle/foot or less commonly direct trauma to the lateral foot. The patient tends to have mechanical pain with activity at the plantar lateral border of the foot at the level of the cuboid tunnel, which may radiate proximally toward the fibula or distally into the plantar foot.

On exam, the patient may have a normal or cavovarus foot type [2]. Anecdotally, it is rare to see a flatfoot with this particular pathology. The patient can have tenderness and swelling along the peroneal tendons and usually the point of maximal tenderness is located at the cuboid tunnel or peroneal tubercle of the calcaneus. There may be varying degrees of pain and weakness with resisted eversion and pronation of the foot and/or pain with inversion of the foot.

Radiographic Evaluation

Plain radiographs consisting of three weightbearing views of the ankle and foot are usually quite helpful in diagnosing os peroneum pathology when combined with a careful physical exam. Fractures of the os peroneum are more commonly diagnosed on plain films compared to MRI. CT scan can also be helpful in diagnosing subtle fractures [2]. The os peroneum can be fractured (Fig. 17.1) with or without diastasis or enlarged and sclerotic with degenerative changes [1, 2]. The os peroneum may be multipartite or show evidence of a remote fracture, which makes clinical correlation important. It is not uncommon to see changes of the os peroneum on X-rays, which are simply incidental findings, and the patient is asymptomatic. The os peroneum may also be seen to be retracted proximally through fracture diastasis or the entire os peroneum [2, 10]. In an acute trauma scenario with the appropriate physical exam, significant retraction on plain films can be diagnostic, and MRI is unnecessary. Retraction can be dramatic even to level of the distal fibula.

MRI is commonly obtained and can be helpful in diagnosing concomitant pathology of the lateral ligaments, osteochondral lesions, peroneus brevis pathology, and the extent of the longus pathology. Interestingly, fractures of the os peroneum are often difficult to visualize on MRI scan (Fig. 17.2). MRI can also show edema of the os peroneum, which can be helpful in the absence of fracture [2].

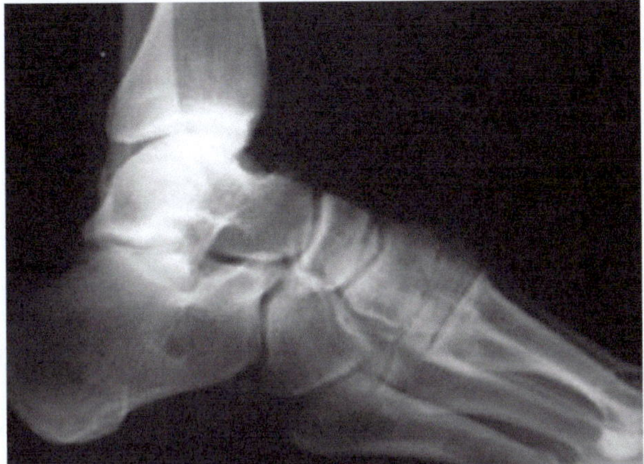

Fig. 17.1 Fracture of the os peroneum seen on radiograph

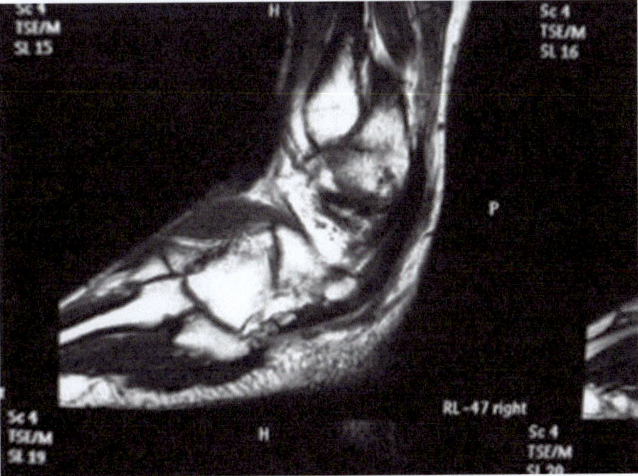

Fig. 17.2 Same patient as Fig. 17.1, showing fracture of the os peroneum on preoperative MRI

In experienced hands, ultrasound can be useful to diagnose peroneal disease, especially when real-time evaluation is needed such as intrasheath subluxation or entrapment of the os peroneum at the cuboid tunnel or peroneal tubercle [5].

Not unlike other tendons in our body, there is a wide spectrum of severity of the pathology of the peroneus longus ranging from tendinitis or tenosynovitis, partial tear, to complete tear or disruption. The presence of an os peroneum adds fracture as an additional type of pathology, which can be encountered.

Conservative Treatment

The presentation and functional demands of the patient will often dictate the treatment approach. Nonsurgical management should be attempted in all, but the complete rupture in a highly functional patient. Patients should be educated on the possibility that the tendon pathology may progress and become more degenerative over time. They should understand that surgical management may be needed if conservative measures fail to improve their symptoms.

Nonsurgical treatment for tenosynovitis, partial tears, or even fractures of the os peroneum without complete disruption of the peroneus longus tendon may include variable periods of weightbearing immobilization from 2 to 6 weeks in a cast, boot, or brace. Other modalities including NSAIDs, lateral posting orthotics, activity modifications, and physical therapy may also be helpful [1–3]. Nonsurgical management of complete disruption of the peroneus longus tendon is always an option in the elderly low-demand patient who is a poor surgical candidate. In that situation, if there are functional symptoms of weakness, persistent pain, or instability, an ankle-foot orthosis may be needed long term.

There has been increasing use of platelet-rich plasma (PRP) injections for the treatment of various types of tendinosis, fasciitis, arthritis, and osteochondral injuries [11–14]. To my knowledge, there is currently no support in evidence-based literature specifically for peroneal tendon PRP injections, but many clinicians are performing this with reports of good outcomes on websites. The basic science does support its use in tendinosis in general [14], but studies specifically looking at its use for peroneal tendons are needed.

Surgical Treatment

This chapter is focusing on pathology of the os peroneum, and thus, the surgical management of more proximal tears is discussed elsewhere. The pathology of the peroneus longus tendon at the level of the peroneal tubercle of the calcaneus and at the cuboid tunnel involving the os peroneum is often intimately related. Os peroneum fractures (Fig. 17.3) and partial tears at the level of the tubercle are often seen together. Depending on the chronicity of the disease, there can be variable stages of healing response with scar tissue and callous that causes enlargement of the tendon

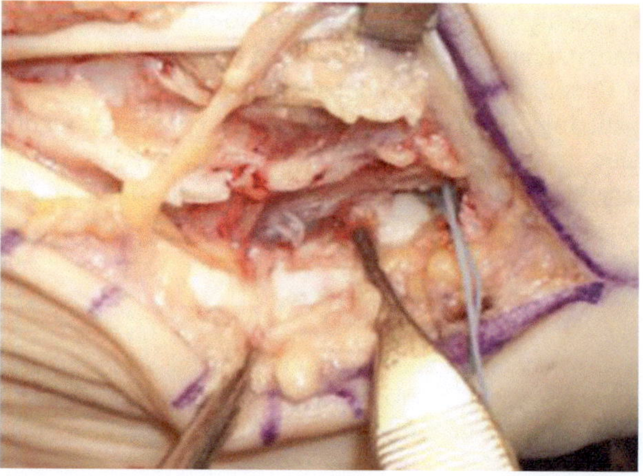

Fig. 17.3 Intraoperative photo with forceps pointing to a fracture through the os peroneum

and os peroneum at these levels. This can cause entrapment or prevent excursion at the level of the cuboid tunnel or peroneal tubercle rendering the peroneus longus tendon essentially nonfunctional [1, 2].

Reported operative techniques for peroneus longus tears with os peroneum pathology include excision of all or part of the os peroneum with primary repair or grafting of the tendon gap, excision of the os peroneum with tenodesis of the peroneus longus to the brevis, and internal fixation of the fractured os peroneum [4]. Most of the publications describing surgical treatment of this particular pathology are either single case reports or small series of 2–5 patients [2].

Stockton and Brodsky reported good results on 12 patients with os peroneum pathology, all treated with excision of the damaged segment of the peroneus longus including the fractured (Fig. 17.4) or enlarged os peroneum (Figs. 17.5 and 17.6), followed by peroneus longus tenodesis to the peroneus brevis. The proximal tenodesis was performed in a side-to-side fashion between the tip of the fibula and the

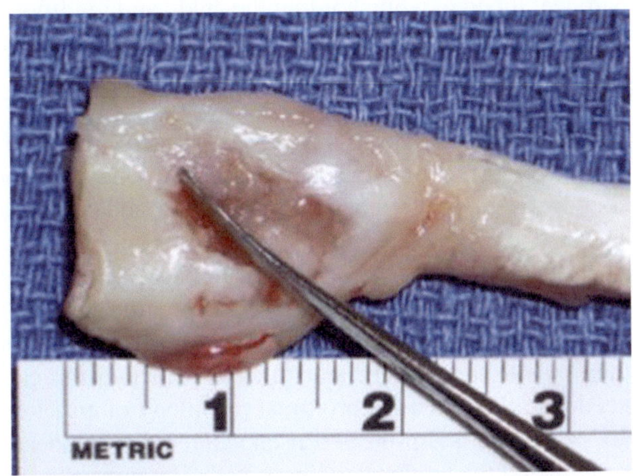

Fig. 17.4 Excised specimen of same patient in Fig. 17.3, showing fractured os peroneum with attached peroneus longus tendon

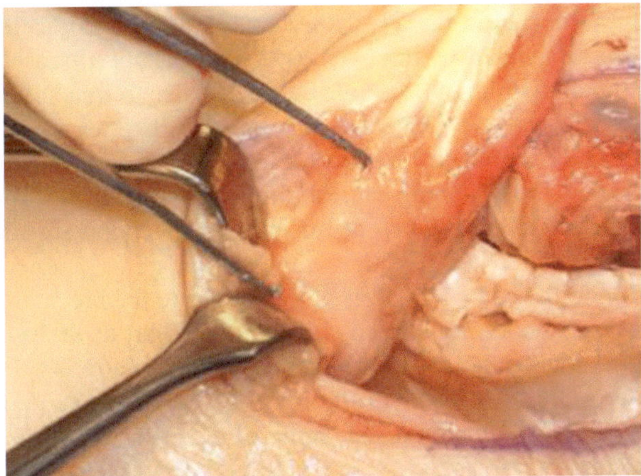

Fig. 17.5 Intraoperative photo showing torn, fibrotic, and thickened segment of the distal peroneus longus tendon, which is demarcated by change in color, texture, and thickness

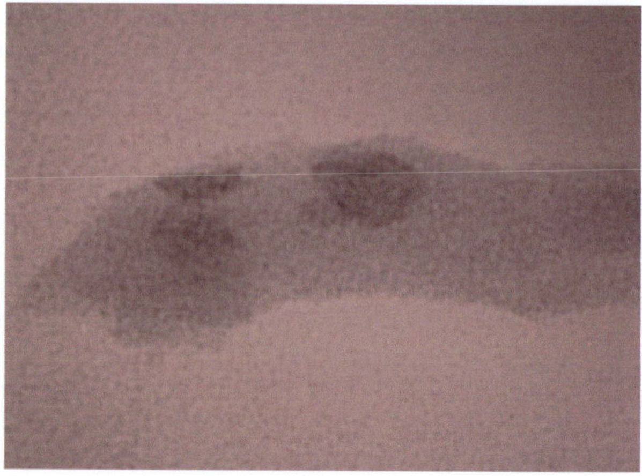

Fig. 17.6 Fluoroscopic scan of the excised segment of the peroneus longus tendon from the patient in Fig. 17.5 showing the separated fragments of the os peroneum within the tendon

peroneal tubercle while holding the ankle and hindfoot in a neutral position. If possible, the distal stump of the peroneus longus was tenodesed at or just proximal to the cuboid tunnel. Concomitant repair of the peroneus brevis was required in 9 of the 12 cases [2].

Sobel reported on eight operatively treated cases with os peroneum fractures, two of which underwent excision of the os peroneum and primary tendon repair, while six underwent excision of the os peroneum and peroneus longus to brevis tenodesis. The classic paper coined the term painful os peroneum syndrome (POPS) [1].

In surgery, the patient is positioned lateral with the operative side up. A bean bag or chest rolls can be used for positioning at the surgeon's discretion. A thigh tourniquet is used. The surgical approach starts with a curvilinear incision from the tip of the fibula to the fifth metatarsal base. This incision can be extended proximally if needed to address more proximal pathology of either tendon. Sural nerve branches are mobilized and protected if encountered. The sheath is opened in the proximal wound, and the tendons are inspected. The inferior peroneal retinaculum is opened carefully off the peroneal tubercle to mobilize the longus tendon, and it is followed into the cuboid tunnel. If the tubercle is pathologically hypertrophied (Fig. 17.7) and thought to be involved as a cause of the disease process, then it is resected smooth with the wall of the calcaneus. The retinaculum can be interposed over the resected bone or bone wax can be used. If a tenodesis is performed, the peroneal tubercle should be resected regardless of its size in order to prevent the combined tendon from rubbing on it and potentially causing future tears. Tenosynovium is excised, and the os peroneum and longus tendon are addressed. If the tendon is not salvageable, then resection of the pathologic os peroneum and damaged longus tendon followed by tenodesis of the longus to the brevis is performed. The tenodesis is usually done in a side-to-side fashion distal to the tip of the fibula and at or just proximal to the peroneal tubercle. If the tendon is salvageable, excision of the os peroneum and repair of the longus tendon can be performed. If tenodesis is performed and enough distal stump of the peroneus longus tendon is available, it can

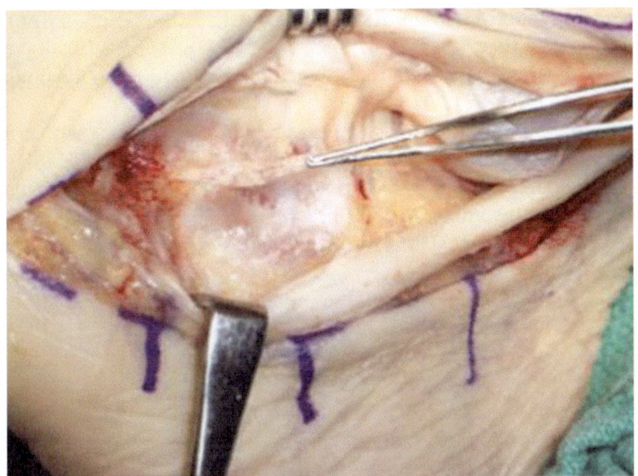

Fig. 17.7 Intraoperative photo showing an example of a pathologically hypertrophied peroneal tubercle of the calcaneus prior to resection

be tenodesed at the level of the cuboid tunnel. If the superior peroneal retinaculum was opened, it should be meticulously repaired with the appropriate tension to prevent subluxation or dislocation of the tendons from behind the fibular groove but allow for easy tendon excursion. The distal sheath is left open, and the wound is closed in layers. The patient is placed in a well-padded non-weightbearing short leg splint with the ankle in neutral position.

The patient is seen at 2 weeks postoperatively, sutures are removed, and they can be placed in a weightbearing short leg cast for 4 additional weeks. At 6 weeks postoperatively, they can be placed in a tall boot and begin physical therapy with weaning of the boot and gradual advancement of activities over the next 4 weeks.

Surgically addressing the peroneus longus and os peroneum pathology along with concomitant cavovarus foot reconstruction is a decision that must be made with the patient. A formal discussion with the patient is needed. In most cases, adding the cavovarus reconstruction changes the postoperative recovery significantly. If the patient has a very severe deformity and/or neuromuscular disease, cavovarus reconstruction is warranted. The dilemma arises when the patient has a mild to moderate deformity without neuromuscular disease. Certainly, it is intuitive to believe that in these cases, cavovarus reconstruction will protect the peroneal reconstruction in the future, but this is difficult to quantify.

References

1. Sobel M, Pavlov H, Geppert MJ, et al. Painful os peroneum syndrome: a spectrum of conditions responsible for plantar lateral foot pain. Foot Ankle. 1994;15(3):112–24.
2. Stockton KG, Brodsky JW. Peroneus longus tears associated with pathology of the os peroneum. FAI. 2014;35(4):346–52.
3. Sammarco GJ. Peroneus longus tendon tears: acute and chronic. FAI. 1995;16(5):245–53.
4. Peacock KC, Resnick EJ, Thorder JJ. Fracture of the os peroneum with rupture of the peroneus longus tendon. A case report and review of the literature. CORR. 1986;202:223–6.

5. Coughlin MJ, Mann RA, Saltzman CL, editors. Surgery of the foot and ankle, vol. 1. 8th ed: Mosby Elsevier, Philadelphia, PA; 2007. p. 1184, 1192–8.
6. Edwards M. The relations of the peroneal tendons to the fibula, calcaneus, and cuboideum. Am J Anat. 1988;42:213–53.
7. Brandes CB, Smith RW. Characterization of patients with primary peroneus longus tendinopathy: a review of twenty-two cases. FAI. 2000;21(6):462–8.
8. Heckman DS, Gluck GS, Parekh SG. Tendon disorders of the foot and ankle, part 1, peroneal tendon disorders. Am J Sports Med. 2009;37(3):614–25.
9. Thompson FM, Patterson AH. Rupture of the peroneus longus tendon. J Bone Joint Surg Am. 1989;71(2):293–5.
10. Sammarco VJ, Cuttica DJ, Sammarco GJ. Lasso stitch with retinaculoplasty for repair of fractured os peroneum. Clin Orthop Relat Res. 2010;468:1012–7.
11. Monto RR. Platelet-rich plasma efficacy versus corticosteroid injection treatment for chronic severe plantar fasciitis. FAI. 2014;35(4):313–8.
12. Gormeli G, Karakaplan M, Gormeli CA, et al. Clinical effects of platelet-rich plasma and hyaluronic acid as an additional therapy for talar osteochondral lesions treated with microfracture surgery: a prospective randomized clinical trial. FAI. 2015;36(8):891–900.
13. Fukawa T, Yamaguchi S, Akatsu Y, et al. Safety and efficacy of intra-articular injection of platelet-rich plasma in patients with ankle osteoarthritis. FAI. 2017;38(6):596–604.
14. Monto RR. Platelet rich plasma treatment for chronic Achilles tendinosis. FAI. 2012;33(5):379–85.

Attritional Rupture of Peroneus Brevis and Peroneus Longus Tendons: Allograft Reconstruction

Andrew E. Hanselman and James A. Nunley

Introduction

Tearing of the Peroneus brevis and/or peroneus longus can be a cause of lateral ankle pain and dysfunction. Like other foot and ankle pathologies, numerous treatment options exist, both nonoperative and operative. In the setting of acute injuries, the tendon can often be tubularized or repaired directly; however, this is not often the case with attritional injuries. In the setting of chronic peroneal tendon tears, intercalary allograft reconstruction is the author's preferred method of treatment when clinically appropriate. Although the data are limited, early cadaveric and clinical studies, along with anecdotal experience, have demonstrated good clinical outcomes by restoring the muscle-tendon unit and patient function. Allograft reconstruction provides the surgeon with several different graft options, while limiting donor site morbidity and decreased functionality that may accompany other treatment options, such as tenodesis and autograft tendon transfers.

Anatomy

The peroneus longus originates on the fibular head and the proximal one-half to two-thirds of the fibular shaft. The Peroneus brevis originates more distally on the inferior two-thirds of the lateral fibular shaft. Both muscles are supplied by the superficial peroneal nerve and blood supply comes from the peroneal artery. The musculotendinous junction of the peroneus longus is more proximal than that of the Peroneus brevis. As the tendons course distally, they run along the retrofibular groove. At this point, the peroneal brevis is more ovoid in shape, lying directly posterior to the fibula, while the peroneus longus is more circular in shape and lies

A. E. Hanselman (✉) · J. A. Nunley
Duke University Department of Orthopaedics, Durham, NC, USA
e-mail: Andrew.hanselman@duke.edu; james.nunley@duke.edu

© Springer Nature Switzerland AG 2020
M. Sobel (ed.), *The Peroneal Tendons*,
https://doi.org/10.1007/978-3-030-46646-6_18

posterior to the Peroneus brevis. At the distal tip of the fibula, the tendons are tethered by the superior peroneal retinaculum, which extends from the distal fibular tip to the calcaneus. Passing through this deep fascial layer, the tendons lie superficial to the calcaneofibular ligament (CFL). The tendons are then encased by another deep fascial layer, the inferior peroneal retinaculum, at which point the peroneal brevis lies superior and the peroneal longus lies inferior to the peroneal tubercle on the lateral aspect of the calcaneus. The peroneal brevis continues distally to its insertion site at the inferolateral aspect of the fifth metatarsal base, while the peroneal longus courses plantar to the cuboid before inserting on the plantar aspect of the medial cuneiform and first metatarsal.

Pathogenesis

Peroneal tendon tears are often categorized as acute or chronic, a description related more to the mechanism of injury, as opposed to the chronicity. Acute injuries tend to be a result of traumatic rupture and are less common than chronic injuries, which tend to be more gradual and attritional [1]. Although the exact pathogenesis of chronic peroneal tendon tears is unclear, two aspects of these tears have been supported in the literature. First, Peroneus brevis tears are more common than peroneus longus tears [2]. Second, the Peroneus brevis is most commonly torn in the retrofibular groove, whereas the peroneus longus is more commonly torn in two different regions, the area surrounding the peroneal tubercle and also the area coursing around the cuboid [3, 4].

Several theories or associated pathologies have been proposed. Some believe that the location of the Peroneus brevis musculotendinous junction, specifically a low-lying muscle belly, may lead to inflammation, increased pressure in the retrofibular space, and even tendon subluxation [5]. Other studies have contradicted this. A recent study by Housley et al. demonstrated, using a cadaveric model, that a more proximal muscle belly extension was associated with increased Peroneus brevis tears. They hypothesized that a lack of muscle belly distally resulted in instability of the retrofibular region [6]. The blood supply of the peroneal tendon has also been called into question. Peterson et al. performed a cadaveric study looking at the blood supply to both tendons. The Peroneus brevis had a relative avascular zone as it passed through the retrofibular groove while the peroneus longus had two relatively avascular zones, one extending from the tip of the distal fibula to the peroneal tubercle and another as it coursed around the cuboid [3]. These avascular zones are consistent with what is seen clinically. The peroneus quartus is an accessory muscle that most often arises from the Peroneus brevis and has shown an association with lateral ankle pathology. Bilgili et al. performed a cadaveric study showing a prevalence of 5.2% and a statistically significant association with the presence of a peroneus quartus and peroneal brevis degeneration [7]. The os peroneum is another pain generator that surgeons should be aware of. Studies have demonstrated a prevalence of an os peroneum in 4–30% of the population [8]. Stockton et al. reviewed 12 cases of patients with symptomatic os peroneum. Eight had peroneus longus tears associated with fractures of the os peroneum, while the remaining four had an enlarged and entrapped os peroneum that was preventing full excursion of the peroneus longus. Nine of the patients had partial tears of the Peroneus brevis [9].

History and Exam

Patients may report a history of recurrent ankle sprains, lateral ankle pain, swelling, and/or instability. On exam, common findings are lateral tenderness, lateral swelling, weakness with eversion, and pain with passive hindfoot range of motion.

On exam, several key findings may help guide the surgeon with both evaluation, as well as future treatment options. Integrity of the flexor hallucis longus (FHL) with manual muscle strength testing is important, as it sometimes used for tendon transfer and reconstruction purposes. Lower extremity alignment should also be a major focus, as a fixed hindfoot varus deformity may need to be addressed in order to prevent repair or reconstruction failure. Anterior drawer testing should be performed to evaluate the integrity of the anterior talofibular ligament (ATFL) and CFL, as ligament reconstruction at the time of the reconstruction may be needed if instability is present. Peroneal tunnel compression testing may be beneficial for evaluation of peroneal brevis tears [10].

Imaging/Studies

Weightbearing foot and ankle X-rays should be obtained to evaluate for fracture, degenerative disease, nonunion, and hindfoot alignment. Some cases may warrant plain film knee imaging if there is concern for knee misalignment. Computed tomography (CT) imaging is generally not beneficial, unless there is concern for further evaluation of degenerative pathology or alignment issues. Ultrasonography (US) imaging has the benefit of being noninvasive and can evaluate the peroneal tendon integrity. Studies have shown that it can identify peroneal tendon tears with 90–100% accuracy, 100% sensitivity, and 85–100% specificity but is limited by operator experience and familiarity [11]. Magnetic resonance imaging (MRI) is often the most common second-line imaging modality. Common findings are tendon thickening, sheath fluid, fissuring, stenosis, and/or scarring. Newer studies have used MRI to evaluate the amount of fatty infiltration in the peroneal muscle bellies for predicting tears. Res et al. retrospectively looked at 30 patients with confirmed MRI findings of peroneal brevis tears compared to 30 patients with MRI findings of no peroneal brevis tears and compared the amount of fatty infiltration using the Goutallier classification. The study group demonstrated statistically significant higher Goutallier grading compared to the control group, leading them to believe that MRI may be beneficial to evaluate the more proximal muscle substance in order to predict severity of tear [12]. Surgeons should also be aware of the magic angle phenomenon, as the tendons take a curvilinear course around the distal fibula, which may misrepresent normal tendon tissue as pathologic [13].

Differential

The surgeon should be aware of other causes of lateral ankle pain and instability. These include, but are not limited to, fracture (fibula, lateral process of talus, cuboid, fifth metatarsal, anterior process of the calcaneus), ligamentous injury (ATFL/CFL), subtalar sprain, syndesmotic injury, impingement lesions, osteochondral lesions, tarsal coalition, sinus tarsi syndrome, calcaneocuboid syndrome, neuritis, accessory muscle/bone, and degenerative joint disease.

Allograft Use in Orthopedics

According to the American Association of Tissue Banks, musculoskeletal grafts make up the largest component of all tissue grafts distributed in the United States, at 71% in 2015 [14]. Allograft reconstruction allows the surgeon to address length/size deficits encountered in surgery while avoiding further surgery, additional surgical incisions, and/or donor site morbidity. This allows for shorter surgical times and has a lower likelihood to limit the function of donor or local tendons [15].

Along with the known benefits of allograft utilization, surgeons need to be aware that there may be concerns with their use. Transmission of disease, although low, is often a concern expressed by patients. In 2005, the Centers for Disease Control and Prevention (CDC) reported an allograft tissue infection incidence of 0.0004% over a 5-year period, based on estimates of 900,000 allografts per year [16]. In 2011, a report published by Project NOTIFY, led by the World Health Organization, stated that there were no reported cases of viral contamination for musculoskeletal tissues over an 11-year period due to improved quality and reliability of testing [17]. Bacterial contamination, on the other hand, is more commonly seen with allograft transplant, although the incidence is still low. In 2002, the CDC reported on 650,000 musculoskeletal allografts. Only 26 recipients were found to have bacterial infection due to the graft [18]. A recent study by Yu et al. looked at contamination rates of patients undergoing anterior cruciate ligament (ACL) reconstruction with both processed and nonprocessed allografts. Analyzing over 10,000 patients, they reported a deep infection rate of only 0.15% [19]. Other issues to be aware of when utilizing musculoskeletal allograft are cost, as well as availability. Surgeons should check with their respective surgical centers prior to surgery, in regard to the type and condition of their available allografts.

Operative Technique

Positioning and Limb Preparation

Lateral decubitus, modified lateral, or supine positioning may be utilized depending on surgeon preference. A bean bag support or towel bumps may be needed to help with positioning. Administer preoperative antibiotics. Apply pneumatic tourniquet around mid-thigh. Perform preferred skin preparation and draping of surgical site. Elevate the operative limb, use an esmarch bandage for exsanguination, and then inflate tourniquet.

Surgical Approach

Make a longitudinal surgical incision over the course of the peroneal tendons, starting approximately 1 cm posterior and 1 cm proximal to the distal tip of the fibula and extending down to the base of the fifth metatarsal. The surgeon should utilize caution with this approach, specifically in regard to the presence of the lesser saphenous vein and sural nerve. These are often identified subcutaneously in the distal portion of the wound, just posterior to the incision.

Examination and Debridement of the Peroneal Tendons

Next, use blunt dissection to locate the peroneal tendon sheath (Fig. 18.1). Open the sheath carefully using a scalpel blade and then complete the process using Metzenbaum scissors. Proximally, the sheath should be opened to the level of the musculotendinous junction. Distally, the sheath should be opened to the level of the remaining tendon stump or the fifth metatarsal base. This will be based on the site of allograft fixation later in the procedure (Fig. 18.2). Once the tendon ends have been identified, free up any surrounding tissue and debride the ends back to healthy tendinous tissue. During this step, it is important to examine for any other potential pathological processes that may prohibit healing and future function, such as an accessory peroneal muscle, tenosynovitis, crowding within the fibular groove, and the status of the superior peroneal retinaculum (Fig. 18.3).

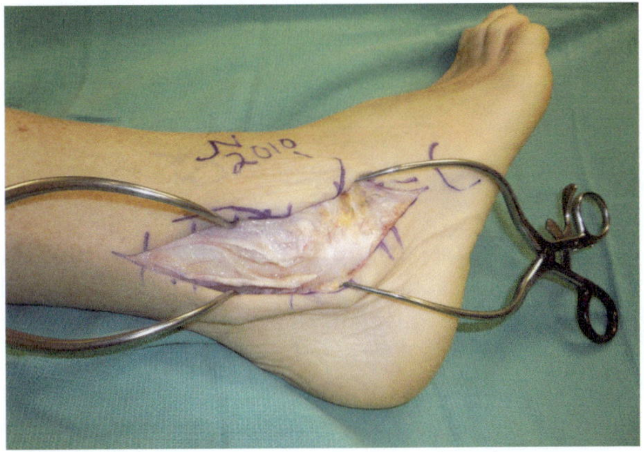

Fig. 18.1 Lateral exposure of the entire peroneal tendon sheath from musculotendinous junction to cuboid tunnel

Fig. 18.2 Shredded peroneus longus and brevis tendon

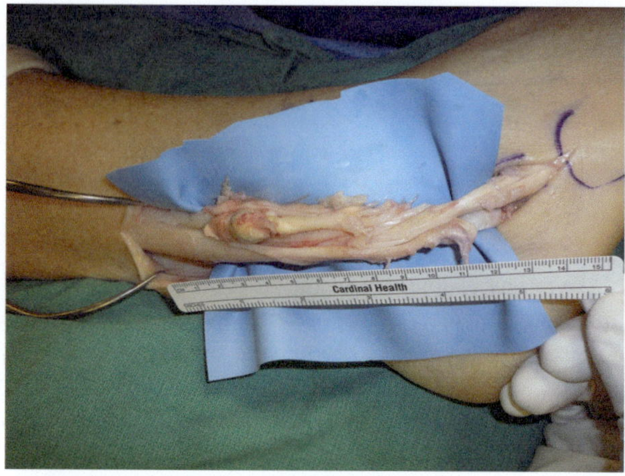

Fig. 18.3 Excision of degenerative tendon distally with shredded proximal tendons

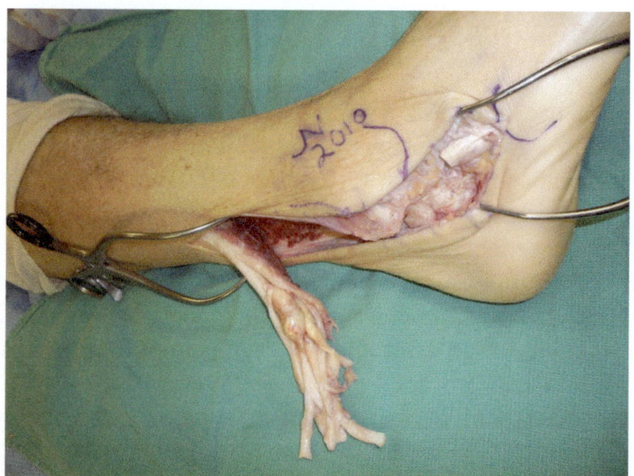

Measuring the Defect and Preparing Allograft

Measure the tendon defect length and select an appropriately sized frozen peroneal tendon allograft or semitendinosus allograft to thaw (Fig. 18.4).

Distal Allograft Fixation

Most often, we find that there is enough distal tendon stump that remains attached to the fifth metatarsal base [20]. Secure the distal portion of the allograft to the remaining stump using a Pulvertaft weave with a braided, nonabsorbable suture (Fig. 18.5). If there is not enough native distal stump remaining for reattachment, you may use suture anchor fixation by preparing a bleeding bone bed at the anatomic footprint of the fifth metatarsal base and attaching the graft via a 3.5-mm suture anchor.

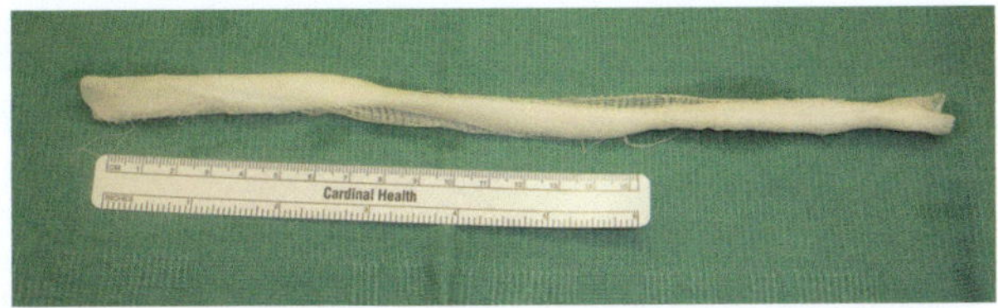

Fig. 18.4 Peroneus longus allograft

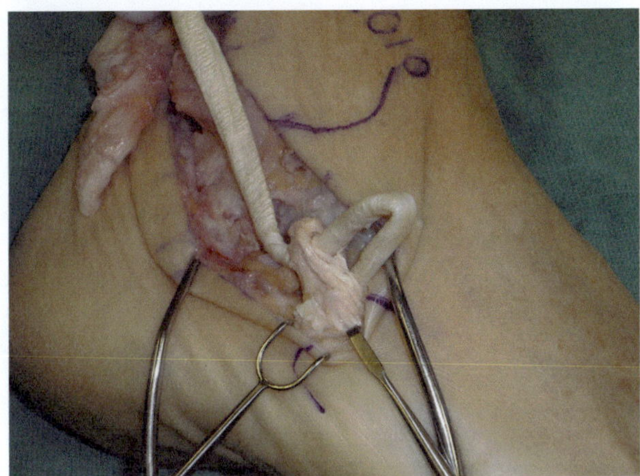

Fig. 18.5 Weaving of allograft into distal Peroneus brevis tendon stump

Proximal Allograft Fixation

Before securing the allograft proximally, it is important to approximate the muscle-tendon unit tension. This is best achieved by placing the foot in neutral inversion/eversion, as well as neutral dorsiflexion. Next, grasp the proximal muscle stump and gently pull it distally. Take note of the amount of excursion achieved during this step. When setting the final allograft length, you want it to be approximately 50% of this excursion length. Hold the proximal native tendon at this length (50% of full excursion) and secure the proximal allograft in a similar fashion as before, using a Pulvertaft weave with braided, nonabsorbable suture (Figs. 18.6, 18.7, and 18.8).

Closure

Close the peroneal tendon sheath using braided, absorbable suture (Fig. 18.9). If there is insufficiency of the superior peroneal retinaculum, we make an attempt at soft tissue mobilization over the tendons, often a combination of remaining retinaculum and periosteum. We then secure this reconstruction with suture anchors. Sometimes, this is not possible and a variety of other options have been described in the literature, including but not limited to, local tendon graft and autograft

A. E. Hanselman and J. A. Nunley

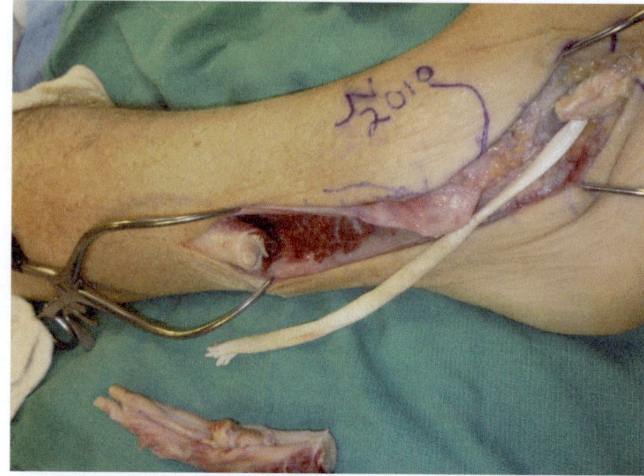

Fig. 18.6 Allograft in retrofibular groove preparing for pulvertaft weave into proximal peroneal tendon and muscle

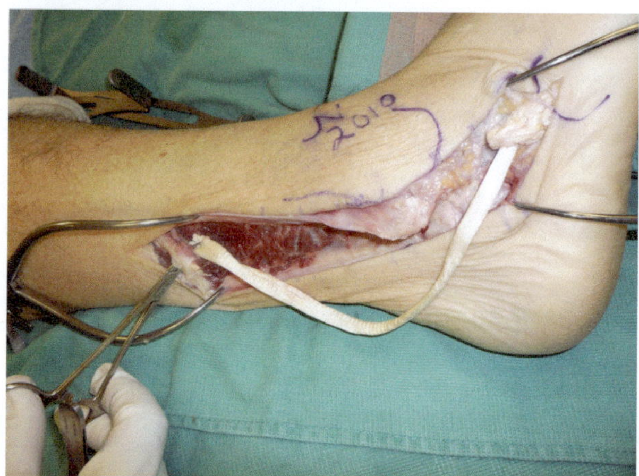

Fig. 18.7 Pulvertaft weave into proximal peroneal muscle

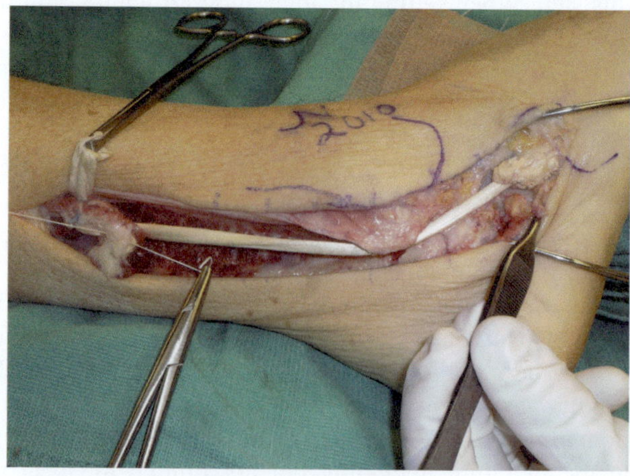

Fig. 18.8 Suturing the tendon and allograft together at correct tension

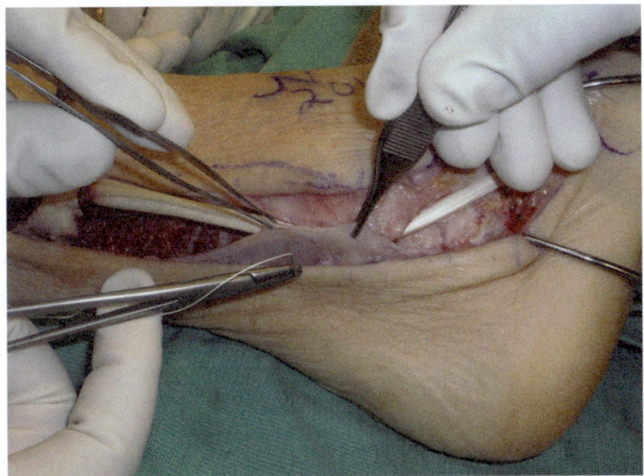

Fig. 18.9 Allograft in position and closure of the superior peroneal retinaculum

reconstruction. In this instance, some surgeons may prefer a groove deepening procedure to help maintain the reduction of the peroneals within the retrofibular groove. Again, various techniques have been described in the literature. Our two most common techniques are the "trap door" technique and the "retrograde drilling" technique. With the "trap door", we make a small cortical window in the posterior fibula, hinge open the cortex, remove underlying cancellous bone, and then gently tamp the cortical window back down into place. With the "retrograde drilling" technique, we run a 2.0mm drill bit, starting at the distal tip of the fibula, just below the posterior fibular cortical surface. Using fluoroscopy, we subsequently increase drill diameters until an adequate amount of underlying cortex is removed. We then gently tamp down the posterior cortex, thus deepening the groove. At this point, close the remaining wound in layers over a drain. Apply a sterile dressing and bulky splint.

Postoperative Care

Our normal postoperative course involves suture removal at approximately 2 weeks postop. If there are concerns about wound healing, sutures may be left in place longer. We then apply a non-weightbearing short leg fiberglass cast. At 4 weeks postop, we remove the cast and start to progress the patient to full weightbearing in a controlled ankle motion boot. Patients are allowed to remove the boot for hygiene and range of motion (dorsiflexion/plantarflexion only). We still limit inversion/eversion at this point. At 6 weeks postop, we transition the patient out of the boot and into an Aircast stirrup (DJO, Vista, Ca). At this point, they are also allowed to start working on inversion/eversion range of motion. At 12 weeks postop, the patient is enrolled into a physical therapy-guided strengthening program and transitioned to unprotected shoe wear.

Outcomes

A retrospective case series by Mook et al. evaluated 14 patients undergoing peroneal tendon allograft reconstruction with a mean follow-up of 17 months showing improvements in both clinical and physical exam findings. Average Short Form-12 (SF-12) Physical Health Survey score improved to 48.8, average Lower Extremity Functional Scores (LEFS) improved to 86.4, and average Visual Analog Scale (VAS) decreased. Average postoperative eversion strength was 4.8/5 (MRC grading) with 9/14 patients achieving full 5/5 strength. All patients returned to their preinjury activity levels [20].

Nunley et al. performed a cadaveric study comparing Peroneus brevis to peroneus longus tenodesis versus allograft reconstruction for isolated Peroneus brevis tears. Using normal cadaveric feet with intact tendons as a control, allograft reconstruction demonstrated statistically significantly better tension restoration compared to tenodesis at a variety of physiological loads (both 50% and 100%) and at a variety of foot positions (inversion/eversion and plantarflexion/dorsiflexion) [21].

Complications

The most common complications unique to this type of surgical reconstruction are wound healing issues, sural nerve injury, and lack of adequate allograft tensioning. In their retrospective study, Mook et al. had no postoperative wound healing complications, infections, tendon reruptures, or reoperations. Four patients had sural nerve sensory numbness, two of them were transient [20].

References

1. Brodsky JW, Zide JR, Kane JM. Acute peroneal injury. [cited 2018 Sep 15]; Available from: https://doi.org/10.1016/j.fcl.2017.07.013.
2. Dombek MF, Lamm BM, Saltrick K, Mendicino RW, Catanzariti AR. Peroneal tendon tears: a retrospective review. J Foot Ankle Surg [Internet]. [cited 2018 Sep 16];42(5):250–8. Available from: http://www.ncbi.nlm.nih.gov/pubmed/14566716.
3. Petersen W, Bobka T, Stein V, Tillmann B. Blood supply of the peroneal tendons: Injection and immunohistochemical studies of cadaver tendons. Acta Orthop Scand [Internet]. 2000 [cited 2018 Sep 15];71(2):168–74. Available from: http://www.ncbi.nlm.nih.gov/pubmed/10852323.
4. Lamm BM, Myers DT, Dombek M, Mendicino RW, Catanzariti AR, Saltrick K. Magnetic resonance imaging and surgical correlation of peroneus brevis tears. J Foot Ankle Surg [Internet]. 2004 [cited 2018 Sep 16];43(1):30–6. Available from: http://linkinghub.elsevier.com/retrieve/pii/S1067251603004186.
5. Mirmiran R, Squire C, Wassell D. Prevalence and role of a low-lying peroneus Brevis uscle belly in patients with peroneal tendon pathologic features: a potential source of tendon subluxation. J Foot Ankle Surg [Internet]. 2015 [cited 2018 Sep 15];54(5):872–5. Available from: http://www.ncbi.nlm.nih.gov/pubmed/25998478.
6. Housley SN, Lewis JE, Thompson DL, Warren G. A proximal fibularis brevis muscle is associated with longitudinal split tendons: a cadaveric study. J Foot Ankle Surg [Internet]. 2017 [cited 2018 Sep 16];56(1):34–6. Available from: http://www.ncbi.nlm.nih.gov/pubmed/27989344.

7. Gökhan Bilgili M, Kaynak G, Botanlıog H, Serdar ·, Basaran H. Peroneus quartus: prevalance and clinical importance. Arch Orthop Trauma Surg [Internet]. 2014 [cited 2018 Sep 16];134:481–7. Available from: https//link-springer-com.proxy.lib.duke.edu/content/pdf/10.1007%2Fs00402-014-1937-4.pdf.

8. Sobel M, Pavlov H, Geppert MJ, Thompson FM, DiCarlo EF, Davis WH. Painful Os peroneum syndrome: a spectrum of conditions responsible for plantar lateral foot pain. Foot Ankle Int [Internet]. 1994 [cited 2018 Sep 16];15(3):112–24. Available from: http://journals.sagepub.com/doi/10.1177/107110079401500306.

9. Stockton KG, Brodsky JW. Peroneus Longus Tears Associated With Pathology of the Os Peroneum. Foot Ankle Int [Internet]. 2014 [cited 2018 Sep 16];35(4):346–52. Available from: http://journals.sagepub.com/doi/10.1177/1071100714522026.

10. Sobel M, Geppert MJ, Olson EJ, O Bohne WH, Arnoczky SP. The dynamics of peroneus brevis tendon splits: a proposed mechanism technique of diagnosis, and classification of injury [Internet]. 1992 [cited 2018 Sep 9]. Available from: http://journals.sagepub.com.proxy.lib.duke.edu/doi/pdf/10.1177/107110079201300710.

11. Molini L, Bianchi S. US in peroneal tendon tear. J Ultrasound [Internet]. 2014 [cited 2018 Sep 14];17(2):125–34. Available from: http://www.ncbi.nlm.nih.gov/pubmed/24883136.

12. Res LCS, Dixon T, Lubberts B, Vicentini JRT, van Dijk PA, Hosseini A, et al. Peroneal Tendon Tears. J Am Acad Orthop Surg [Internet]. 2018 [cited 2018 Sep 15];1. Available from: http://www.ncbi.nlm.nih.gov/pubmed/30138295.

13. Wang X-T, Rosenberg ZS, Mechlin MB, Schweitzer ME. Normal variants and diseases of the peroneal tendons and superior peroneal retinaculum: MR imaging features. RadioGraphics [Internet]. 2005 [cited 2018 Sep 16];25(3):587–602. Available from: http://www.ncbi.nlm.nih.gov/pubmed/15888611.

14. Working Together for Life [Internet]. [cited 2018 Sep 14]. Available from: https://www.aatb.org/sites/default/files/sites/default/files/private/AATB2017AnnualReport.pdf.

15. Xu X, Hu M, Liu J, Zhu Y, Wang B. Minimally invasive reconstruction of the lateral ankle ligaments using semitendinosus autograft or tendon allograft. Foot Ankle Int [Internet]. 2014 [cited 2018 Sep 14];35(10):1015–21. Available from: http://journals.sagepub.com/doi/10.1177/1071100714540145.

16. CEnters for Disease Control and Prevention, Food and Drug Administration, and Health Resources and Services Administration, Department of Health and Human Services convene the Workshop on Preventing Organ and Tissue Allograft-Transmitted Infection: Priori [Internet]. [cited 2018 Sep 14]. Available from: https://www.cdc.gov/transplantsafety/pdfs/BOOTS-Workshop-2005-final-report.pdf.

17. Hinsenkamp M, Muylle L, Eastlund T, Fehily D, Noël L, Strong DM. Adverse reactions and events related to musculoskeletal allografts: reviewed by the World Health Organisation Project NOTIFY. Int Orthop [Internet]. 2012 [cited 2018 Sep 14];36(3):633–41. Available from: http://link.springer.com/10.1007/s00264-011-1391-7.

18. Centers for Disease Control and Prevention (CDC). Update: allograft-associated bacterial infections--United States, 2002. MMWR Morb Mortal Wkly Rep [Internet]. 2002 [cited 2018 Sep 16];51(10):207–10. Available from: http://www.ncbi.nlm.nih.gov/pubmed/11922189.

19. Yu A, Prentice HA, Burfeind WE, Funahashi T, Maletis GB. Risk of infection after allograft anterior cruciate ligament reconstruction: are nonprocessed allografts more likely to get infected? A cohort study of over 10,000 allografts. Am J Sports Med [Internet]. 2018 [cited 2018 Sep 16];46(4):846–51. Available from: http://www.ncbi.nlm.nih.gov/pubmed/29298084.

20. Mook WR, Parekh SG, Nunley JA. Allograft reconstruction of peroneal tendons: operative technique and clinical outcomes. Foot Ankle Int [Internet]. [cited 2018 Sep 3];34(9):1212–20. Available from: http://journals.sagepub.com.proxy.lib.duke.edu/doi/pdf/10.1177/1071100713487527.

21. 2016 IFFAS Award for Excellence Winner. [cited 2018. Sep 9]; Available from: http://journals.sagepub.com.proxy.lib.duke.edu/doi/pdf/10.1177/1071100716658469.

Attritional Rupture of Peroneus Brevis and Peroneus Longus Tendons: Flexor Digitorum Longus Transfer

19

Nick Casscells, Tom Sherman, and Lew Schon

Introduction

Peroneal tendinopathy is a well-recognized source of lateral ankle pain and dysfunction [1–3]. Injury to both tendons invariably leads to loss of normal function. Impaired peroneal function results in a mechanical imbalance of the foot and ankle. Symptoms related to peroneal tendon dysfunction due to attritional ruptures are likely to include hindfoot and ankle instability, which manifests as complaints of lateral ankle pain, difficulty traversing uneven terrain, and recurrent ankle sprains.

Most typically, injury to the peroneals is due to extrinsic, repetitive mechanical insult. To this end, Basset and Spear reported their findings of peroneus brevis tears in a cohort of patients undergoing lateral ankle ligament reconstruction. The authors hypothesized that the tears occurred due to repetitive impingement of the peroneus brevis on the fibular groove due to excessive anteriorly directed pressure applied by the peroneus longus. They reported that when the foot was specifically positioned in 15 to 25 degrees of plantarflexion, the tendons were at greatest risk for injury due to the peroneus brevis becoming draped over the posterior ridge of the fibula that defines the peroneal groove [1]. Likewise, others have demonstrated that pressure increases between the peroneal tendons and fibula groove in certain ankle positions [4]. It is possible, that with repetitive loading, the resultant increased pressure causes attritional wear to the tendons. In support of this theory, Sobel and colleagues [5] reported their findings of a cadaveric study that found longitudinal split tears of the peroneus brevis reliably corresponded to the area of the distal aspect of the posterior fibular groove. Concomitant injury to the peroneus longus seemed to result from

N. Casscells (✉)
Medstar Georgetown University Hospital, Washington, DC, USA

T. Sherman
Orthopedic Associate of Lancaster, Lancaster, PA, USA

L. Schon
Mercy Medical Center, Baltimore, MD, USA

impingement of the longus tendon against the distal fibula through the split tear of the peroneus brevis tendon.

Given that it is the repetitive impingement of the tendons against the fibular groove that propagates attritional injury, it stands to reason that certain concomitant anatomic and mechanical factors may exacerbate this process. For instance, some have proposed that a low-lying muscle belly of the peroneus brevis inherently increases pressure in the region of the fibular groove, as the volume of this area is relatively constant by virtue of the rigid fibula and relatively stout peroneal retinaculum in the same area [6, 7]. However, this concept remains a controversial one, as others have challenged this theory, finding no association between the distal extent of the muscle and the presence of tears [8, 9]. Similarly, the presence of a peroneus quartus has been espoused as a contributing factor in the development of attritional injury to the tendons. The mechanism by which this occurs has been suggested to result from relative hypertrophy of the peroneal tubercle, where the quartus typically inserts, thus causing increased pressure and mechanical irritation to the brevis and longus tendons [9]. Redundancy of the peroneal superior retinaculum may also precipitate attritional injury to the peroneal tendons by allowing the tendon's greater excursion over the bony ridge of the fibula that defines the fibular groove [3].

Histologic analysis of the peroneal tendon tears has revealed fibroblastic and vascular proliferation in the areas of the tear with thickening of the peritenon and tenosynovium, but little evidence of inflammation [10]. The authors concluded that the tears were the result of a repetitive mechanical injury rather than chronic inflammation or avascular atrophy. However, Petersen and colleagues reported the presence of heterogeneity in the vascularity of the peroneal tendons based on their study, in which they characterized the blood supply to the tendons using injection and immunohistochemical techniques. The authors reported a nearly avascular zone in the intratendinous bloody supply of the peroneus brevis as it traverses the fibula groove, the same area where tears are typically located. They also reported relative avascularity in the peroneus longus in the region of the peroneal tubercle and at the level of the cuboid [11].

Thus, it is the authors' belief that attritional injury to the peroneal tendons is most typically due a repetitive mechanical mechanism. In the case of peroneus brevis tears, it is repetitive pressure conferred by the posterior bony ridge of the fibula that causes tear propagation (Fig. 19.1).

Factors such as low-lying muscle belly, attenuated retinaculum, a cavus foot posture, and/or shallow fibular groove likely contribute to attritional wear. As tears become more extensive, the peroneus longus, which lies posterior to the brevis, will also impinge on the fibula resulting in longitudinal split tears. Peroneus longus pathology may also result from impingement at the peroneal tubercle or from an accessory os peroneum at the level of the cuboid bone [12]. Relative avascularity of tendons in these regions impedes their healing potential, resulting in the tendency for tears to become chronic. It should be noted as well, that other extrinsic factors have been hypothesized to confer risk to chronic tendon pathology or rupture, such as inflammatory arthropathies (gout, rheumatoid arthritis, and psoriatic arthritis), diabetes, hyperparathyroidism, and local steroid injections to the tendons [13–15].

The surgical management of peroneal tendon dysfunction is dictated by multiple factors including the size, location, and severity of the tears, as well as which tendon

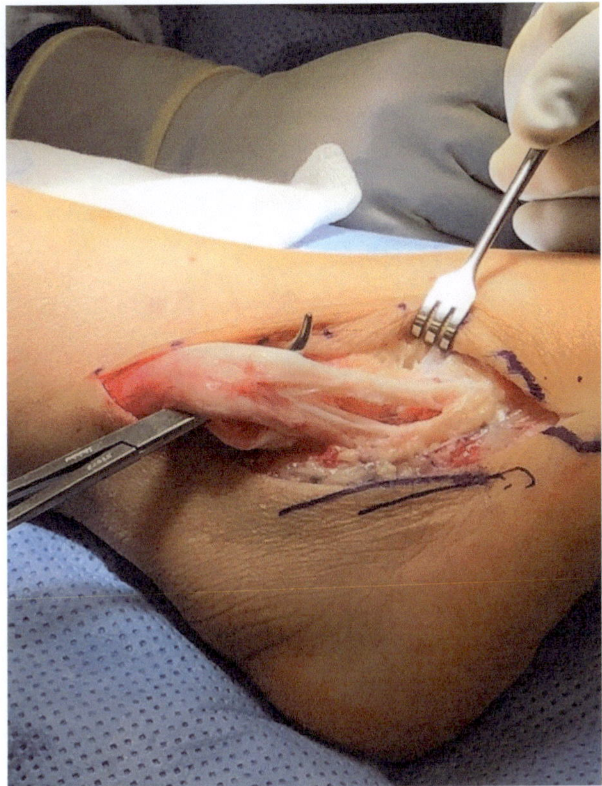

Fig. 19.1 Intraoperative photograph demonstrating significant thickening of the peroneus brevis tendon proximally (left) and a large split tear of the peroneus brevis at the level of the distal fibula

or tendons are involved. Maintaining and restoring normal anatomy is the most preferable option when possible in cases in which both the peroneus brevis and longus tendons are pathologic [16]. However, debridement and repair are not a feasible option when there is extensive involvement of both tendons, such as with fibrosis and complex tears, involving more than 50% of the cross-sectional areas of the tendons. Options of surgical management of extensive tendinopathy involving both the peroneus brevis and longus tendons, to the extent that they are functionally disabled, are limited (Fig. 19.2).

In such situations, the tendon that is not reconstructable may be tenodesed to a repaired portion of the other tendon. This technique, however, creates a nonanatomic tendon configuration, and there is a dearth of literature detailing its outcomes. Others have advocated for tendon allograft reconstruction in cases in which the tendons cannot be salvaged; however, the success of this technique may be compromised when there has been prolonged scarring of the peroneal tendons, which may render the respective muscles atrophic and contracted [17]. In such situations, the tendons' respective muscle bellies may undergo significant degeneration rendering them unamenable to tendon allograft reconstruction. Fatty degeneration of the respective muscle bellies can be visualized on MRI T1 imaging, and is useful for surgical planning purposes (Fig. 19.3). Peroneal dysfunctions as a result of neurologic etiology, such as a proximal superficial peroneal nerve lesion, common

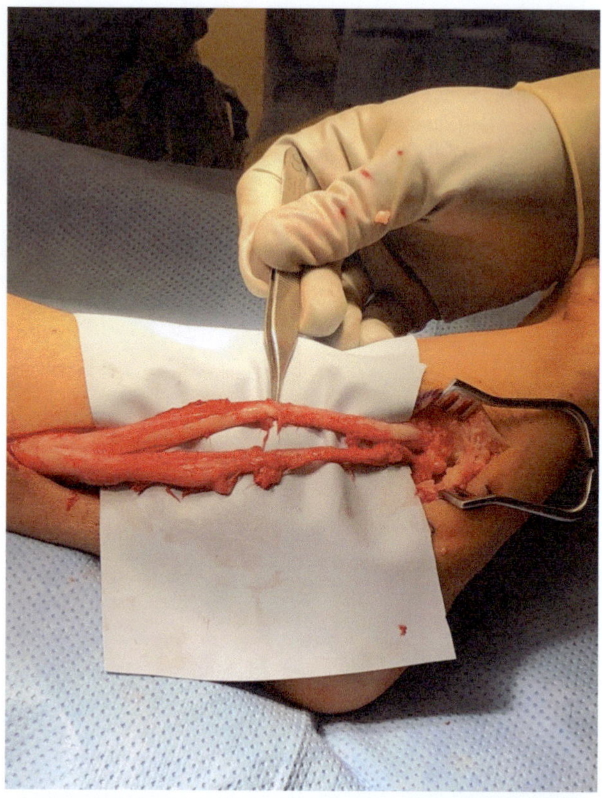

Fig. 19.2 Intraoperative photograph of the peroneus longus and brevis tendons with marked thickening, fibrosis, and split tears of both tendons

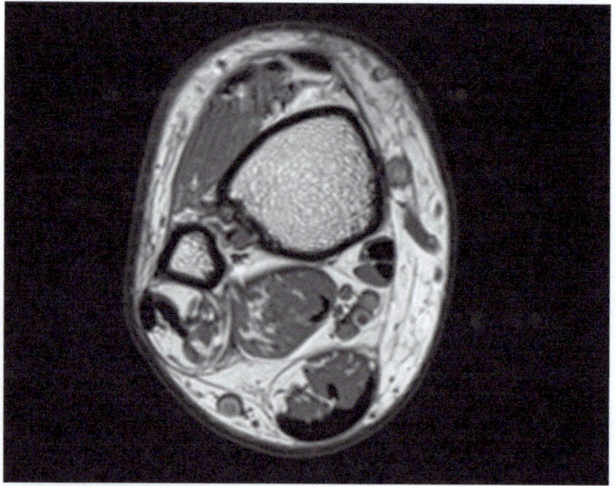

Fig. 19.3 Axial T1 weighted images above the level of the ankle demonstrating significant fatty atrophy of the peroneal muscles

peroneal nerve lesion, or hereditary peripheral neuropathy such as Charcot–Marie–Tooth are also contraindications to allograft reconstruction.

A viable surgical option for the management of severe tendon disease of both the peroneus brevis and the peroneus longus is lateral transfer of the flexor digitorum longus (FDL) or flexor hallucis longus (FHL) to the lateral foot, most typically the fifth metatarsal base [2, 18–20]. The FDL has a similar excursion distance and work percentage to that of the peroneus brevis, making it a reasonable option for transfer [21]. The first description of the FDL to the lateral foot for the management of unrepairable peroneal tendinopathy was provided by Borton and colleagues, in which two patients with transverse tears of both peroneal tendons were managed with FDL transfer to the lateral foot [2]. At final follow-up for each patient, 6 and 8 years, respectively, the authors reported that each patient was asymptomatic and had excellent restoration of near normal function and were able to return to playing competitive golf [2]. Jockel and Brodsky reported the results of eight patients in whom either the FHL or FDL tendon was transferred to the lateral foot for nonreconstructable tears of both the peroneus brevis and peroneus longus tendons. At a mean follow-up of 58 months, all patients had improved AOFAS hindfoot scores, less pain, and expressed overall satisfaction with their treatment [18]. Subsequently, Redfern and Myerson further defined the utility of tendon transfer for peroneal tendinopathy (2004). They advocated for lateral tendon transfer in situations in which both peroneal tendons were diseased with no muscle belly excursion proximally, or in situations where there was significant tendon bed scarring. Four patients in their cohort of 28 patients underwent an FDL tendon transfer, and the authors reported improvement in AOFAS scores in each patient [19].

Seybold and colleagues reported their outcomes of nine patients who underwent lateral transfer of either the FHL or FDL tendon for concomitant peroneus brevis and peroneus longus tears. Five patients underwent transfer of the FHL tendon and four underwent transfer of the FDL tendon using disparate fixation techniques; eight of nine patients had additional procedures to correct underlying pathologic posture of the foot contributing to tendinopathy. The outcomes of eight of the nine patients included assessment by the short-form (SF-12) and foot function index (FFI), while seven also returned for range of motion assessment, balance tests, and power evaluation at a mean follow-up of 35.7 months. The authors reported that all patients were satisfied. The authors did note three instances of sural neuritis and two of tibial neuritis, the latter of which they hypothesized was due to transfer of the tendon posterior to the neuromuscular bundle [20].

In a retrospective analysis of 15 of our own patients from 2009 to 2015 with 53.7 months mean follow-up and who underwent FDL transfer to the base of the fifth metatarsal, 76.5% of the patients were "very satisfied." Compared to preoperative function, there were no additional self-reported limitations following surgery and only four patients endorsed intermittent use of an ankle support brace postoperatively. Eight patients (53.3%) had on average a 58% reduction in their eversion motion arc compared to the nonoperative side. Nine patients (60%) showed an average loss of 28% of inversion arc of motion compared to the nonoperative side. Both isometric peak torque and isotonic peak velocity were decreased by 38.4% and 28.8%, respectively, compared to the nonoperative side. On average, power in the operative limb was diminished by 56%. These results are consistent with those of Seybold et al. [20]. All patients were able to return to their desired activities and had significant reduction in their pain level as measured by preoperative and postoperative Visual Analogue Scale (VAS) scores. Additional clinical assessment provided by the Foot and Ankle Ability Measure (FAAM), Foot Function Index (FFI), and

Short Musculoskeletal Function Assessment (SMFA) demonstrated favorable scores regarding pain and disability postoperatively. There was one complication in this series, which was a wound infection that resolved without long-term sequelae. There were no instances of tibial nerve injury.

The indications for a flexor digitorum transfer are largely based on surgical assessment of the peroneal tendons. A lateral foot FDL tendon transfer is appropriate for management of tears involving greater than 50% of the cross-sectional areas of both the peroneus brevis and longus tendons of previously failed peroneal tendon surgical procedures, extensive scarring of the peroneal tendons to the peroneal sheath, and scarring or fibrosis of the peroneal muscle bellies.

Technique

The patient is generally positioned with a large bump under the ipsilateral hip so as to internally rotate the operative limb or alternatively in the lateral decubitus position. The surgery may be performed with or without the use of tourniquet.

The peroneal tendons are exposed using a convex posterior curvilinear incision over the peroneal tendons. If previous peroneal tendon surgery has been performed, the previous incision is used. Exposure should be extensive enough to fully debride or excise the diseased tendons. The peroneal muscle bellies should be assessed for scarring and fibrosis by pulling tension on the musculotendinous unit. There should be "springiness" or a natural recoil when tension is released. If the muscle is completely fibrosed, there will be little or no excursion or recoil of both tendons and an allograft reconstruction or tenodesis is of little utility (Fig. 19.4).

Underlying hindfoot varus positioning should be corrected simultaneously, as failure to do so will result in increased tension of the transferred tendon and compromise its durability. These procedures should be completed prior to the tendon transfer so as to allow for appropriate tensioning of the transferred tendon and mitigate injury to it. Consideration should be given to a lateralizing calcaneal tuberosity osteotomy with or without a lateral closing wedge component. This may be performed through the same incision or with a separate incision more posteriorly (Fig. 19.5).

The lateral tuberosity of the calcaneus is exposed via an oblique incision just posterior to the sural nerve. An oscillating saw is used to perform a lateral to medial osteotomy. Care is taken to avoid overpenetration of the medial cortex so as to mitigate risk to the neurovascular bundle. Constant irrigation is used to mitigate thermal necrosis. Consideration may also be given to a minimally invasive technique using a speed-limiting burr [22]. Removal of laterally based wedge is based upon surgeon preference, but is typically 5–10 mm in width. A lamina spreader is useful to distract the osteotomy site and facilitate lateral translation through relaxation of the soft tissue. The tuberosity fragment is translated laterally and compressed against the body of the calcaneus to restore a neutral conformity (Fig. 19.6). The foot should be dorsiflexed to assist with compression of the osteotomy and closure of any resected wedge. Additional compression and fixation is achieved with one or two cannulated partially threaded screws oriented perpendicular to the osteotomy.

Fig. 19.4 Example of peroneus brevis lacking "springiness" in the muscle belly

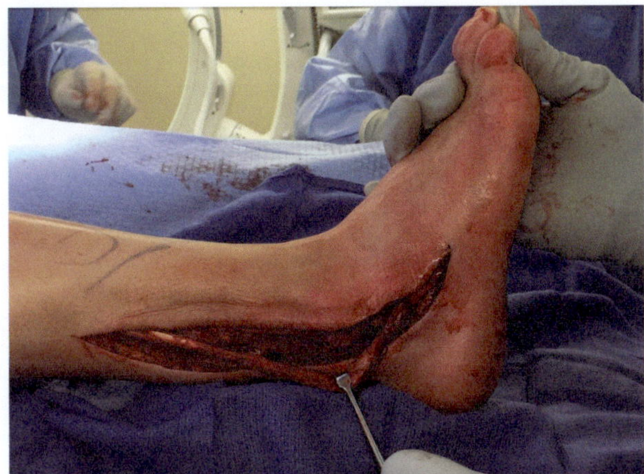

Fig. 19.5 Intraoperative photograph demonstrating a 5-mm lateral closing wedge osteotomy made through a separate incision posterior to that used to approach the peroneal tendons

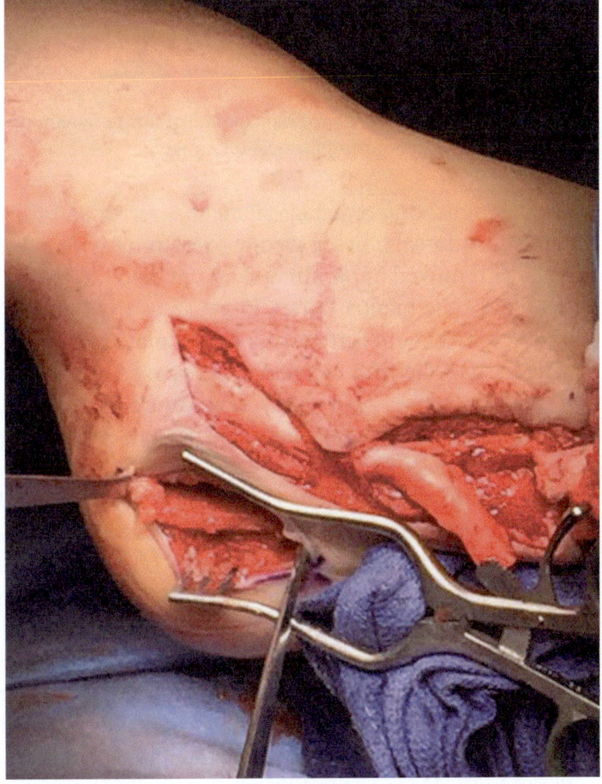

A dorsiflexion closing wedge osteotomy of the first metatarsal may also be necessary to correct forefoot-driven varus. This is determined based upon preoperative Coleman block test and can be confirmed intraoperatively. This is approached through a dorsal incision based over the proximal first metatarsal. The extensor

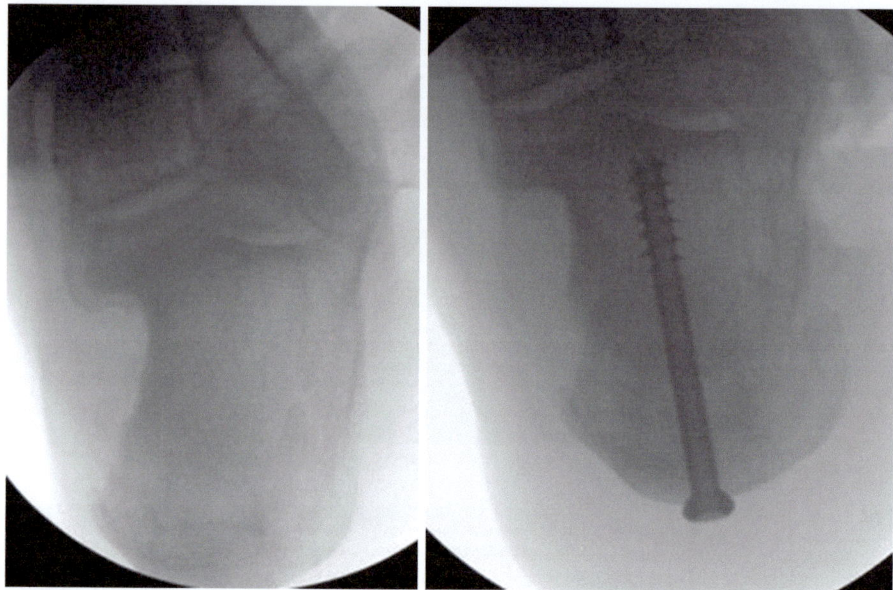

Fig. 19.6 Intraoperative fluoroscopy demonstrating preoperative hindfoot varus of the calcaneus and lateral translation of the calcaneal tuberosity

hallucis longus, dorsomedial cutaneous nerve, and tibialis anterior tendon must be protected. A dorsal closing wedge osteotomy with a 3–5 mm dorsally based wedge of bone is removed approximately 1 cm distal to the first tarsometatarsal joint with care to leave the plantar cortex intact so as to hinge closed the osteotomy. Fixation can be achieved with screws or a dorsal plate.

The base of the fifth metatarsal is exposed at the insertion of the peroneus brevis to permit insertion of a corkscrew suture anchor deep into metaphyseal bone. Intraoperative fluoroscopy should be used to ensure proper placement of the anchor (Figs. 19.7 and 19.8).

Harvesting of the FDL or FHL tendon is facilitated by removal of the bean bag or ipsilateral bump so as to externally rotate the limb and expose the medial foot. The FDL tendon can be harvested either plantarly or medially.

In the plantar approach, an incision is made in line with the plantar crease obliquely from proximal medial to distal lateral. Blunt dissection is made down to the plantar fascia (Fig. 19.9).

The plantar fascia is then incised in line with its fibers. The muscle belly of the Flexor Digitorum Brevis (FDB) is exposed and retracted medially. The medial plantar nerve may also be encountered and should be protected and retracted medially with the FDB. Deep to the FDB muscle belly lies the decussation of FDL and FHL (Fig. 19.10).

The FDL is confirmed through simultaneous flexion and extension of the lesser toes. The tendon should be tagged with a suture before the FDL is ligated as the tendon can retract proximally out of view once cut (Fig. 19.11).

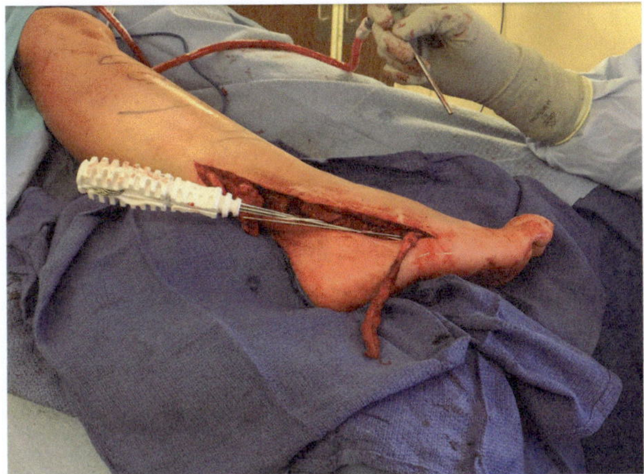

Fig. 19.7 Clinical photograph of corkscrew anchor placement at the base of the fifth metatarsal

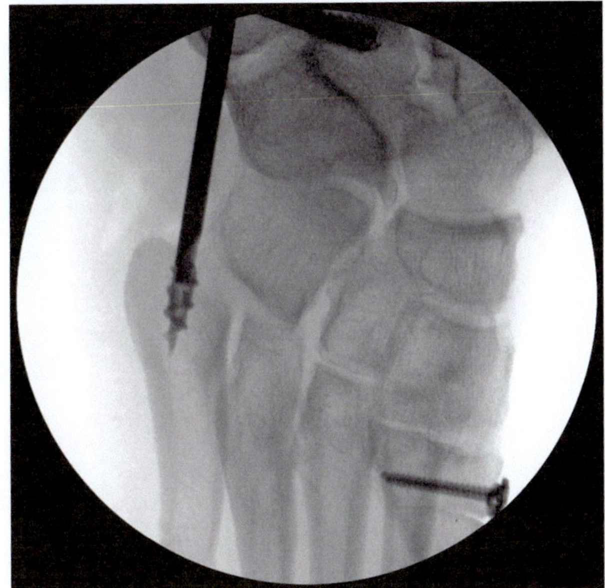

Fig. 19.8 Intraoperative fluoroscopy of placement of a corkscrew anchor at the base of the fifth metatarsal

The FDL tendon is harvested just proximal to the master knot of Henry. The distal stump of FDL may be tenodesed to the FHL tendon if desired for select patient populations, such as athletes.

Alternatively, the FDL can be harvested from the medial arch of the foot. An incision is made in the plantar–medial aspect of the arch obliquely in the direction of FDL. The incision should be superior to the level of the abductor hallucis from the medial pole of the navicular toward the head of the first metatarsal. The interval between the abductor hallucis muscle belly and the first metatarsal is developed, reflecting the abductor plantarly. Hemostasis must be maintained while dissecting

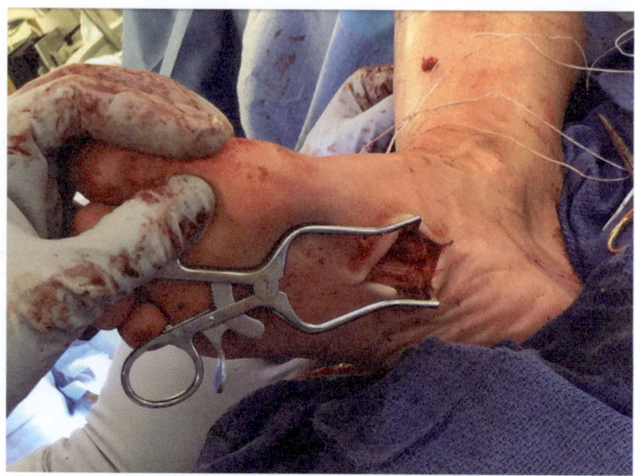

Fig. 19.9 Intraoperative photograph demonstrates a plantar oblique incision with exposure of the plantar fascia

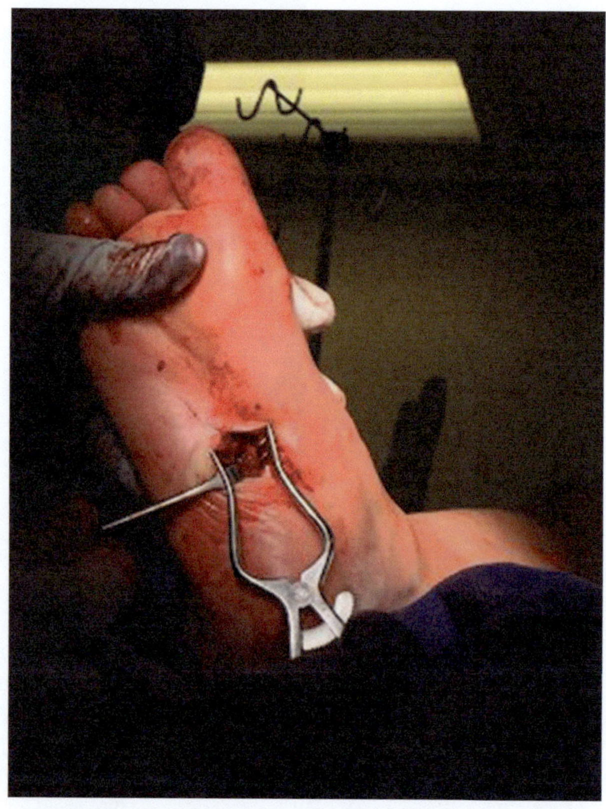

Fig. 19.10 Intraoperative photograph of exposure of the FDL and FHL tendons

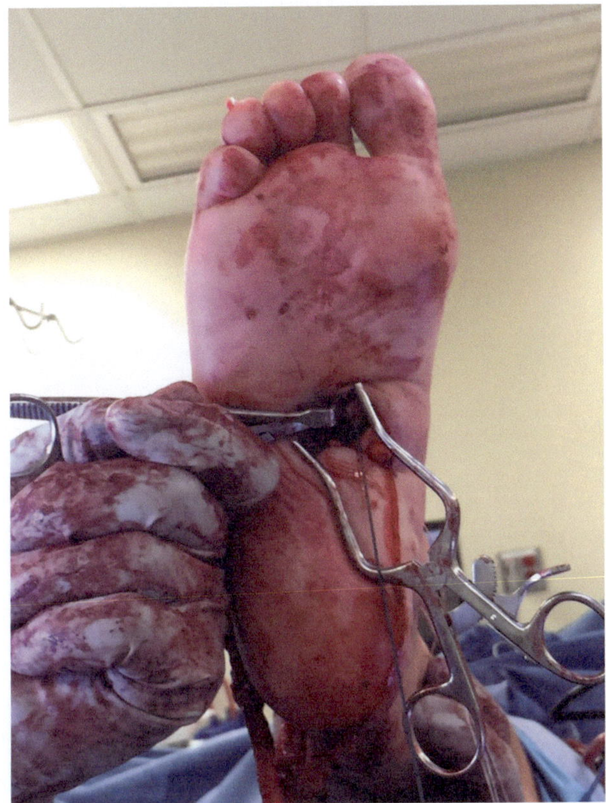

Fig. 19.11 Intraoperative photograph of FDL being tagged before it is ligated

through this hypervascular area. Identification of the FDL is facilitated by partially releasing the origin of the Flexor Hallucis Brevis. The FDL is palpable and confirmed through simultaneous flexion and extension of the lesser toes. Once exposed, the tendon should be retracted out of the wound with a right-angled clamp to confirm the FDL has been isolated (Fig. 19.12).

The neurovascular structures sit just plantar to the long flexor tendons beneath, and thus it is important to stay within the second muscular layer of the foot during dissection. The tendon should be tagged with a suture before the FDL is ligated as the tendon can retract proximally out of view once cut. The FDL tendon is harvested just proximal to the master knot of Henry (Fig. 19.13).

Any adhesions along the FDL tendon should then be released. A 3-cm proximal medial incision is made 7 cm above the medial malleolus. The FDL is identified in

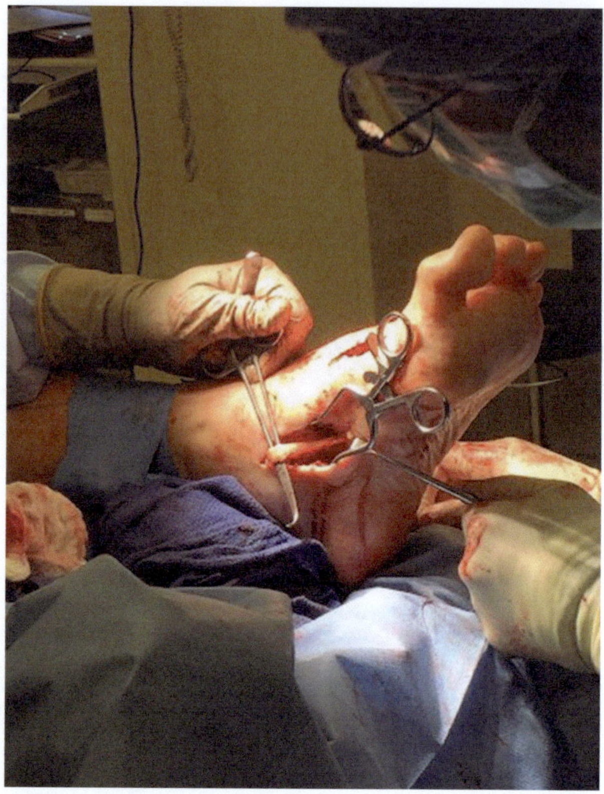

Fig. 19.12 Intraoperative photograph of isolation of the FDL tendon

the deep posterior compartment and pulled proximally preserving any distal muscle belly (Fig. 19.14). A Kelly clamp is passed from the medial incision immediately posterior to the tibia and fibula until the peroneal sheath is entered. If this clamp is not exposed through the lateral incision, a new incision is made where the clamp penetrates. A second Kelly clamp is connected to the first through the lateral incision and the tip of the clamp is delivered into the medial wound. The clamp is then used to pull the FDL tendon to the lateral side (Fig. 19.15).

The FDL is passed through the peroneal sheath and distally must be passed deep to the sural nerve. The length of the tendon is assessed with the tendon taut, and the foot and ankle held in maximum eversion and 20 degrees of plantar flexion. Any excess tendon is resected.

A modified Krackow technique using one arm of the #0 or #2 suture from the anchor placed into the base of the fifth metatarsal is then woven through the FDL up one side and down the other. The other suture strand is then used to advance the tendon to the tuberosity and tied securely. The reconstruction can be reinforced with additional suture into the remnant peroneus brevis tendon stump. Alternatively, if preferred, the FDL can be anastomosed to a distal tendon stump directly. Care must be taken to make sure the anastomosis site is not going to be too bulky or in the retrofibular region resulting in an impediment to tendon gliding.

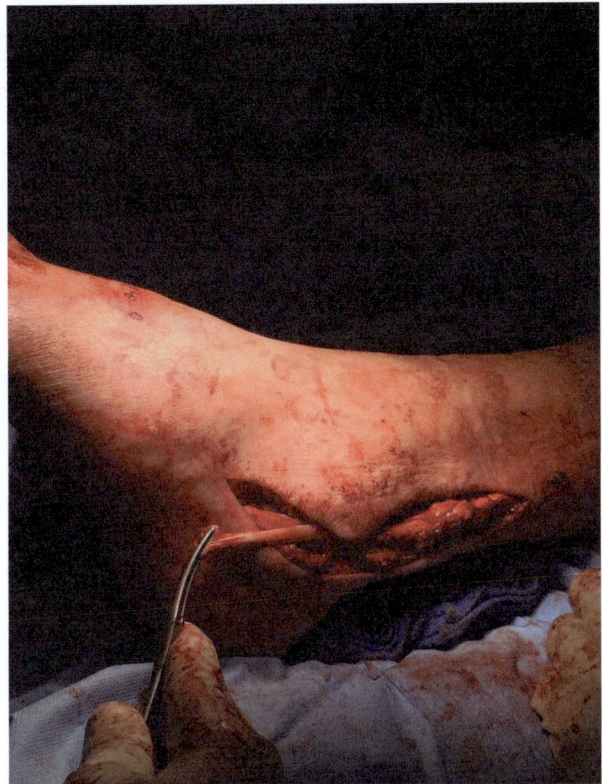

Fig. 19.13 Intraoperative photograph of the harvested FDL tendon through the medial approach

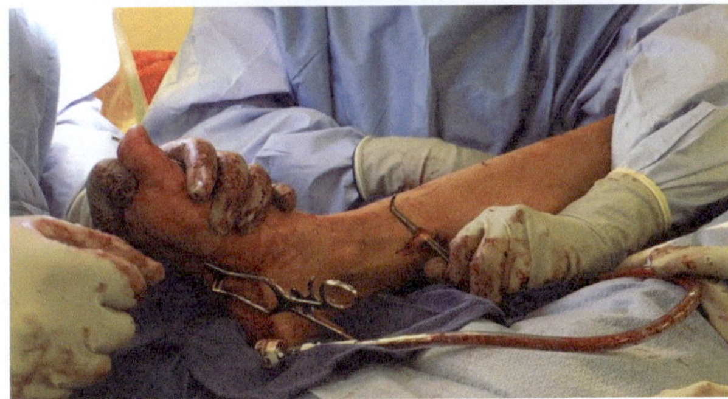

Fig. 19.14 A Kelly clamp is used to isolate the FDL tendon proximally and pull the tendon out of the medial incision

The incisions are then irrigated and closed with the foot and ankle in a relaxed plantar flexed and everted position. Sterile dressings are applied and a bulky splint with U and posterior plaster slabs is applied in this relaxed 20-degree plantar flexed and everted position.

Postoperatively, the patient is kept non-weight bearing for 6 weeks. The splint and sutures are removed at 2 weeks and gentle range of motion exercises are begun to minimize tendon adhesion. The patient is placed in a removable boot brace in 20

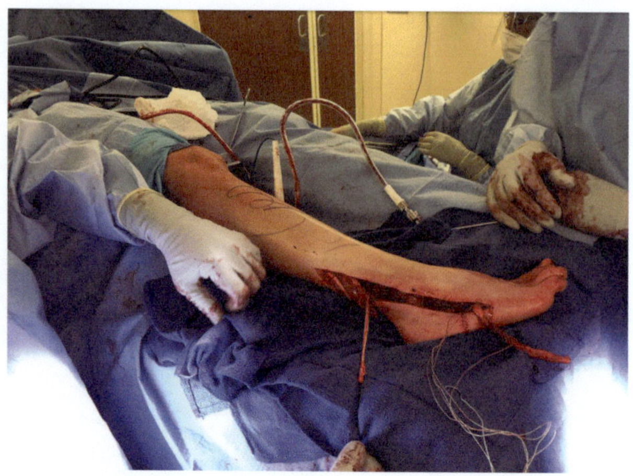

Fig. 19.15 The tendon is then delivered into the peroneal sheath passing behind the tibia and the fibula

degrees of equinus for the next 4 weeks. Passive eversion is encouraged, but active eversion is limited for 6 weeks. The patient should also avoid dorsiflexion past 10 degrees of equinus and 10 degrees of inversion. At 6 weeks, the boot brace's hinge is changed to allow 0–20 degrees of plantar flexion and weight bearing in the brace is initiated. A progressive weight-bearing protocol is utilized allowing an additional 20 LBS every other day until full weight bearing is achieved. At 10–12 weeks post-operatively, the patient may transition into a supportive lace-up ankle brace. Full range of motion and resisted eversion is now permitted as well as unrestricted walking activities. At 6 months from surgery, the patient may start jogging as tolerated.

Single-stage FDL transfer for chronic severe tears of both peroneal tendons is a safe and successful procedure, which restores function and reliably decreases pain. Further prospective, comparative studies of tendon transfer and allograft reconstruction are needed to better define indications and outcomes for peroneal reconstruction.

References

1. Bassett FH 3rd, Speer KP. Longitudinal rupture of the peroneal tendons. Am J Sports Med. 1993;21(3):354–7.
2. Borton DC, Lucas P, Jomha NM, Cross MJ, Slater K. Operative reconstruction after transverse rupture of the tendons of both peroneus longus and brevis. Surgical reconstruction by transfer of the flexor digitorum longus tendon. J Bone Joint Surg Br. 1998;80(5):781–4.
3. Krause JO, Brodsky JW. Peroneus brevis tendon tears: pathophysiology, surgical reconstruction, and clinical results. Foot Ankle Int. 1998;19(5):271–9.
4. Title CI, Jung HG, Parks BG, Schon LC. The peroneal groove deepening procedure: a biomechanical study of pressure reduction. Foot Ankle Int. 2005;26:442–8.
5. Sobel M, Geppert MJ, Olson EJ, et al. The dynamics of peroneus brevis tendon splits: a proposed mechanism, technique of diagnosis, and classification of injury. Foot Ankle. 1992;13(7):413–22.
6. Freccero DM, Berkowitz MJ. The relationship between tears of the peroneus brevis tendon and the distal extent of its muscle belly: an MRI study. Foot Ankle Int. 2006;27:236–9.

7. Geller J, Lin S, Cordas D, Vieira P. Relationship of a low-lying muscle belly to tears of the peroneus brevis tendon. Am J Orthop. 2003;32:541–4.
8. Unlu MC, Bilgili M, Akgun I, et al. Abnormal proximal musculotendinous junction of the peroneus brevis muscle as a cause of peroneus brevis tendon tears: a cadaveric study. J Foot Ankle Surg. 2010;49:537–40.
9. Athavale SA, Swathi V. Anatomy of the superior peroneal tunnel. J Bone Joint Surg Am. 2011;93:564–71.
10. Sobel M, DiCarlo EF, Bohne WH, Collins L. Longitudinal splitting of the peroneus brevis tendon: an anatomic and histologic study of cadaveric material. Foot Ankle. 1991;12:165–70.
11. Petersen W, Bobka T, Stein V, Tillmann B. Blood supply of the peroneal tendons: injection and immunohistochemical studies of cadaver tendons. Acta Orthop Scand. 2000;71(2):168–74.
12. Sobel M, Pavlov H, Geppert MJ, et al. Painful os peroneum syndrome: a spectrum of conditions responsible for plantar lateral foot pain. Foot Ankle Int. 1994;15:112–24.
13. Jahss M. Tendon disorders of the foot and ankle. In: Jahss M, editor. Disorders of the foot and ankle: medical and surgical management. 2nd ed. Philadelphia: WB Saunders; 1991. p. 1461–512.
14. Truong DT, Dussault RG, Kaplan PA. Fracture of the os peroneum and rupture of the peroneus longus tendon as a complication of diabetic neuropathy. Skelet Radiol. 1995;24:626–8.
15. Borland S, Jung S, Hugh IA. Complete rupture of the peroneus longus tendon secondary to injection. Foot (Edinb). 2009;19:229–31.
16. Demetracopoulos CA, Vineyard JC, Kiesau CD, Nunley JA 2nd. Long-term results of debridement and primary repair of peroneal tendon tears. Foot Ankle Int. 2014;35(3):252–7. Epub 2013 Dec 6.
17. Mook WR, Parekh SG, Nunley JA. Allograft reconstruction of peroneal tendons: operative technique and clinical outcomes. Foot Ankle Int. 2013;34(9):1212–20.
18. Jockel JR, Brodsky JW. Single-stage flexor tendon transfer for the treatment of severe concomitant peroneus longus and brevis tendon tears. Foot Ankle Int. 2013;34(5):666–72.
19. Redfern D, Myerson M. The management of concomitant tears of the peroneus longus and brevis tendons. Foot Ankle Int. 2004;25(10):695–707.
20. Seybold JD, Campbell JT, Jeng CL, Short KW, Myerson MS. Outcome of lateral transfer of the FHL or FDL for concomitant peroneal tendon tears. Foot Ankle Int. 2016;37(6):576–81.
21. Silver RL, de la Garza J, Rang M. The myth of muscle balance. A study of relative strengths and excursions of normal muscles about the foot and ankle. J Bone Joint Surg Br. 1985;67(3):432–7.
22. Sherman TI, Guyton GP. Minimal incision/minimally invasive medializing displacement calcaneal osteotomy. Foot Ankle Int. 2018;39(1):119–28.

Staged Reconstruction for Chronic Rupture of Both Peroneal Tendons Using Hunter Rod and Flexor Hallucis Longus Tendon Transfer

20

Christy M. Christophersen, Osama Elattar,
and Keith L. Wapner

Introduction

Chronic lateral ankle pain can have many different etiologies. Peroneal tendon pathology is a major cause [2, 3, 12, 15, 19, 20, 23–25, 27–29, 31–34, 38]. Fissuring and longitudinal splitting of the peroneus brevis and longus tendons have been reported as an etiology of chronic lateral ankle pain and functional instability. The etiology of longitudinal fissures of the peroneal tendons has not been clearly identified, and several theories have been postulated [15, 18, 24]. Histologic evaluation of these splits has shown chronic wear with cystic and myxoid degeneration of the tendon. Frey and Shereff [9] proposed a zone of critical hypovascularity as a source of tendon splitting [9]. However, Sobel et al. [30, 31] have shown no correlation between the sites of tendon splitting and hypovascularity. They believe that there is a mechanical impingement from the fibular groove [30, 31]. Other authors suggested incompetence of the superior peroneal retinaculum, the presence of a sharp posterior fibular ridge, or dynamic compression between the peroneus longus and brevis tendons [6, 7, 22, 29, 31–35].

When recognized early, direct repair usually is possible with good results [1, 3–5, 8, 13, 14, 17, 21, 24, 35]. However, when these lesions become chronic or involve both tendons, the results of surgery are less favorable. Redfern and Myeron [42] proposed an algorithm for surgical treatment of peroneal tendon tears based upon the state of the tendons. A direct repair was proposed if both tendons were grossly intact, while tenodesis was proposed, if one tendon was still considered functional.

C. M. Christophersen
Department of Orthopaedic Surgery, Mayo Clinic, Rochester, MN, USA

O. Elattar
Department of Orthopaedic Surgery, University of Toledo Medical Center, Toledo, OH, USA

K. L. Wapner (✉)
Department of Orthopaedic Surgery, Penn Medicine, Philadelphia, PA, USA
e-mail: twinsons1@comcast.net

© Springer Nature Switzerland AG 2020
M. Sobel (ed.), *The Peroneal Tendons*,
https://doi.org/10.1007/978-3-030-46646-6_20

If both tendons were considered nonfunctional, then a tendon graft or tendon transfer using flexor digitorum longus to peroneus brevis was done; they performed a staged procedure using a silicon rod if there was considerable scarring [42]. Mook et al. [43] described a single-stage allograft tendon for reconstruction of an intercalary segment defect involving the peroneal tendons using appropriately sized peroneal tendon or semitendinosus allograft. Barton et al. [44] proposed surgical reconstruction by transfer of the flexor digitorum longus tendon for transverse rupture of the peroneal tendons. However, there is a paucity of literature on surgical treatment for patients with advanced pathology who have failed both primary repair and anastomosis of peroneus brevis and longus. These cases present a surgical challenge, especially in young active patients where the goal is to achieve pain relief, dynamic stabilization of the ankle, and to restore peroneal tendon function.

Wapner et al. [41] described a technique of staged reconstruction with excision of the remaining portion of the peroneal tendons and reconstruction with a Hunter rod and flexor hallucis longus (FHL) transfer. The patient cohort involved seven patients, with chronic ruptures of both peroneal tendons, who had a minimum of two previously failed attempts at surgical repair. Before involvement in this study, all patients in this series were told that they would need either full-time bracing or possibly surgical fusion of their hindfoot. Evaluation by MRI, of their patient cohort, demonstrated chronic thickening, fissuring, and stenosis of the remaining peroneal structures [41]. This presented two problems for salvage: the loss of an adequate tendon sheath and the lack of adequate remaining tendon tissue. Borrowing from techniques in the hand literature, these tendons were reconstructed using a staged procedure of excising the remaining tendon, placing a Hunter rod to form a new tendon sheath [10, 40], and transfer of the FHL into the newly formed sheath 3 months later. This technique involves insertion of the FHL tendon into the residual stump of the peroneus brevis tendon and restores its function. The distal portion of the peroneus longus tendon has been found to be too enmeshed in scar to serve as a viable insertion point for the FHL tendon, and further dissection into the plantar lateral aspect of the foot to retrieve the distal portion of the peroneus longus tendon would create greater morbidity than benefit [41]. Follow-up has shown no measurable morbidity from the loss of active peroneus longus tendon function, including a lack of cavus or varus deformity; this is likely secondary to the distal portion of the peroneus longus tendon being scarred down producing a tenodesis effect that counteracted the pull of the invertor tendons [41].

Operative Technique

The first stage of reconstruction consists of debridement of the remaining peroneal tendon tissue and tendon sheath, and implanting a 6-mm Hunter rod into the bed of the peroneal sheath (Figs. 20.1 and 20.2). The Hunter rod was sutured to the remaining stump of the peroneus brevis tendon distally and the proximal end remained free

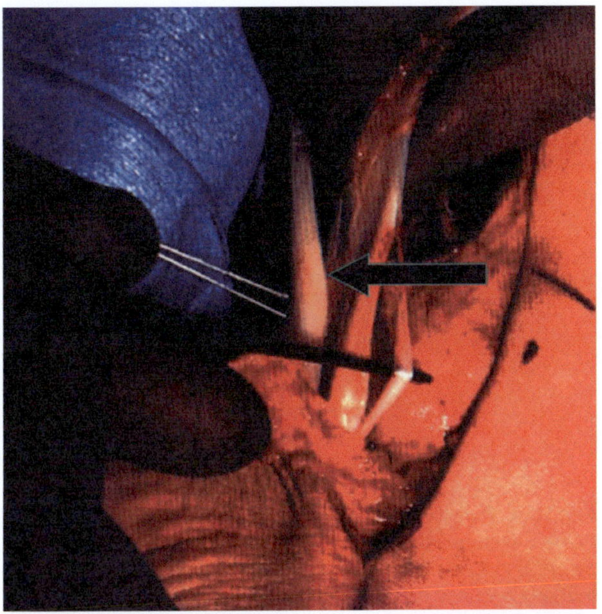

Fig. 20.1 Intraoperative photograph of a longitudinal peroneus brevis tear. (With permissions from Wolters Kluwer Health)

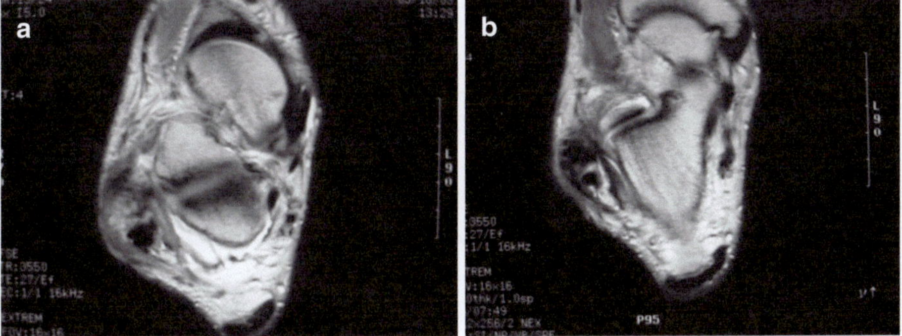

Fig. 20.2 Axial T2 MRI image demonstrating (**a**) a tear in the peroneal tendon and (**b**) fluid around the tendon sheath. (With permissions from Wolters Kluwer Health)

in the sheath (Fig. 20.3). The sheath is then trimmed of any redundancy and closed over the Hunter rod.

Transfer of the FHL tendon occurs 3 months later. The FHL is harvested in the traditional fashion (Fig. 20.4) [36, 37]. Once the FHL is harvested, a small incision is made at the proximal aspect of the previously made lateral incision overlying the proximal aspect of the Hunter rod, staying proximal to the lateral malleolus. The FHL is transferred from medial to lateral into this incision (Fig. 20.5). The proximal portion of the Hunter rod is identified, and the FHL is attached to the rod (Fig. 20.6).

Fig. 20.3 The peroneal incision is identified from over the peroneals to the base of the fifth metatarsal. (With permissions from Wolters Kluwer Health)

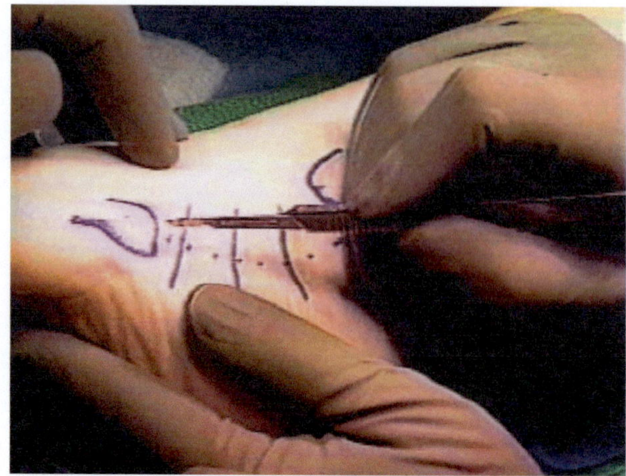

Fig. 20.4 Extensive scar tissue is seen overlying the peroneal tendons in this multiply operated patient (With permissions from Wolters Kluwer Health)

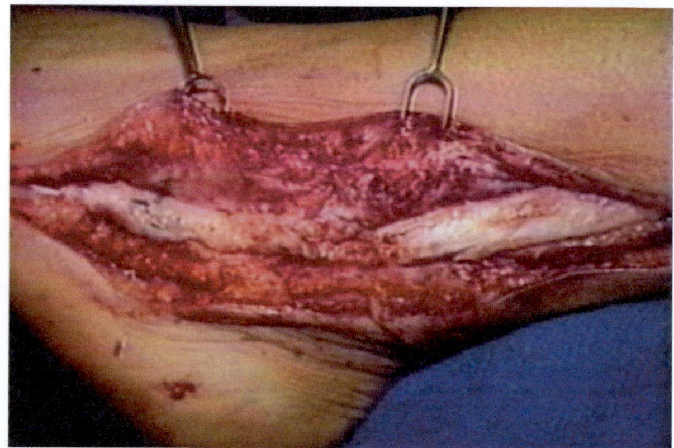

Fig. 20.5 The peroneal tendon sheath and tendon are debrided. (With permissions from Wolters Kluwer Health)

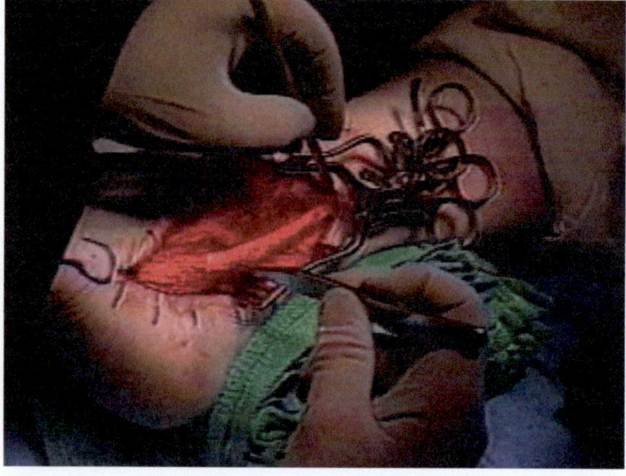

Fig. 20.6 A 6-mm Hunter rod is placed into the bed of the peroneal sheath. The Hunter rod is sutured into the remaining stump of the peroneal brevis tendon distally with nonabsorbable suture. Proximally, the rod remains free in the sheath. (With permissions from Wolters Kluwer Health)

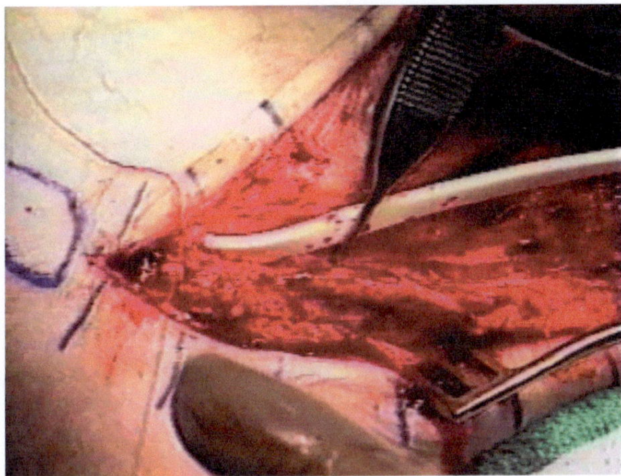

Fig. 20.7 The sheath is trimmed of any redundancy and closed over the Hunter rod. (With permissions from Wolters Kluwer Health)

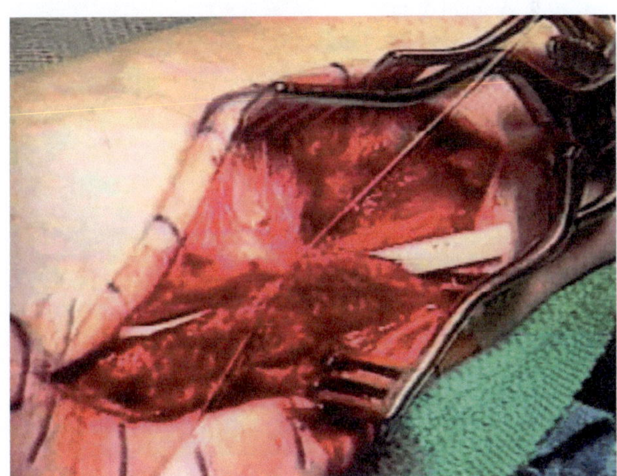

A small distal incision is made over the distal suture site of the Hunter rod and the remaining portion of the peroneus brevis tendon. The Hunter rod is released from this suture site and then pulled distally, allowing the FHL tendon to slide into the newly formed tendon sheath (Fig. 20.7). The FHL is then attached to the remaining stump of the peroneus brevis tendon using a Pulvertaft weave (Figs. 20.8, 20.9, and 20.10).

Postoperatively, the patients are allowed partial weight bearing for 3 weeks and then advanced to full weight bearing in a removable walking cast. They should be instructed to begin active and passive range-of-motion exercises of the ankle and hindfoot in all planes of motion. Home strengthening exercises should begin at 6 weeks, and the patients are advanced to an ankle stirrup at 8–10 weeks based on their strength. Formal physical therapy for functional rehabilitation of the ankle should start at 8 weeks.

Fig. 20.8 After the flexor halluces longus is released from the plantar surface of the foot, it is identified in the deep posterior compartment at its origin on the posterior fibula. It is then pulled into the lateral incision. (With permissions from Wolters Kluwer Health)

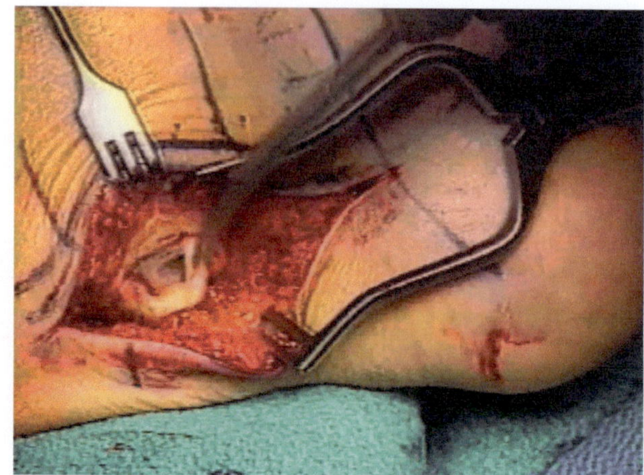

Fig. 20.9 A small distal incision is made over the distal suture site of the Hunter rod and the remaining portion of the peroneus brevis. (With permissions from Wolters Kluwer Health)

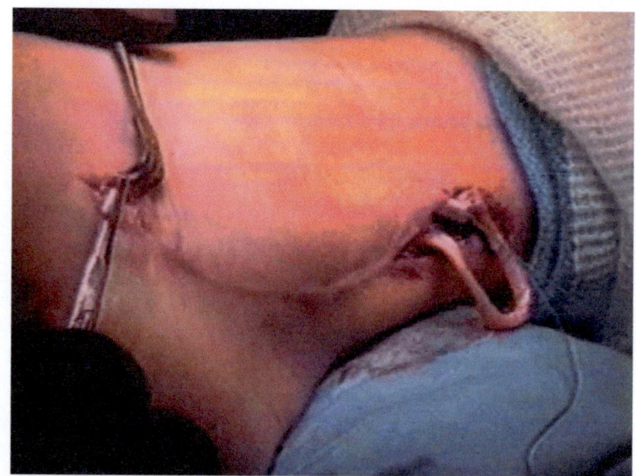

Fig. 20.10 The flexor halluces longus is attached to the remaining stump of the peroneus brevis tendon using a Pulvertaft weave. (With permissions from Wolters Kluwer Health)

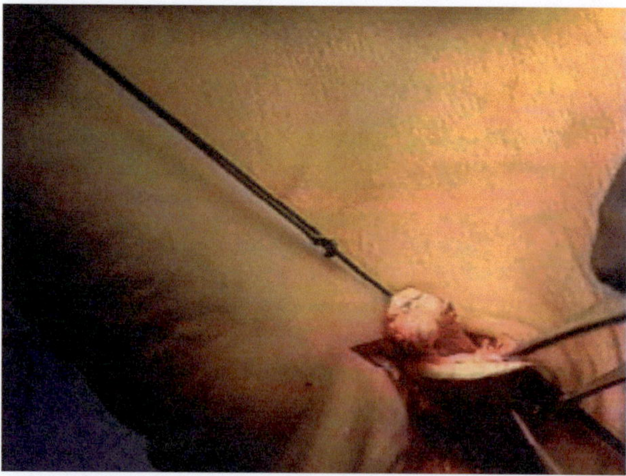

Discussion

Chronic lesions of the peroneal tendons represent a surgical dilemma. Several surgical solutions have been proposed; however, there is a paucity of literature for treatment of chronic tears involving both tendons in active young patients. The technique delineated by Wapner et al. provides a solution with satisfactory outcomes in this patient demographic.

Of the seven patients involved in the cohort, none developed wound complications. Patients ranged in age from 30 to 57 years, with an average age of 38 years. All were women. At average follow-up of 8.5 (range 5.5–11.9) years, six patients reported complete resolution of pain. The only patient with pain was the one workers' compensation patient in the group. This patient was the only patient requiring the use of an ankle support (molded polypropylene ankle foot orthosis), all other patients walked without assistive devices. The same six patients had symmetric, painless range of motion bilaterally at the ankle, subtalar, and transverse tarsal joints. Four had symmetric 5/5 motor strength of the peroneals on manual muscle testing. Two had 4+/5 motor strength, and the one workers' compensation patient had 3/5 strength. All patients except the one workers' compensation patient could perform single-heel rise and walk on their tiptoes without instability or pain. One patient required a Brostrom ankle ligament repair 2 years after surgery after a new injury. She remained free of pain at 62 months after surgery. All patients except the workers' compensation patient returned to full-time employment, one as a school bus driver, one as a college volleyball coach, one as a high school teacher, and three as office workers. These six patients were satisfied with their results and stated that they would have the surgery again and would recommend the surgery to a friend. Based on this evaluation, the authors rated the results as five excellent, one good, and one poor result.

For successful reconstruction, it is important to create a viable tendon sheath that allows free movement of the new tendon, with re-establishment of the stability of the peroneal retinaculum and to find a suitable motor unit to provide a dynamic replacement for the peroneal tendons. In chronic peroneal tendon ruptures, the peroneal muscles are atrophied, resulting in decreased excursion, and do not provide a reliable source of a viable motor unit. The use of a Hunter rod recreates a viable tendon sheath; the principle of implantation of a silicone rubber rod and subsequent reimplantation of a tendon transfer has been well documented with studies demonstrating a mesothelial cell-lined pseudosheath. The fluid formed resembles synovial fluid and lubricates the gliding motion of the newly transferred tendon [10, 11, 16, 39].

The success of the use of FHL transfer in the treatment of chronic Achilles tendon repair is well documented as a suitable motor unit [36, 37]. The FHL has a strength percentage of 3.6 and could be a substitute for the peroneus brevis muscle-tendon unit, which has a strength percentage of 2.6 as determined by Silver et al. [26]. The length of the FHL tendon provides adequate tissue for transfer. The FHL is an in-phase muscle with an axis of contracture similar to the peroneal muscle–tendon unit as it arises off of the posterior fibula (18). Previous work using the FHL for Achilles tendon reconstruction demonstrated minimal donor morbidity [36, 37].

Conclusion

There were a few weaknesses of the study, the biggest being its retrospective nature. This is an infrequent problem and the collection of data extended over 6 years with only seven patients. No standardized preoperative collection of objective and subjective data was done other than the information being gathered by the senior author (KLW) in his assessment of the patients clinically. Wapner et al. relied upon patient's physical examinations and subjective responses at the time of follow-up for outcome measures. We recognize that this does not provide statistically significant data, but with the small sample size, statistically significant data would have been unlikely.

Nonetheless, with the available number of patients, we believe the clinical results and patient satisfaction level demonstrate that staged reconstruction of chronic degeneration of both peroneal tendons with a Hunter rod and FHL tendon transfer provides a satisfactory result for this difficult clinical problem. Six of our seven patients were pain free at average follow-up of 8.5 years and were working full time without complaints.

References

1. Bassett F, Speer K. Longitudinal rupture of the peroneal tendons. Am J Sports Med. 1993;21:354–7.
2. Brage ME, Hansen ST. Traumatic subluxation/dislocation of peroneal tendon. Foot Ankle. 1992;13:423–31.
3. Burman M. Stenosing tendovaginitis of the foot and ankle studies with special reference to the stenosing tendovaginitis of the peroneal tubercle. AMA Arch Surg. 1953;67:686–98.
4. Cox D, Paterson F. Acute calcific tendonitis of the peroneus longus. J Bone Joint Surg. 1991;73-B:342.
5. Davies J. Peroneal compartment syndrome secondary to rupture of the peroneus longus. J Bone Joint Surg. 1979;61-B:783–4.
6. Eckert WR, Davis EA Jr. Acute rupture of the peroneal retinaculum. J Bone Joint Surg. 1976;58:A:670–2.
7. Edwards ME. The relations of peroneal tendon to the fibula, calcaneus, and cuboideum. Am J Anal. 1928;42:213–53.
8. Evans J. Subcutaneous rupture of the tendon of the peroneus longus: a case report. J Bone Joint Surg. 1966;48:B:507–9.
9. Frey C, Shereff M, Greenidge N. Vascularity of posterior tibial tendon. J Bone Joint Surg. 1990;72-A:884–8.
10. Hunter JM, Salisbury R. Flexor Tendon reconstruction in severely damaged hand: a Two Stage Procedure using a Silicone-Dacron reinforced Gliding prosthesis prior to tendon Grafting. J Bone Joint Surg. 1971;53-A:829–58.

11. Imbriglia JE, Hunter J, Rennie W. Secondary Flexor Tendon Reconstruction. Hand Clin. 1989;5:395–413.
12. Karlsson J, Brandsson S, Kalebo P, Eriksson BI. Surgical treatment of concomitant chronic ankle instability and longitudinal rupture of the peroneus brevis tendon. Scand J Med Sci Sports. 1998;8(1):42–9.
13. Kilkelly FX, McHale KA. Acute rupture of the peroneal longus tendon in a runner: a case report and review of the literature. Foot Ankle Int. 1994;15:567–9.
14. Krause JO, Brodsky JW. Peroneus Brevis tears: pathophysiology and surgical reconstruction and clinical results. Foot Ankle Int. 1998;19:271–9.
15. Larsen E. Longitudinal rupture of the peroneus brevis tendon. J Bone Joint Surg. 1987;69-B:340–1.
16. La Salle WB, Strickland JW. An evaluation of two stage flexor tendon reconstruction technique. J Hand Surgery. 1983;8:263–7.
17. Le Melle DP, Janis R. Longitudinal rupture of the peroneus brevis tendon: a study of eight cases. J Foot Surg. 1989;28:132–6.
18. Meyer AW. Further evidence of attrition in the human body. Am J Anat. 1924;34:324–67.
19. Munk RL, Davis PH. Longitudinal rupture of the peroneus brevis tendon. J Trauma. 1976;16:803–6.
20. Parvin RW, Fort TL. Stenosing tenosynovitis of the common peroneal tendon sheath. J Bone Joint Surg. 1956;38-A:1352–7.
21. Pelet S, Saglini M, Garofalo R, Wettstein M, Mouhsine E. Traumatic rupture of both peroneal longus and brevis tendons. Foot Ankle Int. 2003;24:721–3.
22. Purnell ML, Drummond DS, Engber WO, Breed AL. Congenital dislocation of peroneal tendon. J Bone Joint Surg. 1983;65-B:316–9.
23. Regan TP, Hughston JC. Chronic ankle sprain secondary to anomalous peroneal tendon. Clin Orthop. 1977;123:52–4.
24. Sammarco GJ, DiRaimondo CV. Chronic peroneus brevis tendon lesions. Foot Ankle. 1989;9:163–70.
25. Sammarco GJ, DiRaimondo CV. Surgical treatment of lateral ankle instability. Am J Sports Med. 1988;16:501–11.
26. Silver RL, deLa Garza J, Rang M. The myth of muscle balance: A study of relative strength and excursions of normal muscle about the foot and ankle. J Bone Joint Surg. 1985;67-B:432–7.
27. Sobel M, Bohne WHO, Markisz JA. Cadaver correlation of peroneal tendon changes with magnetic resonance imaging. Foot Ankle. 1991;11:384–8.
28. Sobel ML, DiCarlo EF, Bohne WHO, Collins L. Longitudinal splitting of peroneus brevis tendon: An anatomic and histologic study of cadaveric material. Foot Ankle. 1991;12:165–70.
29. Sobel M, Geppert MJ. Repair of concomitant lateral ankle ligament instability and peroneus brevis split through a posteriorly modified Brostom Gould. Foot Ankle. 1992;13:224–5.
30. Sobel M, Geppert MJ, Hannafin JA, Bohne WH, Arnoczky SP. Microvascular anatomy of the peroneal tendons. Foot Ankle. 1992;13:469–72.
31. Sobel M, Geppert MJ, Olson E, Bohne WH, Arnoczky SP. The dynamics of peroneus brevis tendon splits: a proposed mechanism, techniques of diagnosis, and classification of injury. Foot Ankle. 1992;13:413–22.
32. Sobel M, Levy M, Bohne WH. Congenital variations of peroneus quartus muscle: an anatomic study. Foot Ankle. 1990;11:81–9.
33. Sobel M, Levy M, Bohne WH. Longitudinal attrition of peroneus brevis tendon in the fibular groove: an anatomic study. Foot Ankle. 1990;11:124–8.
34. Sobel M, Warren RF, Brourman S. Lateral ankle instability associated with dislocation of peroneal tendon treated by a modified Chrisman-Snook procedure: a new technique and review of literature. Am J Sports Med. 1990;18:539–43.
35. Thompson F, Patterson A. Rupture of the peroneus longus tendon: report of three cases. J Bone Joint Surg. 1989;71-A:293–5.

36. Wapner KL, Pavlock GS, Hecht PJ, Naselli F, Walther R. Repair of Chronic Achilles Tendon Rupture with Flexor Hallucis Longus Tendon Transfer. Foot Ankle. 1993;14:443–9.
37. Wapner KL, Dalton GP. Repair of chronic Achilles tendon rupture with flexor hallucis longus transfer. Op Tech Orthop. 1994;4:132–6.
38. Webster FS. Peroneal tenosynovitis with pseudotumor. J Bone Joint Surg. 1968;50-A:153–7.
39. Wehbe MA, Mawr B, Hunter JM, Schneider LH, Goodwyn BL. Two-stage flexor tendon reconstruction. J Bone Joint Surg. 1986;68- A:752–63.
40. Weinstein SL, Sprague BL, Flatt AE. Evaluation of two stage flexor tendon reconstruction in severely damaged digits. J Bone Joint Surg. 1976;58A:786–91.
41. Wapner KL, Taras JS, Lin SS, Chao W. Staged reconstruction for chronic rupture of both peroneal tendons using Hunter rod and flexor hallucis longus tendon transfer: a long-term followup study. Foot Ankle Int. 2006;27(8):591–7.
42. Redfern D, Myerson M. The management of concomitant tears of the peroneus longus and brevis tendons. Foot Ankle Int. 2004;25(10):695–707.
43. Mook WR, Parekh SG, Nunley JA. Allograft reconstruction of peroneal tendons: operative technique and clinical outcomes. Foot Ankle Int. 2013;34(9):1212–20.
44. Borton DC, Lucas P, Jomha NM, Cross MJ, Slater K. Operative reconstruction after transverse rupture of the tendons of both peroneus longus and brevis: surgical reconstruction by transfer of the flexor digitorum longus tendon. J Bone Joint Surg. British volume. 1998;80(5):781–4.

Immobilization and Rehabilitation After Surgical Treatment of Peroneal Tendon Tears and Ruptures

21

P. A. D. Van Dijk, A. Tanriover, C. W. DiGiovanni, G. R. Waryasz, and Peter Kvarda

Introduction

Peroneal tendon disorders are a common cause of posterolateral ankle pain specifically after trauma. Since early return to activity is of great importance in treatment outcome, surgical repair only marks the beginning of a long recovery period: adequate rehabilitation is purported as an important aspect of the clinical success of any surgically treated tendon disorder, facilitating healing, minimal scarring, and early return to preinjury level of activity or sports.

To date, evidence lacks randomized controlled trials or other high level of evidence studies on rehabilitation after operative treatment of peroneal tendon injuries. In general, peroneal surgery is followed by both non-weight-bearing immobilization

P. A. D. Van Dijk (✉)
Department of Orthopedic Surgery, Academical University Medical Centers, Amsterdam, The Netherlands

Surgical Department, Onze Lieve Vrouwe Gasthuis, Amsterdam, The Netherlands
e-mail: p.a.vandijk@amc.uva.nl

A. Tanriover
Department of Orthopedic Surgery, Massachusetts General Hospital, Harvard Medical School, Boston, MA, USA

C. W. DiGiovanni · G. R. Waryasz
Department of Orthopedic Surgery, Massachusetts General Hospital, Harvard Medical School, Boston, MA, USA

Department of Orthopedic Surgery, Newton-Wellesley Hospital, Newton, MA, USA
e-mail: cwdigiovanni@partners.org; gwaryasz@partners.org

P. Kvarda
Department of Orthopedic Surgery, Massachusetts General Hospital, Harvard Medical School, Boston, MA, USA

Department of Orthopedics and Traumatology, University Hospital of Basel, Basel, Switzerland

© Springer Nature Switzerland AG 2020
M. Sobel (ed.), *The Peroneal Tendons*,
https://doi.org/10.1007/978-3-030-46646-6_21

347

(NWB) and weight-bearing immobilization (WB) to facilitate optimal healing while preventing reinjury [1]. While there is no consensus on optimal immobilization time [1], early range of motion (ROM) is commonly recommended based on the concept that tendons tend to form adhesions between the repaired tissue and surrounding scar tissue after surgical repair [2]. In peroneal tendon injuries, progression to full weight bearing depends on both the nature of the pathology and the type of treatment (conservative, tendoscopic, open with or without repair of the superior peroneal retinaculum (SPR)).

In this chapter the authors propose a rehabilitation protocol after surgical treatment of peroneal tendon injuries, based on the best available evidence. It is important to keep in mind that the proposed protocol should be adjusted to every specific patient in order to optimize recovery.

Phases of Rehabilitation

Rehabilitation is typically based on the mechanism and timeframe of both intrinsic and extrinsic healing combined with the specific surgical procedure and each patient's personal characteristics. There is a wide variation of peroneal tendon's rehabilitation protocols, confirming that there is no consensus among foot and ankle providers. Based on best available evidence, peroneal rehabilitation is generally divided into four phases:

1. Immobilization (non-weight, partial weight, or full weight bearing)
2. Active ROM
3. Exercises and proprioceptive training
4. Patient (and sports) specific training

Immobilization

Promoting early return to activity and sports is key in patients treated for peroneal tendon injuries. While current literature lacks peroneal-specific studies, many rehabilitation recommendations have been published regarding flexor tendons of the hand [2]. Flexor tendons are known to form adhesions between the repaired tendon and the surrounding tissue(s), possible leading to scar formation, loss of ROM, and limitation in gliding of the tendon. Therefore, in order to prevent the formation of adhesions, early ROM is recommended and immobilization time is kept to a minimum [3–6].

Recently, this theory has been passed over to the tendons of the foot and ankle. For example, several authors advocated early postoperative ROM after Achilles tendon surgery [7–11]. While peroneal literature shows a wide variation in the total immobilization period after surgical treatment (0–13 weeks) [1], there also seems to be a recent trend toward early ROM exercises after peroneal tendon surgery [12, 13]. For example, two recently published studies described a change in their postoperative management based on latest research [12–14]. While initially immobilizing patients 6 weeks in a lower leg cast, Demetracouplos et al changed their postoperative protocol aiming early ROM after 4 weeks of immobilization [12]. Karlsson et al immobilized patients for 6 weeks in earlier research but shortened this period in a study published 4 years later to only 2 weeks of immobilization followed by a weight-bearing-air cast brace to provide early ROM training [13, 14].

The international ESSKA-AFAS consensus statement on peroneal tendon pathology proposed that for optimal immobilization time, one must distinguish whether or not the SPR was repaired. In case the SPR is not repaired, rehabilitation should be rather goal instead of time based, focusing on the promotion of early mobilization and ROM. In situ repair of the peroneal tendons (sheath opened only distal to the tip of the fibula) can undergo early ROM in all planes without extra risk of dislocation. Peroneal tendoscopic repairs can also undergo early ROM given the lack of damage to the SPR. When a SPR repair is performed, immobilization should consist of 2 weeks NWB in a lower leg cast, followed by 4 weeks of WB in a cast or a walker boot [15]. The rehabilitation restriction in certain planes of motion is to ensure that the tendons do not dislocate and that the SPR repair can heal.

Rehabilitation Exercises

After immobilization (see section 'Immobilization'), physical therapy is initiated in order to restore ROM and peroneal strength. No high level of evidence is available with regard to best exercises in the rehabilitation of surgically treated peroneal tendon injuries. Based on the evaluation of available protocols in today's literature as well as personal experience, in 2016, the authors of this chapter published an evidence-based algorithm for the rehabilitation of after peroneal surgery [1]. Within the algorithm, several types of exercises are recommended.

Range-of-Motion Exercises

During ankle plantar flexion, dorsiflexion, and inversion, the peroneal tendons are secured within the retromalleolar groove by the SPR. Since only limited loading is put on the tendons during these movements, they are generally started early after surgery. Eversion of the ankle stretches the SPR, which is contraindicated in case the SPR is repaired during surgery. To protect the repaired SPR, eversion should therefore be delayed. If the SPR was not violated to repair the tendons, early eversion can be performed, as there is no effective risk of peroneal dislocation because the SPR was kept intact.

Peroneal Strengthening Exercises

After immobilization and ROM exercises, depending on the nature of surgery and patient characteristics, isometric and isotonic exercises are started. During the initial immobilization period, electric stimulation can already be used to prevent muscle atrophy. Forced eversion of foot with a plantar-flexed ankle is the main exercise to strengthen peroneal muscles (Figs. 21.1 and 21.2). Subsequently, isometric exercises (forced plantar flexion of the foot against a fixed object), and eccentric exercises (peroneal muscle length increases but muscle contracts against inverting force) are recommended, ensuring that the retinacular repair is not violated.

Calf and Foot Strengthening Exercises

An important part of rehabilitation after surgery of peroneal tendons is calf and foot strengthening exercises. Due to the immobilization and NWB period, the gastrocnemius and intrinsic foot muscles lose strength and flexibility. In order to restore a stable walking pattern, calf, foot strength and flexibility are required. While intrinsic foot exercises can be started immediately after surgery, calf strengthening should be started with WB (Figs. 21.3 and 21.4).

Proprioceptive Exercises

As the patient starts weight bearing, the walking pattern should be closely observed. Depending on the procedure, proprioceptive training is given on both the ground and unstable surfaces (Figs. 21.5, 21.6, 21.7, and 21.8). As the patient weans from crutches, (s)he starts partial weight bearing, full weight bearing on two legs, single leg weight bearing, and lastly full weight bearing on unstable surfaces consecutively. During this period, walking exercises in the swimming pool or seated strengthening exercises are helpful.

Schematic Overview Rehabilitation Process

In 2018, the international ESSKA-AFAS consensus statement on peroneal tendon pathology proposed an algorithm to guide optimal immobilization time after surgical treatment of peroneal tendon pathology (Table 21.1) [15]. Based on a review by van Dijk et al, a schematic timeline of ROM and exercise is proposed after the initial immobilization in Table 21.2 [1].

Figs. 21.1 and 21.2 Eversion against resistance with ankle plantarflexed. This exercise may be done both sitting and lying

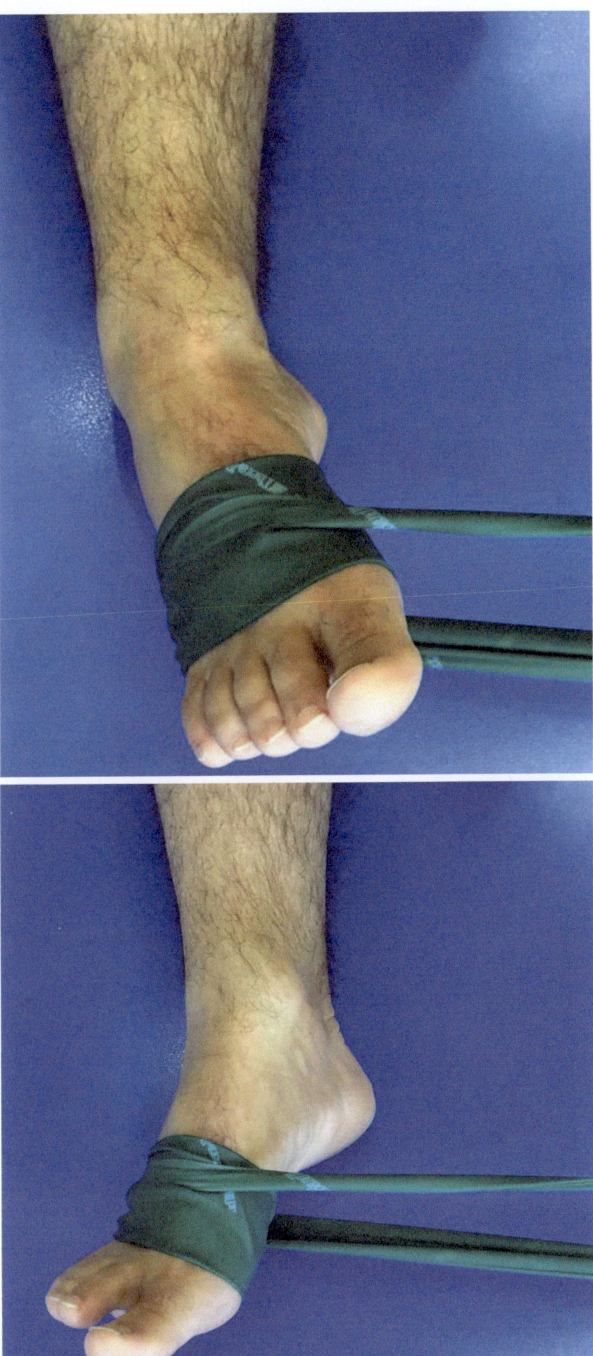

Figs. 21.3 and 21.4 Calf strengthening exercises are important due to atrophy after immobilization

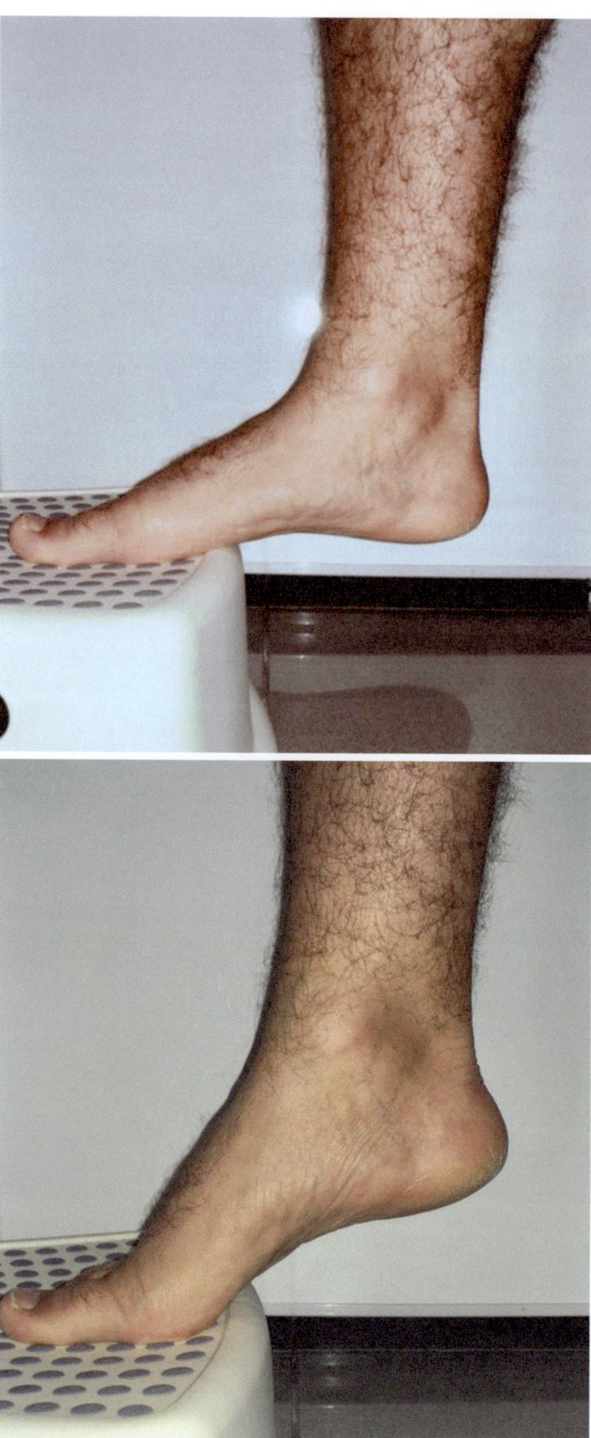

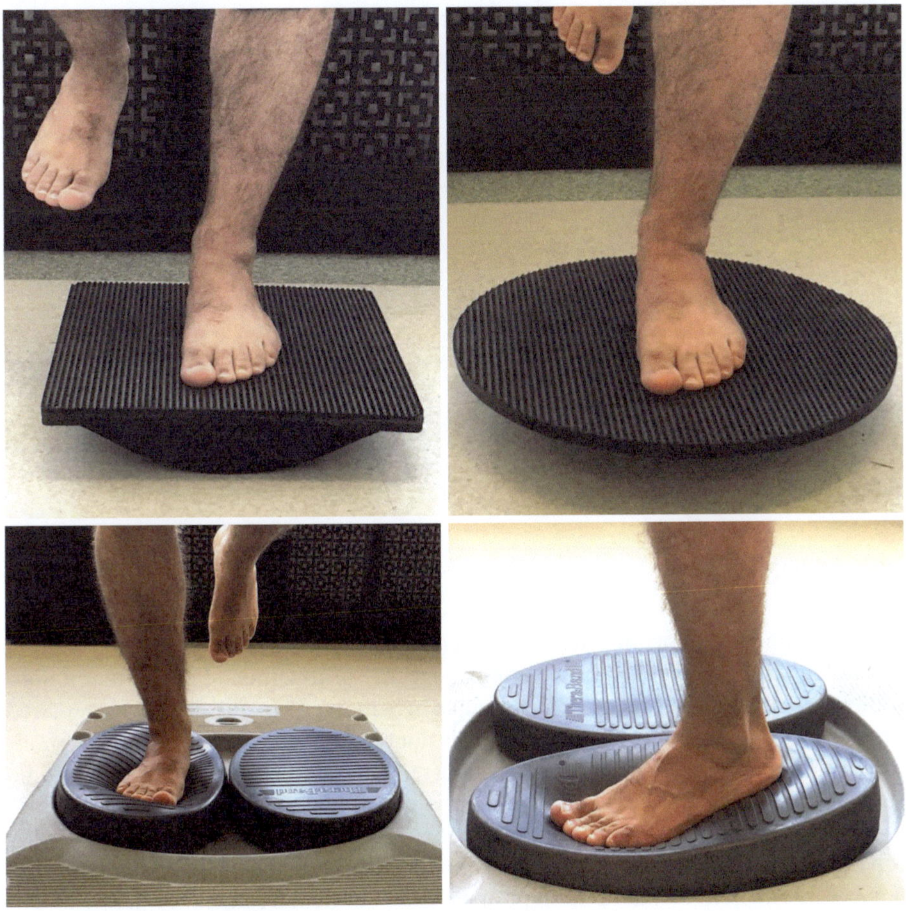

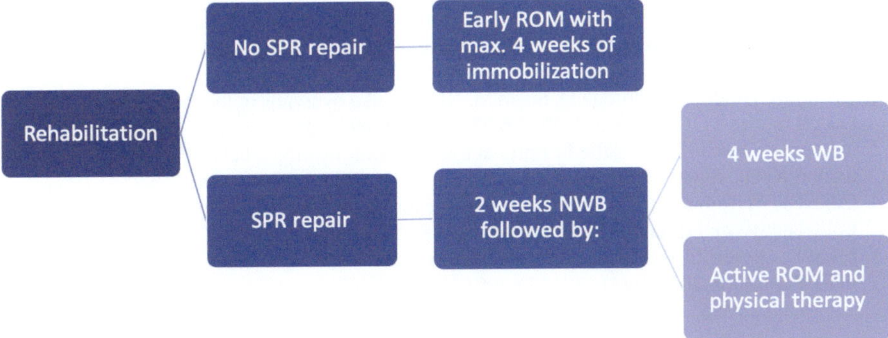

Figs. 21.5, 21.6, 21.7, and 21.8 Proprioceptive exercises are the most important component of peroneal tendon surgery rehabilitation. Single-leg training on unstable and stable surfaces starting from single plane to multiplanar unstable exercises is demonstrated

Table 21.1 Overview optimal immobilization time after peroneal surgery

Table 21.2 Schematic overview ROM and exercise after initial immobilization

	0–2 weeks*	2–4 weeks*	6–8 weeks*	8–12 weeks*	12–24 weeks*	>24 weeks*
Active ROM		X	X			
Strength exercises			X			
Proprioceptive training			X	X		
Eccentric/ concentric exercises				X	X	
Running						X
Sport-specific training						X
Provocation peroneal tendons						X

*Number of weeks after operation
ROM range of motion

Conclusion

Since peroneal tendon injuries are typically diagnosed in the active population, proper rehabilitation is key in the clinical success of treatment. For optimal immobilization time, surgeons must distinguish whether or not the SPR was repaired during the surgical procedure; if the SPR is not repaired, NWB time should be minimalized to prevent tethering of the tendon(s), aiming an immobilization period no longer than 4 weeks. In case a SPR repair is performed, the ankle should be immobilized for a minimum of 2 weeks. After initial NWB, the patient is allowed WB combined with physical therapy and supervised ROM to allow peroneal movement.

In this chapter, a rehabilitation protocol after surgical treatment of peroneal tendon injuries is proposed, based on best available evidence. It is important to keep in mind that the proposed protocol should be adjusted to every specific patient in order to optimize recovery.

References

1. van Dijk PA, Lubberts B, Verheul C, DiGiovanni CW, Kerkhoffs GM. Rehabilitation after surgical treatment of peroneal tendon tears and ruptures. Knee Surg Sports Traumatol Arthrosc. 2016;24(4):1165–74. PMC4823352.
2. Griffin M, Hindocha S, Jordan D, Saleh M, Khan W. An overview of the management of flexor tendon injuries. Open Orthop J. 2012;6:28–35.3293389.
3. Becker H, Orak F, Duponselle E. Early active motion following a beveled technique of flexor tendon repair: report on fifty cases. J Hand Surg Am. 1979;4(5):454–60.
4. Cullen KW, Tolhurst P, Lang D, Page RE. Flexor tendon repair in zone 2 followed by controlled active mobilisation. J Hand Surg Br. 1989;14(4):392–5.
5. Elliot D, Giesen T. Avoidance of unfavourable results following primary flexor tendon surgery. Ind J Plast Surg. 2013;46(2):312–324.3901913.

6. Savage R, Risitano G. Flexor tendon repair using a "six strand" method of repair and early active mobilisation. J Hand Surg Br. 1989;14(4):396–9.

7. Jielile J, Badalihan A, Qianman B, et al. Clinical outcome of exercise therapy and early postoperative rehabilitation for treatment of neglected Achilles tendon rupture: a randomized study. Knee Surg Sports Traumatol Arthrosc. 2015. https://doi.org/10.1007/s00167-015-3598-4.

8. Kangas J, Pajala A, Ohtonen P, Leppilahti J. Achilles tendon elongation after rupture repair: a randomized comparison of 2 postoperative regimens. Am J Sports Med. 2007;35(1):59–64.

9. Motta P, Errichiello C, Pontini I. Achilles tendon rupture. A new technique for easy surgical repair and immediate movement of the ankle and foot. Am J Sports Med. 1997;25(2):172–6.

10. Solveborn SA, Moberg A. Immediate free ankle motion after surgical repair of acute Achilles tendon ruptures. Am J Sports Med. 1994;22(5):607–10.

11. Uchiyama E, Nomura A, Takeda Y, Hiranuma K, Iwaso H. A modified operation for Achilles tendon ruptures. Am J Sports Med. 2007;35(10):1739–43.

12. Demetracopoulos CA, Vineyard JC, Kiesau CD, Nunley JA. Long-term results of debridement and primary repair of peroneal tendon tears. Foot Ankle Int. 2014;35(3):252–7.

13. Karlsson J, Wiger P. Longitudinal Split of the Peroneus Brevis Tendon and Lateral Ankle Instability: Treatment of Concomitant Lesions. J Athl Train. 2002;37(4):463–6. Pmc164378.

14. Karlsson J, Brandsson S, Kalebo P, Eriksson BI. Surgical treatment of concomitant chronic ankle instability and longitudinal rupture of the peroneus brevis tendon. Scand J Med Sci Sports. 1998;8(1):42–9.

15. van Dijk PA, Miller D, Calder J, et al. The ESSKA-AFAS international consensus statement on peroneal tendon pathologies. Knee Surg Sports Traumatol Arthrosc. 2018. epub ahead of print.

Peroneal Tendon Injury Associated with the Cavus Foot

Gregory P. Guyton

Peroneal tendon pathology and the cavovarus foot shape are closely aligned. Excessive weight-bearing on the lateral column of the foot yields, in turn, excessive strains on the peroneal tendons and the potential for acute or degenerative tears. The deformity is also commonly associated with lateral ankle ligament laxity. The simultaneous correction of the cavovarus foot, peroneal tendon pathology, and the lateral ankle ligament laxity presents unique challenges of surgical access and decision-making.

The Cavovarus Foot

Who Needs Correction?

The most fundamental question is also the most difficult to answer: what degree of cavovarus deformity requires correction in the presence of peroneal pathology? Even assessing the cavus foot is often a qualitative exercise. Traditionally, an effort has been made to describe these feet as being driven by *forefoot* or *hindfoot* cavus as well as being *rigid* or *flexible*.

Forefoot Cavus

Forefoot cavus implies a deformity in which the first metatarsal is plantarflexed relative to the axis of the talus. It is assessed on the lateral weight-bearing radiograph as a talo-first metatarsal angle that varies from zero. Typically, the apex of the

G. P. Guyton (✉)
Department of Orthopaedic Surgery, MedStar Union Memorial Hospital,
Baltimore, MD, USA

© Springer Nature Switzerland AG 2020
M. Sobel (ed.), *The Peroneal Tendons*,
https://doi.org/10.1007/978-3-030-46646-6_22

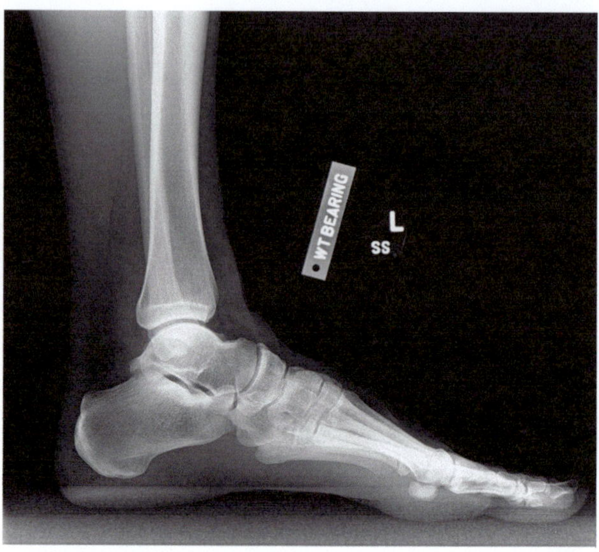

Fig. 22.1 Lateral radiograph showing cavovarus deformity

deformity occurs at the level of the first tarsometatarsal joint or at the naviculocuneiform joint (Figs. 22.1 and 22.2).

Forefoot cavus is the hallmark of Charcot-Marie-Tooth disease, a group of inherited neurologic disorders in which the anterior and lateral compartment musculature of the leg is typically weakened relative to that of the posterior compartments [1, 2]. Most cases of the disorder exhibit relative sparing of peroneus longus function, likely due to a more direct pathway of innervation for that muscle [3]. In these cases, the overpull of the intact peroneus longus against the weakened anterior tibialis plantarflexes the first ray; the hindfoot falls into varus passively. The most common form, CMT 1-A, accounts for 60% of cases and involves a focal trisomy of a segment of chromosome 17 [4]. The duplicated segment contains the gene for peripheral myelin protein-22, a myelin sheath constituent. Numerous other point mutations in several genes can also produce the CMT phenotype. While the disease is heritable, roughly 50% of clinical cases represent new mutations or chromosomal rearrangements. This is an important point; previously undiagnosed patients do occasionally present for their foot and ankle complaints. Charcot-Marie-Tooth disease is relatively rare, with a prevalence of 1:2500 [1]. While most clinical cases involving a plantarflexed first ray are, in fact, idiopathic, making the diagnosis of CMT when evaluating a cavus foot is critical because it represents a *progressive* disorder. In addition to the bony correction of the cavus foot, appropriate tendon transfers in CMT can eliminate the worsening deforming forces. Typically, this involves transferring the still-functioning peroneus longus to the weakened peroneus brevis.

Hindfoot Cavus

Hindfoot cavus implies a deformity with a fixed vertical angulation of the calcaneus. The angle subtended by the long axis of the calcaneus relative to floor, the calcaneal pitch, is increased. In this case, the forefoot deformity is compensatory.

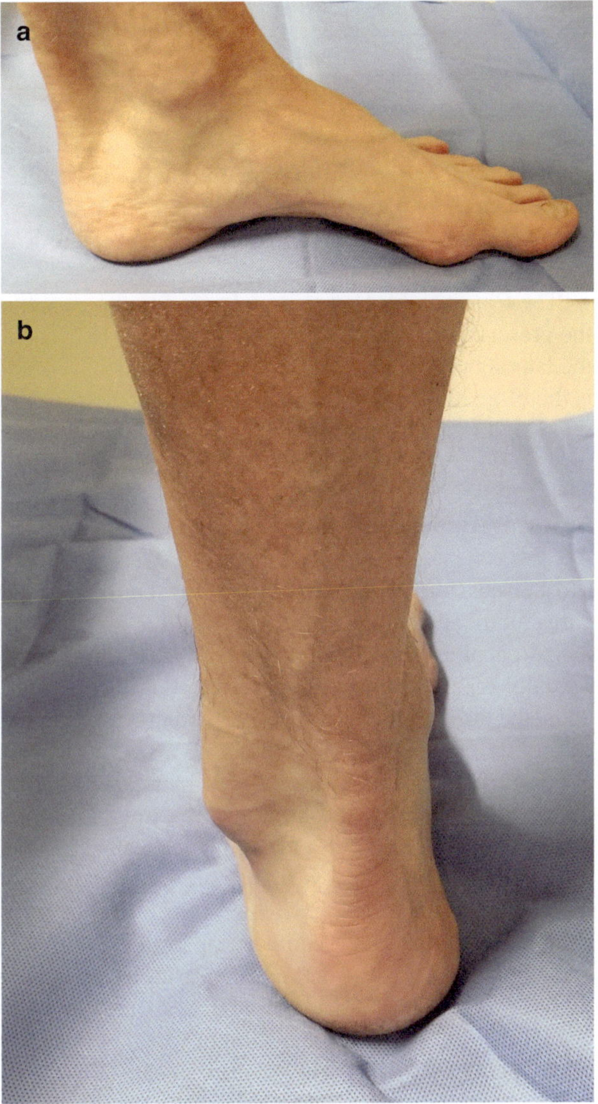

Fig. 22.2 Clinical photographs showing lateral view (**a**) and hindfoot varus (**b**)

Hindfoot cavus is classically associated with poliomyelitis and can be seen in profound neuromuscular conditions with preferential loss of the foot intrinsics [5]. With the absence of polio in modern practice, pure hindfoot cavus is rarely encountered.

Although the dichotomy between hindfoot and forefoot cavus provides a useful framework from which to approach the cavus foot, the majority of clinical situations in which the cavus foot is encountered in conjunction with reconstructable peroneal tendons are idiopathic in nature and have a mixture of elements.

Rigidity

The degree of rigidity in a cavus foot depends upon a number of elements: the severity of the deformity, whether or not it is congenital or acquired, the length of time it has been present, and the nature of any underlying neuromuscular condition. Rigidity is best viewed along a continuum, and either or both of the hindfoot and forefoot components can become fixed. In practice, correction of a rigid plantarflexed medial column can readily be corrected; it is most important to detect a contracture of the hindfoot.

The Coleman block test was devised to detect subtalar joint contracture even in the presence of a fixed plantarflexed first ray [6]. The patient is asked to stand with the lateral border of the heel and forefoot resting on an elevated block. The first ray is therefore allowed to drop, and the heel is viewed from behind. A mobile hindfoot will result in a normal valgus position of the heel; a rigid one will not move.

Metatarsus Adductus

Most discussions of the cavovarus foot focus on the cavus, but it is in fact the sudden varus moments applied to the hindfoot that give the most potential for pathology of the peroneal tendons. Metatarsus adductus is a developmental deformity thought to partially result from molding of the foot during intrauterine life. The forefoot is adducted through the level of the tarsometatarsal joints, typically with each metatarsal falling off medially more than the one to its lateral side to create a windswept appearance on X-ray. Most cases of metatarsus adductus slowly improve over the course of growth. For those that do not, mild deformities either manifest no symptoms or as mild irritation at the first metatarsal head. Severe deformities can have major implications, however. They are rare in adulthood and are almost completely overlooked in the literature. Because the center of pressure in the forefoot is moved medially, excessive load is placed on both the lateral metatarsals and the hindfoot. Fifth metatarsal stress fractures and insertional peroneal pathology may result.

The Peroneal Tubercle

The peroneal tubercle is a prominence of bone found on approximately 90% of calcanei that can have a variety of morphologies [7, 8]. It serves as an insertion point for the inferior peroneal retinaculum and divides the peroneus longus and brevis into separate distal sheaths. Additionally, it is the most common insertion point for the accessory peroneus quartus, a variation that is associated with hypertrophy of the tubercle [9]. Enlarged peroneal tubercles have been associated with tears of the peroneus longus secondary to a stenosing tenosynovitis [10–12]. There is no evidence that the incidence of an enlarged tubercle is higher in the cavus foot than its neutral or planus counterparts, but the forces on the peroneus longus are greater and the corresponding risk of tear is likely higher. A high index of suspicion should be generated for the enlarged peroneal tubercle as a source of pathology when a cavovarus foot is examined.

Radiographic Evaluation

Lateral X-Ray

The lateral weight-bearing radiograph readily allows the apex of the cavus deformity to be identified. The talo-first metatarsal angle is drawn down the long axis of the talus and ordinarily passes down the long axis of the first metatarsal. The boundaries of normal in the population remain ill defined, but traditionally the normally no angulation is present and a 4-degree drop in the first ray is considered to represent cavus [13]. The calcaneal pitch can also be visually referenced on the lateral view.

Qualitatively, the minimal overlap between the talus and calcaneus is evident in a cavus foot; the tarsal canal is well visualized as a round passageway between the two bones in the sinus tarsi.

AP Foot X-Ray

The AP foot view demonstrates relative collinearity between the long axis of the talus and the calcaneus. Care must be taken when interpreting this AP talo-calcaneal angle; standard radiographic views allow limited visualization of the two bones. Even among expert reviewers the inter-rater 95% confidence interval for measurement was 20 degrees [14].

Importantly, however, the AP foot view also allows the assessment of metatarsus adductus. The metatarsus adductus angle (MAA) is the most reliable and reproducible measurement. One line is drawn connecting the proximal point of the medial navicular to the distal point of the medial aspect of the first cuneiform. Another is drawn along the lateral border of the cuboid from its proximal to distal aspects. The midpoints of these lines are then connected to essentially define the horizontal axis of the midfoot (Fig. 22.3). This axis is then compared with the long axis of the second metatarsal. Metatarsus adductus is considered to be present if the value is above 20 degrees [15].

Hindfoot Alignment View

Efforts have been made to evaluate the overall alignment of the hindfoot by long AP or PA radiographs. The hindfoot alignment view popularized by Saltzman is most commonly used. A posterior-to-anterior view with the source centered on the ankle and oriented 20 degrees down the floor is shot with the film normal to the beam. The weight-bearing line of the tibia falls within 8 mm of the lowest point of the calcaneus in 80% of subjects [16].

Fig. 22.3 Radiograph
showing metatarsus
adductus angle (arrow)

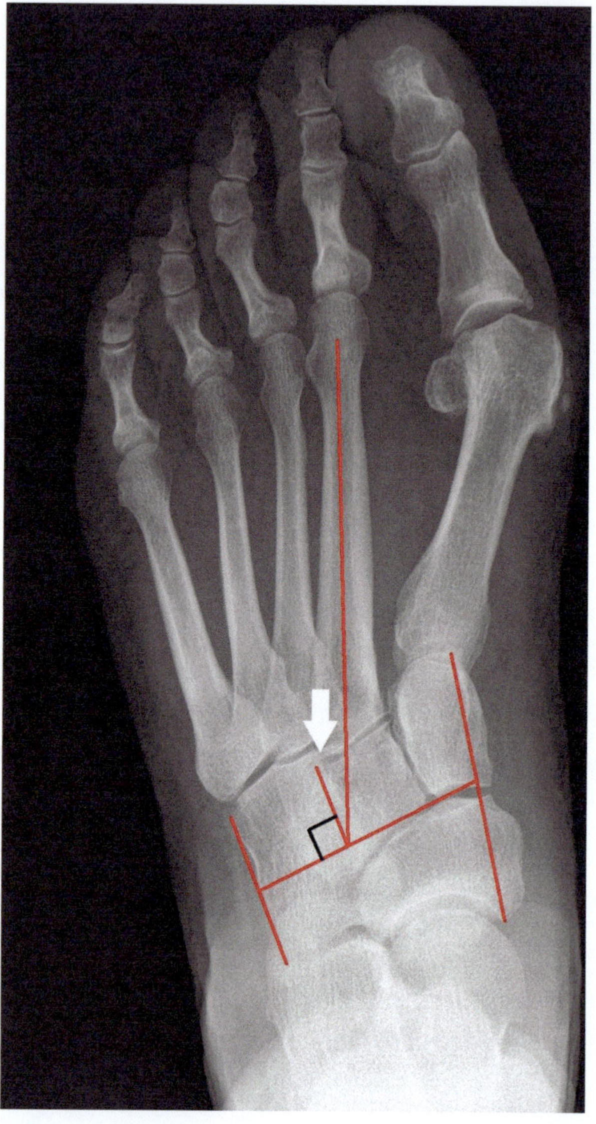

Recent interest in other variants of hindfoot alignment views has suggested that the method of Meary may demonstrate greater inter-rater reliability [17]. This view is essentially a mortise view of the ankle with a flexible wire applied as a stirrup around the hindfoot. The long axis of the tibia is compared to the center of the radiographic footprint of the soft tissue around the hindfoot. Normal values exhibit a slight valgus alignment of 3.9 ± 3.5 degrees. The reliability of both Saltman and Meary views has been reported as relatively poor, however [18].

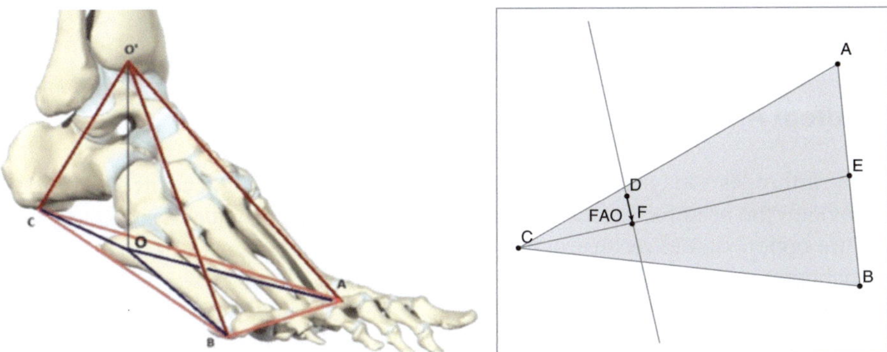

Fig. 22.4 Foot and ankle offset

Weight-Bearing CT Scans

Weight-bearing CT scans have recently come into clinical use. They offer an opportunity to automate the process of measuring the alignment of the medial column and the hindfoot. Several candidate measurements based upon the measurement of anatomic points on CT have been proposed. Most common in current use is the Foot and Ankle Offset, a measurement based upon the weighted center of triangle defined by the weight-bearing points of the calcaneus, the first metatarsal head, and the fifth metatarsal head compared to the axial position of the highest and centermost point on the talar dome (Fig. 22.4) [19]. The value is then normalized to the size of the foot and reported as a percentage. Normal values are 2.3% ± 2.9%. Most importantly, the interobserver reliability has been reported as 0.99, a very significant improvement over standard X-ray. To date, large-scale clinical studies correlating the outcomes of surgical procedures utilizing weight-bearing CT data have not been reported.

Criteria for Bony Correction with Peroneal Pathology

No clear data exist that clearly correlate the failure of peroneal tendon repair or reconstruction with the failure to reconstruct any particular magnitude of a cavovarus or metatarsus adductus deformity. In their absence, the criterion most appropriately used should be that also associated with lateral ankle ligament reconstruction; the presence of any appreciable calcaneal varus deformity should be corrected to prevent excessive force on the repaired lateral soft tissues.

Metatarsus adductus is generally better tolerated in its milder forms. As a general rule, only deformities with very significant metatarsus adductus angles far greater than 20 degrees should be considered for correction in conjunction with peroneal repair. Additionally, the presence of chronic stress fractures of the lateral metatarsals is a relative indication for bony reconstruction.

Surgical Strategies for Concurrent Bony Correction with Peroneal Repair/Reconstruction

Hindfoot Arthrodesis

Triple arthrodesis may represent the only option for severe, rigid cavus deformities. It obviates the need for functioning peroneal tendons and provides a secondary procedure option should reconstruction fail. The peroneal tendons can be resected in conjunction with a triple arthrodesis. In addition to the immediate negative clinical effects of hindfoot stiffness, however, triple arthrodesis does carry long-term risk of adjacent joint arthritis, particularly involving the ankle [20]. It should be considered a salvage procedure.

There are circumstances in which isolated subtalar arthritis mandates fusion of the subtalar joint alone. Correction of varus deformity through a subtalar fusion can be accomplished; in addition to removing a laterally based wedge of bone from the joint, care must be taken to allow the talar head to rotate medially and diverge as the deformity is corrected. Fusion of the subtalar joint does not eliminate the need for functional peroneal tendons; if the tendons are resected the unopposed pull of the posterior tibialis may still lead to further abduction deformity through the transverse tarsal joint.

Spasticity and Tendon Rebalancing

Cavovarus deformities associated with spasticity may present in conjunction with peroneal pathology; care in each case must be individualized to the pattern of disease.

Spasticity associated with cerebrovascular accident most typically results in tonic activity of the anterior tibialis tendon due to involvement of the motor cortex supplied by the middle cerebral artery [21]. The traditional approach has been to consider a split transfer of the anterior tibialis tendon to the cuboid, but a whole tendon transfer to the third cuneiform is more effective and carries no risk of overcorrection [22].

Spasticity of the posterior tibialis is commonly associated with cerebral palsy and may be subtle. Some patients with severe disease may be better served by triple arthrodesis, but rebalancing is mandated in conjunction with peroneal procedures if a dynamic inversion force is intractable. This may take the form of Botulinum toxin injections in milder cases [23]. Fractional lengthening of the posterior tibialis at the myotendinous junction can be performed in more severe cases without fixed deformity [24].

Dorsiflexion Osteotomy of First Ray/First TMT Fusion

The mainstay of the treatment for a plantarflexed first ray is the dorsiflexion osteotomy of the first metatarsal [19]. The surgery is easily accomplished with a greenstick osteotomy hinging on the plantar cortex made parallel and approximately 1 cm distal to the tarsometatarsal joint. The degree of deformity correction required dictates the degree of wedge resection required, but 4–5 mm inclusive of the kerf of the saw blade is typically removed. Fixation may be undertaken in many ways, but a dorsally based T-plate prebent to accommodate the desired dorsiflexion is easily applied.

The desired correction can also be easily accomplished through fusion of the first tarsometatarsal joint if arthritis or severe deformity is present. The joint is deeper than commonly appreciated, with a vertical dimension of approximately 30 mm. Any wedge cuts accomplished in conjunction with fusion must take this into account.

Lateralizing Calcaneal Osteotomy

Several variants of lateralizing calcaneal osteotomy may be used to bring the weight-bearing surface of the calcaneus laterally in the commonly encountered situation of a still-mobile subtalar joint but inadequate hindfoot eversion to allow the heel to come out of varus [25].

The Dwyer osteotomy is a simple laterally based oblique wedge resection of the calcaneus that provides correction through a hinged closure of the bone. The additional correction associated with wedge correction is often unnecessary, and a simple lateral sliding osteotomy will often suffice. For maximal correction, a lateralizing wedge and slide may be combined [20].

The Malerba osteotomy represents an additional option for lateralization. A step-cut is made in the calcaneus from a lateral approach and a wedge resected from the horizontal limb. A recent biomechanical study has demonstrated no additional corrective force for the Malerba osteotomy beyond that afforded by the Dwyer osteotomy combined with lateral displacement [26]. Given that this osteotomy also requires extensive dissection underneath the bed of the peroneal tendons, it is not recommended in conjunction with peroneal reconstruction.

Regardless of the technique of lateralizing osteotomy chosen, there is potential for compression of the tarsal tunnel as the tuberosity is shifted. This was initially demonstrated through the use of MRI to measure the volume of the tarsal canal in cadavers following the procedures [27]. Limited clinical data are available; one small series has reported a risk of tibial nerve dysfunction as high as 34% [28]. Notably, however, no protective effect was associated with a prophylactic tarsal tunnel release [28].

Incision Planning for Multiple Procedures

Managing peroneal pathology in conjunction with the cavus foot almost always involves multiple procedures. Relatively long incisions over the fibula must be made to accomplish augmented lateral ankle ligament reconstruction or fibular groove deepening procedures. Calcaneal osteotomies cannot be performed through this approach without exposure and retraction of the sural nerve. A single-incision approach to all procedures on the lateral hindfoot is not appropriate.

This then begs the question: How closely can parallel incisions be safely made? Limited data exist to provide guidance. Most well studied are incisions for fractures of the tibial plafond. For many years, a 7-cm parallel incision rule was propagated in the literature [29]. The origin of the rule could be traced not to an evidence-based determination but to expert opinion in the original A-O manual [30]. A subsequent prospective evaluation of the procedure failed to demonstrate an effect of incision distance on wound healing despite an average skin bridge between incisions of 5.9 cm [31].

The Minimal-Incision Lateralizing Calcaneal Osteotomy

The peroneal angiosome passes between the incisions for lateral ankle reconstruction and that for calcaneal osteotomy [30]. This likely provides an element of safety, but it is still prudent to minimize the extent of the calcaneal osteotomy incision to the extent possible. Minimal incision techniques now offer an alternative to the open incision that may be applied to the multiple-procedure hindfoot to obviate the issue entirely.

Calcaneal osteotomies can readily be performed using a minimal incision with the Shannon burr [32]. A learning curve is required to use the technique and the resultant osteotomy yields an irregular cut with a typical kerf of 3 mm [33, 34]. The following minimal incision technique utilizing both a microsagittal saw and a micro-reciprocating saw offers an alternative that relies upon more commonly available equipment and creates a smooth cut without the use of a jig.

The patient is placed in a full lateral or floppy lateral position. Critical to the technique is the ability to obtain high-quality perfect lateral images of the ankle and hindfoot. The center of the calcaneal tuberosity is marked at a point 11 mm or less anterior to a line connecting the plantar fascia origin and the superoposterior apex of the calcaneus on the lateral view. While this approach point cannot guarantee complete avoidance of the small lateral calcaneal sensory branches, it has been demonstrated to consistently avoid the main trunks of the sural nerve laterally and medial and lateral plantar nerves medially [35].

A 5-mm oblique incision is made in line with the anticipated osteotomy (Fig. 22.5) and a small periosteal elevator is passed dorsally and plantarly to free the tissue over the site. A 1.6-mm K-wire is placed normal to the osteotomy and trimmed just above the skin to mark the center point of the osteotomy. This is then checked on lateral and axial fluoroscopic views (Fig. 22.6).

A 5-mm microsagittal saw blade is placed to a depth of 5–8 mm against the templating K-wire. It is then released from the handle and a lateral fluoroscopic image is used to confirm the angle of the blade matches the desired angle of cut (Fig. 22.7). The saw is then reloaded and driven across the calcaneus to create a channel in the center of cut.

Fig. 22.5 Photograph showing oblique incision

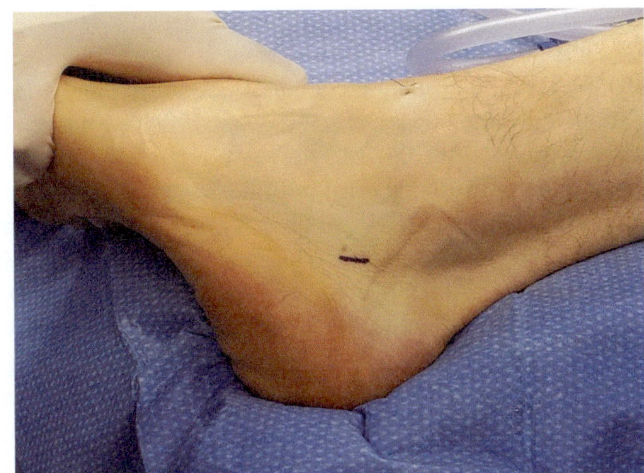

Fig. 22.6 A 1.6-mm K-wire placed normal to the osteotomy and trimmed just above the skin

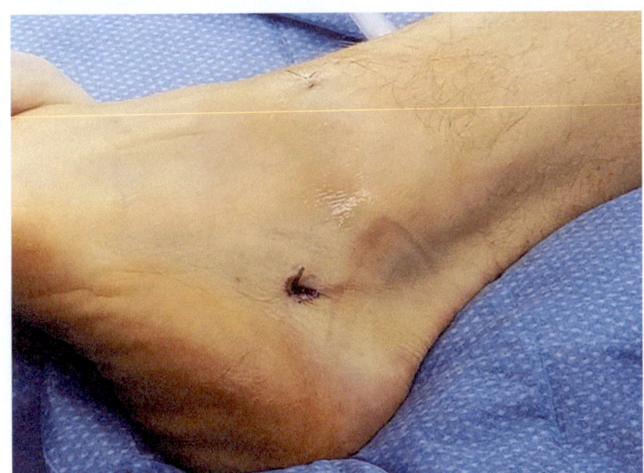

Fig. 22.7 Photograph showing saw blade used to confirm that angle of the blade matches the desired angle of cut

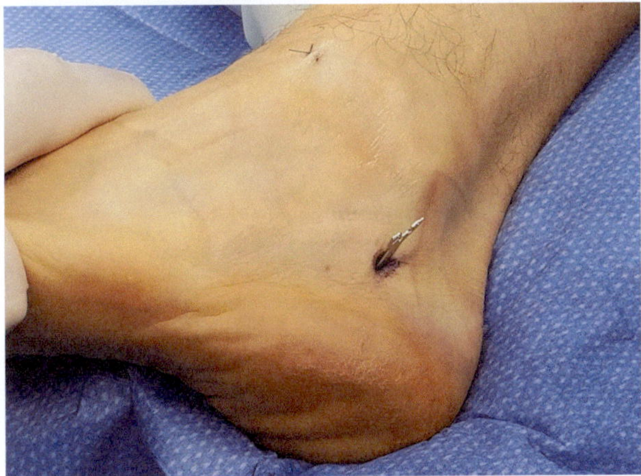

A micro-reciprocating saw is now placed down the channel created by the first cut. It is first used to complete the cut inferiorly by pivoting through the small lateral incision (Fig. 22.8). Unlike a burr, once started in the narrow channel created by the sagittal saw, the flat reciprocating saw blade would naturally follow the initial path to create a flat cut (Fig. 22.9). After completing the inferior cut, the blade is simply inverted and the dorsal portion of the osteotomy completed.

If necessary, a small Freer elevator can be placed in the completed osteotomy site to loosen the two fragments. Medial or lateral displacement is easily achieved. Axial screw fixation is then placed percutaneously (Fig. 22.10). Typically, a shift of 8 mm is achievable; more anterior osteotomy placement allows for greater displacement but places the sural and tibial nerves at a greater risk. The completed osteotomy incision is typically 5–50 mm, and larger parallel incisions for peroneal tendon reconstruction can easily be made with regard to spacing (Fig. 22.11).

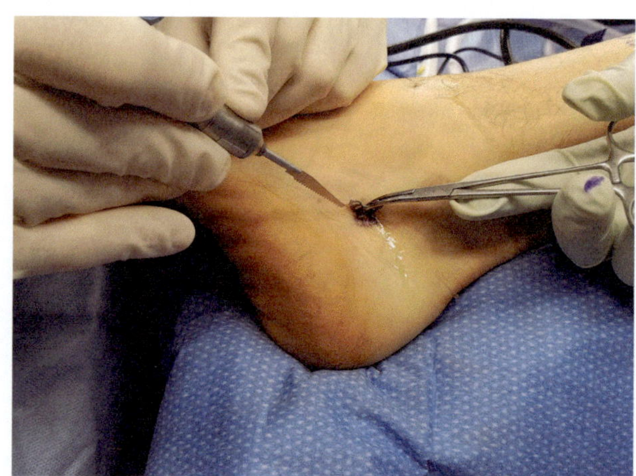

Fig. 22.8 Photograph showing cut being placed inferiorly by pivoting through the small lateral incision

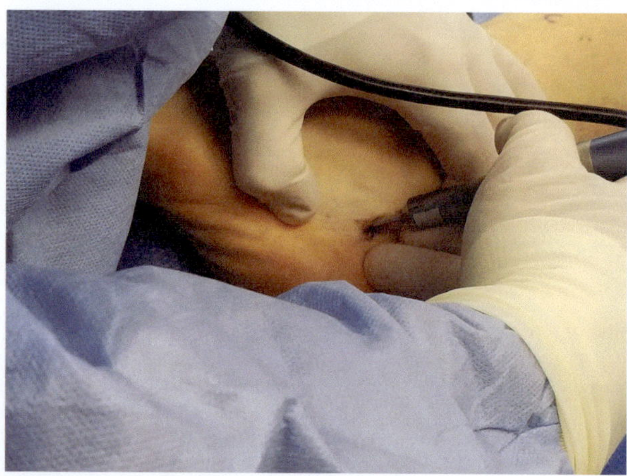

Fig. 22.9 The flat reciprocating saw blade naturally follows the initial path to create a flat cut

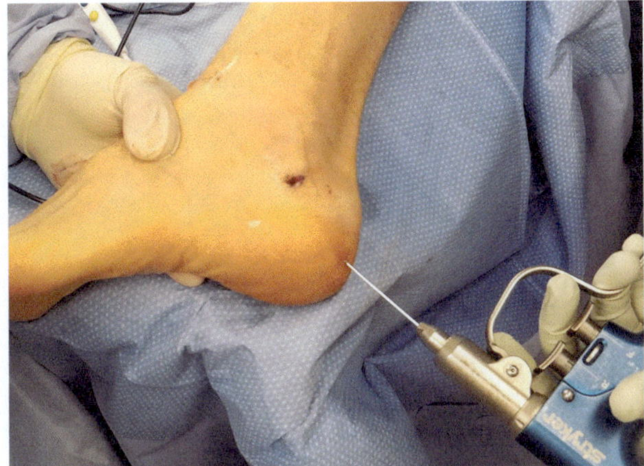

Fig. 22.10 Axial screw fixation done percutaneously

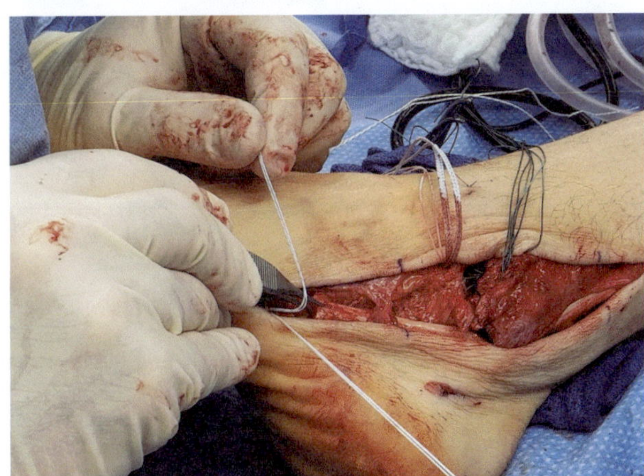

Fig. 22.11 Percutaneous lateralizing calcaneal osteotomy performed with peroneal debridement, longus transfer to the fifth metatarsal base, and Brostrom procedure

Surgical Correction of Severe Metatarsus Adductus

Metatarsus adductus is usually considered in conjunction with its effects on hallux valgus correction [15, 36]. In its severe variants, it becomes an important contributor to lateral foot pathology, including stress fractures of the lateral metatarsals and insertional peroneal pathology [37]. These severe cases are rare, and no evidence currently exists connecting any given magnitude of the deformity with outcomes of peroneal surgery.

When surgery for metatarsus adductus in an adult is indicated, arthritic changes in the medial column are common along with chronic stress reactions of the lateral rays. Severe deformities can only be corrected through surgery on all five metatarsals. One combination that appears well tolerated is fusion of the first, second, and third tarsometatarsal joints and osteotomies of the fourth and fifth metatarsals as required (Fig. 22.12). The procedure is challenging and requires individualized

Fig. 22.12 Radiograph showing severe metatarsus adductus. The right foot has undergone arthrodesis of the first, second, and third tarsometatarsal joints with osteotomies of the fourth and fifth metatarsals

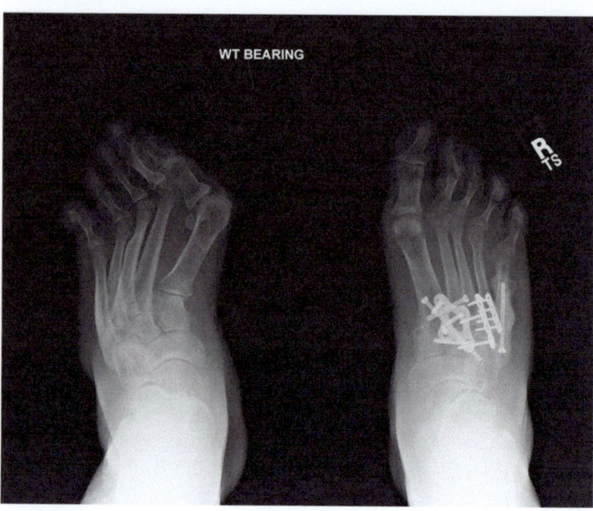

aligning cuts at the base of each metatarsal to reduce the deformity. Care must be taken to correct any elevation or depression of the medial column as well; both may be encountered.

References

1. Guyton GP. Current concepts review: orthopaedic aspects of Charcot-Marie-Tooth disease. Foot Ankle Int. 2006;27(11):1003–10.
2. Guyton GP, Mann RA. The pathogenesis and surgical management of foot deformity in Charcot-Marie-Tooth disease. Foot Ankle Clin. 2000;5(2):317–26.
3. Guyton GP. Peroneal nerve branching suggests compression palsy in the deformities of Charcot-Marie Tooth disease. Clin Orthop Relat Res. 2006;451:167–70.
4. Vance JM, Barker D, Yamaoka LH, Stajich JM, Loprest L, Hung WY, et al. Localization of Charcot-Marie-Tooth disease type 1a (CMT1A) to chromosome 17p11.2. Genomics. 1991;9(4):623–8. Epub 1991/04/01.
5. Schwend RM, Drennan JC. Cavus foot deformity in children. J Am Acad Orthop Surg. 2003;11(3):201–11. Epub 2003/06/28.
6. Deben SE, Pomeroy GC. Subtle cavus foot: diagnosis and management. J Am Acad Orthop Surg. 2014;22(8):512–20. Epub 2014/07/27.
7. Hyer CF, Dawson JM, Philbin TM, Berlet GC, Lee TH. The peroneal tubercle: description, classification, and relevance to peroneus longus tendon pathology. Foot Ankle Int. 2005;26(11):947–50. Epub 2005/11/29.
8. Agarwal AK, Jeyasingh P, Gupta SC, Gupta CD, Sahai A. Peroneal tubercle and its variations in the Indian calcanei. Anat Anz. 1984;156(3):241–4.
9. Sobel M, Levy ME, Bohne WH. Congenital variations of the peroneus quartus muscle: an anatomic study [published erratum appears in Foot Ankle. 1991;11(5):342]. Foot Ankle. 1990;11(2):81–9.
10. Palmanovich E, Laver L, Brin YS, Kotz E, Hetsroni I, Mann G, et al. Peroneus longus tear and its relation to the peroneal tubercle: a review of the literature. Muscles Ligaments Tendons J. 2011;1(4):153–60. Epub 2011/10/01.

11. Brandes CB, Smith RW. Characterization of patients with primary peroneus longus tendinopathy: a review of twenty-two cases. Foot Ankle Int. 2000;21(6):462–8.
12. Sammarco GJ. Peroneus longus tendon tears: acute and chronic. Foot Ankle Int. 1995;16(5):245–53.
13. Gould N. Graphing the adult foot and ankle. Foot Ankle. 1982;2:213–9.
14. Saltzman CL, Brandser EA, Berbaum KS, DeGnore L, Holmes JR, Katcherian DA, et al. Reliability of standard foot radiographic measurements. Foot Ankle Int. 1994;15(12):661–5.
15. Aiyer A, Shub J, Shariff R, Ying L, Myerson M. Radiographic recurrence of deformity after hallux valgus surgery in patients with metatarsus adductus. Foot Ankle Int. 2016;37(2):165–71. Epub 2015/11/15.
16. Saltzman CL, el-Khoury GY. The hindfoot alignment view. Foot Ankle Int. 1995;16(9):572–6.
17. Neri T, Barthelemy R, Tourne Y. Radiologic analysis of hindfoot alignment: comparison of Meary, long axial, and hindfoot alignment views. Orthop Traumatol Surg Res. 2017;103(8):1211–6. Epub 2017/10/03.
18. Dagneaux L, Moroney P, Maestro M. Reliability of hindfoot alignment measurements from standard radiographs using the methods of Meary and Saltzman. Foot Ankle Surg. 2019;25(2):237–41. Epub 2018/02/08.
19. Lintz F, Welck M, Bernasconi A, Thornton J, Cullen NP, Singh D, et al. 3D biometrics for hindfoot alignment using weightbearing CT. Foot Ankle Int. 2017;38(6):684–9. Epub 2017/02/12.
20. Saltzman CL, Fehrle MJ, Cooper RR, Spencer EC, Ponseti IV. Triple arthrodesis: twenty-five and forty-four-year average follow-up of the same patients. J Bone Joint Surg Am. 1999;81(10):1391–402.
21. Deltombe T, Gilliaux M, Peret F, Leeuwerck M, Wautier D, Hanson P, et al. Effect of the neuro-orthopedic surgery for spastic equinovarus foot after stroke: a prospective longitudinal study based on a goal-centered approach. Eur J Phys Rehabil Med. 2018;54(6):853–9. Epub 2018/06/16.
22. Henderson CP, Parks BG, Guyton GP. Lateral and medial plantar pressures after split versus whole anterior tibialis tendon transfer. Foot Ankle Int. 2008;29(10):1038–41.
23. Choi JY, Jung S, Rha DW, Park ES. Botulinum toxin type A injection for spastic equinovarus foot in children with spastic cerebral palsy: effects on gait and foot pressure distribution. Yonsei Med J. 2016;57(2):496–504. Epub 2016/02/06.
24. Altuntas AO, Dagge B, Chin TY, Palamara JE, Eizenberg N, Wolfe R, et al. The effects of intramuscular tenotomy on the lengthening characteristics of tibialis posterior: high versus low intramuscular tenotomy. J Child Orthop. 2011;5(3):225–30. Epub 2011/07/23.
25. An TW, Michalski M, Jansson K, Pfeffer G. Comparison of lateralizing calcaneal osteotomies for varus hindfoot correction. Foot Ankle Int. 2018;39(10):1229–36. Epub 2018/07/17.
26. Cody EA, Kraszewski AP, Conti MS, Ellis SJ. Lateralizing calcaneal osteotomies and their effect on calcaneal alignment: a three-dimensional digital model analysis. Foot Ankle Int. 2018;39(8):970–7. Epub 2018/04/05.
27. Bruce BG, Bariteau JT, Evangelista PE, Arcuri D, Sandusky M, DiGiovanni CW. The effect of medial and lateral calcaneal osteotomies on the tarsal tunnel. Foot Ankle Int. 2014;35(4):383–8.
28. Taylor GI, Pan WR. Angiosomes of the leg: anatomic study and clinical implications. Plast Reconstr Surg. 1998;102(3):599–616.
29. Thordarson DB. Complications after treatment of tibial pilon fractures: prevention and management strategies. J Am Acad Orthop Surg. 2000;8(4):253–65. Epub 2000/08/22.
30. Muller ME, Allgower M, Schneider R. Fractures of the shaft of the tibia. In: Manual of internal fixation: techniques recommended by the AO Group. Berlin Heidelberg: Springer Verlag; 1979. p. 278.
31. Howard JL, Agel J, Barei DP, Benirschke SK, Nork SE. A prospective study evaluating incision placement and wound healing for tibial plafond fractures. J Orthop Trauma. 2008;22(5):299–305; discussion -6. Epub 2008/05/02.
32. VanValkenburg S, Hsu RY, Palmer DS, Blankenhorn B, Den Hartog BD, DiGiovanni CW. Neurologic deficit associated with lateralizing calcaneal osteotomy for cavovarus foot correction. Foot Ankle Int. 2016;37(10):1106–12. Epub 2016/06/25.

33. Gutteck N, Zeh A, Wohlrab D, Delank KS. Comparative results of percutaneous calcaneal osteotomy in correction of hindfoot deformities. Foot Ankle Int. 2018;9:1071100718809449. Epub 2018/11/11.
34. Guyton GP. Minimally invasive osteotomies of the calcaneus. Foot Ankle Clin. 2016;21(3):551–66. Epub 2016/08/16.
35. Talusan PG, Cata CE, Tan EW, Parks BG, Guyton GP. Safe zone for neural structures in medial displacement calcaneal osteotomy: a cadaveric and radiographic investigation. Foot Ankle Int. 2015;36(12):1493–8.
36. Sharma J, Aydogan U. Algorithm for severe hallux valgus associated with metatarsus adductus. Foot Ankle Int. 2015;36(12):1499–503. Epub 2015/07/15.
37. Karnovsky SC, Rosenbaum AJ, DeSandis B, Johnson C, Murphy CI, Warren RF, et al. Radiographic analysis of National Football League Players' fifth metatarsal morphology relationship to proximal fifth metatarsal fracture risk. Foot Ankle Int. 2019;40(3):318–22. Epub 2018/11/08.

Peroneal Tendon Pathology Associated with Calcaneus Fractures

23

Rull James Toussaint, Nicholas P. Fethiere, and Dominic Montas

Anatomy

The peroneal tendons reside within a fibro-osseous tunnel and traverse the lateral calcaneus distally and serve to aid the peroneus longus and brevis muscles in pronating and everting the foot, aiding in foot stability and resisting inversion with ambulation [1]. The fibro-osseous tunnel is composed of the retrofibular groove, peroneal sheath, and superior peroneal retinaculum (SPR) at the ankle. At the hindfoot, it includes the lateral aspect of the calcaneus, the calcaneofibular and posterior talofibular ligaments, and the inferior peroneal retinaculum. The SPR is a thickening of the peroneal sheath and is the principal structure responsible for preventing subluxation of the peroneal tendons. The SPR runs from the distal tip of the fibula to the lateral wall of the calcaneous and the anterior portion of the achilles tendon sheath. It has been implicated in the relationship of calcaneus fractures and peroneal tendon subluxation [1, 2].

The original version of this chapter was revised. The correction to this chapter can be found at
https://doi.org/10.1007/978-3-030-46646-6_26

R. J. Toussaint (✉)
The Orthopaedic Institute, Gainesville, FL, USA

N. P. Fethiere
University of Florida College of Medicine, Gainesville, FL, USA
e-mail: nfethiere@ufl.edu

D. Montas
University of Florida, Gainesville, FL, USA
e-mail: dmontas@ufl.edu

373

Epidemiology

The calcaneus is the most frequently fractured tarsal bone and constitutes approximately 2% of all fractures seen in emergency departments [3–5]. The majority of which (approximately 75–80%) are intra-articular fractures involving the posterior facet or subtalar joint [4, 6]. Fractures of the calcaneus generally involve sustaining a high-energy force oriented axially which drives a primary fracture line as the talus lyses the calcaneus into anteromedial and posterolateral fragments with several classification systems describing the fracture pattern of the secondary fracture lines [4, 6]. One of the complications that may accompany calcaneus fractures but is often underdiagnosed and thus undertreated is peroneal tendon displacement (PTD), which includes subluxation or dislocation of the tendons [3, 4]. To date, the largest multicenter study investigating the relationship of PTD and calcaneus fractures found that 28% (118 out of 422 cases) of intra-articular calcaneus fractures had CT evidence of peroneal tendon displacement. However, only 10% of the 118 cases were acknowledged by radiologists and only 5.9% of the cases were treated by surgeons when performing open reduction and internal fixation of the associated calcaneus fractures [4]. A systematic review and meta-analysis involving nine studies identified a 29.3% prevalence of PTD (range 23.7–39.7%) in association with calcaneus fractures [3]. In addition, the prevalence of PTD increased with the severity of the fracture according to the Sanders Classification (Table 23.1).

Table 23.1 Association of calcaneus fracture classification and peroneal tendon displacement

	Number of cases	% with evidence of PTD on CT scan	
All cases included in study	422	28.0%	
"Fleck" sign on X-ray	44	84.1%	$p < 0.001$
Essex Lopresti classification			
Joint depression	321	30.8%	$p < 0.001$
Tongue type	100	19.0%	
Unclassifiable (gun shot wound)	1	0.0%	
Sanders classification			
Type I	44	4.5%	
Type II	169	16.0%	
Type III	138	34.8%	
Type IV	60	58.3%	Bonferroni $p < 0.002$
Unclassifiable (no coronal reformats available)	11	–	

The presence of the "fleck" sign, joint depression and greater fracture severity according to the Sanders classification was associated with a greater risk of peroneal tendon displacement (subluxation or dislocation)

Reprinted with permission from Wolters Kluwer Health, Inc. (Toussaint et al. [1])

History and Physical Examination

Calcaneus fractures are typically the result of high-energy mechanisms such as falls from a height or a motor vehicle collision. As such, these fractures commonly have associated injuries such as trauma to the spine and ipsilateral or contralateral extremity. Patients with calcaneus fractures should be subject to a thorough secondary survey to limit the delayed diagnosis and treatment of associated injuries.

The most common presentation for a patient with an isolated calcaneus fracture will involve pain, swelling, and ecchymosis at the injured hindfoot. Patients with concomitant PTD injuries may have similar complaints to those with isolated calcaneal fractures. Thus, a high index of suspicion will be necessary to diagnosis an associated peroneal tendon injury. Patients with a history of a high-energy mechanism are more likely to have PTD [4]. In addition, increased swelling over the lateral malleolus will also warrant further evaluation. During the examination, the surgeon may also palpate and manually reduce the dislocated tendons or ask the patient to actively evert the injured foot against resistance in an attempt to demonstrate dynamic peroneal instability.

Diagnostic Tests

A thorough physical examination is the standard for diagnosing isolated PTD. However, in the setting of an acute calcaneus fracture, physical examination findings may be limited by pain and swelling. A combination of preoperative and intraoperative diagnostic modalities is recommended to minimize the rate of missed diagnoses as well as false positives. Rosenberg et al. suggest that plain radiographs often inadequately define overlapping tarsal structures and underestimate the degree of posterior calcaneal facet displacement [6]. Plain radiographs clearly lack soft-tissue detail but highlight soft-tissue swelling. Wong-Chung et al. found that plain films to be a helpful diagnostic aid and should raise the clinician's index of suspicion when swelling is denoted at the level of the lateral malleolus [7]. The radiographic fleck sign represents an avulsion fracture of the distal fibula at the attachment site of the superior peroneal retinaculum and is largely considered pathognomonic for PTD [4] (Fig. 23.1). The fleck sign highly specific for the presence of the peroneal tendon displacement considering over 84% of cases with a fleck sign was shown to have peroneal tendon displacement in the presence of intra-articular calcaneus fractures. That said, its absence does not rule out the possibility of PTD, given that the fleck sign is only seen in 54.7% of cases with PTD [3].

Two reasons that PTD accompanying intra-articular calcaneus fractures may go unnoticed are the lack of soft-tissue detail present in plain radiographs and the limitations posed by the physical examination. Magnetic resonance imaging is the standard method for evaluating tendon disorders [8]. However, a CT scan is generally seen as a mandatory part of preoperative planning for all intra-articular calcaneus fractures. A paper by Ho et al. proposes a method for standardizing the diagnosis of

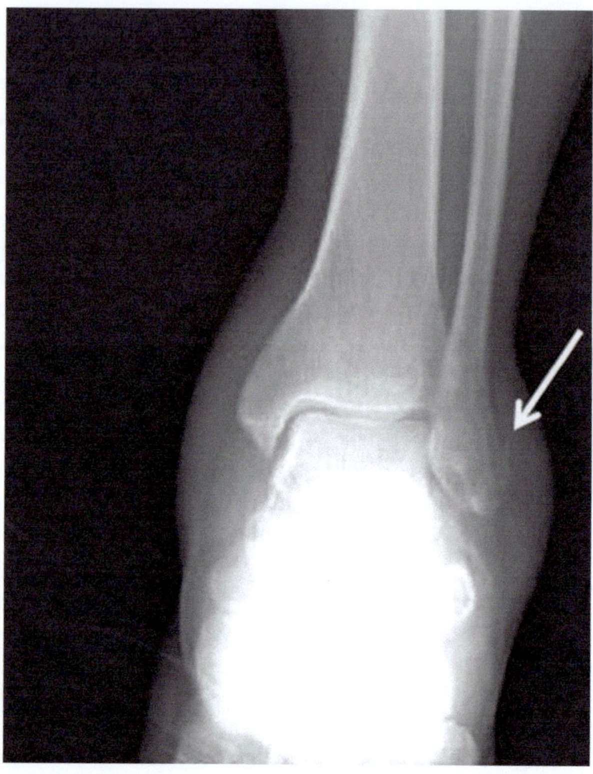

Fig. 23.1 An anteroposterior radiograph showing lateral ankle soft-tissue swelling and a subtle distal fibular avulsion fracture or fleck sign (arrow). (Reprinted with permission from Wolters Kluwer Health, Inc. (Toussaint et al. [1]))

peroneal tendon dislocation on CT imaging, thus making MRI imaging unnecessary in this case [9]. Ho et al. describe a three-step method utilizing a "triangle" of structures that should surround the peroneal tendons: the posterolateral margin of the distal fibula (anterolateral border), the superior peroneal retinaculum (posterolateral border), and the calcaneofibular ligament (anteromedial border). The second and third steps require finding the fibular groove, where the tendon sheath should lie, and a distal fibular avulsion fracture, which is indicative of retinacular damage or peroneal tendon dislocation [9] (Fig. 23.2).

Despite the aforementioned diagnostic advantage of a CT scan, Ketz et al. assert that the position of the peroneal tendons on preoperative imaging is of minimal importance [10]. In the absence of a clinically confirmed superior peroneal retinacular disruption, the displaced position of the peroneal tendons on a static CT image may overestimate the true prevalence of peroneal tendon instability, given that the problem is dynamic in nature [10]. In light of this, Ketz et al. conducted a study comparing the preoperative evaluation of peroneal tendon dislocation on CT imaging utilizing the technique described by Ho et al. and the detection of dislocation intraoperatively after fixing the calcaneal fracture with an extensile lateral approach. A Freer elevator was placed into the peroneal sheath to the level of the malleolus and anterior pressure to the instrument. Displacement of the elevator anterior to the malleolus is indicative of injury to the superior peroneal retinaculum and peroneal tendon instability [10].

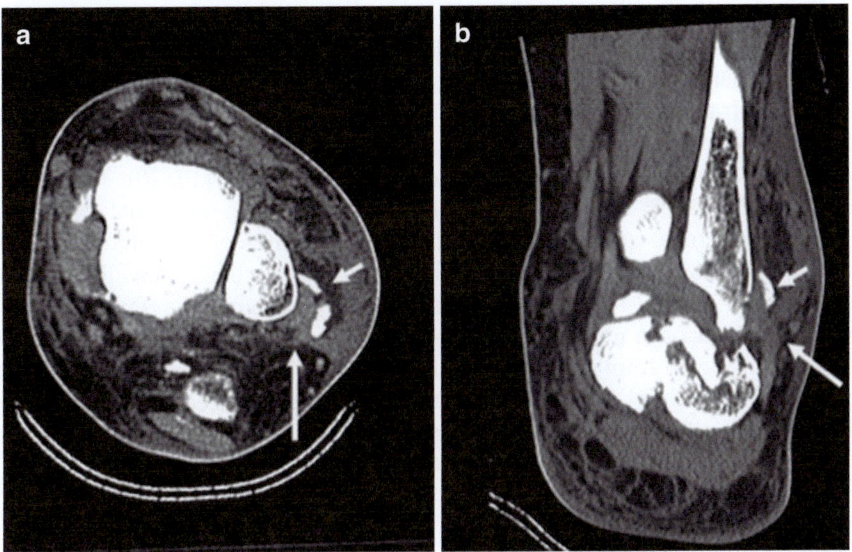

Fig. 23.2 Axial (**a**) and coronal (**b**) CT images acquired with the use of a soft-tissue algorithm. The short arrow indicates the fibular avulsion fracture or fleck sign, and the long arrow indicates the dislocated peroneal tendons. (Reprinted with permission from Wolters Kluwer Health, Inc. (Toussaint et al. [1]))

Surgical Treatment

Untreated isolated peroneal tendon disorders can lead to persistent lateral ankle pain and functional deficits [2]. In the case of acute isolated peroneal dislocation, surgery or temporary immobilization may be offered, although surgery is recommended for high-demand individuals and to limit the risk of recurrence. Surgery is preferred for symptomatic chronic isolated peroneal dislocations in order to achieve a satisfactory outcome [11, 12]. Although no studies exist comparing the outcomes of patients with and without surgical treatment of PTD after intra-articular calcaneus fractures, failure to treat PTD will likely lead to worse outcomes.

A number of surgical techniques have been described to treat patients with isolated peroneal tendon dislocation, including direct or indirect repair of the SPR, with or without addressing the retrofibular groove and tissue transfer techniques to reinforce the SPR [13–18]. However, patients with a combined calcaneus fracture and PTD will have limitations placed on the surgical approaches to treat the PTD due to the incisions utilized to address the calcaneus fracture.

Extensile Lateral Approach

The extensile lateral approach as described by Zwipp et al. and popularized by Benirschke has been utilized for decades as a utilitarian approach to calcaneus fractures. However, limitations of this approach include poor visualization of the peroneal tendons and wound-healing issues. Of particular importance is the vulnerability of the vascular supply to the lateral flap. The cadaveric study by Borelli highlights the importance of the lateral calcaneal artery (LCA) as the main arterial supply to the apex of the lateral soft-tissue flap overlying the calcaneus [19]. When performing the extensile approach to calcaneus fractures, the author addresses the peroneal tendon dislocation in the manner described by Ketz et al. and Ehrlichman et al. [10, 20]. This method minimizes the risk of vascular injury to the flap by avoiding additional incisions as required by alternate approaches [21, 22]. The vertical limb of the approach is made anterior to the lateral edge of the Achilles tendon to preserve the LCA while also avoid exposing the Achilles. The horizontal limb is at the junction of glabrous and nonglabrous skin. After open reduction and fixation of the calcaneus, the peroneal tendons are partly dissected from the flap at the level of the SPR. Care is taken not to over dissect and devascularize the flap. The tendons are then reduced within the groove, and the SPR is either repaired directly or reconstructed indirectly by creating a suture bridge of tissue attached to the lateral plate with absorbable suture.

Sinus Tarsi Approach

The sinus tarsi approach to calcaneus fractures has the advantage of allowing the surgeon to directly visualize the peroneal tendons. An incision is made overlying the sinus tarsi extending from the base of the fourth metatarsal distally and curving proximally along the posterior border of the fibula. Great care should be taken not to cause further injury to the peroneal tendons, since the dislocated tendons will be located laterally and relatively superficial to the malleolus. After open reduction and fixation of the calcaneus is completed, the author will extend the proximal aspect of the incision to allow visualization and repair of the SPR with either absorbable suture or anchors as needed.

Chronic Peroneal Tendon Injuries

The patient with a remote intra-articular calcaneus fracture will often present with lateral hindfoot pain. In this setting, the lead item on the differential diagnosis will be post-traumatic subtalar arthritis. However, surgeons should have a high index of suspicion to identify chronic peroneal pathology as another potential cause for the patient's pain. Rosenberg et al. found that impingement on the tendons by bony fragments correlated with the subsequent development of peroneal tenosynovitis in long term follow-up [23]. As a result, the clinician should consider a CT scan and/ or an MRI to further evaluate the integrity of the peroneal tendons and superior peroneal retinuculum prior to settling on an isolated diagnosis of subtalar arthritis. Depending on the imaging findings, the surgeon should be prepared to perform various procedures to address the peroneal tendon pathology. In addition to a subtalar joint fusion, a lateral calcaneal wall decompression, peroneal tendon debridement, reduction behind the fibular groove and reconstruction of the SPR may be necessary.

References

1. Tresley J, Subhawong TK, Singer AD, Clifford PD. Incidence of tendon entrapment and dislocation with calcaneus and pilon fractures on CT examination. Skelet Radiol. 2016;45(7):977–88.
2. Heckman DS, Reddy S, Pedowitz D, Wapner KL, Parekh SG. Operative treatment for peroneal tendon disorders. JBJS. 2008;90(2):404–18.
3. Mahmoud K, Mekhaimar MM, Alhammoud A. Prevalence of peroneal tendon instability in calcaneus fractures: a systematic review and meta-analysis. J Foot Ankle Surg. 2018;57:572–8.
4. Toussaint RJ, Lin D, Ehrlichman LK, Ellington JK, Strasser N, Kwon JY. Peroneal tendon displacement accompanying intra-articular calcaneal fractures. JBJS. 2014 Feb 19;96(4):310–5.
5. O'connell F, Mital MA, Rowe CR. Evaluation of modern management of fractures of the os calcis. Clin Orthop Relat Res. 1972 Mar 1;83:214–23.
6. Rosenberg ZS, Feldman F, Singson RD. Intra-articular calcaneal fractures: computed tomographic analysis. Skelet Radiol. 1987 Feb 1;16(2):105–13.
7. Wong-Chung J, Marley WD, Tucker A, O'Longain DS. Incidence and recognition of peroneal tendon dislocation associated with calcaneal fractures. Foot Ankle Surg. 2015 Dec 1;21(4):254–9.
8. Mitchell M, Sartoris DJ. Magnetic resonance imaging of the foot and ankle: an updated pictorial review. J Foot Ankle Surg. 1993 May-Jun;32(3):311–42.
9. Ho RT, Smith D, Escobedo E. Peroneal tendon dislocation: CT diagnosis and clinical importance. Am J Roentgenol. 2001 Nov;177(5):1193.
10. Ketz JP, Maceroli M, Shields E, Sanders RW. Peroneal tendon instability in intra-articular calcaneus fractures: a retrospective comparative study and a new surgical technique. J Orthop Trauma. 2016 Mar 1;30(3):e82–7.
11. Selmani E, Gjata V, Gjika E. Current concepts review: peroneal tendon disorders. Foot Ankle Int. 2006 Mar;27(3):221–8.
12. Porter D, McCarroll J, Knapp E, Torma J. Peroneal tendon subluxation in athletes: fibular groove deepening and retinacular reconstruction. Foot Ankle Int. 2005 Jun;26(6):436–41.
13. Kelly RE. An operation for the chronic dislocation of the peroneal tendons. Br J Surg. 1920;7:502–4.
14. Mason RB, Henderson JP. Traumatic peroneal tendon instability. Am J Sports Med. 1996 Sep-Oct;24(5):652–8.
15. Micheli LJ, Waters PM, Sanders DP. Sliding fibular graft repair for chronic dislocation of the peroneal tendons. Am J Sports Med. 1989 Jan-Feb;17(1):68–71.
16. Ogawa BK, Thordarson DB, Zalavras C. Peroneal tendon subluxation repair with an indirect fibular groove deepening technique. Foot Ankle Int. 2007;28(11):1194–7.
17. Stein RE. Reconstruction of the superior peroneal retinaculum using a portion of the peroneus brevis tendon. A case report. J Bone Joint Surg Am. 1987 Feb;69(2):298–9.
18. Walther M, Morrison R, Mayer B. Retromalleolar groove impaction for the treatment of unstable peroneal tendons. Am J Sports Med. 2009 Jan;37(1):191–4.
19. Borrelli J Jr, Lashgari C. Vascularity of the lateral calcaneal flap: a cadaveric injection study. J Orthop Trauma. 1999 Feb 1;13(2):73–7.
20. Ehrlichman LK, Toussaint RJ, Kwon JY. Surgical relocation of peroneal tendon dislocation with calcaneal open reduction and internal fixation: technique tip. Foot Ankle Int. 2014 Sep;35(9):938–42.
21. Clare MP. Acute and chronic peroneal tendon dislocations. Tech Foot Ankle. 2009;8:112–8.
22. Mak MF, Tay GT, Stern R, Assal M. Dual-incision approach for repair of peroneal tendon dislocation associated with fractures of the calcaneus. Orthopedics. 2014 Feb;37(2):96–100.
23. Rosenberg ZS, Feldman F, Singson RD, Price GJ. Peroneal tendon injury associated with calcaneal fractures: CT findings. AJR Am J Roentgenol. 1987;149(1):125–9.

Peroneal Tendon Injury in the Elite Athlete

24

Robert B. Anderson, Eric Folmar, Michael Gans, and Mark Sobel

Introduction

Peroneal tendon problems can be divided into three categories, which often overlap: (1) peroneal tendonitis or tendinosis, (2) peroneal tendon tears (splits) or ruptures, and (3) peroneal tendon subluxation or dislocation [4]. Pain and swelling in the posterolateral aspect of the ankle or lateral hindfoot are the main presenting complaints. The presence of chronic lateral ankle instability, and/or a cavovarus deformity, may predispose the patient to peroneal tendon pathology [5–9].

Peroneal tendon disorders occur in one of three anatomic zones as described by Smith et al. [10]. The three zones are shown in Fig. 24.1.

The original version of this chapter was revised. The correction to this chapter can be found at https://doi.org/10.1007/978-3-030-46646-6_26

R. B. Anderson (✉)
Titletown Sports Medicine and Orthopedics, Green Bay, WI, USA

Associate Team Physician, Green Bay Packers, WI, USA

E. Folmar
Department of Physical Therapy, Movement & Rehabilitation Sciences, Northeastern University, Boston, MA, USA
e-mail: e.folmar@northeastern.edu

M. Gans
PTSMC Orthopedic Residency Program, West Hartford, CT, USA

Physical Therapy and Sports Medicine Centers, Guilford, CT, USA

M. Sobel
Lenox Hill Hospital - Northwell Health, Orthopaedic Surgery, New York, NY, USA
e-mail: msobelmd@comcast.net

© Springer Nature Switzerland AG 2020, corrected publication 2020
M. Sobel (ed.), *The Peroneal Tendons*,
https://doi.org/10.1007/978-3-030-46646-6_24

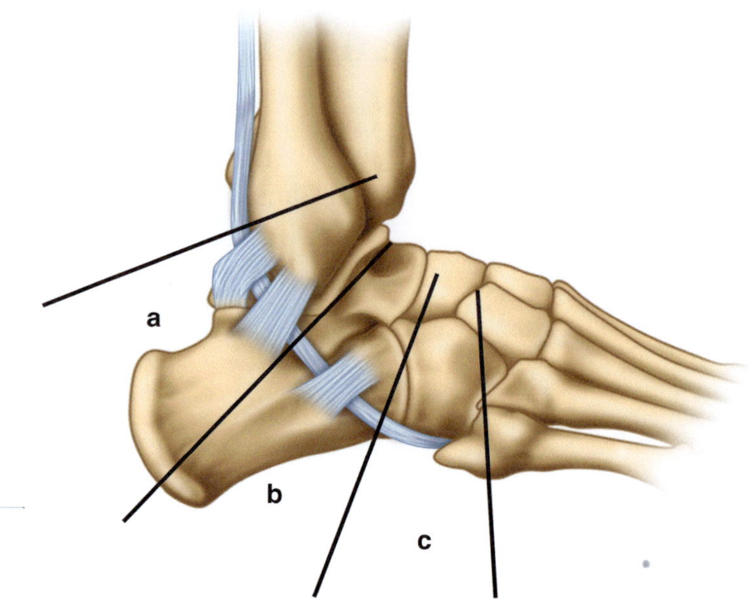

Fig. 24.1 Lateral view of the foot highlighting the three anatomic zones through which the peroneus longus tendon passes. Zone A is the region of the tip of the lateral malleolus and includes the area covered by the superior peroneal retinaculum. Zone B is the region of the lateral calcaneal trochlear process and covered by the inferior peroneal retinaculum. Zone C is the region of cuboid notch where the peroneus longus tendon turns to cross the plantar aspect of the foot [10]

In zone A, the region of the superior peroneal retinaculum (SPR), the peroneus brevis tendon can be torn or split longitudinally, as depicted in Fig. 24.2 [11, 12]. There is also the possibility of a low-lying peroneus brevis muscle belly or anomalous peroneus quartus causing encroachment within the fibular groove in this zone [13, 14]. These issues are often present in conjunction with tendon subluxation [15]. In zone B, along the lateral wall of the calcaneus, the presence of an enlarged peroneal tubercle can contribute to stenosing tenosynovitis of the peroneus longus tendon and one may see further splitting, tearing, or even frank rupture of the peroneus brevis tendon in this zone [16–18]. Zone C encompasses the cuboid tunnel, where the peroneus longus can rupture in an area of thinning and attenuation created by the os peroneum and its articulation with the cuboid. Injury to the os peroneum itself can include fracture of the os peroneum, shown in Fig. 24.3, or diastasis of an enlarged multipartite os peroneum, much like a hallux sesamoid [19, 20].

In the professional or elite athlete, an accurate and timely diagnosis is crucial, and accordingly, one must have a high index of suspicion for these injuries in those who present with pain along the posterolateral ankle and lateral hindfoot region. A thorough history and physical examination can be diagnostic. In addition, one should have a low threshold for rapid use of ancillary tests, such as MRI and high-resolution ultrasound. MRI can identify the pathology and help in planning an appropriate surgical treatment should nonoperative management be unsuccessful.

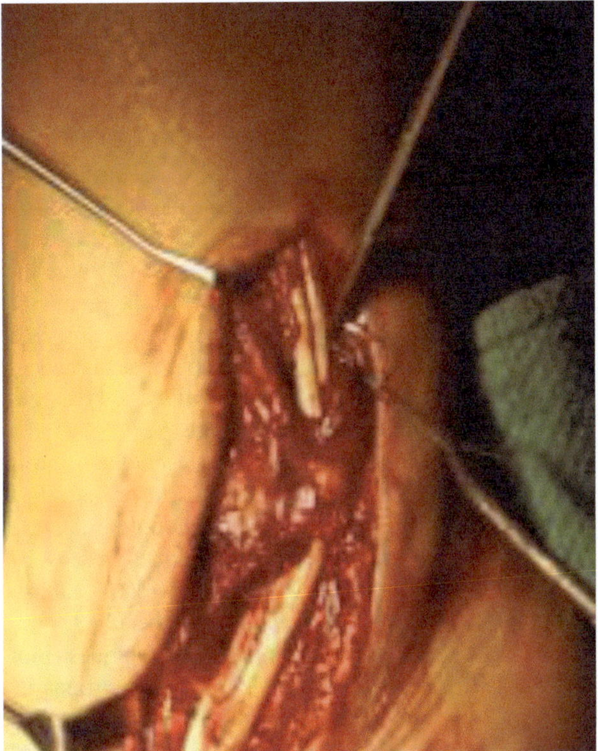

Fig. 24.2 Zone 1 Injuries. Associated with peroneal tendon dislocation, subluxation with split tears, and vice versa, tendon rupture, and lateral ankle ligament instability

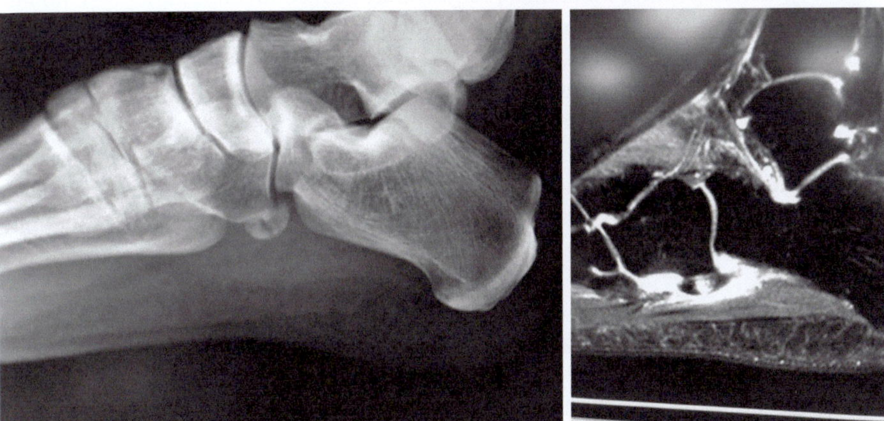

Fig. 24.3 Fractured os peroneum in zone C

However, unlike ultrasound, it is a static study and not helpful for tendon hypermobility, where dynamic ultrasound would be [21].

Various surgical procedures have been described and recommended depending on the specific pathology found at the time of surgery. These include tendon debridement or tubularization, removal of low-lying peroneus brevis muscle belly or anomalous peroneus quartus tendon, tenodesis, tendon transfer or graft, superior peroneal retinaculum repair +/− fibular groove deepening, and lateralizing calcaneal osteotomy or dorsiflexion osteotomy of the first metatarsal [1, 2, 4, 22–44].

Peroneal tenosynovitis often improves with conservative measures, such as rest with immobilization and injection with PRP, with surgery reserved for refractory cases. In contrast, surgical treatment is frequently required for peroneal tendon subluxation and includes anatomic repair or reconstruction of the superior peroneal retinaculum, typically with fibular groove deepening [34, 35, 45, 46]. Surgical treatment for peroneal tendon tears (splits) is based on the remaining viable tendon. Primary repair and tubularization is recommended for tears involving <50–60% of the tendon, and tenodesis is indicated for tears of the peroneus longus that are not repairable [4, 47]. It is now our preference to perform an interposition allograft reconstruction for complex tears and ruptures of the peroneus brevis [25]. Calcaneus and metatarsal osteotomies are considered in those with significant cavovarus [31, 48].

The mechanism of injury for these peroneal tendon disorders is quite variable, some do to acute forces while others present from chronic overuse [49, 50]. Given the forces generated, athletes are at more risk for both. In addition, hockey and baseball players are exposed to direct trauma along the lateral side of the ankle from errant pucks and baseballs. The surgical techniques employed for these peroneal tendon disorders are similar regardless of the individual's athletic involvement. Nonoperative modalities are initially attempted in both the athlete and non-athlete. This will include relative rest, immobilization, injection techniques (biologics), physical therapy, and orthoses. What does differ between the two groups is the duration of conservative treatment and postoperative care/rehabilitation. Given the player's schedule, a smaller window for conservative modalities is often the case. When performance limiting and refractory to nonoperative modalities, surgery may be recommended after 3–4 months so as not to interfere with consecutive seasons of sport participation.

This chapter wishes to illustrate the different injuries to the peroneal tendons in elite and "career" athletes, and the surgical procedures indicated with the rehab protocols recommended. In that light, the mechanism of injury may be the same for "elite" athletes and recreational ones, but given the high energy imparted with the elite athlete, the injuries are more common and dramatic. There may also be a relationship to the field surface and the cleat–turf interaction, as excessive torque may occur when a shoe fails to release.

History and Physical Examination

A detailed review of when and how the pain and swelling began is helpful. In acute situations, the athlete may recall a specific maneuver, perhaps ankle inversion or forced dorsiflexion against active plantar flexion. Chronic situations will require a discussion of what treatment methods have already been initiated. It is important to determine what maneuvers reproduce the pain, its location, and whether or not there is a feeling of subluxation.

The exam begins with a careful assessment of the entire lower extremity, evaluating the overall alignment with comparison to the contralateral. Genu varum and cavovarus are associated with lateral overload issues. Heel and toe walking is observed, along with one-legged maneuvers. Is pain or tendon subluxation reproduced with a single limb heel rise? The sitting exam determines areas of fullness, localized tenderness, skin or soft tissue changes, as well as continuity and function of the peroneal tendons. Resistance testing helps to assess for strength as well as for the presence of tendon hypermobility, intra-sheath snapping, tendon subluxation, and gross dislocation [49–51]. Ankle and hindfoot joints are tested for pain and instability, with careful comparison to the contralateral.

Imaging

Ankle and foot radiographs are performed routinely for all patients presenting with a potential peroneal tendon problem. As shown in Fig. 24.4, three views of the ankle are recommended as the oblique view better identifies abnormalities to the posterolateral rim of the distal fibula (fleck sign).

Foot X-rays help to highlight avulsions as well as the overall posture of the foot. The oblique view best demonstrates the presence of an os peroneum. Hindfoot alignment views assist with evaluation of the associated cavovarus posture.

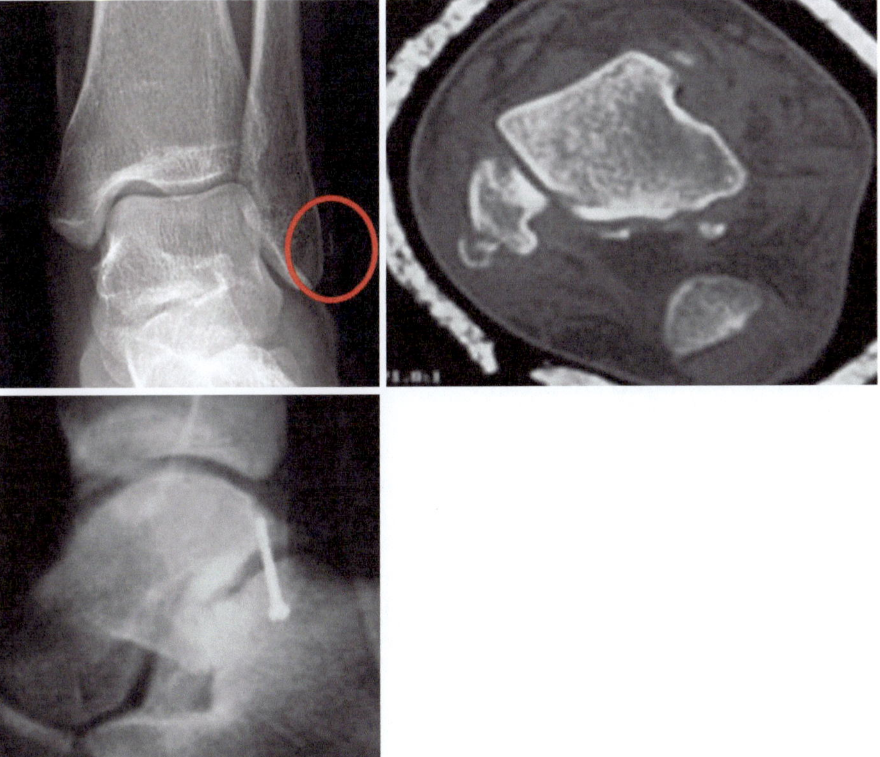

Fig. 24.4 Example of a peroneal tendon dislocation in a professional football player. SPR avulsion with a "fleck sign" (Type 3) was noted. ORIF was performed as the fragment was of adequate size

MRI is routinely ordered for those patients failing to improve with conservative care. Soft tissues are assessed, as well as any associated intra-articular pathology. The peroneal tendons are examined for tenosynovitis, tears, ruptures, and dislocation. However, it should be noted that longitudinal split tears can be difficult to identify on even the best MRI units. In addition, there is a phenomenon of the "magic angle." When a tendon changes direction, as the peroneals do, thinning and partial ruptures can be overdiagnosed. In addition, T2 weighted signals can overread ruptures, and the physician needs to consider this when embarking on surgical intervention. Ultrasound is another imaging modality useful in suspected peroneal tendon issues. Although technologist and reader dependent, this dynamic study helps to define the size of the tendon, its location, and whether it subluxes through various maneuvers.

Conservative Treatment Management

Nearly all peroneal tendon problems encountered are initially managed with nonoperative modalities: immobilization, relative rest, ice, compression, antiinflammatory medications, and eventually, strengthening. Cast immobilization, even for 1–2 weeks, is very beneficial for acute tenosynovitis/tendonitis. A cast ensures compliance over a boot, despite the inconveniences. Formal physical therapy is initiated once acute pain and swelling have subsided, with emphasis on peroneal tendon strengthening. Those with cavovarus will eventually be transitioned to a custom orthoses with a lateral heel wedge and forefoot posting. Associated lateral ankle instability is best treated with a brace that limits inversion. The entities not treated with initial nonoperative management are those with acute dislocation of the peroneals, dislocatable peroneals, and rupture of the peroneus brevis. Failing stage 1 management, other modalities to consider include injection of a biologic material. Cortisone can further weaken a diseased tendon and therefore is avoided for fear of rupture. However, amniotic tissue derivatives and PRP/stem cells can be considered.

Surgically Managed Disorders

As mentioned above, there are several peroneal tendon disorders that will require surgical intervention. Many of these may also need to address associated ankle ligament pathology and an overlying cavovarus [6–8, 48]. It is recommended that an MRI be performed prior to surgery to determine the need for arthroscopic evaluation of the ankle at the same setting. The surgeon needs to be prepared for all reconstruction options, i.e., allograft, hardware, and biologics. The postoperative course and rehabilitation are dependent on the pathology addressed.

Acute Peroneal Tendon Dislocation

It is very difficult to manage an unstable peroneal tendon (Fig. 24.5) nonoperatively. Both acute and chronic types typically require a fibular groove deepening and SPR repair. Multiple techniques for deepening are reported below.

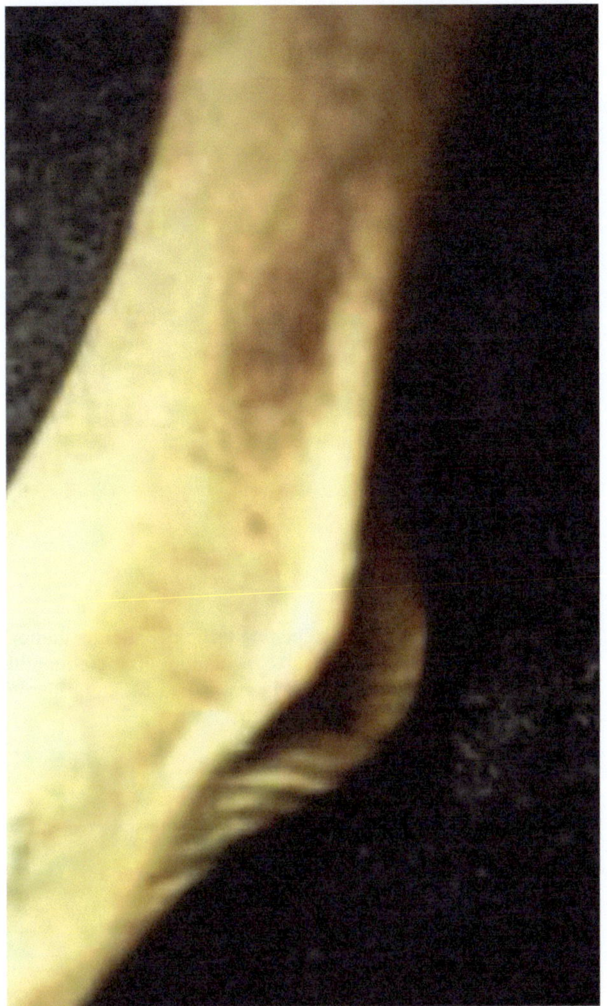

Fig. 24.5 Peroneal tendon dislocation

While a J-pad may be utilized to try to "buy" time, it will not suffice long term and could even place the patient at risk for split tears and frank ruptures of the peroneus brevis tendon. When embarked upon, surgical repair will nearly always necessitate deepening of the fibular groove [1, 45].

An isolated repair of the (SPR) should only be considered in the professional athlete, if it is an acute peroneal tendon dislocation and the patient is found to have a concave sulcus on imaging [49].

The most predictable manner in which to stabilize the tendons is to deepen the groove, as shown in Fig. 24.6, particularly in late presentations [45]. There are a number of different techniques described for fibular groove deepening [1, 35, 45]. Our preference has been to avoid an osteotomy or to create a bed of denuded bleeding bone that could lead to tenodesis and adhesions, thus the "indirect" method was employed [45]. Figures 24.7, 24.8, and 24.9 show the "indirect" groove deepening technique. First, we start with a small diameter drill at the origin of the CFL and

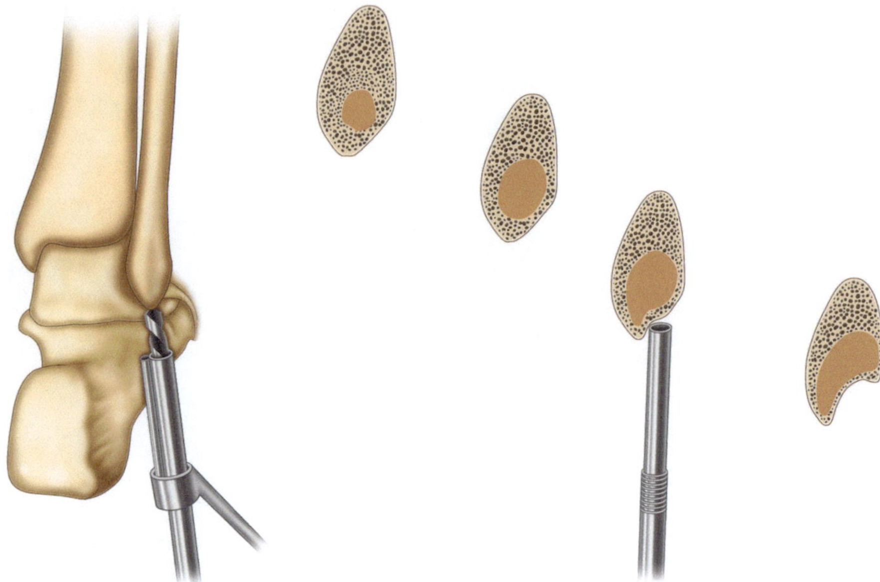

Fig. 24.6 "Indirect" groove deepening technique. Senior author's preferred technique since 1993 as benefits of a "minimally invasive" technique in the elite athlete. Advantages = an "eggshell" procedure. Impaction technique. Maintains soft tissue on peroneal floor. No osteotomy to heal. Good results reported at 2 years [45]

Fig. 24.7 Indirect deepening. Start with small diameter drill at the origin of the CFL and gradually increase diameters, thinning the cortical bone along the posterior aspect of the distal fibula [45]

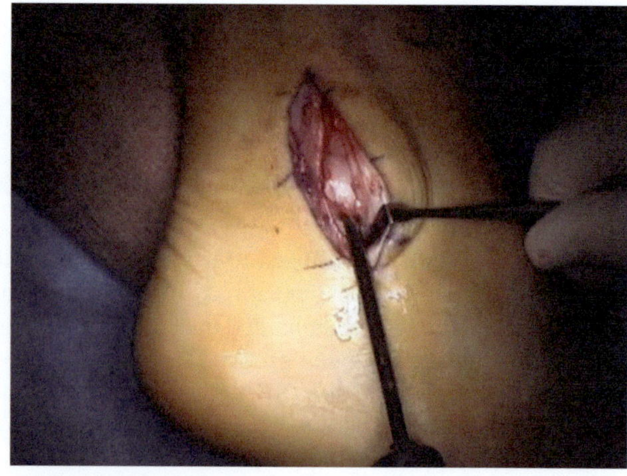

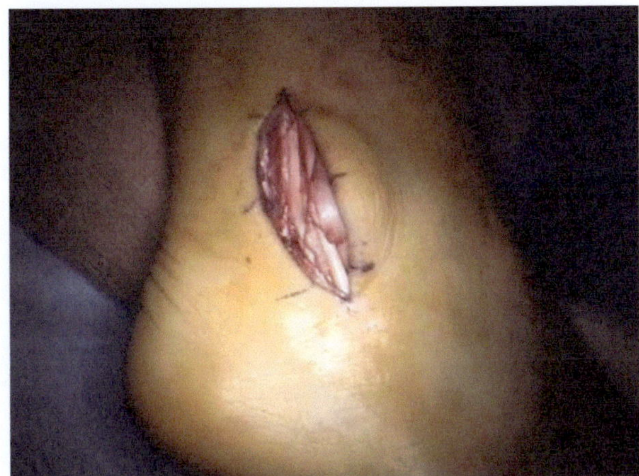

Fig. 24.8 Once the groove deepening is adequate, as assessed by coverage of both peroneal tendons in a neutral position, the SPR is repaired via drill holes in the posterolateral fibula

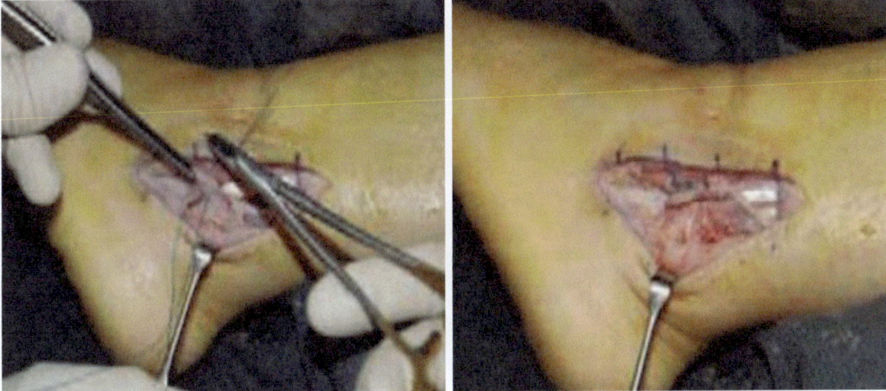

Fig. 24.9 Regardless of type, always add SPR repair. Preference is to do with drill holes in the posterolateral fibula

gradually increase diameters, thinning the cortical bone along the posterior aspect of the distal fibula [45]. Once the groove deepening is adequate, as assessed by coverage of both peroneal tendons in a neutral position, the SPR is repaired via drill holes in the posterolateral fibula.

This technique creates an eggshell of the distal fibula that allows the groove to be impacted inwardly, therefore accentuating the posterior rim. It is inherently stable, requires no bone healing, and maintains the natural floor of the groove [45]. In addition, the procedure includes removal of any excessive soft tissue in the sulcus, such as low-lying brevis muscle, or anomalous peroneal tendons (peroneus quartus). By doing so, there is more space to maintain the peroneus brevis and longus tendons posteriorly. Any split tears are identified and repaired. The SPR is excised of any redundancy and then secured back to drill holes in the posterolateral fibula, further stabilizing the tendons but avoiding a stenosis as well. This repair provides

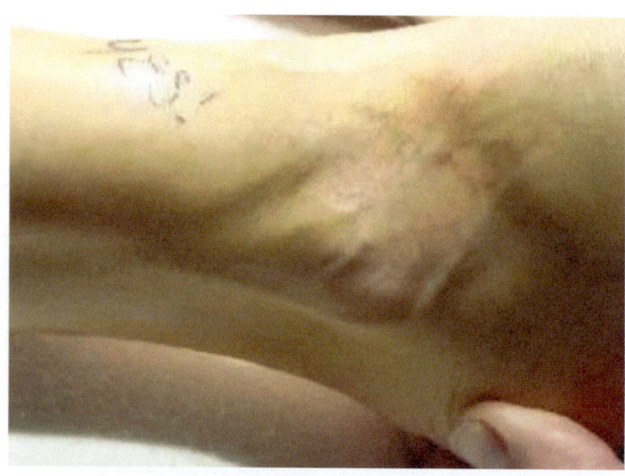

Fig. 24.10 Case example – peroneal subluxation

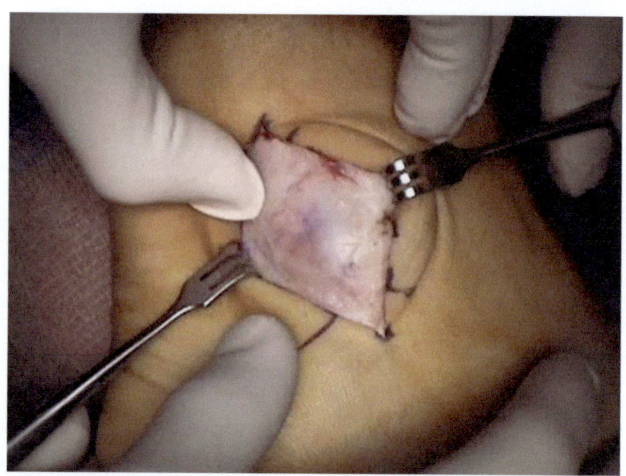

Fig. 24.11 Attenuated SPR

immediate stabilization of the tendons. Thereafter, the postoperative course consists of 2 weeks non-weightbearing in a splint, then weightbearing in a boot for 6 weeks. During this time, gentle active dorsiflexion and plantarflexion are initiated. Straight line running activity commences at 8 weeks and cutting maneuvers by 12 weeks. The athlete is then cleared for all on-field or court activities and returns to full athletic participation when functional recovered.

Figures 24.10, 24.11, and 24.12 show a case example of peroneal subluxation gradually worsening with pain. Upon surgical exploration, the SPR was attenuated. The low lying and hypertrophic peroneus brevis was debrided and debulked.

Figure 24.13 depicts the MRI results of an 18-year-old basketball player with inversion injury. The patient presented with chronic lateral ankle pain and swelling. While the X-rays were negative, MRI results show peroneal tendon dislocation. Figures 24.14 and 24.15 show the indirect groove deepening technique being utilized to repair the torn tendon.

Fig. 24.12 Debride/
debulk low-lying and
hypertrophic
peroneus brevis

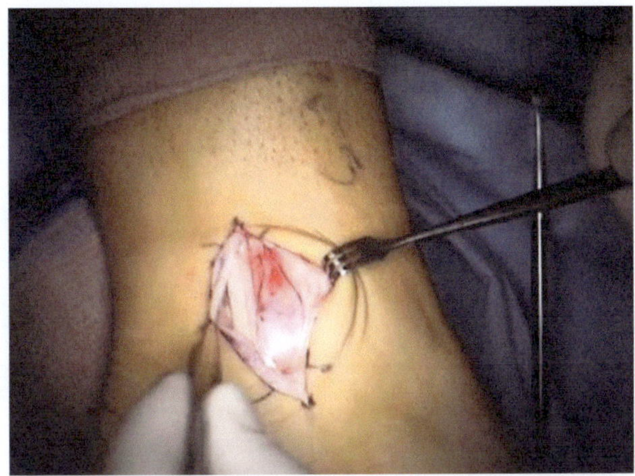

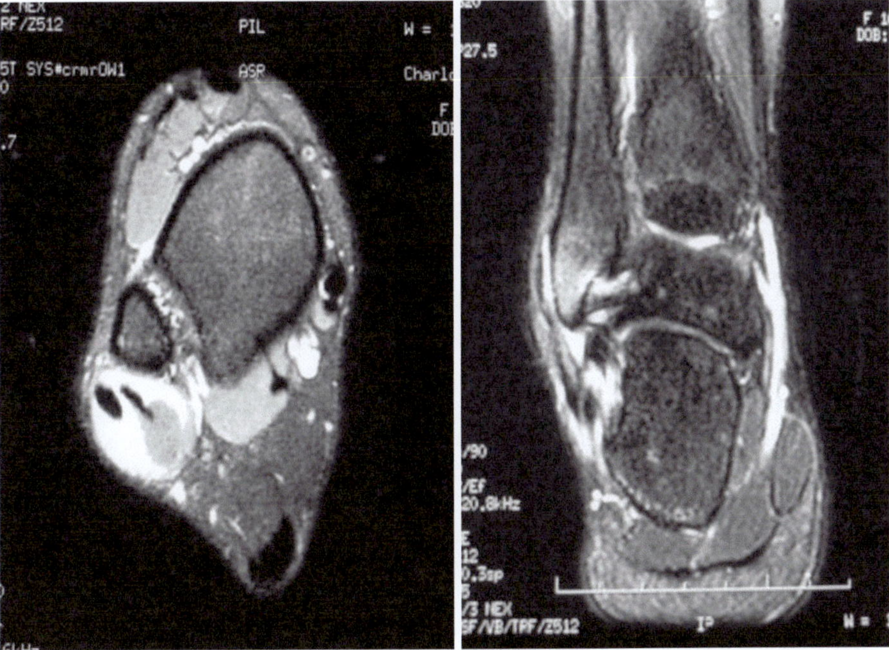

Fig. 24.13 MRI on an elite basketball player confirming peroneal dislocation

Peroneus Longus Rupture/Os Peroneum Syndrome

A number of athletes sustaining these injuries are relatively pain free and functional after 4–6 weeks of immobilization and relative rest. However, those who have persistent pain and swelling in the Zone 3/C region of the hindfoot may require surgical intervention. This is particularly true in those with underlying cavovarus (Fig. 24.16).

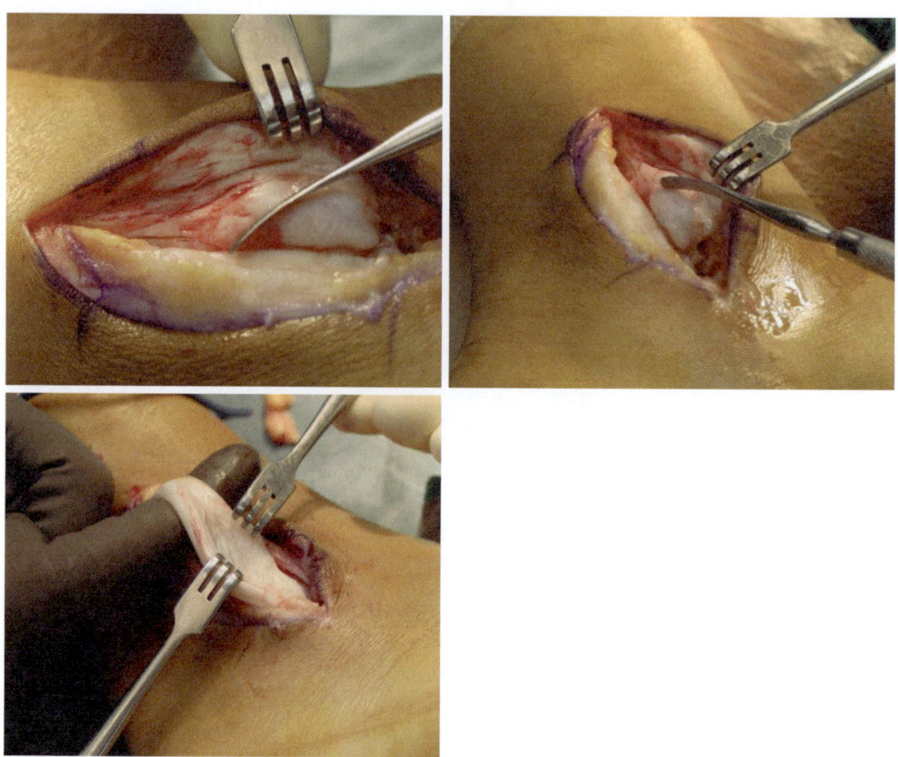

Fig. 24.14 Peroneal subluxation with tear

It is extremely difficult, and unsatisfying, to attempt a repair of a peroneus longus rupture in that location. Even maintaining a longus tendon while exercising a diseased os peroneum is problematic. Therefore, these situations are best addressed with a side-to-side tenodesis to the peroneus brevis tendon [19].

Figures 24.17 and 24.18 show a series of images treating a cavovarus patient with peroneus longus rupture in zone 3. A first metatarsal long oblique dorsiflexion osteotomy is performed with bicortical screw fixation, given the underlying cavovarus (Fig. 24.17). The peroneus longus rupture is then managed with debridement, and tenodesis to the brevis tendon (Fig. 24.18).

The anastomosis is performed with distal retraction on the longus to obtain appropriate tension. In the event the longus is still in continuity, it is best to create the tenodesis prior to excising the diseased distal portion. The peroneal tubercle is removed to avoid placing pressure on the anastomosis. Amniotic tissue products are often utilized in an effort to lessen adhesions. A non-weightbearing splint is applied in the operating room and the patient can be advanced to a weightbearing boot at 2 weeks. Gentle range of motion (ROM) is initiated but resistance exercises are avoided until 8 weeks postoperative. Most athletes can return to full participation by 16 weeks.

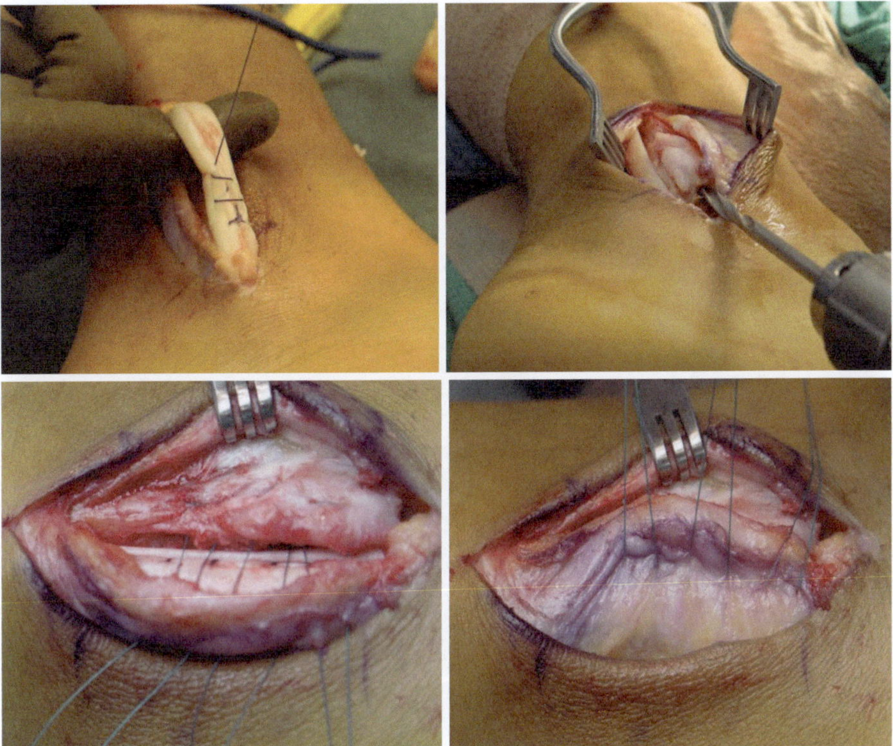

Fig. 24.15 Repair of tear with groove deepening and repair of SPR

Peroneus Brevis Split Tear in Association with Chronic Lateral Ankle Instability

Split tears of the peroneus brevis can occur in conjunction with subluxation, as previously mentioned, or with chronic lateral ankle instability, or both [6–9]. These tears can be located centrally, in the periphery, or may be complex in nature. Central tears can be debrided and repaired with a running suture, typically a PDS or proline type. Peripheral tears of even 60% can be excised and tapered [47]. As shown in Fig. 24.19, a tear less than 50% is excised and tubularized.

Some complex tears can be salvaged with debridement and tuberization, while others may require excision with tenodesis or allograft interposition. The associated lateral ankle instability can be managed with any technique the surgeon feels comfortable with. This may be a modified Brostrom-Gould procedure, an artificial ligament augmentation, or allograft/autograft hamstring tendon weave. Given the already compromised peroneal tendon, an augmentation or transfer utilizing that structure is not recommended. The postoperative course is dependent on the extent

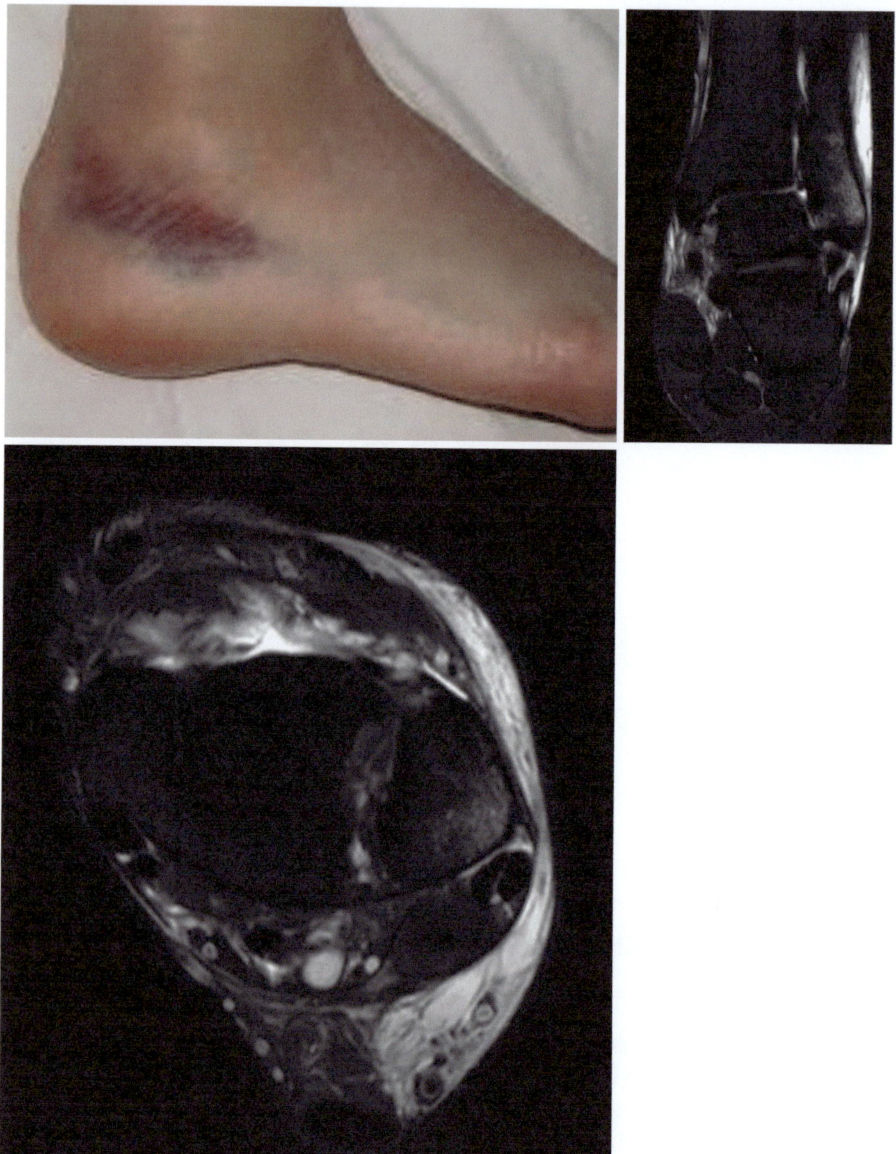

Fig. 24.16 Peroneal tendon rupture in professional football player with cavovarus. MRI often difficult to assess degree and extent

of the peroneal repair and durability of the lateral ligament reconstruction. To avoid tendon adhesions, gentle dorsiflexion and plantar flexion are initiated by 2–3 weeks, with weightbearing in a boot until 8–10 weeks postoperative. At that time, peroneal strengthening can be initiated while avoiding inversion until 14–16 weeks postoperative.

Fig. 24.17 A first metatarsal long oblique dorsiflexion osteotomy is performed with bicortical screw fixation, given the underlying cavovarus

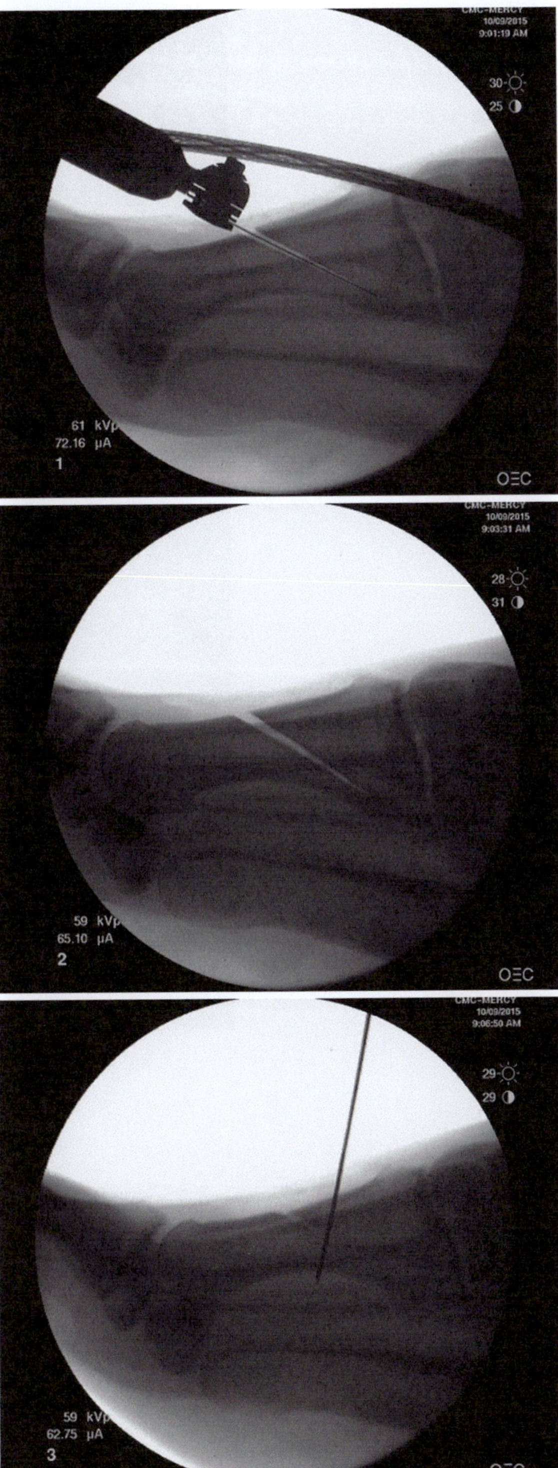

Fig. 24.17 (continued)

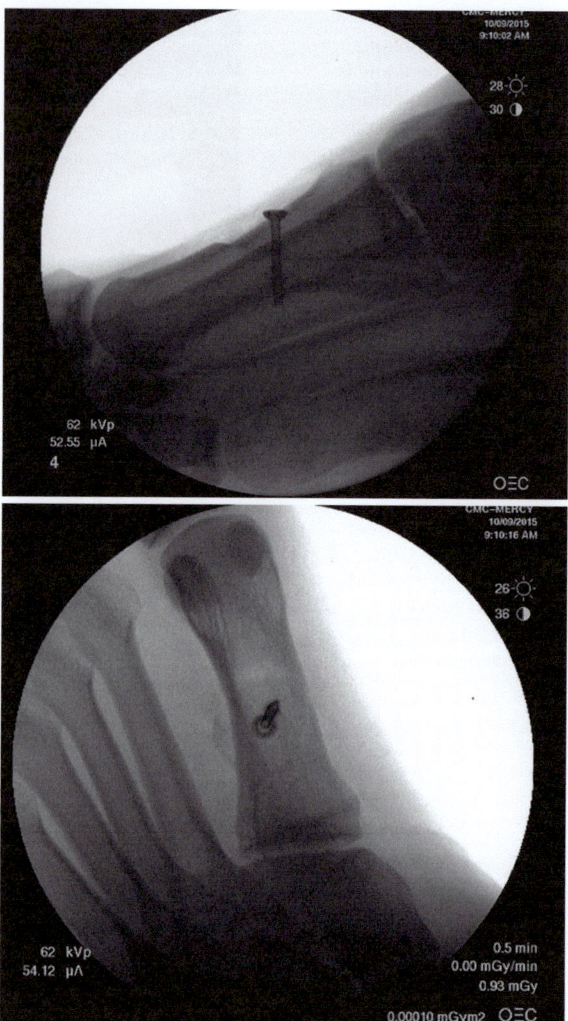

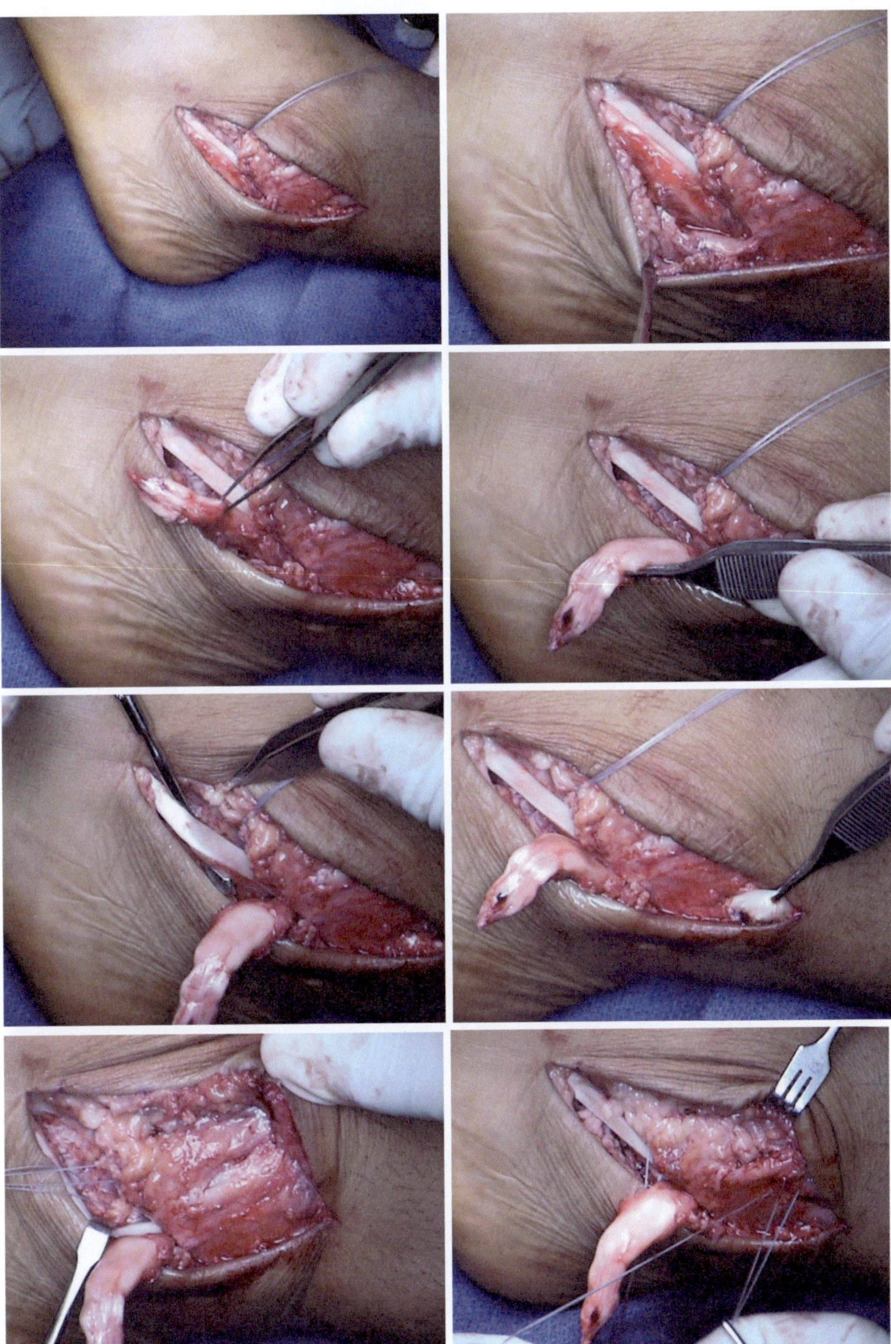

Fig. 24.18 Peroneus longus rupture in zone 3(C) managed with debridement, and tenodesis to the brevis tendon

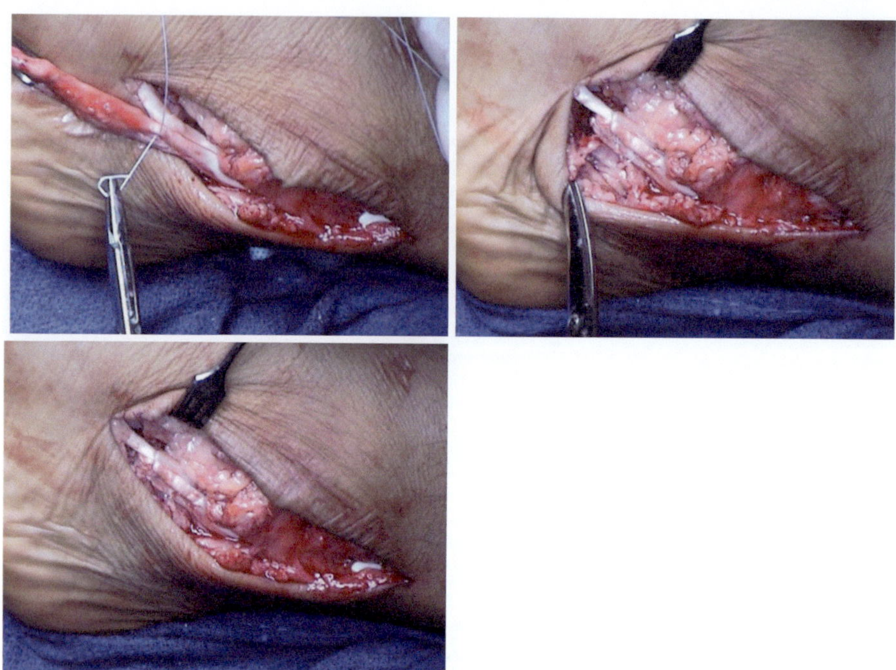

Fig. 24.18 (continued)

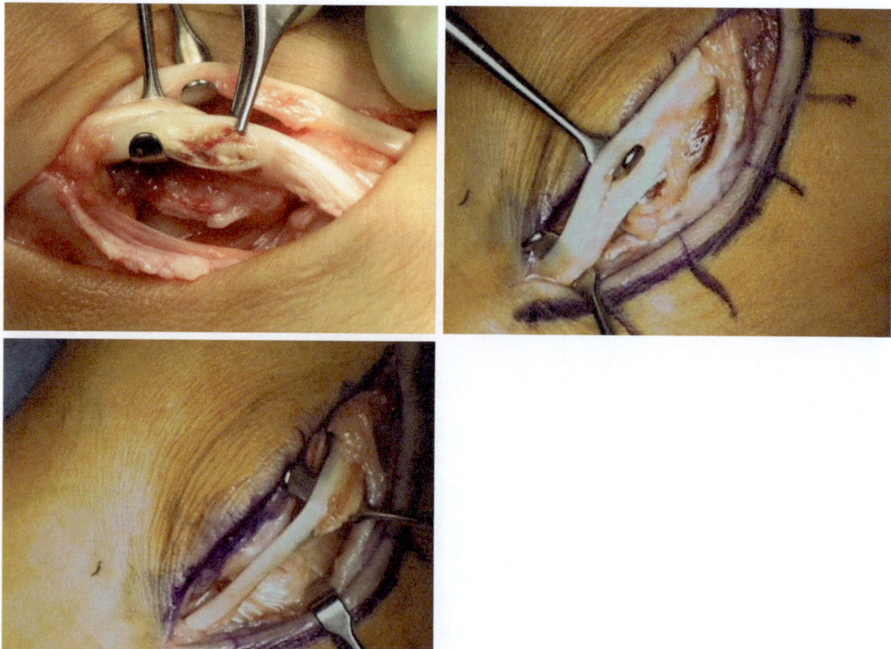

Fig. 24.19 Dislocation with tendon tears. Brevis or longus split tear from inversion

Isolated Peroneus Brevis Rupture

Maintaining integrity and function of the peroneus brevis is paramount in the athlete, particularly in the face of cavovarus. In the case of a rupture, options include tenodesis to the peroneus longus or allograft replacement. In the athlete, it is likely best to maintain the function of both tendons independently, thus avoiding a tenodesis. Unlike the distally located rupture of the longus, the brevis will rupture in zone 2/B and is amenable to salvage with an interposition allograft [25]. Hamstring autografts and allografts work well for this purpose. A pulvertaft weave is performed proximally and then the distal end can then be woven through the remaining stump of the brevis or secured to the base of the fifth metatarsal with an anchor or endobutton, similar to that of repairing a distal biceps rupture. It is important to adequately tension the reconstruction, typically maximum tension with the foot in eversion. It is rare to ever create too tight of a situation. Figure 24.20 shows an MRI of a complex brevis rupture and exemplifies the gracilis tendon allograft for its management. Postoperatively, a non-weightbearing splint is utilized for 2–3 weeks, and then, gentle motion of the ankle is initiated to create a protected excursion of the brevis. The patient weight bears in a boot until 8 weeks postoperative. It is recommended to avoid inversion for 8–10 weeks.

Combined Peroneus Brevis and Peroneus Longus Tendon Rupture

This is a very difficult scenario in any individual, especially the athlete and is magnified with underlying cavovarus. Rarely will a debridement and creation of one tendon unit provide adequate function for the active individual. Assuming that the ruptures are relatively acute (<6 months), the proximal musculature should be

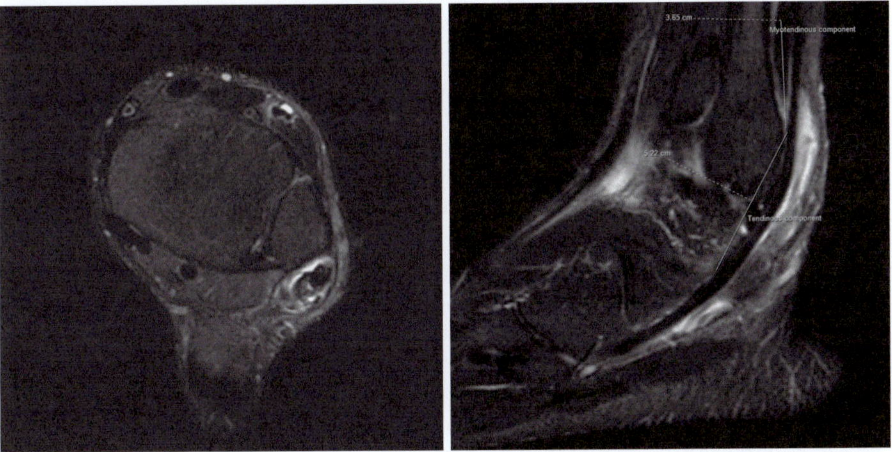

Fig. 24.20 MRI of elite athlete with peroneal tendon rupture. Example of using gracilis tendon allograft for management of this complex brevis rupture

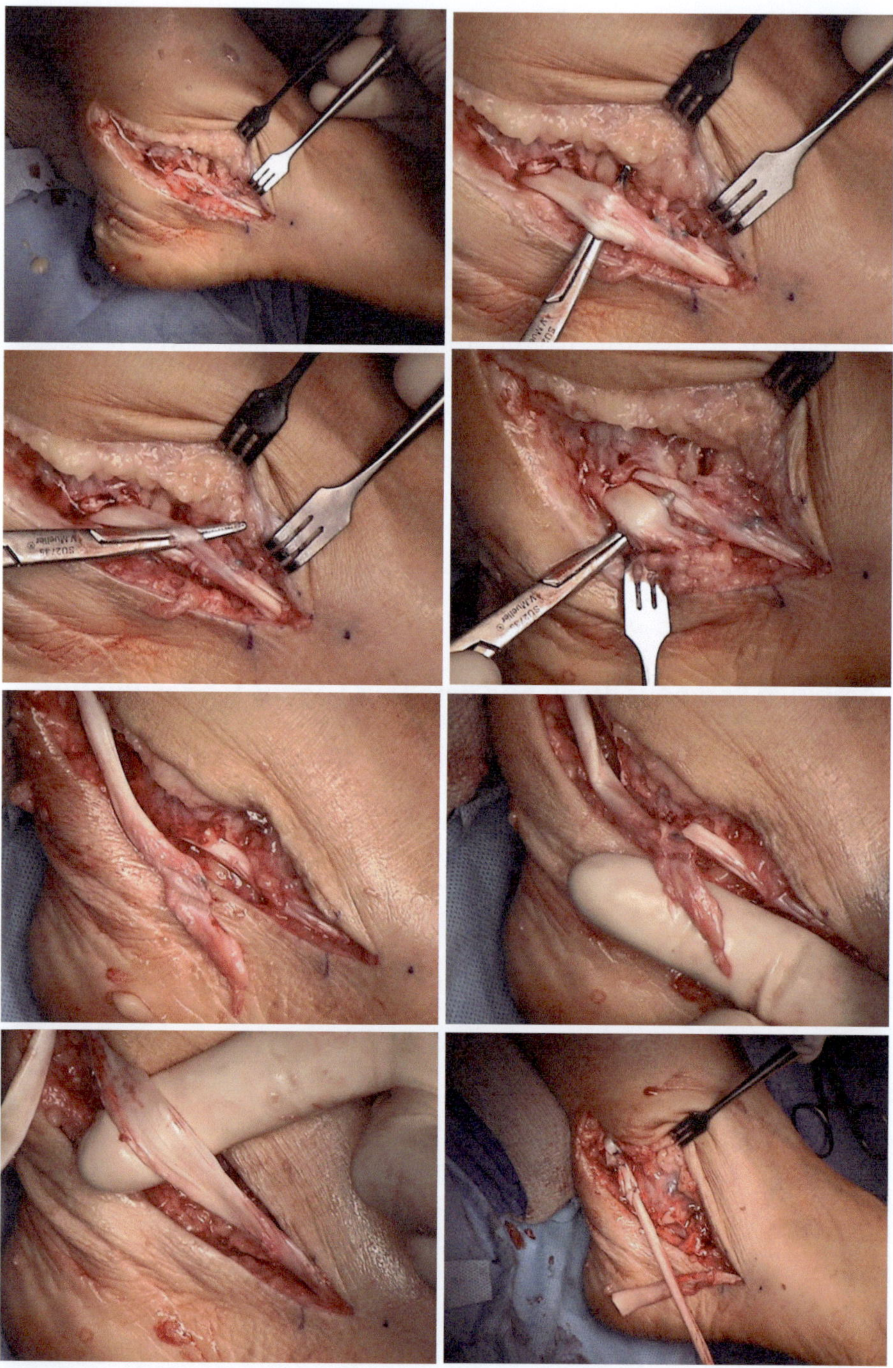

Fig. 24.20 (continued)

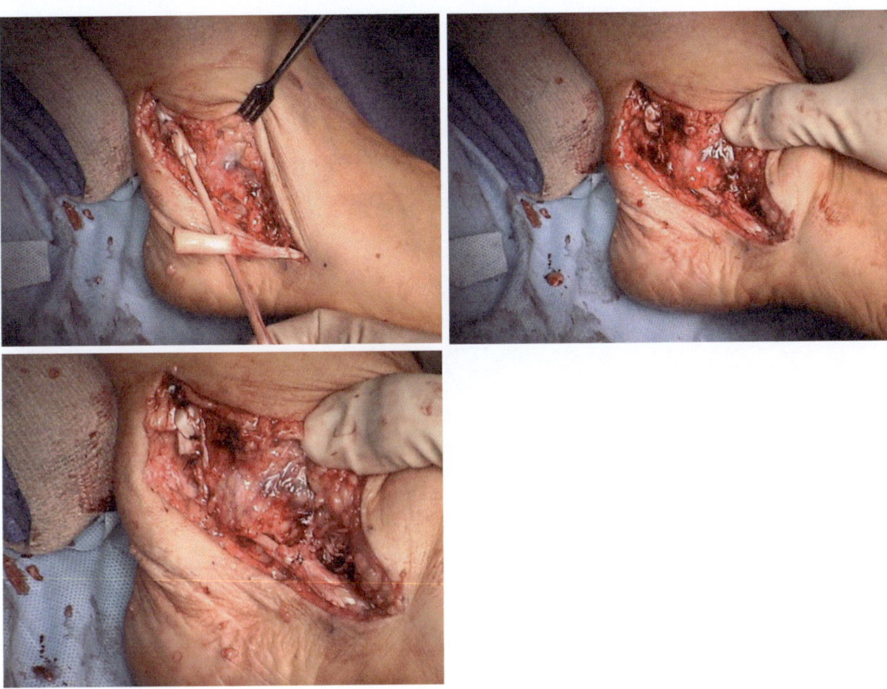

Fig. 24.20 (continued)

healthy and functional, thus allowing for salvage with hamstring allograft interposition to each tendon, if possible. Figure 24.21 shows a case of rupture of both tendons in a 26-year-old professional football player. An allograft tendon interposition was used for both tendons, with indirect groove deepening.

In the event that the proximal muscles are fibrotic and nonfunctional, then a tendon transfer should be considered [24, 52, 53]. I prefer the FHL tendon as opposed to the FDL, due to ease of harvest and improved strength characteristics. Adequate length can be obtained by harvesting the tendon at the plantar aspect of the hallux and then locating it at the master knot of Henry. If necessary, a third incision is placed at the posteromedial ankle to identify and transfer along the posterior aspect of the joint. However, it is possible to identify and redirect the FHL from the posterolateral exposure used for the peroneal tendon exposure, bringing it into the lateral hindfoot region where is it anastomosed to the distal peroneus brevis with maximum tension applied. The postoperative course is similar to that outlined for the isolated brevis rupture and reconstruction. The patient needs to appreciate preoperatively that this is not a substantial transfer and may not rehab to a point that allows for return to a high level of athletic participation. In fact, a few will fail with ongoing inversion tendencies and may eventually require salvage via a subtalar arthrodesis. When faced with the situation where a patient has undergone tendon salvage surgery but has not improved functionally, one may wish to perform a

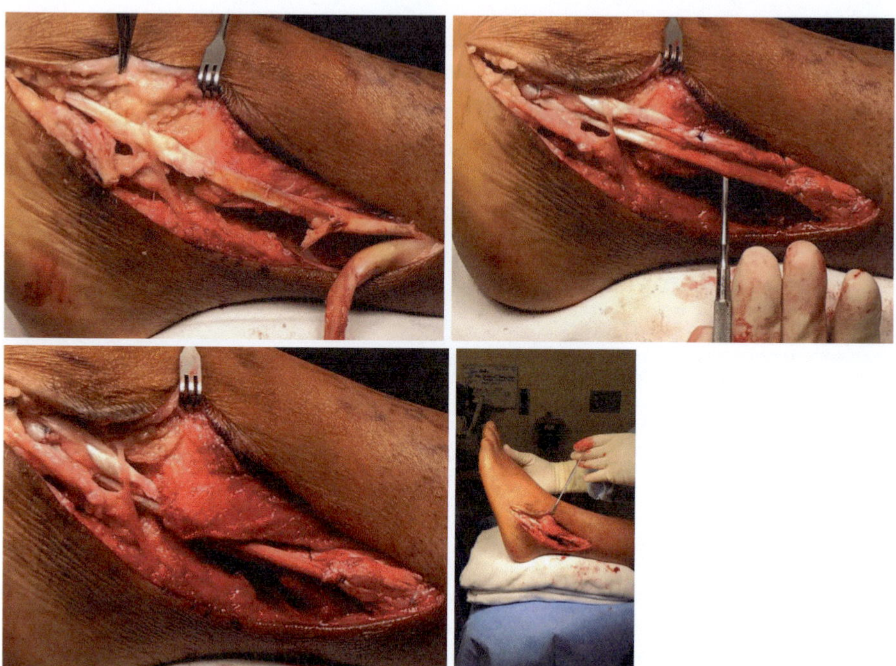

Fig. 24.21 Case: A 26-year-old professional football player. Chronic dislocation and ruptured both tendons. Allograft tendon interposition used for both tendons, with indirect groove deepening

Biodex quantitative strength test to determine whether adequate and successful rehab has been obtained. A baseline study can be followed by a second evaluation 12 weeks later to assess improvements.

Concominent Cavovarus Foot

As has been mentioned, frequently, the cavovarus foot plays a major role not only in the pathophysiology of peroneal tendon and lateral ankle disorders but also in the management and outcome [31]. Any soft tissue reconstruction performed on the lateral ankle and hindfoot region needs to be protected for the best long-term results. Based on careful preoperative evaluation, which includes a Coleman block test, either a lateralizing calcaneal or dorsiflexion 1st metatarsal osteotomy (or both) should be considered in the individual with a cavovarus presentation [48]. I prefer those techniques that include a substantial bone surface, compress with weightbearing forces and allow for screw fixation (i.e., bicortical in the 1st metatarsal). Figure 24.22 depicts an osteotomy for cavovarus. This is not for athletes in the primary situation. These osteotomies are generally protected from weightbearing forces for 3–4 weeks postoperative, after which weightbearing and tendon strengthening are advanced. The long oblique osteotomy and bicortical fixation are biomechanical advantages.

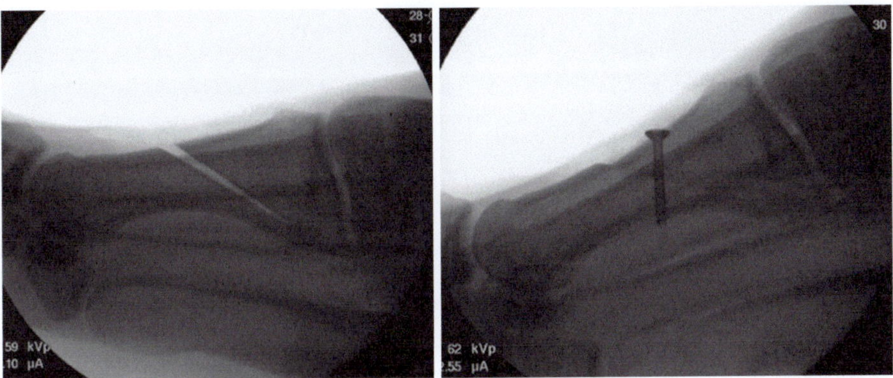

Fig. 24.22 First metatarsal long oblique osteotomy for cavovarus

Role for Peroneal Tendoscopy

Van Djik and others have advocated tendoscopy, particularly for the peroneal tendons. This minimally invasive procedure has been shown to be advantageous in diagnosing split tears and subtle subluxation (intra-sheath) where MRI may not [54, 55]. It is also very useful in the case of tenosynovitis, providing adequate working space to perform a thorough tenosynovectomy. There is a learning curve to this technique, and obvious limitations when dealing with frank tendon dislocation and tendon ruptures.

Postsurgical Rehabilitation

Rehab Protocol

Standardization of any rehabilitation protocol is difficult in any patient population. It is inherently critical that tissue healing, tissue stress, and consideration of concomitant procedures are taken into account when implementing a rehab protocol. However, there has been a shift in rehab philosophy over the recent years to more criterion-based protocols. This shift allows for a progressive approach, allowing for gradient increases in progression based upon the individual's abilities as well as respect for tissue stress and healing. In the athletic population, a detailed understanding of sport-specific demands is crucial to appropriately determine a return-to-sport plan. Figures 24.23 and 24.24 demonstrate an example of postsurgical protocols. Timeframes serve primarily as a reference.

Phase I - Immobilization

There is no consensus in today's literature with regard to an ideal postoperative immobilization time or initiation of range-of-motion exercises [3]. Postoperative

Phase I (0-2 weeks)
Goals

- Rest
- Control swelling and pain
- Activities of daily living

Guidelines

- Non weight bearing in cast or boot
- Sutures removed at 14 to 21 days
- Education: surgery, healing time, anatomy, phases of rehabilitation
- Encourage activities of daily living
- Rest and elevation to control swelling
- Control pain
- Hip and knee active range of motion
- Intrinsic foot muscle activation (per procedure)

Phase II: Week 3-6
Goals

- Full weight bearing in cast or boot with no swelling (early stage)

Guidelines

- Shower without boot
- Elevation to control swelling
- Start to weight bearing
- Massage for swelling
- Submaximal isometrics progressing to full isometric to active range of motion (AROM) ankle and foot: plantarflexion / dorsiflexion / inversion
- NO active eversion/NO Passive inversion
- Progress to stationary bicycle
- Hip strengthening in non-weightbearing

Phase III: Week 7-10
Goals

- Full weight bearing without boot
- Full plantar flexion and dorsiflexion

Guidelines

- Wean from walker boot by ± week 8
- Use an ankle brace during daytime (as indicated)
- Control swelling with elevation and modalities as required
- Stationary bike
- Active range of motion ankle and foot in all directions: gentle inversion & eversion
- Mobilization of foot and ankle in directions that do not directly stress repair (continue to avoid aggressive active eversion and passive inversion)
- Muscle stimulation to intrinsics, invertors, and evertors as necessary
- Implementation of progressive resistive exercise program
- Proprioceptive activities (NWB to WB as able)

Phase IV: Week 11-12
Goals

- Full active range of motion ankle and foot
- Normal gait pattern

Guidelines

- Manual mobilization
- Progression of proprioception and balance
- Continue Phase III rehab

Phase V: Week 13-16
Goals

- Full functional range of motion all movements in weight bearing
- Good balance on surgical side on even surface
- Near full strength lower extremity

Guidelines

- Emphasize proprioception: single leg stance on even surfaces, then progressing to single leg even surface with resistance to arms. Double leg stance on wobble board, Fitter, then progress to single leg stance on wobble board.
- Strength: Calf raises, lunges, squats, plyometrics, and agility drills including jumping and hopping (14+ weeks), running (14+ weeks)
- Manual mobilization to attain normal glides and full physiological range of motion

Phase VI: Week 16+
Goals

- Full function • Good endurance

Guidelines

- Continue building endurance, strength and proprioception
- Plyometric training
- Sport specific training

Fig. 24.23 Sample postsurgical rehab protocol

rehabilitation programs should be designed around the individual patient's goals and prior level of function, pathology addressed, and the surgical technique performed to optimize recovery and reduce the risk of re-injury.

Immobilization and non-weightbearing period varies depending on the severity of the injury and surgical technique. General recommendations for immobilization timeframes and weightbearing restrictions are made with each surgery type. Of note, as the procedure allows, it may be advantageous to have patients start activities

	0–2 weeks[a]	2–4 weeks[a]	6–8 weeks[a]	8–12 weeks[a]	12–24 weeks[a]	>24 weeks[a]
Weight bearing:						
1. Non-weight bearing	x					
2. Partial weight bearing		x	x			
3. Full weight bearing				x	x	x
Active Range of Motion			x			
Strength exercises			x			
Proprioceptive training			x	x		
Eccentric/concentric exercises				x	x	
Isotonic exercises				x	x	
Running					x	x
Sport specific training						x
Provocation peroneal tendons						x

[a] Number of weeks after operation

Fig. 24.24 Overview of the proposed rehabilitation protocol of surgically treated peroneal tendon disorders, based on the evaluation of available protocols in literature. (Reprinted from Van Dijk et al. [3])

	Group A: primary repair ($n = 28$)	Group B: tenodesis ($n = 21$)	Group C: grafting ($n = 16$)	Group D: end-to-end suturing ($n = 7$)
Total immobilization in weeks	Median 6.0 (range 0–12)	Median 7.0 (range 3.0–13)	Median 6.3 (range 3.0–13)	Median 8.0 (range 6.0–11)
NWB in weeks	Median 3.5 (range 0–6.4)	Median 4.3 (range 0–8.0)	Median 4.0 (range 0–8.0)	Median 4.0 (range 2.0–8.0)
WB in weeks	Median 2.3 (range 0–8.0)	Median 3.0 (range 0–8.0)	Median 2.8 (range 0–10)	Median 4.0 (range 0–6.0)
Start ROM in weeks	$n = 23$[a]	$n = 20$[a]	$n = 15$[a]	$n = 4$[a]
	Median: 4.0 (range 2.0–12)	Median: 4.5 (range 0–12)	Median: 4.0 (range 0–12)	Median: 5.5 (range 2.0–8.0)

Fig. 24.25 Overview of the non-weight-bearing and weight-bearing immobilization period and ROM initiation. (Reprinted from Van Dijk et al. [3])

such as toe crunches/wiggling, toe spreading, foot doming as able in the immobilizer. The aim is to maintain proprioceptive capacity, minimize atrophy, and potentially improve fluid movement.

Phase II – Early Mobility/Weightbearing

A recent change to early ROM exercises can be found in operatively treated patients with peroneal tendon injuries [6, 43]. Demetracouplos et al. and Karlsson et al. have recently described a change in their postoperative management based on this information. In contrast to a previous protocol of 6 weeks cast immobilization followed by physical therapy, Demetracouplos et al. [43] implemented a postoperative protocol aiming at early ROM after 4 weeks of WB and NWB immobilization. Karlsson et al. [6] immobilized the patient 6 weeks in a plaster cast, but shortened the period in a study published 4 years later to 2 weeks plaster cast followed by a WB air cast brace to provide early ROM training. Figure 24.25 shows an overview of the non-weight-bearing and weight-bearing immobilization period and ROM initiation based upon the procedure performed.

Gentle early passive ROM is implemented in this phase. The program should focus on the protection of the surgical site and range of motion first, which will help to avoid postoperative adhesion of the peroneal tendons to the retinaculum and surrounding tissues. Gentle early muscle activation can occur in this phase with submaximal isometric contractions. Ideally, this is done concurrently with the initiation of the protected weightbearing in a boot. In a cast or boot, isometric contraction takes place (i.e., no change of muscle length and therefore no forced pull on the tendons) [56]. Early active motion helps to reduce swelling, stiffness, atrophy, pain, and muscle guarding following surgery.

Gentle active ROM can also be initiated. Exercises can be focused on ankle plantar flexors, dorsiflexors and inverters, as well extrinsic and intrinsic foot/toe musculature. Care should be taken to avoid active ankle eversion due to the healing repair. The peroneal tendons are ankle plantar flexors in addition to being everters. Since this is a secondary function, they may report some pulling in the lateral compartment of the leg with plantarflexion. Cardiovascular exercise can be initiated on the stationary bike, but the patient should remain in the boot when performing this activity until week 7.

Phase III – Full Weightbearing/Progressive Exercise

During the third phase of treatment, the patient should be weaned from the boot. Gait mechanics have been altered for the past 2 months with the boot, so it is very important to normalize gait biomechanics as quickly as possible. In order to ensure proper step and stride length, the patient should have full ankle dorsiflexion and plantarflexion by this phase of treatment. It is also important to recognize compensatory movements if ankle ROM is limited. These may include excessive mobility and toe out posturing in the foot and excessive frontal and transverse movement in the knee and hip. Additionally, asymmetric weightbearing from surgical to nonsurgical side can create additional risk in other areas. If ROM is not full, initiate joint mobilizations for dorsiflexion or plantarflexion at this time. Joint mobilizations should only be performed that do not directly stress the repair. Stationary bike can be performed without the boot and gentle active ankle eversion can be performed. If the patient is having difficulty initiating peroneal muscle contraction, electrical stimulation can be used.

Progressive resistive exercises are initiated in this phase, with emphasis on selective stress to each of the muscle groups of the lower limb. Band exercises, balance exercise, and proprioceptive exercises are all included here (Fig. 24.26). In this particular subset of athletes, peroneal tendon injuries often are associated with ankle sprains and chronic ankle instability. It is imperative to identify proprioceptive deficits associated with these injuries. Alteration in gait kinematics, particularly during the early stance phase of gait, has been demonstrated by individuals with chronic ankle instability [57–59]. Overly inverted ankle position is a particular deficit that can lead to recurrent ankle sprains. This position shifts the center of mass laterally,

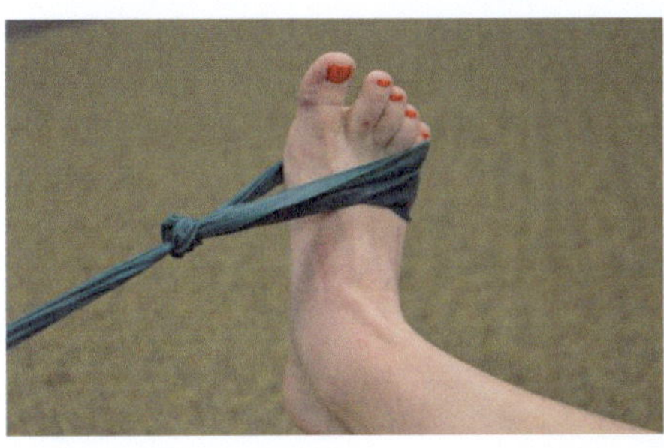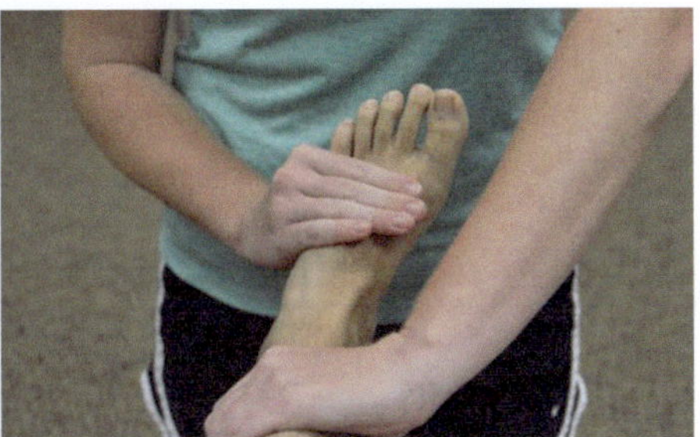

Fig. 24.26 Progressive resistive exercises of the peroneal muscle group. Left picture demonstrates with an elastic band, whereas the right picture demonstrates manual graded resistance

Fig. 24.27 1-lb weight was placed on the dorsal–lateral side of the foot as a perturbation. (Reprinted from Yen et al. [60])

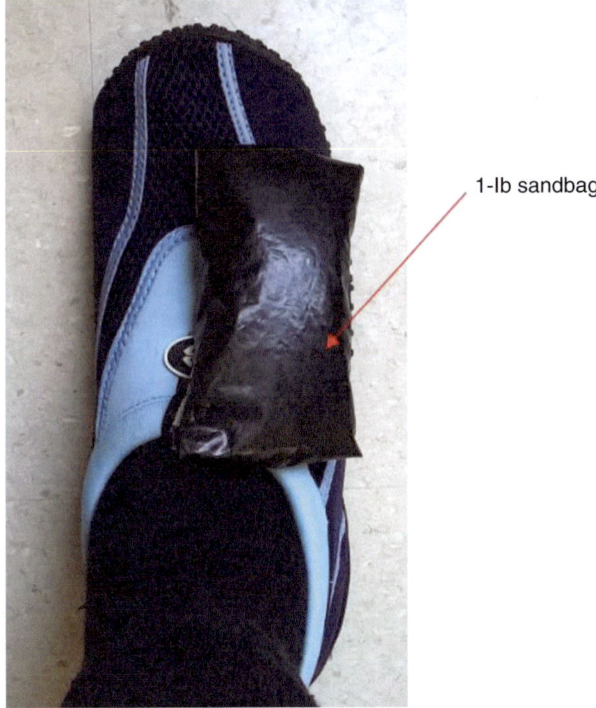

creating potential increased inversion torque during loading response [59]. Efforts at improving inversion positioning during this phase may lead to a reduction in ankle sprain risk. A variety of proprioceptive and gait retraining strategies can be used to improve this. Additionally, taping strategies to influence a more everted position may be beneficial [59]. Error-driven approaches to gait retraining have demonstrated some success as well [60]. Figure 24.27 demonstrates the use of a lightweight on the dorsal lateral aspect of the foot during walking to improve eversion positioning.

By the start of phase four around 3 months, the patient should have normal gait pattern, full ankle range of motion, and the remainder of rehabilitation is focused on strength, balance, proprioception, and return to physical activity.

Phase IV – Optimize Gait/Balance/Proprioception

During this phase of the rehabilitation process, the athlete should demonstrate normal gait mechanics. Any deviations in gait need to be addressed before the implementation of plyometric, agility, and running activities can begin. Additionally, once balance and strength are within approximately 75% of the uninvolved side, functional testing/training can be performed.

Progression of strengthening and balance training are the primary focal points of this phase. Exercises should look to challenge muscle strength throughout the full ROM and muscle endurance.

After surgery, afferent pathways can be impaired, affecting joint proprioception and neuromuscular reaction time. Improving reaction time improves dynamic stabilization of the ankle and surrounding joints, minimizes stress to the surgically repaired tissues, and prevents further injury. Balance activities should progress through variations in surface and environmental challenges. Y-balance testing and star excursion balance tests are objective single-leg balance measures that can be utilized [61]. Progressions include unilateral weightbearing, use of multiplanar surfaces, and perturbation training. Attempts should be made to challenge systems by altering information obtained through visual, vestibular, and somatosensory systems. Replication of sports-specific sensory inputs may be useful as return to sport progressions is made.

Phase V – Full Functional Activity

Initiation of plyometric and agility activities is primary in this stage. Training with focus on impact control, symmetrical limb loading, and multiplanar movements serve as precursors to sport specific training. Plyometric training should be progressing, with attention being paid to its component parts: speed, intensity, volume, and frequency. Progressions should have sport-specific demands in mind. They should incorporate moving from single leg, to double leg, involve varying jumping heights, and incorporate multiplanar movements. Agility activities should follow similar progressions, with consideration given to both acceleration and deceleration activities.

As the athlete demonstrates the ability to accept and manage impact loads effectively, a return-to-running program can be initiated. Return-to-running programs exist in a variety of forms in literature.

General recommendations for return to running are as follows:

- Body weight-supported treadmills (i.e., Alter-G Anti Gravity Treadmill™) is a useful tool to resume running activity, as impact load can be matched to the patient's ability and can be used to incrementally progress loading in a forward running progression.

- Initiation of running requires full sagittal plane ankle ROM. Functional testing for readiness may include a forward step down off an 8″ step to ensure adequate weightbearing dorsiflexion ROM.
- Progression rates of no more than 10% distance per week to allow tissues to attenuate to stress loads.
- Avoid consecutive days of running. Cross-training strategies should be utilized to prevent overuse/stress-related issues.

Phase VI – Return to Sport-Specific Activity

The final phase of rehabilitation involves continued strength, endurance, plyometric, and agility training, leading to sport-specific training. Return to sport training is not currently well defined in the literature with regard to peroneal tendon surgeries. It is acknowledged that both physical readiness and psychological readiness are significant factors in determining a successful return to prior level of sport function. Literature is not specific to peroneal tendon surgeries for return to sport testing. Return to sport functional and psychological testing is well studied in the postoperative anterior cruciate ligament rehabilitation. Though mechanics of surgery and injury are different, principles may be applied to testing after peroneal tendon surgery to optimize objective and safe return to sport testing.

Functional testing for safe return to sport are being utilized to assist the clinician, physician, trainers, and patient in making safe return to sport decisions. Functional hop testing, balance testing, strength assessments, and movement quality assessments, in addition to subjective outcome measures, are available to assist in this process. Figure 24.28 demonstrates the functional hop testing [62]. Collaboration

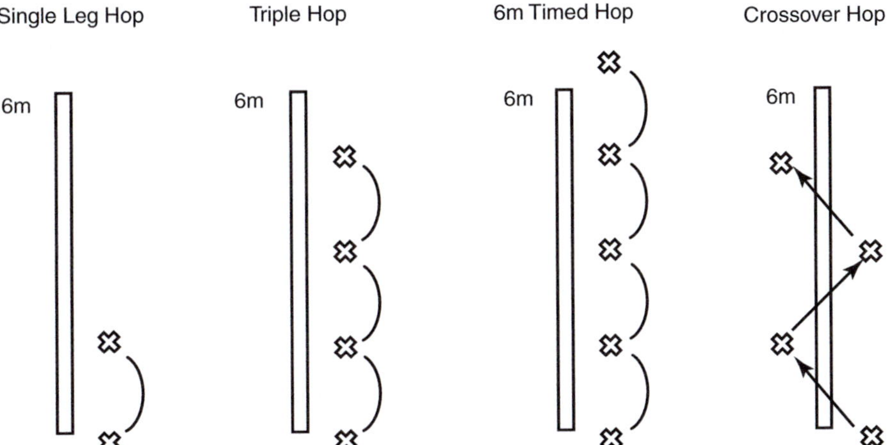

Fig. 24.28 Diagrammatic representation of 4 commonly used hop tests to determine asymmetries

among providers and coaches involved in the athlete's care is crucial in this phase of the rehabilitation process. Successful return after clearance for return will require graded exposure back to full participation with close monitoring.

Psychological readiness has been demonstrated to be a significant factor in the return to sport decision-making process, particularly in the postoperative ACL population [63]. Anxiety and fear can have a significant impact on the rehabilitation process, especially in traumatic injuries such as ACL injury and fractures. In the case of peroneal injuries, there is not necessarily significant trauma associated with the initial injury. Psychological readiness for return may be influenced by the nature of the initial injury.

Surgical factors will also influence return to sport timeframes. Timeframes have been reported with averages from 3 to 5 months [64]. The nature of the surgery will have significant influence on the return to sport time as well as the rate of successful return to prior level of competition. Superior retinacular repairs, groove deepening, tendon repair, etc. can all influence return to sport. Concomitant procedures such as lateral ankle ligament reconstruction can further complicate return to sport rehabilitation.

The single-leg hop requires 1 maximal jump landing on the same limb. Failure to land without falling over or "bouncing forward" requires the test to be retaken. The triple hop assesses maximal distance for 3 hops in a rebounding pattern. A stable landing must also be demonstrated for the final hop. The 6-m timed hop positions timing gates at 0 and 6 m asks subjects to hop on 1 limb as fast as they can for the total distance, thus reporting the outcome of time. The crossover hop requires 3 maximal hops (for distance) in a diagonal pattern. A stable landing must also be demonstrated on the final hop (reprinted from Bishop et al. [62]).

Summary

Successful outcomes in surgical management and subsequent rehabilitation of athletes involve many factors and extensive collaboration among providers. Nature of injury, surgical procedure, sport demands, and even timing of a particular event can all influence return to sport rate. Training should be targeted at sport-specific demands as the healing process allows.

References

1. Porter D, Mccarroll J, Knapp E, Torma J. Peroneal tendon subluxation in athletes: fibular groove deepening and retinacular reconstruction. Foot Ankle Int. 2005;26:436–41.
2. Steel MW, Deorio JK. Peroneal tendon tears: return to sports after operative treatment. Foot Ankle Int. 2007;28:49–54.
3. Dijk PADV, Lubberts B, Verheul C, Digiovanni CW, Kerkhoffs GMMJ. Rehabilitation after surgical treatment of peroneal tendon tears and ruptures. Knee Surg Sports Traumatol Arthrosc. 2016;24:1165–74.

4. Heckman DS, Pedowitz D, Parekh SG, Reddy S, Wapner K. Operative treatment for peroneal tendon disorders. J Bone Joint Surg Am. 2008;90:404–18.

5. Sobel M, Geppert MJ, Warren RF. Chronic ankle instability as a cause of peroneal tendon injury. Clin Orthop Relat Res. 1993;296:187–91.

6. Karlsson J, Wiger P. Longitudinal split of the peroneus brevis tendon and lateral anlkle instability: treatment of concomitant lesions. J Athl Train. 2002;37:463–6.

7. Karlsson J, Brandsson S, Kälebo P, Eriksson BI. Surgical treatment of concomitant chronic ankle instability and longitudinal rupture of the peroneus brevis tendon. Scand J Med Sci Sports. 2007;8:42–9.

8. Bonnin M, Tavernier T, Bouysset M. Split lesions of the peroneus brevis tendon in chronic ankle laxity. Am J Sports Med. 1997;25:699–703.

9. Digiovanni BF, Fraga CJ, Cohen BE, Shereff MJ. Associated injuries found in chronic lateral ankle instability. Foot Ankle Int. 2000;21:809–15.

10. Brandes CB, Smith RW. Characterization of patients with primary peroneus longus tendinopathy: a review of twenty-two cases. Foot Ankle Int. 2000;21:462–8.

11. Sobel M, Bohne WH, Levy ME. Longitudinal attrition of the peroneus brevis tendon in the fibular groove: an anatomic study. Foot Ankle. 1990;11:124–8.

12. Davis WH, Sobel M, Deland J, Bohne WH, Patel MB. The superior peroneal retinaculum: an anatomic study. Foot Ankle Int. 1994;15:271–5.

13. Mick CA, Lynch F. Reconstruction of the peroneal retinaculum using the peroneus quartus. A case report. J Bone Joint Surg. 1987;69:296–7.

14. Sobel M, Bohne WHO, Obrien SJ. Peroneal tendon subluxation in a case of anomalous peroneus brevis muscle. Acta Orthopaedica Scan. 1992;63:682–4.

15. Sobel M, Geppert MJ, Olson EJ, Bohne WHO, Arnoczky SP. The dynamics of peroneus brevis tendon splits: a proposed mechanism, technique of diagnosis, and classification of injury. Foot Ankle. 1992;13:413–22.

16. Palmanovich E, Laver L, Brin YS, Kotz E, Hetsroni I, Mann G, Nyska M. Peroneus longus tear and its relation to the peroneal tubercle: A review of the literature. Muscles Ligaments Tendons J. 2012;1:153–60.

17. Bruce WD, Christoferson MR, Phillips DL. Stenosing tenosynovitis and impingement of the peroneal tendons associated with hypertrophy of the peroneal tubercle. Foot Ankle Int. 1999;20:464–7.

18. Pierson JL, Inglis AE. Stenosing tenosynovitis of the peroneus longus tendon associated with hypertrophy of the peroneal tubercle and an os peroneum. JBJS Am. 1992;74:440–2.

19. Sobel M, Pavlov H, Geppert MJ, Thompson FM, Dicarlo EF, Davis WH. Painful os peroneum syndrome: a spectrum of conditions responsible for plantar lateral foot pain. Foot Ankle Int. 1994;15:112–24.

20. Stockton KG, Brodsky JW. Peroneus longus tears associated with pathology of the os peroneum. Foot Ankle Int. 2014;35:346–52.

21. Raikin SM, Elias I, Nazarian LN. Intrasheath subluxation of the peroneal tendons. J Bone Joint Surg Am Vol. 2008;90:992–9.

22. Alanen J, Orava S, Heinonen OJ, Ikonen J, Krista M. Peroneal tendon injuries. Ann chir gynaecol. 2001;90:43–6.

23. Heckman DS, Gluck GS, Parekh SG. Tendon disorders of the foot and ankle, part 1: peroneal tendon disorders. AmJSports Med. 2009;37:614–25.

24. Wapner KL, Taras JS, Lin SS, Chao W. Staged reconstruction for chronic rupture of both peroneal tendons using hunter rod and flexor hallucis longus tendon transfer: a long-term followup study. Foot Ankle Int. 2006;27:591–7.

25. Mook WR, Parekh SG, Nunley JA. Allograft Reconstruction of Peroneal Tendons. Foot Ankle Int. 2013;34:1212–20.

26. Brodsky JW, Zide JR, Kane JM. Acute peroneal Injury. Foot Ankle Clin. 2017;22:833–41.

27. Sammarco G, Mangone P. Diagnosis and treatment of peroneal tendon injuries. Foot Ankle Surg. 2000;6:197–205.

28. Sammarco GJ, Diraimondo CV. Chronic peroneus brevis tendon lesions. Foot Ankle. 1989;9:163–70.
29. Krause JO, Brodsky JW. Peroneus brevis tendon tears: pathophysiology, surgical reconstruction, and clinical results. Foot Ankle Int. 1998;19:271–9.
30. Redfern D, Myerson M. The management of concomitant tears of the peroneus longus and brevis tendons. Foot Ankle Int. 2004;25:695–707.
31. Manoli A, Graham B. The subtle cavus foot, "the Underpronator," a review. Foot Ankle Int. 2005;26:256–63.
32. Sobel M, Mizel MS. Peroneal Tendon Injury. In: Pfeffer GB, Frey CC, editors. Current practice in foot and ankle surgery. New York: McGraw-Hill, Health Professions Division; 1993.
33. Dombek MF, Lamm BM, Saltrick K, Mendicino RW, Catanzariti AR. Peroneal tendon tears: a retrospective review. J Foot Ankle Surg. 2003;42:250–8.
34. Ogawa BK, Thordarson DB, Zalavras C. Peroneal tendon subluxation repair with an indirect fibular groove deepening technique. Foot Ankle Int. 2007;28:1194–7.
35. Khazen GE, Adam N, Wilson MD, Schon LC (2005) Peroneal groove deepening via a posterior osteocartilaginous flap: a retrospective analysis. presented at the 21st Annual American Orthopaedic Foot and Ankle Summer Meeting, Boston, 15–17 July 2005
36. McGarvey W, Clanton T. Peroneal tendon dislocations. Foot Ankle Clin. 1996;1:325–42.
37. Bassett FH III, Speer KP. Longitudinal rupture of the peroneal tendons. Am J Sports Med. 1993;21:354–7.
38. Saxena A, Pham B. Longitudinal peroneal tendon tears. J Foot Ankle Surg. 1997;36:173–9.
39. Saxena A, Cassidy. Peroneal tendon injuries: an evaluation of 49 tears in 41 patients. J Foot Ankle Surg. 2003;42:215–20.
40. Squires N, Myerson MS, Gamba C. Surgical treatment of peroneal tendon tears. Foot Ankle Clin. 2007;12:675–95.
41. Mason RB, Henderson IJP. Traumatic peroneal tendon instability. Am J Sports Med. 1996;24:652–8.
42. Dijk PAV, Miller D, Calder J, et al. The ESSKA-AFAS international consensus statement on peroneal tendon pathologies. Knee Surg Sports Traumatol Arthrosc. 2018;26:3096–107.
43. Demetracopoulos CA, Vineyard JC, Kiesau CD, Nunley JA 2nd. Long-term results of debridement and primary repair of peroneal tendon tears. Foot Ankle Int. 2013;35:252–7.
44. Selmani E, Gjata V, Gjika E. Current concepts review: peroneal tendon disorders. Foot Ankle Int. 2006;27:221–8.
45. Shawen SB, Anderson RB. Indirect groove deepening in the management of chronic peroneal tendon dislocation. Tech Foot Ankle Surg. 2004;3:118–25.
46. Coughlin MJ, Schon LC. Chapter 24, Disorders of Tendons. In: Coughlin MJ, Saltzman CL, Anderson RB, editors. Mann's surgery of the foot and ankle, vol. 24. Philadelphia: Saunders, an imprint of Elsevier Inc; 2014. p. 1232–75.
47. Wagner E, Wagner P, Ortiz C, Radkievich R, Palma F, Guzmán-Venegas R. Biomechanical cadaveric evaluation of partial acute peroneal tendon tears. Foot Ankle Int. 2018;39:741–5.
48. Krause FG, Guyton GP. Chapter 26, Pes Cavus. In: Coughlin MJ, Saltzman CL, Anderson RB, editors. Mann's surgery of the foot and ankle, vol. 24. Philadelphia: Saunders, an imprint of Elsevier Inc; 2014. p. 1362–82.
49. Eckert W, Davis E. Acute rupture of the peroneal retinaculum. J Bone Joint Surg. 1976;58:670–2.
50. Maffulli N, Ferran NA, Oliva F, Testa V. recurrent subluxation of the peroneal tendons. Am J Sports Med. 2006;34:986–92.
51. Raikin SM, Elias I, Nazarian LN. Intrasheath subluxation of the peroneal tendons. J Bone Joint Sur Am Vol. 2008;90:992–9.
52. Jockel JR, Brodsky JW. Single-stage flexor tendon transfer for the treatment of severe concomitant peroneus longus and brevis tendon tears. Foot Ankle Int. 2013;34:666–72.
53. Seybold JD, Campbell JT, Jeng CL, Short KW, Myerson MS. Outcome of lateral transfer of the FHL or FDL for concomitant peroneal tendon tears. Foot Ankle Int. 2016;37:576–81.

54. Dijk CV, Kort N. Tendoscopy of the peroneal tendons. J Arthroscopy Related Surg. 1998;14:471–8.
55. Bare A, Ferkel RD. Peroneal tendon tears: associated arthroscopic findings and results after repair. Arthroscopy. 2009;25:1288–97.
56. Espinosa N, Maurer M. Peroneal tendon dislocation. Eur J Trauma Emerg Surg. 2015;41(6):631–7.
57. Delahunt E, Monaghan K, Caulfield B. Altered neuromuscular control and ankle joint kinematics during walking in subjects with functional instability of the ankle joint. Am J Sports Med. 2006;34(12):1970–6.
58. Monaghan K, Delahunt E, Caulfield B. Ankle function during gait in patients with chronic ankle instability compared to controls. Clin Biomech (Bristol, Avon). 2006;21(2):168–74.
59. Yen SC, Folmar E, Friend KA, Wang YC, Chui KK. Effects of kinesiotaping and athletic taping on ankle kinematics during walking in individuals with chronic ankle instability: A pilot study. Gait Posture. 2018;66:118–23.
60. Yen SC, Gutierrez GM, Wang YC, Murphy P. Alteration of ankle kinematics and muscle activity during heel contact when walking with external loading. Eur J Appl Physiol. 2015;115(8):1683–92.
61. Gribble PA, Bleakley CM, Caulfield BM, et al. 2016 consensus statement of the International Ankle Consortium: prevalence, impact and long-term consequences of lateral ankle sprains. Br J Sports Med. 2016;50(24):1493–5.
62. Bishop C, Turner A, Jarvis P, Chavda S, Read P. Considerations for selecting field-based strength and power fitness tests to measure asymmetries. J Strength Cond Res. 2017;31:2635–44.
63. Webster KE, Nagelli CV, Hewett TE, Feller JA. Factors associated with psychological readiness to return to sport after anterior cruciate ligament reconstruction surgery. Am J Sports Med. 2018;46(7):1545–50.
64. Van Dijk PA, Gianakos AL, Kerkhoffs GM, Kennedy JG. Return to sports and clinical outcomes in patients treated for peroneal tendon dislocation: a systematic review. Knee Surg Sports Traumatol Arthrosc. 2016;24(4):1155–64.

Synthetic Graft Augmentation (Polyurethane Urea) for Reconstruction of Peroneal Tendon Injury

Steven K. Neufeld, Daniel J. Cuttica, and Syed H. Hussain

Background/Introduction

Autograft and allograft currently remain the gold standard for peroneal tendon reconstructions. However, a disadvantage of these grafts is rapid loss of strength and elasticity due to tissue necrosis and resorption [1]. During remodeling, these avascular grafts are eliminated through phagocytosis, followed by revascularization, cellular infiltration, and matrix remodeling via collagen type 1 production to restore mechanical strength and elasticity. These grafts lose up to 90% of their strength during early remodeling, while ligaments and tendons take 12–24 months to reach maturation and restored functional capacity [2].

Reinforcement devices made from xenografts, polytetrafluoroethylene (PTFE), polyethylene terephthalate (Dacron), polypropylene, polyethylene degradable polydioxanone (PDS), and carbon fibers have all been used clinically for soft-tissue repair and subsequently abandoned due to high stiffness, stress shielding, and ultimately device and repair failure [3–9].

Artelon® (Artelon, Marietta, GA) is made from fibers of polycaprolactone-based polyurethane urea (PUUR) that have been knitted into textile patches and strips for optimal mechanical properties and ease of use (Fig. 25.1). PUUR has many desirable qualities for soft-tissue reinforcement and peroneal tendon reconstructions. It is inert and less reactive than common biomaterials such as titanium and polystyrene [10]. It is strong and creep resistant to protect the repair during acute healing.

S. K. Neufeld (✉) · D. J. Cuttica
The Orthopaedic Foot and Ankle Center, Center for Advanced Orthopedics,
Falls Church, VA, USA
e-mail: sneufeld@cfaortho.com

S. H. Hussain
Wake Orthopaedics, Raleigh, NC, USA

© Springer Nature Switzerland AG 2020
M. Sobel (ed.), *The Peroneal Tendons*,
https://doi.org/10.1007/978-3-030-46646-6_25

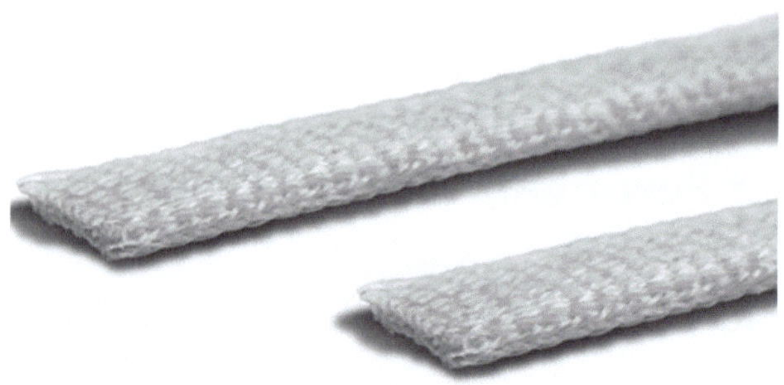

Fig. 25.1 Polyurethane urea (Artelon) graft

However, it is also hyperelastic to permit loading and stimulation of the tissues during late remodeling [11, 12]. It integrates into the repair site without necrosis or foreign body reaction, maintains its strength for 4–6 years, and is eliminated benignly through hydrolytic degradation [13]. These characteristics permit PUUR graft to function as a synthetic provisional matrix, rather than a simple mechanical reinforcement, accelerating the formation of mature and organized tissue in the damaged peroneal tendon.

There are extensive scientific data to support the use of PUUR in soft-tissue reconstruction. Peterson [14] reported on PUUR for ACL reconstruction in a long-term multicenter RCT with over 200 patients and 12 years of follow-up. Patients who received the PUUR implant had equivalent safety outcomes as patients who received autograft alone, with 92% survivorship of the implants at 12 years postoperative, and demonstrated improved rotational stability (pivot-shift test) vs. the control group. Biopsy and histology from 1 to 6 years postoperatively demonstrated excellent integration of the implant without immune reaction and remodeling of organized ligament tissue.

Giza et al. [11] conducted a biomechanical study with PUUR graft to reinforce Achilles tendon repairs. Using cadaveric limbs, Achilles tendons were severed in the watershed area, 2 cm proximal to the calcaneal insertion. Half of the tendons were repaired with Krakow style sutures alone, and half were reinforced with a tubularized patch of PUUR graft. Using a cyclic mechanical loading device, specimens were stressed to failure. The reinforced repairs showed a 49% increase in ultimate load to failure and a 51% decrease in creep. These differences were statistically significant. The authors believe that this type of reinforcement would permit their patients to begin rehabilitation earlier than without reinforcement.

Recent research on the use of PUUR graft in foot and ankle reconstruction has been promising. Shoaib and Mishra [19] performed a series of seven tendon repairs which incorporated a V-Y plasty reinforced with PUUR graft to repair chronic ruptured Achilles tendons with gaps of 5 cm or greater. After 29 months, they found no evidence of infection or rejection and no complications related to the tendon augmentation. All patients showed significant improvement on both the AOFAS and Achilles Tendon Total Rupture Score (ATRS).

Sanders et al. reported on a case series utilizing PUUR graft in acute tibialis anterior tendon repairs, with an average follow-up of 6.5 months. At an average follow-up of 6.5 months, all patients had AOFAS scores demonstrating good function and low levels of pain and dysfunction with a high patient satisfaction rate. No complications, infections, or reruptures occurred [20].

More recently, McKenna et al. reported on a series of 28 patients who underwent lateral ankle ligament reconstruction utilizing a PUUR graft. Their series demonstrated a high success rate and low complication rate with the use of PUUR graft, as the reconstruction retained correction in all but one patient [21].

Thus, there is a strong scientific and clinical evidence to suggest that a Synthetic Provisional Matrix strategy utilizing a PUUR implant is useful, safe, and effective for reconstruction of peroneal tendons.

Indications/Contraindications

Indications for the use of a PUUR graft include the surgical treatment of peroneal tendon pathology in patients who have failed nonoperative management. Traditional conservative treatments include immobilization, bracing, physical therapy, medications, and injections.

PUUR grafts are indicated in cases that include the following:

1. Reinforcement of a repair of peroneal brevis or longus tendon degeneration (>50%) tearing in a younger or active patient in whom the surgeon might want to retain the individual function of both tendons by avoiding doing a tenodesis.
2. Repair of a chronic peroneal tendon rupture in which end-to-end repair is not possible due to a large gap.
3. Chronic peroneal tendon subluxation in which the superior peroneal retinaculum has poor tissue quality.
4. Excision of a symptomatic os peroneum where primary repair is not possible.

Contraindications to the use of a PUUR graft include situations as follows:

1. An infected or contaminated wound where placement of a synthetic graft might act as a nidus for infection.
2. A patient in whom severe peripheral vascular disease precludes surgical reconstruction.
3. Chronic peroneal tendon ruptures where there is no tendon excursion. Tendon transfer is indicated in such a situation.
4. Rigid hindfoot or severe degenerative joint disease, where a hindfoot fusion would be more appropriate.

Preoperative Planning

Preoperative planning for treating peroneal tendon pathology should include a complete history and physical examination in conjunction with radiographs and other imaging modalities, in order to make an accurate diagnosis and recognize pathology for which the patient might benefit from a PUUR graft for soft-tissue reconstruction.

The history obtained from the patient should include where the patient's pain is localized, history of acute or prior trauma, and symptoms of instability, snapping, or crepitus. Chronic pain or subluxation in the peroneal tendon region might be indicative of more severe tendon or superior peroneal retinaculum (SPR) degeneration; in such a situation, PUUR might be needed to augment an incompetent tendon or retinaculum or to bridge a chronic gap between tendon ends. History should also take note of what conservative treatment measures have already been pursued, such as immobilization, bracing, physical therapy, medications, and injections.

Physical examination should include assessing heel position and ligamentous stability [15]. Hindfoot varus and lateral ligamentous laxity are findings which can be associated with and exacerbate peroneal pathology, and they might lead to recurrence after surgical intervention if they are not also addressed at the same time as the peroneal tendon pathology. Tenderness to palpation and swelling is often seen with peroneal tenosynovitis, localized along the course of the tendons from behind the fibula down to the brevis insertion on the base of the fifth metatarsal and the longus insertion on the plantar aspect of the foot to the first metatarsal base and the medial cuneiform. Pain with passive inversion and loss of strength in eversion can also be seen with peroneal tendon pathology. It is also important to assess for subluxation or dislocation of one or both of the peroneal tendons over the posterolateral ridge of the fibula with dorsiflexion and eversion.

A 3-view AP, lateral, and mortise series of weight-bearing ankle X-rays as well as AP, lateral, and oblique foot X-rays should be utilized to assess peroneal tendon pathology. It can rule out acute bony trauma, as well as assess for a cavovarus foot, ligamentous laxity, or degenerative joint changes. One can also assess for a fleck sign, which might suggest a superficial peroneal retinacular tear. The os peroneum should also be assessed for fracture, as well as for proximal migration, suggesting tendon rupture which might require PUUR graft reinforcement.

To confirm or further assess peroneal pathology, an MRI can also be utilized. MRI can show various peroneal pathology that might generate pain, including tenosynovitis, low-lying peroneal muscle belly, accessory muscle or tendon, subluxation or dislocation of the peroneal tendons, or an enlarged peroneal tubercle. It can also assess the extent of peroneal tearing and tendinosis. Extensive tendinosis or tenosynovitis on MRI might suggest a high-grade tear for which PUUR can be utilized to bolster a tendon repair.

CT scans can also be utilized to assess bony detail, such as peroneal groove morphology [16].

Ultrasound is another imaging technique that can give the provider a more dynamic assessment of the peroneal tendons, such as to evaluate for peroneal subluxation or dislocation.

After a thorough history and physical examination is obtained along with radiographs and other imaging studies as needed, the provider can make a diagnosis and begin preparing for the appropriate intervention, whether it be continued conservative management, peroneal tendon debridement/repair, SPR repair/reconstruction, lateral ligamentous reconstruction, hindfoot alignment correction, or a combination of the above, utilizing a PUUR graft for soft-tissue reinforcement, where appropriate.

Surgical Techniques Utilizing PUUR (Artelon) Graft

Peroneal Repair

A standard approach to the peroneal tendons is employed. A longitudinal incision is made along the course of the peroneal tendons, beginning just proximal to the distal fibula and extending distally. The sural nerve should be identified and protected. The peroneal tendon sheath is incised, exposing the tendons. Next, the peroneal tendons are inspected, and associated pathology is addressed. Any tenosynovitis is debrided, any low-lying peroneal muscle belly or peroneal quartus is excised, and any hypertrophic peroneal tubercle impinging on the tendons is excised.

Once the peroneal tear is encountered, it is initially repaired in usual fashion. Degenerative tendon at the tear site is sharply excised. Any longitudinal split is repaired with a running 2–0 suture buried core stitch, followed by tubularization of the tendon (Figs. 25.2 and 25.3).

After repair of the peroneal tendon, the PUUR graft is utilized to augment the repair. The graft is sized, ensuring that the length of the graft spans the repair site. Typically, a 0.5 × 8 cm sized graft is used (Fig. 25.4). The graft is then sutured to the peroneal tendon, with 10–20% tension applied to the graft (Fig. 25.5). The peroneal tendon sheath is not closed to prevent postoperative adhesions to the tendon. The superior peroneal retinaculum (SPR) is closed.

Historically, if more than 50% of the tendon was debrided, a tenodesis was required. However, the use of a PUUR graft precludes the need for tenodesis. Its

Fig. 25.2 Longitudinal peroneal brevis tear identified

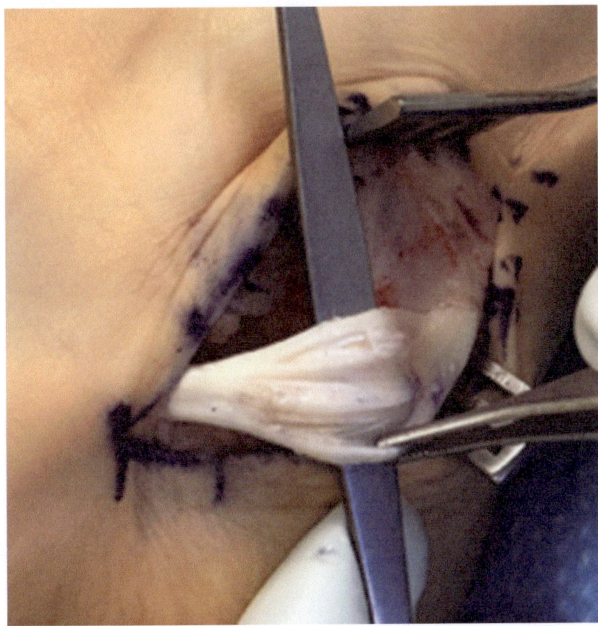

Fig. 25.3 The peroneal tear is repaired with a running suture buried core stitch, followed by tubularization of the tendon

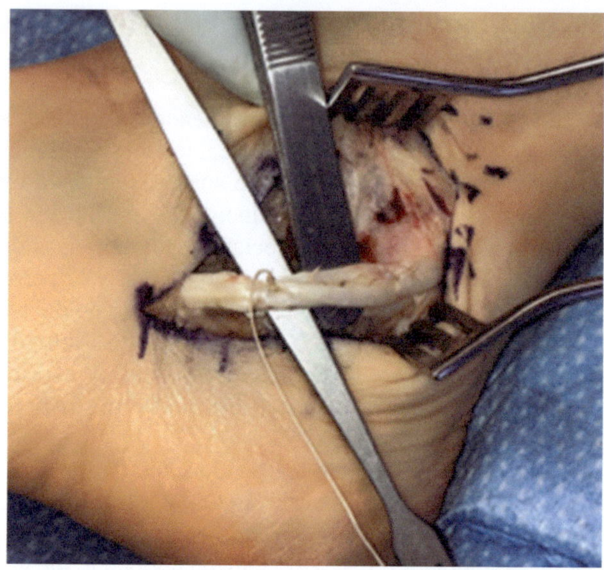

Fig. 25.4 The PUUR graft is sized, ensuring that the length of the graft spans the repair site. Typically, a 0.5 × 8 cm sized graft is utilized

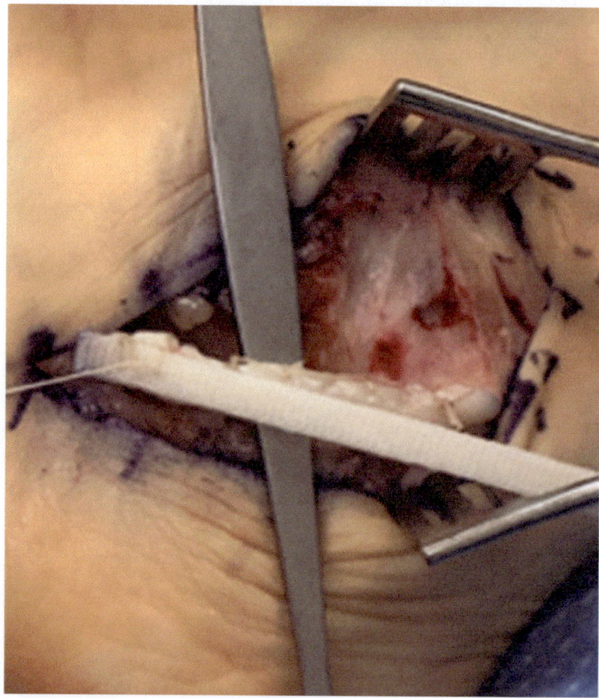

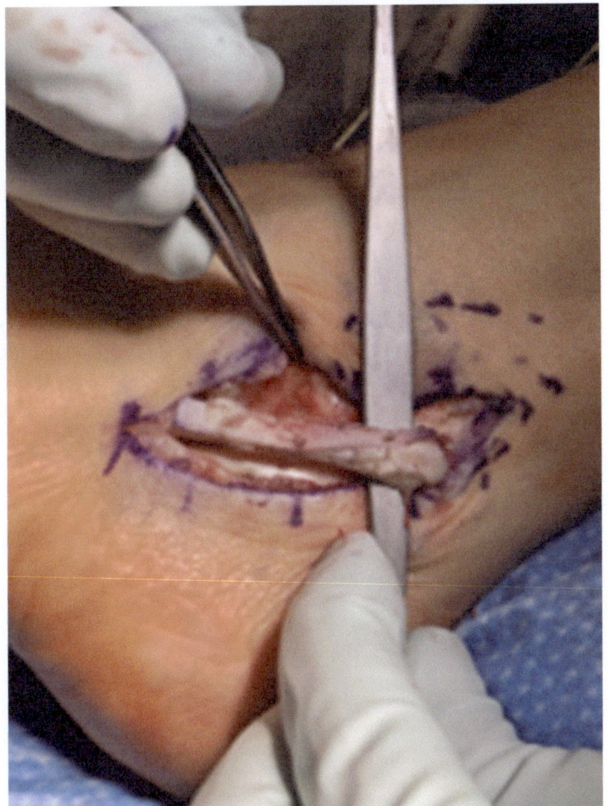

Fig. 25.5 The PUUR graft is sutured to the repaired peroneal tendon, with 10-20% tension applied to the graft

properties allow it to integrate into the repair site and act as a scaffold for new tissue growth, permitting load sharing and rapid tissue remodeling through mechanotransduction, thus strengthening the repair site [17].

Peroneal Tendon Reconstruction for Rupture

In cases of a complete rupture of the peroneal longus or brevis tendons, a direct end-to-end repair is usually not possible as a defect is often present (Fig. 25.6). Therefore, options include tenodesis, allograft reconstruction, or tendon transfer. If tendon excursion is present, we have employed reconstruction utilizing the PUUR dynamic matrix allograft. We prefer reconstruction as it has been shown to be more effective at restoring peroneal tension, compared to a peroneal tendon tenodesis [18].

Prior to reconstruction, all diseased tendon and any adhesions are excised. A 0.5 × 8 cm PUUR graft is sized and cut to bridge the tendon defect. An overlap of the tendon and graft should be approximately 1 cm (Fig. 25.7). The graft is sutured to the proximal tendon stump in a side-to-side manner. The foot is placed in slight

Fig. 25.6 A complete peroneal brevis rupture with retraction of the proximal stump is identified

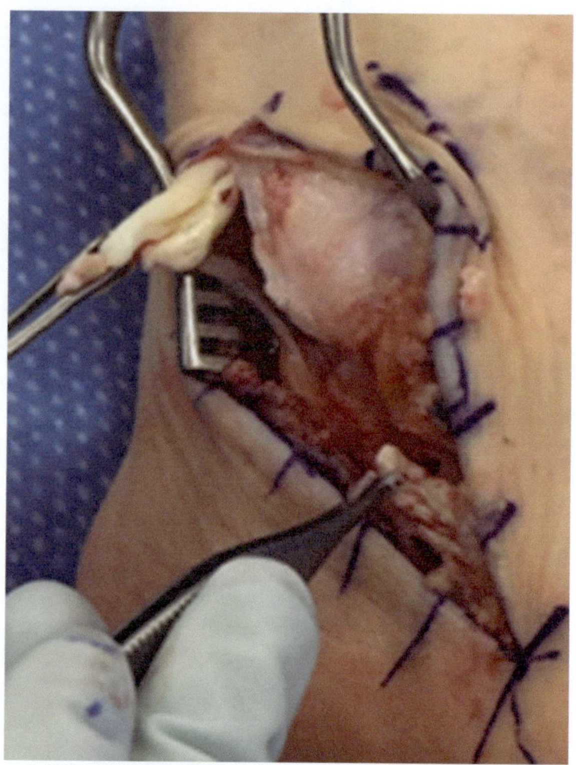

Fig. 25.7 After the diseased tendon and adhesions are excised, the PUUR graft is sized and cut to bridge the tendon defect. The graft is sutured to the proximal tendon stump in a side-to-side manner with an overlap of the tendon and graft of approximately 1 cm

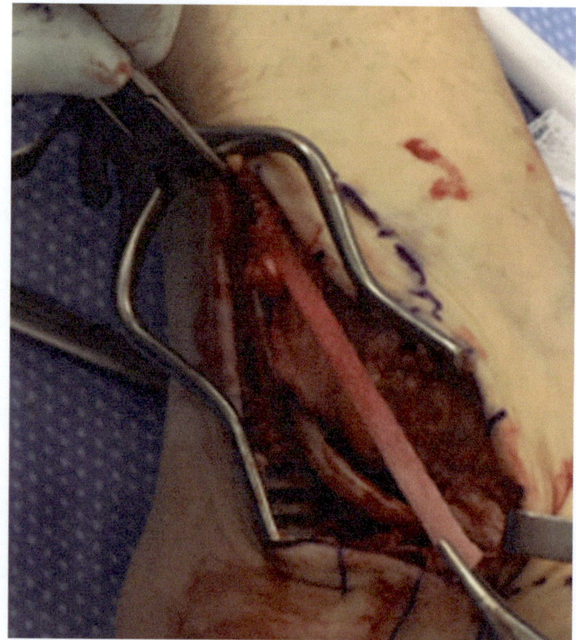

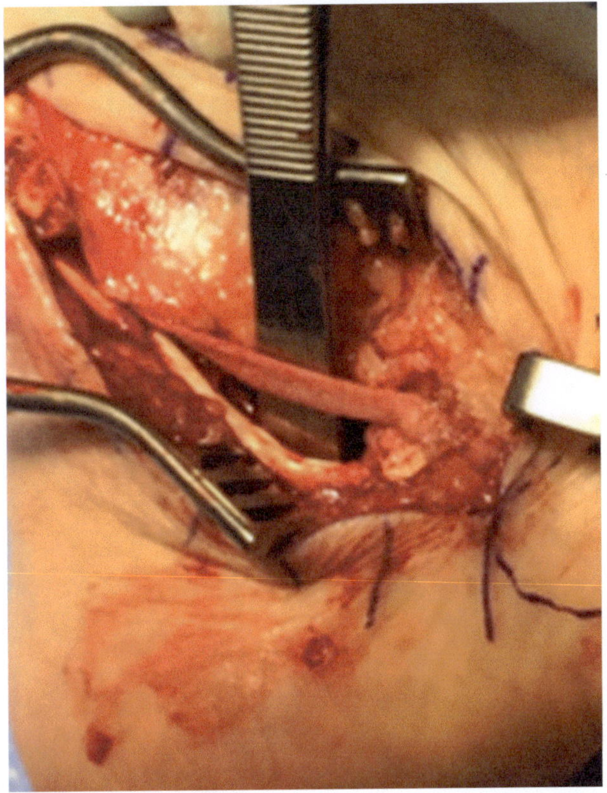

Fig. 25.8 The unattached distal end of the graft is sutured to the distal tendon stump, while applying tension to the distal end of the graft with the foot in slight eversion

eversion, and the unattached distal end is sutured to the distal tendon stump, while applying 10–20% tension to the distal end of the graft (Fig. 25.8). The distal end can alternatively be repaired to the fifth metatarsal base with a suture anchor in a similar manner. The tendons are then reduced, and superior peroneal retinaculum repaired, and the wound is closed in a routine manner.

Os Peroneum Excision

An incision is made over the course of the peroneal tendons in the inframalleolar region (Fig. 25.9). The sural nerve is encountered in this region and should be protected. The peroneal tendons are exposed, and the peroneal longus is traced distally to the cuboid tunnel. At the os peroneum, there is often thickening and tendinosis, and a fragmented os peroneum can also be encountered (Fig. 25.10). The os peroneum is shelled out and excised, often leaving little tendon or a defect for repair. The PUUR graft can be employed to augment and bridge the repair. An appropriately sized graft is measured and cut, to fit and bridge the defect and tendon (Fig. 25.11). The distal portion of the peroneal longus is deep in the cuboid tunnel, making suture placement difficult. Therefore, a suture passer can be used to secure the graft to the distal aspect of the tendon (Figs. 25.12 and 25.13). Next, the

Fig. 25.9 Incision along the peroneal longus

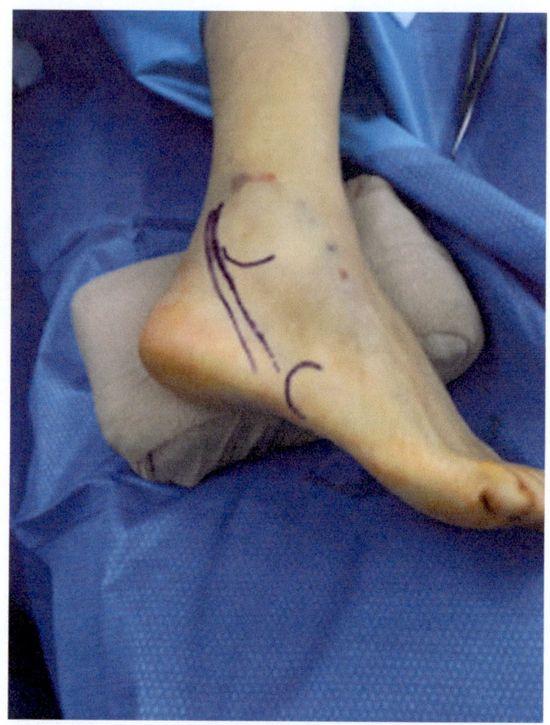

Fig. 25.10 Thickened peroneal longus and excised os peroneum and resulting gap

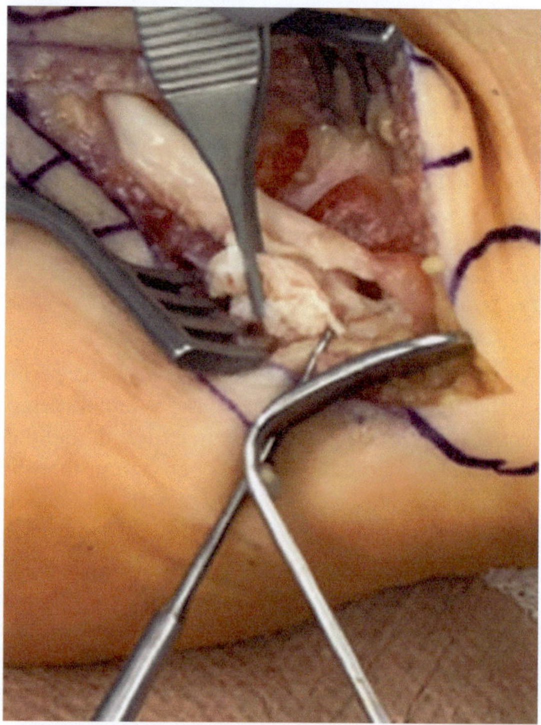

Fig. 25.11 Measuring and cutting the PUUR graft

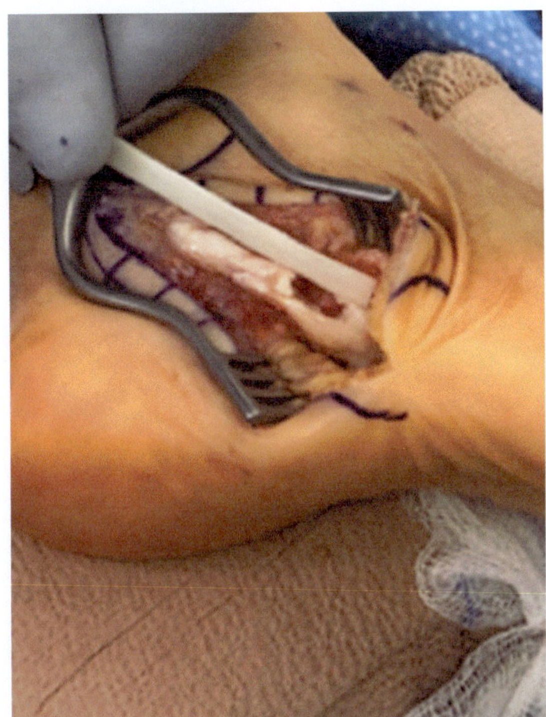

Fig. 25.12 A suture passer is used to attach a non-absorbable suture to the distal peroneal longus remnants

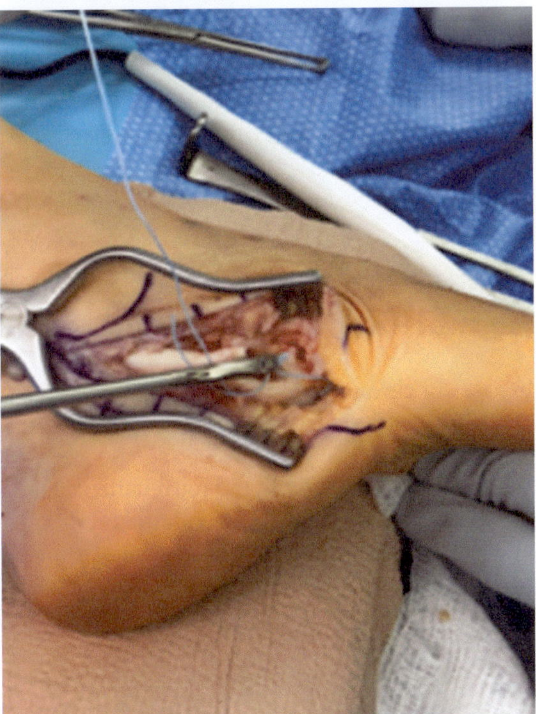

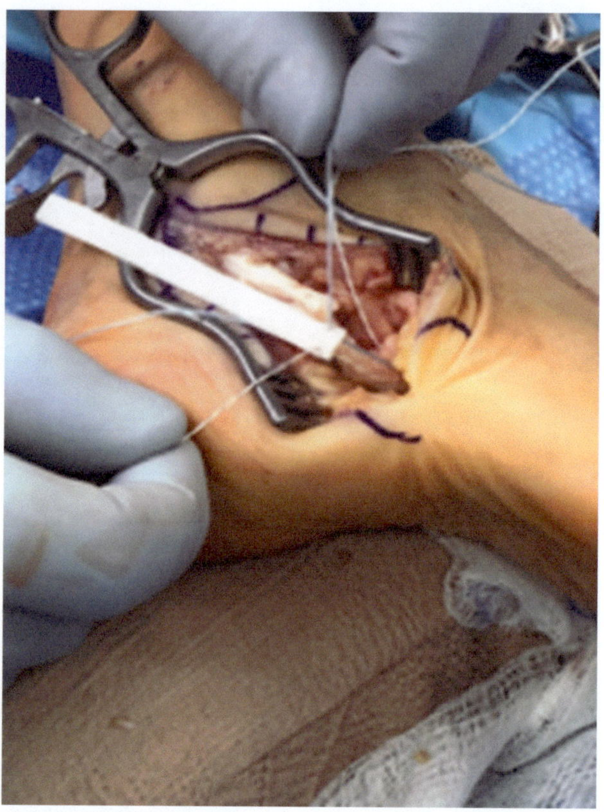

Fig. 25.13 Securing the PUUR graft to the distal peroneal longus tendon

unattached end of the graft is pulled into 10–20% tension and secured directly to the proximal tendon (Fig. 25.14). The reconstructed peroneal longus tendon is then relocated (Fig. 25.15). Range of motion is performed to ensure no tendon or graft entrapments. The incision is closed, and the foot splinted in plantar flexion and eversion.

Superior Peroneal Retinaculum Reconstruction

In cases of chronic peroneal subluxation, a PUUR graft can be useful, especially in chronic cases with poor superior peroneal retinaculum (SPR) quality or in revision procedures.

An incision is made in the retromalleolar region over the peroneal tendons and extended distally. The SPR is identified. It is typically found to be avulsed from its fibular attachment and can be thin and attenuated (Fig. 25.16). The SPR is incised and peroneal tendons are identified. The tendons should be assessed for any tears or other pathology, including a low-lying muscle belly or peroneal quartus, which can contribute to peroneal instability (Fig. 25.17). The fibular groove should also be assessed, and a groove deepening is performed if necessary. When performing the

Fig. 25.14 Secure the PUUR graft and reinforce the proximal peroneal longus tendon

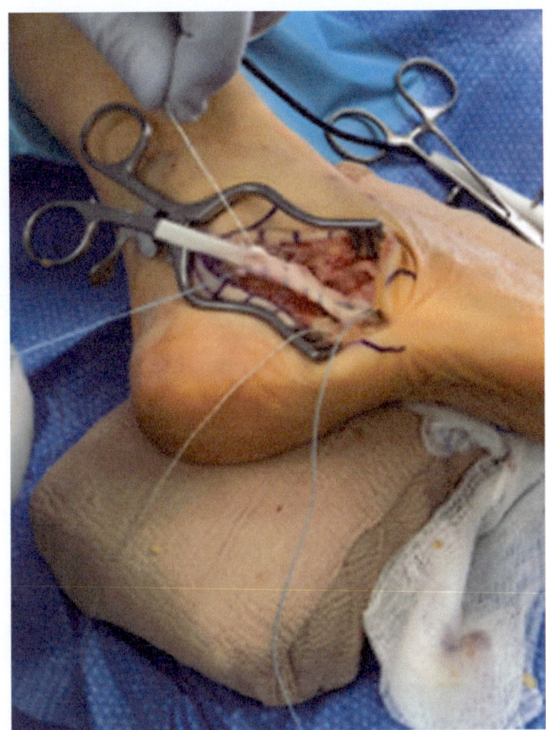

Fig. 25.15 Final repaired peroneal longus tendon attached to the PUUR graft

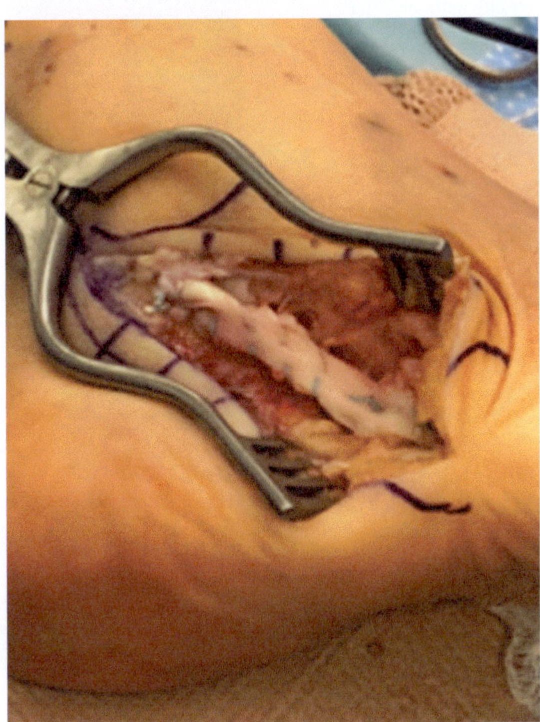

                                                                                                 S. K. Neufeld et al.

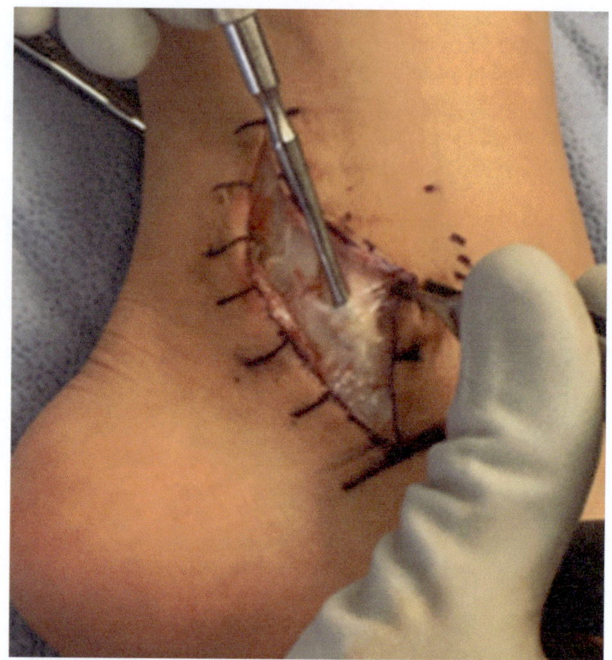

Fig. 25.16 The SPR is identified and is found to be avulsed from its fibula attachment, and thin and attenuated

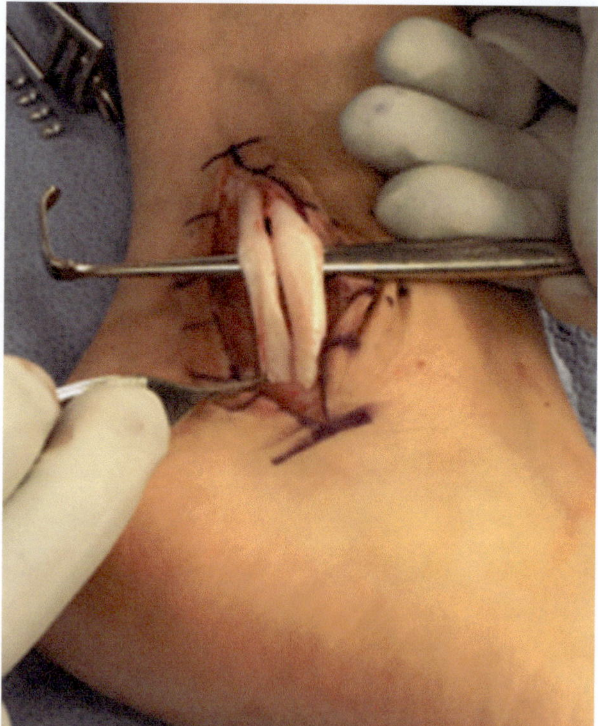

Fig. 25.17 The peroneal tendons should be assessed for any tears or other pathology

SPR reconstruction, the peroneal tendons are reduced, and the SPR is repaired back to its fibula attachment (Fig. 25.18).

Next, the PUUR graft is utilized. A suture anchor is placed into the posterolateral aspect of the fibula at the SPR attachment, and a 0.5 × 8 cm graft is attached (Fig. 25.19). A second suture anchor is placed at the calcaneal attachment of the SPR (Fig. 25.20). The unattached end of the graft is tensioned and secured directly

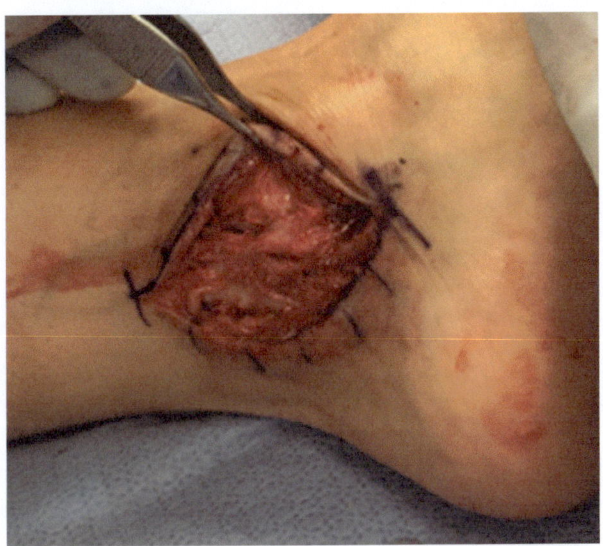

Fig. 25.18 The SPR is repaired back to its fibula attachment

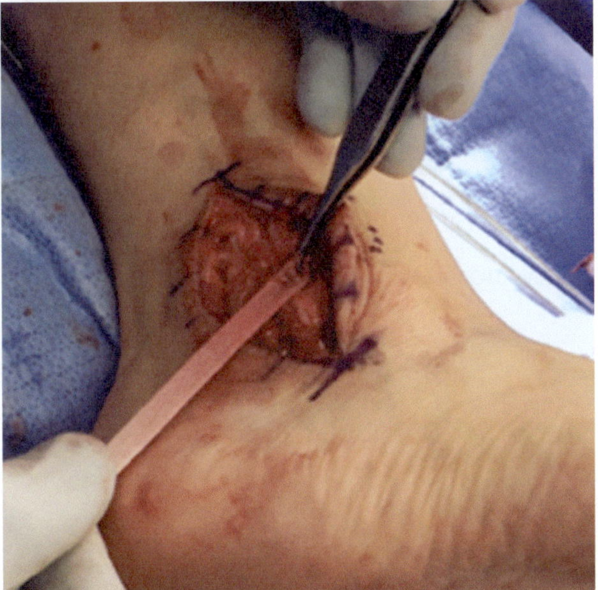

Fig. 25.19 A suture anchor is placed into the posterolateral aspect of the fibula and the PUUR graft is attached

to the lateral calcaneal attachment of the SPR, applying 10–20% tension (Fig. 25.21). The ankle is circumducted to ensure that peroneal tendons are gliding but remain reduced. The incision is then closed in a routine manner, and the foot is placed in a posterior splint.

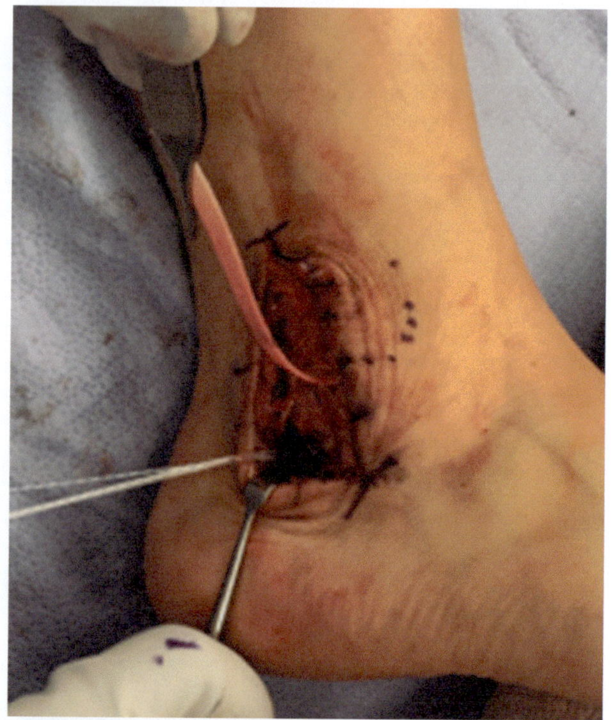

Fig. 25.20 A second suture anchor is placed at the calcaneal attachment of the SPR

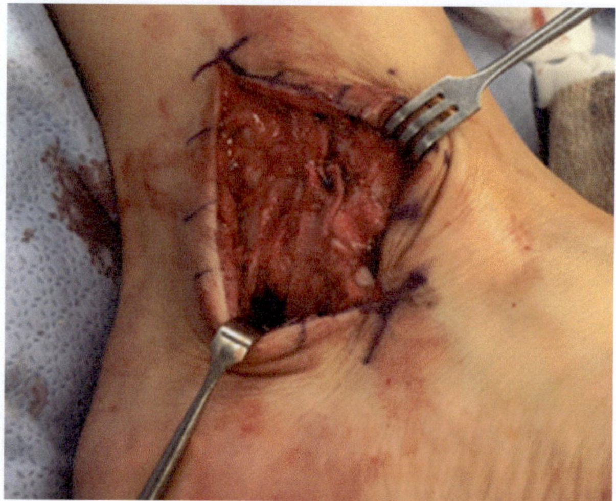

Fig. 25.21 The unattached end of the PUUR graft is tensioned and secured directly to the lateral calcaneal attachment of the SPR, applying 10-20% tension

Potential Complications

- Wound-healing problems
- Retear or rupture
- Sural neuralgia or nerve injury
- Scarring of the tendons, which may lead to chronic pain

Post-op Care

- Patients are initially placed in a well-padded posterior splint for 1 week. At 1 week post-op, the patient is placed into a walking boot and weight bearing is initiated.
- At the 3-week post-op visit, the sutures are removed, and gentle active range-of-motion exercises are started daily to prevent postoperative adhesions.
- At 4 weeks postoperatively, formal physical therapy is prescribed for focus on functional rehabilitation. The patient is gradually weaned out of the boot into a supportive lace-up ankle brace at 6–8 weeks post-op.
- Patients who undergo reconstruction requiring bridging of a tendon defect or superior peroneal retinaculum reconstruction are initially placed in a well-padded posterior splint for 1 week. At 1 week post-op, they are placed into a cast, with protected weight bearing.
- At the 3-week post-op visit, the sutures are removed, and the patient is placed into a walking boot. Gentle active range-of-motion exercises are started daily to prevent postoperative adhesions. However, plantar flexion and inversion are avoided to minimize the risk of disrupting the repair.
- At 6 weeks postoperatively, formal physical therapy is prescribed, for focus on functional rehabilitation. The patient is gradually weaned out of the boot and into a supportive lace-up ankle brace at 8–9 weeks post-op.

Outcomes

Table 25.1 shows the results of our case series of patients with various peroneal tendon pathology treated with the assistance of PUUR graft. There were no incidents of adverse foreign body reaction, graft failure, or need for repeat surgical intervention. One patient did have delayed wound healing which resolved with local wound care. These results are consistent with previous PUUR graft outcome studies, and suggest that PUUR graft is a safe and effective tool for soft-tissue reconstruction in the setting of peroneal tendon pathology [20, 21].

Table 25.1 Outcomes after PUUR graft utilization for peroneal tendon pathology

Procedure	Number of patients receiving procedure	Average follow-up (months)	Adverse events
Peroneal tendon complete rupture repair	2	5.4	None
Peroneal tendon tear repair augmentation	4	4.5	Delayed wound healing resolved with local wound care ($n = 1$)
Superior peroneal retinaculum reconstruction	1	14	None
Excision of painful os peroneum with augmentation of repair of peroneus longus tear	2	4.3	None

References

1. Weiler A, Peters G, Mäurer J, Unterhauser FN, Südkamp NP. Biomechanical properties and vascularity of an anterior cruciate ligament graft can be predicted by contrast-enhanced magnetic resonance imaging. A two-year study in sheep. Am J Sports Med. 2001;29(6):751–61.
2. Clancy WG Jr, Narechama RG, Rosenberg RD, Gmeiner JG, Wisnefske DD, Lange TA. Anterior and posterior cruciate ligament reconstruction in rhesus monkeys. J Bone Joint Surg Am. 1981;63(8):1270–84.
3. Fu F, Bennett CH, Lattermann C, Benjamin C. Current trends in anterior cruciate ligament reconstruction. Part 1: Biology and biomechanics of reconstruction. Am J Sports Med. 1999;27(6):821–30.
4. Rading J, Peterson L. Clinical experience with the Leeds-Keio artificial ligament in anterior cruciate ligament reconstruction. A prospective two-year follow-up study. Am J Sports Med. 1995;23(3):316–9.
5. Wredmark T, Engstrom B. Five-year results of anterior cruciate ligament reconstruction with the Stryker Dacron high-strength ligament. Knee Surg Sports Traumatol Arthrosc. 1993;1(2):71–5.
6. Engström B, Wredmark T, Westblad P. Patellar tendon or Leeds-Keio graft in the surgical treatment of anterior cruciate ligament ruptures. Intermediate results. Clin Orthop Relat Res. 1993;295:190–7.
7. Denti M, Bigoni M, Dodaro G, Monteleone M, Arosio A. Long-term results of the Leeds-Keio anterior cruciate ligament reconstruction. Knee Surg Sports Traumatol Arthrosc. 1995;3(2):75–7.
8. Pattee GA, Friedman M. A review of autogenous intraarticular reconstruction of the anterior cruciate ligament. In: Friedman MJ, Ferkel RD, editors. Prosthetic ligament reconstruction of the knee. Philadelphia: WB Saunders; 1988. p. 22–8.
9. Puddu G, Cipolla M, Cerullo G, Franco V, Giannì E. Anterior cruciate ligament reconstruction and augmentation with PDS graft. Clin Sports Med. 1993 Jan;12(1):13–24.
10. Gretzer C, Emanuelsson L, Liljensten E, Thomsen P. The inflammatory cell influx and cytokines changes during transition from acute inflammation to fibrous repair around implanted materials. J Biomater Sci Polym Ed. 2006;17(6):669–87.
11. Giza E, Frizzell L, Farac R, Williams J, Kim S. Augmented tendon Achilles repair using a tissue reinforcement scaffold: a biomechanical study. Foot Ankle Int. 2011 May;32(5):S545–9.
12. Gisselfält K, Edberg B, Flodin P. Synthesis and properties of degradable poly(urethane urea)s to be used for ligament reconstructions. Biomacromolecules. 2002 Sep-Oct;3(5):951–8.

13. Liljensten E, Gisselfält K, Edberg B, Bertilsson H, Flodin P, Nilsson A, Lindahl A, Peterson L. Studies of polyurethane urea bands for ACL reconstruction. J Mater Sci Mater Med. 2002 Apr;13(4):351–9.
14. Peterson L, Eklund U, Engström B, Forssblad M, Saartok T, Valentin A. Long-term results of a randomized study on anterior cruciate ligament reconstruction with or without a synthetic degradable augmentation device to support the autograft. Knee Surg Sports Traumatol Arthrosc. 2014;22(9):2109–20.
15. Coughlin MJ, Saltzman CL, Anderson RB. Mann's surgery of the foot and ankle. Philadelphia: Saunders/Elsevier; 2014.
16. Ogawa BK, Thordarson DB. Current concepts review: peroneal tendon subluxation and dislocation. Foot Ankle Int. 2007;28(9):1034–40.
17. Gersoff WK, Bozynski CC, Cook CR, Pfeiffer FM, Kuroki K, Cook JL. Evaluation of a novel degradable synthetic biomaterial patch for augmentation of tendon healing in a large animal model. J Knee Surg. 2019;32(5):434–40.
18. Pellegrini MJ, et al. Effectiveness of allograft reconstruction for irreparable peroneal brevis tears: a cadaveric model. Foot Ankle Int. 2016;37(8):803–8.
19. Shoaib A, Mishra V. Surgical repair of symptomatic chronic Achilles tendon rupture using synthetic graft augmentation. Foot Ankle Surg. 2017;23:179–82.
20. Sanders TH, Neufeld SK, Cuttica DJ. Anterior tibial tendon repair with polycaprolactone-based polyurethane urea based graft. Am Orthop Foot Ankle Soc. 33rd Annual Meeting, July 11-14, 2018, Boston, MA.
21. McKenna BJ, et al. Lateral Ankle Stabilization: Anatomic reconstruction for chronic lateral ankle instability utilizing degradable synthetic graft – a case series. Am Coll Foot Ankle Surg Scientific Conference, February 19–22, 2020, San Antonio, TX.

Correction to: The Peroneal Tendons

Mark Sobel

Correction to: M. Sobel (ed.), The Peroneal Tendons, https://doi.org/10.1007/978-3-030-46646-6

This title was recently Published. The title of Chapter 23, was incorrectly published as "Peroneal Tendon Pathology Associated with Calcaneous Fractures".

The correct title should read "Peroneal Tendon Pathology Associated with Calcaneus Fractures".

Also the affiliation of the author Dr. Michael Gans was published incorrectly in Chapters 7 and 24.

The correct affiliation should read, "PTSMC Orthopedic Residency Program, West Hartford, CT Physical Therapy and Sports Medicine Centers, Guilford, CT".

The updated versions of the chapters can be found at
https://doi.org/10.1007/978-3-030-46646-6_7
https://doi.org/10.1007/978-3-030-46646-6_23
https://doi.org/10.1007/978-3-030-46646-6_24

Index

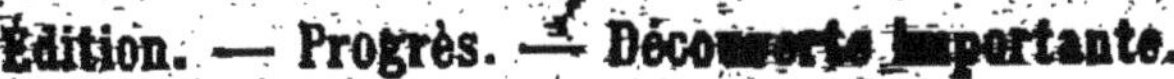

LUTTERBACH.

ART
DE RESPIRER

MOYEN POSITIF
POUR AUGMENTER AGRÉABLEMENT
LA VIE

7me ANNÉE. — 7me PUBLICATION.

PRIX : UN FR.

PARIS

Lacroix-Comond, Librairie Scientifique, Industrielle et Agricole,
Quai Malaquais, 15.

CHEZ L'AUTEUR, OUVRAGES ET DÉMONSTRATIONS
Rue Saint-Honoré, 97.

1857.